Jasjit S. Suri
Aly A. Farag

Deformable Models

Theory and Biomaterial Applications

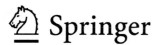 Springer

Jasjit S. Suri
Eigen LLC
Grass Valley, CA 95945
USA
jsuri@comcast.net

Aly A. Farag
Professor of Electrical
  and Computer Engineering
Computer Vision and Image
  Processing Laboratory
University of Louisville
Louisville, KY 40292
USA
aly.farag@louisville.edu

Series Editor

Evangelia Micheli-Tzanakou
Professor and Chair
Department of Biomedical Engineering
Rutgers University
Piscataway, NJ 08854-8014
Etzanako@rci.rutgers.edu

Library of Congress Control Number: 2007925875

ISBN-13: 978-0-387-31204-0   e-ISBN-13: 978-0-387-68343-0

Printed on acid-free paper.

9 8 7 6 5 4 3 2 1

springer.com

PREFACE

This volume carries the same flavor as Volume 1 in covering the theory, algorithms, and applications of level sets and deformable models in medical image analysis.

Chapter 1 describes a new approach that integrates the T-Surfaces model and isosurface generation methods within a general framework for segmentation and surface reconstruction in 3D medical images.

Chapter 2 is a study of active contour models in medical image analysis. Various issues with respect to implantation are discussed.

Chapter 3 also deals with active contours with a primary focus on the application and performance of different types of deformable models for analyzing microscopic pathology specimens.

Chapter 4 focuses on construction of the speed function of level sets as applied to segmentation of tagged MR images.

Chapter 5 presents a parallel computational method for 3D image segmentation based on solving the Riemannian mean curvature flow of graphs. The method is applied to segmentation of 3D echocardiographic images.

Chapter 6 provides a review of the level set method and shows the usage of shape models for segmentation of objects in 2D and 3D within a level set framework via regional information.

Chapter 7 also deals with basic application of deformable models to image segmentation. Various applications of the method are presented.

Chapter 8 employs geometric deformable models/level sets to extract the topology of the shape of breast tumors. Using this framework, several features of breast tumors are extracted and subsequently used for classification of breast disease.

Chapter 9 examines various theoretical and algorithmic details of active contour models and their use for image segmentation.

Chapter 10 uses deformable models to devise a segmentation approach for ultrasound images for the study of prostate cancer.

Chapter 11 proposes a novel variational formulation for brain MRI segmentation that uses J-divergence (symmetrized Kullback-Leibler divergence) to measure the dissimilarity between local and global regions.

Chapter 12 examines the use of shape transformations for morphometric analysis in the brain. A shape transformation is a spatial map that adapts an individual's brain anatomy to that of another.

Chapter 13 proposes a nonlinear statistical shape model for level set segmentation. Various algorithmic details are provided to show the effectiveness of the approach.

Chapter 14 uses the level sets methods for structural analysis of brain white and gray matter in normal and dyslexic people.

Chapter 15 describes an approach for estimating left- and right-ventricular deformation from tagged cardiac magnetic resonance imaging using volumetric deformable models constructed from nonuniform rational B-splines (NURBS).

Chapter 16 is a generalization of the methods presented in Chapter 14 with an emphasis on autism. The 3D distance map is used as a shape descriptor of the white matter, and a novel nonrigid registration approach is used to quantify changes in the corpus callosum of normal and autistic individuals.

Overall, the thirty-one chapters in the two volumes provide an elegant cross-section of the theory and application of variational and PDE approaches in medical image analysis. Graduate students and researchers at various levels of familiarity with these techniques will find the two volumes very useful for understanding the theory and algorithmic implementations. In addition, the various case studies provided demonstrate the power of these techniques in clinical applications.

The editors of the two volumes once again express their deep appreciation to the staff at Springer who made this project a fruitful experience.

Jasjit Suri and Aly Farag
January 2007

CONTENTS

Chapter 7
MEDICAL IMAGE SEGMENTATION BASED ON DEFORMABLE
MODELS AND ITS APPLICATIONS 209
Yonggang Wang, Yun Zhu, and Qiang Guo

Chapter 8
BREAST STRAIN IMAGING:
A CAD FRAMEWORK 261
*Ruey-Feng Chang, Chii-Jen Chen, Chia-Ling Tsai, Wei-Liang Chen,
and Jasjit S. Suri*

Chapter 9
ALTERNATE SPACES FOR MODEL DEFORMATION:
APPLICATION OF STOP AND GO ACTIVE MODELS TO
MEDICAL IMAGES 289
Oriol Pujol and Petia Radeva

Chapter 16
ROBUST NEUROIMAGING-BASED CLASSIFICATION TECHNIQUES
Rachid Fahmi, Ayman El-Baz, Hossam Abd El-Munim, Alaa E. Abdel-Hakim,
Aly A. Farag and Manuel F. Casanova

CONTRIBUTORS

ALAA E. ABDEL-HAKIM
Computer Vision and
Image Processing Laboratory
Department of Electrical and
Computer Engineering
University of Louisville
Louisville, Kentucky, USA

AMIR A. AMINI
Cardiovascular Image Analysis Laboratory
Washington University
St. Louis, Missouri, USA

SWAPNA BANERJEE
Department of Electronics and ECE
Indian Institute of Technology
Kharagpur, India

MANUEL F. CASANOVA
Department of Psychiatry and Behavioral
    Sciences
University of Louisville
Louisville, Kentucky, USA

RUEY-FENG CHANG
Department of Computer Science and
    Information Engineering
Graduate Institute of Networking and
    Multimedia
National Taiwan University
Taipei, Taiwan

CHII-JEN CHEN
Department of Computer Science and
    Information Engineering
National Chung Cheng University
Chiayi, Taiwan

WEI-LIANG CHEN
Department of Computer Science and
    Information Engineering
National Chung Cheng University
Chiayi, Taiwan

DANIEL CREMERS
Department of Computer Science
University of Bonn
Bonn, Germany

BIPUL DAS
Imaging Technology Division
GE India Technology Centre
Bangalore, India

CHRISTOS DAVATZIKOS
Section of Biomedical Image Analysis
Department of Radiology
University of Pennsylvania
Philadelphia, Pennsylvania, USA

MINGYUE DING
Institute for Pattern Recognition and
    Artificial Intelligence
Huazhong University of Science and
    Technology
Wuhan, China

AYMAN EL-BAZ
Bioengineering Department
University of Louisville
Louisville, Kentucky, USA

H. ABD EL-MUNIM
Computer Vision and Image Processing
    Laboratory
Department of Electrical and Computer
    Engineering
University of Louisville
Louisville, Kentucky, USA

N. YOUSSRY EL-ZEHIRY
Computer Vision and Image Processing
    Laboratory
Department of Electrical and Computer
    Engineering
University of Louisville
Louisville, Kentucky, USA

RACHID FAHMI
Computer Vision and Image Processing
    Laboratory
Department of Electrical and Computer
    Engineering
University of Louisville
Louisville, Kentucky, USA

ALY A. FARAG
Computer Vision and Image Processing
    Laboratory
Department of Electrical and Computer
    Engineering
University of Louisville
Louisville, Kentucky, USA

AARON FENSTER
Robarts Research Institute
London, Ontario, Canada

DAVID J. FORAN
Center for Biomedical Imaging
UMDNJ-Robert Woods Johnson Medical
    School
Piscataway, New Jersey, USA

GILSON A. GIRALDI
National Laboratory for Scientific
    Computing
Petropolis, Brazil

QIANG GUO
Institute of Image Processing and Pattern
    Recognition
Shanghai Jiaotong University
Shanghai, China

PHENG ANN HENG
Department of Computer Science and
    Engineering
The Chinese University of Hong Kong
Hong Kong, China

TIANZI JIANG
National Laboratory of Pattern Recognition
Institute of Automation
Beijing, China

WALTER JIMÉNEZ
National Laboratory for Scientific
    Computing
Petropolis, Brazil

HANIF LADAK
Department of Medical Biophysics
The University of Western Ontario
London, Ontario, Canada

XIAOBO LI
National Laboratory of Pattern Recognition
Institute of Automation
Beijing, China

KAROL MIKULA
Department of Mathematics and
    Descriptive Geometry
Slovak University of Technology
Bratislava, Slovakia

ASHRAF MOHAMED
Section of Biomedical Image Analysis
Department of Radiology
University of Pennsylvania
Philadelphia, Pennsylvania, USA

ANTONIO A.F. OLIVEIRA
Federal University
Rio de Janeiro, Brazil

ORIOL PUJOL
Departamento Matemática Aplicada i
    Análisi
Universidad de Barcelona
Barcelona, Spain

YINGGE QU
Department of Computer Science and
    Engineering
The Chinese University of Hong Kong
Hong Kong, China

PETIA RADEVA
Centre de Visió per Computador
Universidad Autónoma de Barcelona
Barcelona, Spain

PAULO S.S. RODRIGUES
National Laboratory for Scientific
    Computing
Petropolis, Brazil

MIKAEL ROUSSON
Department of Imaging and Visualization
Siemens Corporate Research
Princeton, New Jersey, USA

ALESSANDRO SARTI
Dipartmento di Elettronica
Informatica e Sistemistica
University of Bologna
Bologna, Italy

RODRIGO L.S. SILVA
National Laboratory for Scientific
    Computing
Petropolis, Brazil

MILAN SONKA
Department of Electrical and Computer
    Engineering
The University of Iowa
Iowa City, Iowa, USA

EDILBERTO STRAUSS
Federal University
Rio de Janeiro, Brazil

JASJIT S. SURI
Biomedical Research Institute
Idaho State University
Pocatello, Idaho, USA

CHIA-LING TSAI
Department of Computer Science and
    Information Engineering
National Chung Cheng University
Chiayi, Taiwan

NICHOLAS J. TUSTISON
Cardiovascular Image Analysis Laboratory
Washington University
St. Louis, Missouri, USA

YONGGANG WANG
Institute of Image Processing and Pattern
    Recognition
Shanghai Jiaotong University
Shanghai, China

TIEN-TSIN WONG
Department of Computer Science and
    Engineering
The Chinese University of Hong Kong
Hong Kong, China

FUXING YANG
Department of Electrical and Computer
    Engineering
The University of Iowa
Iowa City, Iowa, USA

LIN YANG
Department of Electrical and Computer
    Engineering
Rutgers University
Piscataway, New Jersey, USA

WANLIN ZHU
National Laboratory of Pattern Recognition
Institute of Automation
Beijing, China

YUN ZHU
Institute of Image Processing and Pattern
    Recognition
Shanghai Jiaotong University
Shanghai, China

1

T-SURFACES FRAMEWORK FOR OFFSET GENERATION AND SEMIAUTOMATIC 3D SEGMENTATION

Gilson A. Giraldi, Rodrigo L.S. Silva,
Paulo S.S. Rodrigues, and Walter Jiménez

National Laboratory for Scientific Computing
Petropolis, Brazil

Edilberto Strauss and Antonio A.F. Oliveira

Federal University, Rio de Janeiro, Brazil

Jasjit S. Suri

Biomedical Research Institute, Idaho State
University, Pocatello, Idaho, USA

This chapter describes a new approach that integrates the T-Surfaces model and isosurface generation methods in a general framework for segmentation and surface reconstruction in 3D medical images. Besides, the T-Surfaces model is applied for offset generation in the context of geometry extraction. T-Surfaces is a parametric deformable model based on a triangulation of the image domain, a discrete surface model, and an image threshold. Two types of isosurface generation methods are considered in this work: continuation and marching. The continuation approach is useful during reparameterization of T-Surfaces, while the latter is suitable to initialize the model closer the boundary. First, the T-Surfaces grid and the threshold are used to define a coarser image resolution. This field is thresholded to obtained a 0–1 function that is processed by a marching method to generate

Address all correspondence to: Gilson A. Giraldi, Laboratório Nacional de Computação Científica, Av. Getulio Vargas, 333, Quitandinha, Petropolis, Brazil, CEP: 25651-075. Phone: +55 24 2233-6088, Fax: +55 24 2231-5595. gilson@lncc.br.

1

polygonal surfaces whose interior may contain the desired objects. If a polygonal surface involves more than one object, the resolution is increased in that specific region, and the marching procedure is applied again. Next, we apply T-Surfaces to improve the result. If the obtained topology remains incorrect, we enable the user to modify the topology by an interactive method based on the T-Surfaces framework. Finally, we discuss the utility of diffusion methods and implicit deformable models for our approach.

1. INTRODUCTION

Deformable Models, which include the popular *snake models* [1] and deformable surfaces [2, 3], are well-known techniques for boundary extraction and tracking in 2D/3D images. Basically, these models can be classified into three categories: parametric, geodesic snakes, and implicit models. The relationships between these categories have been demonstrated in several works [4, 5].

Parametric Deformable Models consist of a curve (or surface) that can dynamically conform to object shapes in response to internal (elastic) and external (image and constraint) forces [6]. In geodesic snakes formulations, the key idea is to construct the evolution of a contour as a geodesic computation. A special metric is proposed (based on the gradient of the image field) to let the state of minimal energy correspond to the desired boundary. This approach allows addressing the parameterization dependence of parametric snake models and can be extended to three dimensions through the theory of minimal surfaces [7, 5]. Implicit models, such as the formulation used in [8], consist of embedding the snake as the zero level set of a higher-dimensional function and to solve the corresponding equation of motion. Such methodologies are best suited for the recovery of objects with unknown topologies.

When considering the three mentioned categories, two aspects are fundamental within the context of the present work: user interaction and topological changes. Parametric models are more suitable for user interaction than the others because they use neither the higher-dimensional formulations of Level Sets nor globally defined features, like the metric in the geodesic approach. However, for most parametric methods the topology of the structures of interest must be known in advance since the mathematical model cannot deal with topological changes without adding extra machinery [9, 10].

Recently, McInerney and Terzopoulos [11, 9, 10] proposed the T-Snakes/ T-Surfaces model to add topological capabilities (*splits and merges*) to a parametric model. The resulting method has the power of an implicit approach without requiring a higher-dimensional formulation.

The basic idea is to embed a discrete deformable model within the framework of a simplicial domain decomposition (*triangulation*) of the image domain. In this framework, the reparameterization is based on the projection of the curve/surface over the triangulation and on a *Characteristic Function*, which distinguishes the interior grid nodes of the (closed) curve/surface from the exterior ones. The set of simplices in which the Characteristic Function changes value (*Combinatorial Manifold*) gives a simple way to reparameterize the model.

This reparameterization process allows to reconstruct surfaces with significant protrusions and objects with bifurcations. Furthermore, that process can easily deal with self-intersections of the surface during model evolution. Also, T-Snakes/ T-Surfaces depends on some threshold to define a normal force that is used to drive the model toward the targets [10].

Based on these elements (discrete surface model, simplicial decomposition framework, and threshold), we present in this chapter a semiautomatic segmentation approach for 3D medical images based on isosurface extraction methods and the T-Surfaces model. Among the isosurface methods [12], two types are considered in this chapter: continuation and marching methods.

The continuation methods propagate the surface from a set of seed cells [12, 13]. Unlike these approaches, in the traditional Marching Cubes, each surface-finding phase visits all cells of the volume, normally by varying coordinate values in a triple *for* loop [14]. As we have already demonstrated in previous works [15, 16, 17], continuation methods are useful during both the reparameterization and initialization of the T-Surfaces model if some topological and scale restrictions for the targets are supposed.

In the present work we discard these restrictions. We show that continuation methods remain suitable in the reparameterization process. However, Marching methods should be used to initialize T-Surfaces close to the boundary. These are the key points of this work.

Specifically, in the first stage, the T-Surfaces grid is used to define a coarser image resolution by sampling the image field over the grid nodes. The obtained low-resolution image field is a thresholded to get a binary field, which we call an *Object Characteristic Function*. This field will be searched by the isosurface generation method. The obtained result may be a rough approximation of the target. However, the obtained surfaces are in general not smooth, and topological defects (holes) may occur. Besides, due to inhomogeneities of the image field, some components of the objects may be split as well as merged due to the low image resolution used. The result is improved by using the T-Surfaces model.

The grid resolution is application dependent. However, an important point of our method is its multiresolution/multigrid nature: having processed (segmented) the image in a coarser (grid) resolution, we can detect regions where the grid has to be refined, and then recursively applying the method only over those specific regions.

If the extracted topology remains incorrect, even at the finest resolution, we propose an interactive procedure based on the T-Surfaces framework to force merge and split operations. This method is an extension of the one described in [15, 16].

In the case of noisy images, diffusion methods can improve both the isosurface extraction and the T-Surfaces result. We discuss the utility of 3D image filtering by anisotropic diffusion and implicit deformable models for our approach. Besides, the T-Surfaces framework is applied for offset generation and its utility for Dual approaches is considered [18].

The following section presents some background on deformable surfaces and related works. The T-Surfaces framework is developed in Section 2.1. The key points behind utilization of isosurfaces to initialize T-Surfaces are considered in Section 2.2. Sections 3 and 4 discuss the isosurface generation methods inside the T-Surfaces context. We present our in Section 5. The experimental results are given in Section 6. Finally, the proposed method is compared with related ones and we discuss new perspectives for our method through Level Sets and vector diffusion approaches (Section 7). Conclusions are given in Section 8. Appendix A focuses on diffusion methods for image processing.

2. BACKGROUND AND PREVIOUS WORKS

The use of isosurface methods in initialization of deformable surfaces requires special considerations to guarantee efficiency [19, 20, 17, 21].

To explain the concepts, let us consider the following balloon-like model for closed surfaces [3]:

$$v : \Re^+ \times [0,1] \times [0,1] \rightarrow \Re^3;$$

$$v(t,r,s) = (v_1(t,r,s), v_2(t,r,s), v_3(t,r,s));$$

$$\frac{\partial v}{\partial t} - \omega_{10}\frac{\partial^2 v}{\partial s^2} - \omega_{01}\frac{\partial^2 v}{\partial r^2} + 2\omega_{11}\frac{\partial^4 v}{\partial r^2 \partial s^2} + \omega_{20}\frac{\partial^4 v}{\partial s^4} + \omega_{02}\frac{\partial^4 v}{\partial r^4}$$

$$= F(v) - kn(v); \qquad (1)$$

$$\text{Initial} \quad \text{Estimation} : v(0,r,s) = v_0(r,s)$$

where $n(v)$ is the normal (unitary) field over the surface v, F is the image force field (may be normalized), and k is a force scale factor. The parameters ω_{ij} control the smoothness and flexibility of the model.

By using the internal pressure force $(kn(v))$, the model behaves as a balloon-like object that is inflated passing over regions in which the external force is weaker. Consequently, the model becomes less sensitive to initialization, which is an advantage over more traditional active models [22, 6].

For shape-recovering applications, numerical methods must be considered in order to solve Eq. (1). If Finite Differences are used, the continuous surface $v(r,s)$ is discretized, generating a polygonal mesh. During mesh evolution, self-intersections must be avoided. In general, this is a challenge if we aim to use isosurfaces to define the initial estimation $v_0(r,s)$ in Eq. (1). This happens because isosurfaces are in general both not smooth and irregular for 3D medical images. Also, they may be far from the target in some points. Figure 1 depicts a bidimensional example with such difficulties.

Traditional deformable models [6, 3, 1], including the one defined by the Eq. (1), cannot efficiently deal with self-intersections. This is due to the non-local

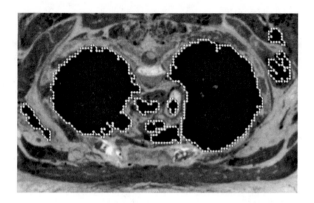

Figure 1. Isocontours for a medical image.

self-intersection dependency, which requires $O\left(N^2\right)$ in the worst case, where N is the number of mesh nodes.

Moreover, the image forces may be not strong enough to push the model toward the object boundary. (Appendix A discusses recent proposals to address this problem.) Even the balloon model in Eq. (1) cannot deal with such problems because it is difficult to predict if the target is inside or outside the isosurface (see Figure 1). This makes it harder to accurately define the normal force field.

Besides, due to image field inhomogeneities, topological defects (holes) may corrupt the extracted surface. Also, the objects may split and/or merge during the isosurface extraction process.

These problems can be addressed through an efficient pre-segmentation. For instance, when reconstructing the geometry of the human cerebral cortex, Prince at al. [19] used a fuzzy segmentation method (*Adaptive Fuzzy C-Means*) to obtain the following elements: a segmented field that provides a fuzzy membership function for each tissue class; the mean intensity of each class; and the inhomogeneity of the image, modeled as a smoothly varying gain field (see [19] and the references therein).

The result can be used to steer the isosurface extraction process as well as the deformable model, which is initialized by the obtained isosurface. We used a similar approach in [20].

In [21], pre-segmentation is done by using the *Image Foresting Transformation* (IFT). The isosurface extraction is then performed. The IFT is a segmentation process based on the idea of mapping an input image into a graph, computing the shortest-path forest in this graph, and outputting an annotated image, which is basically an image and its associated forest. A watershed transform by markers and other connected operators can be efficiently implemented by the image foresting transformation, which emphasizes the capabilities of this technique [23].

In order to reduce computation time, in [21] the IFT algorithm was applied at a lower image resolution. Another advantage of this procedure is that at the lower resolution, small background artifacts become less significant relative to the object(s) of interest. This philosophy, very well known in the field of multi-resolution image processing [24], was also incorporated in our work, as we shall see later.

Recently, in [17], we showed that most of the mentioned problems for initialization of deformable models through isosurfaces are naturally addressed when using the T-Surfaces model. The reparameterization process of this model can deal naturally with self-intersections and also efficiently perform topological changes (merges/splits) over the surface(s) during the evolution process. These capabilities enable automatic corrections of topological defects of the initial isosurface. We next describe the T-Surfaces model.

2.1. T-Surfaces

The T-Surfaces approach is composed of three components [10]: (1) a tetra-hedral decomposition (CF-Triangulation) of the image domain $D \subset \Re^3$; (2) a particle model of the deformable surface; (3) a *Characteristic Function*, χ, defined on the grid nodes that distinguishes the interior $(Int(S))$ from the exterior $(Ext(S))$ of a surface S:

$$\chi : D \subset \Re^3 \to \{0, 1\} \tag{2}$$

where $\chi(p) = 1$ if $p \in Int(S)$ and $\chi(p) = 0$ otherwise, where p is a node of the grid.

Following the classical nomenclature, a vertex of a tetrahedron is called a *node* and the collection of nodes and triangle edges is called the grid Γ_s. A tetrahedron (also called a simplex) σ is a *transverse* one if the characteristic function χ in Eq. (2) changes its value in σ, analogously, for an edge.

In the framework composed by both the simplicial decomposition and the characteristic function, the reparameterization of a surface is done by [10]: (1) computing the intersections points of the surface with the grid; (2) finding the set of transverse tetrahedrons (*Combinatorial Manifold*); (3) choosing an intersection point for each transverse edge; (4) connecting the selected points.

In this reparameterization process, the transverse simplices play a central role. Given such a simplex, we choose in each transverse edge an intersection point to generate the new surface patch. In general, we will obtain three or four transverse edges in each transverse tetrahedron (Figure 5). The former gives a triangular patch, and the latter defines two triangles. So at the end of the step (4), a triangular mesh is obtained. Each triangle is called a *triangular element* [10].

Taking a 2D example, let us consider the characteristic functions (χ_1 and χ_2) relative to the two contours depicted in Figure 2. The functions are defined on the vertices of a CF-triangulation of the plane. The vertices marked are those where $\max\{\chi_1, \chi_2\} = 1$. Observe that they are enclosed by a merger of the contours. This merge can be approximated by a curve belonging to the region obtained by tracing the transverse triangles. The same would be true for more than two contours (and, obviously, for only one).

After the reparameterization process, a suitable evolution scheme must be applied, as described in the following section.

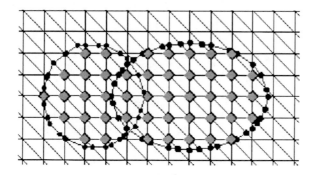

Figure 2. Two snakes colliding with the inside grid nodes and snaxels marked.

2.1.1. Discrete Model

A T-Surface can be seen as a discrete form of the parametric deformable surfaces given by Eq. (1) [10]. It is defined as a closed elastic mesh. Each node is called a *node element*, and each pair of connected nodes v_i, v_j is called a *model element*.

The node elements are linked by springs, whose natural length we set to zero. Hence, a tensile force can be defined by:

$$\vec{\alpha_i} = \sum_j \vec{S}_{ij} \text{where} \vec{S}_{ij} = c(r_{ij}), \tag{3}$$

where c is a scale factor and $r_{ij} = \|v_i - v_j\|$ is the length of the corresponding model element. The model also has a normal force that can be weighted as follows [10]:

$$F_i = k(sign_i) n_i, \tag{4}$$

where n_i is the normal vector at node i, k is a scale factor, and $sign_i = +1$ if $I(v_i) > T$ and $sign_i = -1$ otherwise (T is a threshold of the image I). This force is used to push the model toward image edges until it is opposed by external image forces.

The forces defined by the Eqs. (3)–(4) are internal forces. The external force is defined as an image data function, according to the interested features. Several different approaches have been adopted according to the application [18, 25]. In our case, it can be defined as follows:

$$\text{Image} :: \text{Force} :: f_i^t = -\gamma_i \nabla P; \quad P = \|\nabla I\|^2. \tag{5}$$

The surface evolution is controlled by the following discrete dynamical system:

$$v_i^{(t+\Delta t)} = v_i^t + h_i \left(\overrightarrow{\alpha_i}^t + \overrightarrow{F_i}^t + \overrightarrow{f_i}^t \right), \tag{6}$$

where h_i is an evolution step.

During the T-Surfaces evolution, some grid nodes become interior to the surface. Such nodes are called *burnt nodes*, and their identification is required by update of the characteristic function [10]. To deal with self-intersections, the T-Surfaces model incorporates an entropy condition: *once a node is burnt it stays burnt*. A termination condition is set based on the number of deformation steps in which a simplex has remained a transverse one.

Now, it is important to make considerations about the T-Surfaces model, which will guarantee efficiency by initializing the T-Surfaces through isosurface methods. This is the starting point for our previous works [20, 17].

2.2. Initialization of T-Surfaces

The threshold T, used in the normal force definition (Eq. (4)), plays an important role in the T-Surfaces model [11, 10]. If it was not properly chosen, the T-Surfaces can be frozen in a region far from the target(s) [20, 17].

The choice of T is critical when two target objects are closer, as shown in Figure 3. In this example, the marked grid nodes (spheres) are those whose image intensity falls below threshold T. They belong to the target objects that are the two cells enclosed by the white-colored T-Snake.

For the T-Snakes model to accurately segment the pictured objects, it has to burn the marked grid nodes between the two objects. However, the normal force (given by Eq. (4)) changes its signal while the T-Snakes gets closer. So, the force parameters in Eqs. (3)–(4) should be properly chosen to guarantee advance over the narrow region. However, parameter choice remains an open problem in snake models [26]. One solution is increasing the grid resolution as it controls T-Surface flexibility. However, this increases the computational cost of the method.

To address the tradeoff between model flexibility and computational cost, we proposed in [16, 15] to get a rough approximation of the target surfaces through isosurfaces generation methods and then applying the T-Surfaces model. The topological capabilities of T-Surfaces enable evolving the extracted isosurfaces in

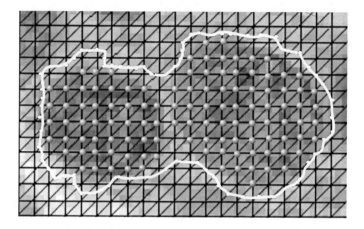

Figure 3. T-Snake (white curve) and the marked grid nodes (spheres).

an efficient manner. Thus, we combined the advantages of a closer initialization (through isosurfaces) and the advantages of using a topologically adaptable deformable model. These are the key ideas of our previous works [16, 15]. Let us now examine some of the details.

At first, a *Local Scale Property* for the targets was supposed: given an object O and a point $p \in O$, let r_p be the radius of a hyperball B_p that contains p and lies entirely inside the object. We assume that $r_p > 1$ for all $p \in O$. Hence, the minimum of these radii (r_{min}) is selected.

Thus, we can use r_{min} to reduce the image's resolution without losing the objects of interest. This idea is shown in Figure 4. In this simple example, we have a threshold ($T < 150$) that identifies the object and a CF triangulation whose grid resolution is 10×10.

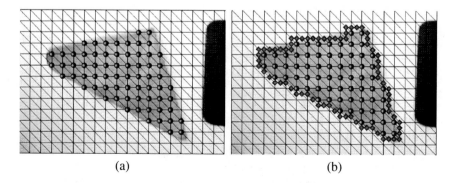

(a)   (b)

Figure 4. (a) Original image and Characteristic Function. (b) Boundary approximation.

Now, we can define a simple function, called an *Object Characteristic Function*, similar to function (2):

$$\chi(p) = 1, \quad if \quad I(p) < T, \tag{7}$$
$$\chi(p) = 0, \quad \text{otherwise},$$

where p is a node of the triangulation (marked grid nodes in Figure 4a).

We can take it a step further, shown in Figure 4b, where we present a curve that belongs to the transverse triangles. Observe that this curve approximates the boundary we seek. This curve (or surface for 3D) can be obtained by isosurface extraction methods and can be used to efficiently initialize the T-Surfaces model, as we pointed out earlier.

If we take a grid resolution coarser than r_{min}, the isosurface method might split the objects. Also, in [16, 15] it is supposed that the object boundaries are closed and connected. These topological restrictions imply that we do not need to search inside a generated connected components.

In this chapter we discard the mentioned scale and topological constraints. As a consequence, the target topology may be corrupted. So a careful approach will be required to deal with topological defects. An important point is the choice of method for isosurfaces generation, which will be discussed next.

3. ISOSURFACE EXTRACTION METHODS

Isosurface extraction is one of the most often-used techniques for visualization of volume data sets. Due to the data type (time-varying or stationary) and the data set size, many works have been done to improve the basic methods in this area [12]. In this chapter we consider two kinds of isosurface generation methods: marching and continuation.

In Marching Cubes, each surface-finding phase visits all cells of the volume, normally by varying coordinate values in a triple *for* loop [14]. As each cell that intersects the isosurface is found, the necessary polygon(s) representing the portion of the isosurface within the cell is generated. There is no attempt to trace the surface into neighboring cells. Space subdivision schemes (like Octree and k-d-tree) have been used to avoid the computational cost of visiting cells that the surface does not cut [27, 12].

Once the T-Surfaces grid is a CF one, the Tetra-Cubes is specially interesting for this discussion [28]. As in the marching cubes, its search is linear: each cell of the volume is visited and its simplices (tetrahedrons) are searched to find surface's patches. Following marching cubes implementations, Tetra-Cubes uses auxiliary structures based on the idea that the topology of the intersections between a plane and a tetrahedron can be reduced to the three basic configurations pictured on Figure 5.

Case 0   **Case 1**   **Case 2**

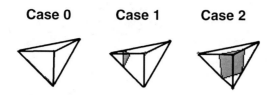

Figure 5. Basic types of intersections between a plane and a simplex in 3D.

Unlike marching methods, continuation algorithms attempt to trace the surface into neighboring simplices [13]. Thus, given a transverse simplex, the algorithm searches its neighbors to continue surface reconstruction. The key idea is to generate the combinatorial manifold (set of transverse simplices) that holds the isosurface.

The following definition will be useful. Suppose that two simplices σ_0 and σ_1, which have a common face and vertices $v \in \sigma_0$ and $v' \in \sigma_1$ both opposite to the common face. The process of obtaining v' from v is called *pivoting*. We now present the basic continuation algorithm [13].

Algorithm 1 PL Generation Algorithm

Find a transverse triangle σ_0
$\sum = \{\sigma_0\}$; $V(\sigma_0) = $ set of vertices of σ_0
while $V(\sigma) \neq \emptyset$ for some $\sigma \in \sum$ **do**
    get $\sigma \in \sum$ such that $V(\sigma) \neq \emptyset$;
    get $v \in V(\sigma)$
    obtain σ' from σ by pivoting v into v'
    if σ' is not transverse **then**
        drop v from $V(\sigma)$
    else

        if $\sigma' \in \sum$ **then**
            drop v from $V(\sigma)$, v' from $V(\sigma')$
        else
            $\sum \Longleftarrow \sum + \sigma'$
            $V(\sigma') \Longleftarrow$ set of vertices of σ'
            drop v from $V(\sigma)$, v' from $V(\sigma')$
        end if
    end if
end while

Different from Tetra-Cubes, once the generation of a component is begun, the algorithm runs until it is completed. However, the algorithm needs a set of seed simplices to be able to generate all the components of an isosurface. This is an important point when comparing continuation and marching methods.

If we do not have guesses about seeds, every simplex should be visited. Thus, the computational complexity of both methods is the same ($O(N)$, where N is the number of simplices). However, if we know in advance that the target boundary is connected we do not need to search inside a connected component. Consequently, the computational cost is reduced if continuation methods are applied.

We have emphasized in previous works that the isosurfaces methods are useful not only for initialization but also for reparameterization of T-Surfaces [16, 15]. In these studies, continuation methods were used for both those steps due to the fact that topological restrictions were supposed for the target. If these constraints are discarded, new considerations must be made to decide the more suitable isosurface method. This is demonstrated in the next section.

4. T-SURFACES AND ISOSURFACE METHODS

The reparameterization of T-Surfaces gives the link between the isosurface generation methods, described above, and the T-Surfaces model. To explain this, let us take the Object Characteristic Function defined in Eq. (7). If we apply tetra-cubes or continuation methods to this field, we get a set of piecewise linear (PL) surfaces that involve the structures of interest. It can be verified that each obtained connected component $\widehat{M}$ has the following properties: (1) the intersection $\sigma_1 \cap \sigma_2$ of two distinct triangles $\sigma_1, \sigma_2 \in \widehat{M}$ is empty, a common vertex or edge of both triangles; (2) an edge $\tau \in \widehat{M}$ is common to at most two triangles of $\widehat{M}$; (3) $\widehat{M}$ is locally finite, that is, any compact subset of $\Re^3$ meets only finitely many cells of $\widehat{M}$.

A polygonal surface with such a property is called a Piecewise Linear Manifold (*PL Manifold*) [13]. From the reparameterization process of Section 2.1, we can see that a T-Surface is also a PL Manifold. Thus, the isosurface extraction methods can be used in a straightforward fashion to initialize T-Surfaces. Besides, the Object Characteristic Function (Eq. (7)) gives the initial Characteristic Function. However, what kind of isosurface method should be used? Based on the discussion about tetra-cubes and PL generation (Section 3), we can conclude that if we do not have the topological and scale restrictions (Section 2.2), marching methods are more appropriate to initialize the T-Surfaces. In this case, it is not worthwhile to attempt to reconstruct the surface into neighboring simplices because all simplices should be visited to find surface patches.

However, for the T-Surfaces reparameterization (steps (1)–(4) of Section 2.1), the situation is different. Now, each connected component is evolved at a time.

Thus, a method that generates only the connected component being evolved is interesting, that is, the PL Generation algorithm.

However, what about the seed points? Our implementation of T-Surfaces uses a hash whose elements are specified by keys composed by two integers: the first one indicates a simplex and the second the connected component that cuts the simplex. There is one entry for each simplex of the triangulation. This structure is simple to implement. There are no additional costs of insertion or removal operations, and the cost of verifying if a transverse tetrahedron has been cut is $O(1)$. In this structure, seed points are found as follows. Let us take an intersection point obtained in step (1) of the reparameterization process. If it belongs to a simplex that is on the hash, the point is stored in a hash entry. Otherwise, we check if that simplex is a transverse one. If true, the point is stored and the simplex becomes a new seed to find another connected component through the PL Generation Algorithm (Section 3). The simplices that are obtained through this algorithm become new entries on the hash. Following this procedure, when the queue of projected points is empty, we can be sure that all the transverse simplices are on the hash. Then, the T-Surfaces components can be obtained by traversing the hash only once.

The next section presents our segmentation framework, which is the main contribution of the present work. It is based on application of isosurface techniques in the context of the T-Surfaces framework. In addition, we take advantage of the T-Surfaces reparameterization process (Section 2.1) to enable offset generation.

5. RECONSTRUCTION METHOD AND OFFSET GENERATION

The segmentation/surface reconstruction method that we propose in this chapter is based on the following steps [17]: (1) extract the threshold T, or a range $[T - \Delta T, T + \Delta T]$ that characterizes the objects of interest; (2) coarser image resolution; (3) define the *Object Characteristic Function*; (4) PL manifold extraction by the tetra-cubes; (5) if needed, increase the resolution and return to step (3); (6) apply the T-Surfaces model; (7) user interaction, if needed.

Step (1) can be performed by a simple inspection or any pre-segmentation step cited in Section 2. It is important to highlight that the T-Surfaces model can deal naturally with the self-intersections that may occur during the evolution of the surfaces obtained by step (4). This is an important advantage of T-Surfaces.

Among the surfaces extracted in step (4), there may be open surfaces that start and end in the image frontiers, small surfaces corresponding to artifacts or noise in the background. The former is discarded by a simple automatic inspection. To discard the later, we need a set of predefined features (volume, surface area, etc.), and corresponding lower bounds. For instance, we can set the volume lower bound as $8\,(r)^3$, where r is the dimension of the grid cells.

Besides, some polygonal surfaces may contain more than one object of interest (see Figure 7). Now, we can use upper bounds for the features. These upper bounds are application dependent (anatomical elements can be used).

The surfaces whose interior has volumes larger than the upper bound will be processed at a finer resolution. It is important to stress that the upper bound(s) is not an essential point for the method. Its role is only to avoid expending time of computation in regions where the boundaries enclose only one object.

When the T-Surface's grid resolution is increased, we just reparameterize the model over the finer grid and evolve the corresponding T-Surfaces. For uniform meshes, as in the Figure 6, this multiresolution scheme can be implemented through *Adaptive Mesh Refinement* data structures [29]. In these structures each node in the refinement level l splits into η^n nodes in level $l + 1$, where η is the refinement factor and n is the space dimension ($\eta = 2$ and $n = 3$ in our case). Such a scheme has also been explored in the context of *Level Sets* methods [30].

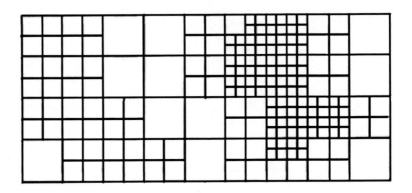

Figure 6. Representation of the multiresolution scheme.

As an example, let us consider Figure 7. In this image, the *outer* scale corresponding to the separation between the objects is finer than the object scales. Hence, the coarsest resolution could not *separate* all the objects. This happens for the bottom-left cells in Figure 7a. To correct that result, we increase the resolution only inside the extracted region to account for more details (Figure 7b).

Instead of using a multiresolution method, we could apply mathematical morphology operators before steps (1)–(4) in order to avoid the problems depicted in Figure 7a. However, even for these approaches, some manual intervention may be required to split the upper-right cells in Figure 7b. Besides, due to inhomogeneities of the image field (supposed graylevel), some objects may be split in step (4). Sometimes, T-Surfaces model are not able to merge them again.

To correct these problems, the user can manually burn some grid nodes to force merges or splits. From the entropy condition, these nodes remain burnt

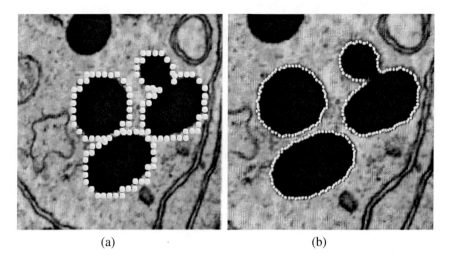

(a)   (b)

Figure 7. (a) PL manifolds for resolution 3×3. (b) Result with the highest (image) resolution.

until the end of the process. This functionality can be implemented by selecting grid nodes with a pointer (e.g., a mouse), through implicitly defined surfaces (see Section 6 below), or through a *virtual* scalpel.

We next we present our offset generation approach. Its background is also the T-Surfaces framework.

5.1. Offset Generation

Offsets have been used for computing levels of detail of a given polygonal object [31], as well as for initialization of Dual Snakes approaches [18]. Offset surfaces can self-intersect, and procedures to address this problem may be computational expensive. The efficiency of T-Surfaces to avoid self-intersections is the main point of using this model for offsets generation.

To describe our approach, let us first assume that we have an oriented and connected PL Manifold S. In this chapter we call an n-offset of S the polygonal surface obtained after n iterations of the T-Surfaces model initialized through S with $\gamma = 0$ in Eq. (5).

Before applying T-Surfaces, we should initialize the Characteristic Function. As the PL Generation Algorithm attempts to trace the surface into neighboring simplices, we do not need to visit all grid nodes to perform this task. In fact, we need only trace the combinatorial manifold whose dual is S. This can be implemented by considering that S is oriented. Thus, given a simplex cut by the surface, we can distinguish the vertices that lie inside from the ones that lie outside S. Henceforth, we reduce the complexity of the initialization step.

The self-intersections that may happen during evolution are easily resolved by the T-Surfaces model. Thus, we can preserve the topology of S. However, there is no correspondence between the points of S and the points of its n-offset because the reparameterization depends on projection of the surface over the grid. This is a disadvantage of this method compared with other offset generation approaches [31].

The n-offset is smoother than the initial surface S due to the elastic forces given by Eq. (3). The evolution can be seen as a curvature diffusion process in which the velocity of each surface point depends on the surface curvature. This kind of surface evolution has been explored in the context of implicit deformable models (*Level Sets*) and applied for shape recovery and mesh generation problems [30]. In Section 6.5 we will analyze the application of n-offsets for geometry extraction.

6. EXPERIMENTAL RESULTS

6.1. Noisy Images

The first point that will be demonstrated is the utility of image diffusion methods in our work. We take a synthetic $150 \times 150 \times 150$ image volume composed of a sphere with radius 30 and an ellipsoid with axes 45, 60, and 30 inside a uniform noise specified by the image intensity range 0–150.

Figure 8 shows the result for steps (1)–(4) from Section 5, applied to this volume after gaussian diffusion (Figure 8a), and anisotropic diffusion (Figure 8d), defined by the following equation:

$$\frac{\partial I}{\partial t} = div \left(\frac{\nabla I}{\left(1 + [\|\nabla I\| / K]^2\right)} \right), \tag{8}$$

where the threshold K can be determined by a gradient magnitude histogram. In this example, K was set to 300, and the number of iterations of the used numerical scheme [32] to solve this equation was set to 4.

Figures 8b and 8e show the cross-section corresponding to slice 40. We observe that with anisotropic diffusion (Figure 8e) the result is closer to the boundary than with the gaussian one (Figure 8b).

Also, the final result is more precise when pre-processing with anisotropic diffusion (Figure 8f). This is expected because, according to Appendix A, Eq. (8) enables one to blur small discontinuities (gradient magnitude below K) as well as to enhance edges (gradient magnitude above K).

Another point becomes clear in this example: the topological abilities of T-Surfaces enable correcting the defects observed in the surface extracted through steps (1)–(4). We observed that, after a few iterations, the method gives two closed components. Thus, the reconstruction is better.

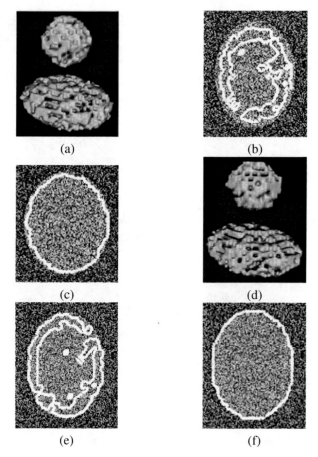

Figure 8. (a) Result for steps (1)–(4) with Gaussian Diffusion. (b) Cross-sections of (a) for slice 40. (c) Cross-section of final solution for slice 40. (d) Result for steps (1)–(4) with Anisotropic Diffusion. (e) Cross-sections of (d) for slice 40. (f) Cross-section of final solution when using anisotropic diffusion (slice 40).

The T-Surface parameters used are: $c = 0.65$, $k = 1.32$, and $\gamma = 0.01$. The grid resolution is $5 \times 5 \times 5$, the freezing point is set to 15, and the threshold $T \in (120, 134)$ in Eq. (4). The number of deformation steps for T-Surfaces was 17. The model evolution can be visualized at http://virtual01.lncc.br/~rodrigo/links/tese/elipse.html.

6.2. User Interaction

We will now demonstrate the potential of the user interaction procedure to force merges.

In this example, we have three spheres of intensity 50 placed in a $150 \times 150 \times 150$ image volume. The spheres were previously extracted by the proposed method

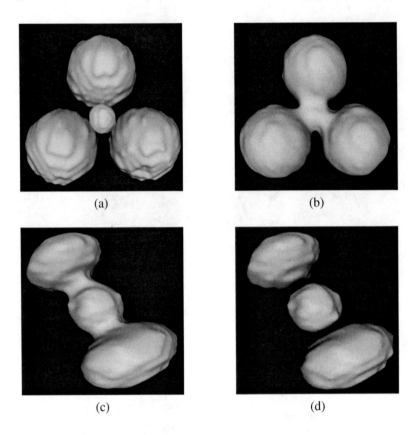

(a)   (b)

(c)   (d)

Figure 9. (a) Original objects. (b) Merge through the user interaction method. (c)Partial result. (d) Solution after manual cut.

with the following parameters: grid $5 \times 5 \times 5$, freezing point = 10, $\gamma = 0.01$, $k = 1.222$; $c = 0.750$. Each sphere has radius 30 (pixels). In this case, the merge is forced through an implicit defined surface placed between the spheres (Figure 9a). Grid nodes inside the surface are easily detected by the surface equation and then burnt. During the evolution, all the four surfaces will merge and the final result is a connected surface (Figure 9b).

Another possibility would be to manually burn a set of grid nodes linking the spheres. The idea in this case is that the new set of burnt grid nodes generates a connected combinatorial manifold.

Let us demonstrate the manual split. Figure 9c shows an example where steps (1)–(6) were not able to complete the segmentation. The 3D image is composed by 2 ellipsoids of radius 30, 45, and 60 and a sphere of radius 30, immersed in a $150 \times 150 \times 150$ noise volume.

The segmentation can be completed by user interaction based on the following steps: (a) define a cutting plane; (b) set to zero the grid nodes belonging to the triangles that the plane cuts and that are interior to the T-Surface; (c) apply steps (4)–(6) above. The grid nodes set to zero become burnt nodes. Thus, the entropy condition will prevent intersections of the surfaces generated. Hence, they will not merge again.

Figure 9d shows the final result. The T-Surface parameters are: $c = 0.65$, $k = 1.32$, and $\gamma = 0.01$. The grid resolution is $5 \times 5 \times 5$, the freezing point is set to 15, and threshold $T \in (120, 134)$ in Eq. (4).

6.3. Artery Segmentation

In this section we demonstrate the advantages of applying T-Surfaces plus isosurface methods. First, we segment an artery from an $80 \times 86 \times 72$ image volume obtained from the Visible Human project. This in an interesting example because the intensity pattern inside the artery is not homogeneous.

Figure 10a shows the result of steps (1)–(4) when using $T \in (28, 32)$ to define the object characteristic function (Eq. (7)). The extracted topology is too different from that of the target. However, when applying T-Surfaces the obtained geometry is improved.

Figure 10b shows the result after the first step of evolution. The merges among components improve the result. After 4 iterations of the T-Surfaces algorithm, the extracted geometry becomes closer to that of the target (Figure 10c).

However, the topology remains different. The problem in this case is that the used grid resolution is too coarse if compared with the separation between branches of the structure. Thus, the flexibility of the model was not enough to correctly perform the surface reconstruction.

The solution is to increase the resolution and take the partial result of Figure 10c to initialize the model at the finer resolution. In this case, the correct result is obtained only with the finest grid $(1 \times 1 \times 1)$. Figure 10d shows the desired result obtained after 9 iterations. We also observe that new portions of the branches were reconstructed due to increasing the flexibility of T-Surfaces obtained through the finer grid. We should emphasize that an advantage of the multiresolution approach is that at the lower resolution, small background artifacts become less significant relative to the object(s) of interest. Besides, it avoids the computational cost of using a finer grid resolution to get closer to the target (see Section 2.2).

The T-Surfaces parameters are $\gamma = 0.01$, $k = 1.222$, and $c = 0.750$. The total number of evolutions is 13. The number of triangular elements is 10104 for the highest resolution, and the CPU time was on the order of 3 minutes.

Sometimes, even the finest resolution may not be enough to get the correct result. Figure 11a depicts such an example.

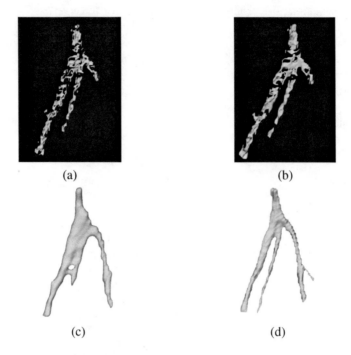

Figure 10. (a) Result of steps (1)–(4) with grid $3 \times 3 \times 3$. (b) T-Surfaces evolution (step 1). (c) Solution for initial grid. (d)Final solution for grid $1 \times 1 \times 1$.

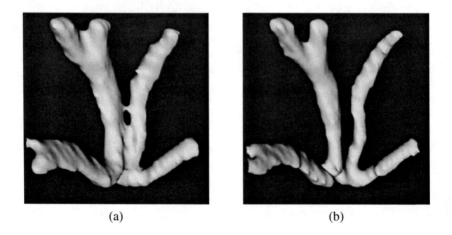

Figure 11. (a) Example showing an incorrect result. (b) Anisotropic diffusion in a pre-processing phase improving the final result.

In this case, we segment an artery from an $155 \times 170 \times 165$ image volume obtained from the Visible Man Project. The T-Surfaces parameters are: $c = 0.75$, $k = 1.12$, $\gamma = 0.3$, grid resolution $4 \times 4 \times 4$, and freezing point set to 10. The result of steps (1)–(6) is depicted in Figure 11a.

Among the proposals to address this problem (relax the threshold, mathematical morphology [33], etc), we have tested anisotropic diffusion [32]. The properties of this method (see Appendix A) enable smoothing within regions in preference to smoothing across boundaries. Figure 11b shows the correct result obtained when pre-processing the image with anisotropic diffusion and then applying steps (1)–(6).

6.4. CT Images

In this section we test our approach for a $150 \times 175 \times 180$ computed tomography image. The structure of interest is the right kidney. Figure 12a shows the result of steps (1)–(4) when using $T \in (205, 255)$ in Eq. (7) as well as the following parameters: $\gamma = 0.01$, $k = 1.222$, and $c = 0.750$. The total number of evolutions was 8. The grid resolution is $3 \times 3 \times 3$.

Like in previous examples, the genus of the extracted surface is not the correct one and some small disconnected components appear (Figure 12a). After 10 iterations of the T-Surfaces algorithm, the geometry extracted becomes that one of the target. Figures 12b and 12c show that the defects (holes) observed in Figure 12a have disappeared and that the final topology is the correct one.

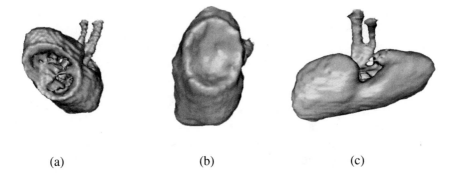

(a)   (b)   (c)

Figure 12. (a) Result for steps (1)–(4) for CT volume images. (b) View of final solution showing that topological defects were corrected. (c) Another view of the final solution.

6.5. Image Segmentation and Offsets

Finally, we demonstrate the potential of the offset generation procedure from Section 5.1. For this goal, we reproduce in Figure 13a the result presented on Figure 11b and take an offset of it. Figure 13b shows the 5-offset of this surface. We observe that the topology was preserved.

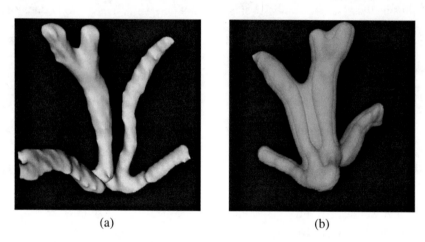

(a)   (b)

Figure 13. (a) Initial surface. (b) Offset generated by T-Surfaces model.

For geometry reconstruction, offsets have been used by some of us in the context of Dual Active Contour Models approaches (see [18] and the references therein). To initialize these models we need two contours (an inner and an outer one), which will evolve toward the boundary through an energy/position balance. In [18], we used a 2D version of the method proposed in Section 5.1 to generate offsets for automatic initialization of our Dual-T-Snakes approach [34, 18]. Dual-T-Snakes can be extended to 3D, through T-Surfaces. Thus, we intend to use surface offsets to initialize it.

7. DISCUSSION AND PERSPECTIVES

It is interesting to compare our approach to that proposed in [11]. In that study, a set of small spherical T-Snakes was uniformly distributed over the image. These curves progressively expand/merge to recover the geometry of interest. The same can be done for 3D.

Our approach can be viewed as an improvement on this method. Our basic argument is that we should use the threshold to get *seeds* closer to the objects of interest. Thus, we avoid expending time on evolving surfaces far from the target geometry. Besides, we have observed an improvement in the performance of the segmentation process if compared with the traditional initialization of T-Surfaces (an implicitly defined surface inside the object) [10]. For instance, when segmenting an object with approximately 7000 triangular elements immersed in a $128 \times 128 \times 25$ synthetic volume, our method takes 33 seconds against the 9 minutes and 12 seconds with the traditional method (see http://virtual01.lncc.br/~rodrigo/links/tese/teste2.html). In this case, the grid resolution was $6 \times 6 \times 2$. Besides, the computational complexity of our method can be compared with that of using just a T-Surfaces initialized through the traditional method. Let us suppose that the inner volume of a structure of interest encompasses C tetrahedrons. In this case, the T-Surfaces has to pass over $O(C)$ simplices to get the target surface when initialized by the implicit surface. Therefore, if C is $O(N)$, where N is the number of simplices of the domain subdivision, then the computational complexity of both our segmentation approach and the traditional T-Surfaces is the same.

The proposed method is adaptive in the sense that we can increase the T-Surfaces grid resolution where it is necessary. As the T-Surfaces grid controls the density of the polygonal surfaces obtained, the number of triangular elements gets larger inside these regions. That density increasing is not due to boundary details but because the outer scale corresponding to the separation between the objects is too fine (like in Figure 7). This is a disadvantage of our approach. Such a problem would be avoided if we could define significant areas along the surfaces, and then apply the refinement only in the regions around them. However, it is difficult to automatically perform this task.

As a consequence, polygonal meshes generated by the T-Surface method may not be efficient for some further application. For instance, for finite-element purposes, small triangles must be removed. Consequently, filtering mesh procedures must be applied in order to improve the surface. Mesh smoothing and denoising filtering methods, like that one proposed in [35], could also be useful in this post-processing step.

We tested the precision of our approach when segmenting a sphere immersed on a uniform noise specified by the image intensity range 0–150. We found a mean error of 1.58 (pixels) with standard deviation of 2.49 for a $5 \times 5 \times 5$ grid resolution, which we consider acceptable in this case. This error is due to the projection of T-Surfaces as well as the image noise. Following [9, 10], when T-Surfaces stops, we can discard the grid and evolve the model without it to avoid errors due to the projections. However, for noisy images, the convergence of deformable models to the boundaries is poor due to the non-convexity of the image energy [26].

Anisotropic diffusion applied to 3D images can improve the result, as already stated in Section 6.3. Vector diffusion techniques can also be applied to generate an image force field that improves the convergence of the model toward the boundary when the grid is turned off (see Appendix A).

We will now consider the following question: Would it be possible to implement the reconstruction method, the user interaction approach, and the offset generation through Level Sets? The relevance of it will be not only the possibility of implementing an alternative formulation for our work, but also to compare Level Sets with T-Surfaces within its context.

To answer this question we must review some details of the Level Sets formulation [8]. The main idea of this method is to represent the deformable surface (or curve) as a zero level set $\{x \in \Re^3 | G(x) = 0\}$ of an embedding function:

$$G : \Re^3 \times \Re^+ \rightarrow \Re, \tag{9}$$

such that the deformable surface (also called the *front* in this formulation), at $t = 0$, is given by a surface S:

$$S(t = 0) = \{x \in \Re^3 | G(x, t = 0) = 0\}. \tag{10}$$

The next step is to find an Eulerian formulation for the front evolution. Following Sethian [8], let us suppose that the front evolves in the normal direction with velocity $\overrightarrow{F}$, where $\overrightarrow{F}$ may be a function of the curvature, normal direction, etc.

We need an equation for the evolution of $G(x, t)$, considering that the surface S is the level set given by:

$$S(t) = \{x \in \Re^3 | G(x, t) = 0\}. \tag{11}$$

Let us take a point $x(t)$, $t \in \Re^+$ of the propagating front S. From its implicit definition given above, we have

$$G(x(t), t) = 0. \tag{12}$$

We can now use the Chain Rule to compute the time derivative of this equation:

$$G_t + F|\nabla G| = 0, \tag{13}$$

where $F = \left\| \overrightarrow{F} \right\|$ is called the *speed function*. An initial condition $G(x, t = 0)$ is required. A straightforward (and expensive) technique to define this function is to compute a signed-distance function as follows:

$$G(x, t = 0) = \pm d, \tag{14}$$

where d is the distance from x to the surface $S(x, t = 0)$ and the signal indicates if the point is interior (–) or exterior (+) to the initial front.

Finite-difference schemes, based on a uniform grid, can be used to solve Eq. (13). The same entropy condition of T-Surfaces (*once a grid node is burnt it stays burnt*) is incorporated in order to drive the model to the desired solution (in fact, T-Surfaces was inspired by the Level Sets model [9]).

In this higher-dimensional formulation, topological changes can be efficiently implemented. Numerical schemes are stable, and the model is general in the sense that the same formulation holds for 2D and 3D, as well as for merges and splits. Besides, the surface geometry is easily computed. For example, the front normal and curvature are given by:

$$\vec{n} = \nabla G\left(x, t\right), \quad K = \nabla \cdot \left(\frac{\nabla G\left(x, t\right)}{\|\nabla G\left(x, t\right)\|}\right), \tag{15}$$

respectively, where the gradient and the divergent ($\nabla \cdot$) are computed with respect to x.

The initialization of the model through Eq. (14) is computationally expensive and not efficient if we have more than one front to initialize [4].

The *narrow-band* technique is much more appropriate for this case. The key idea of this technique comes from the observation that the front can be moved by updating the level set function at a small set of points in the neighborhood of the zero set instead of updating it at all the points on the domain (see [8, 30] for details).

To implement this scheme, we need to pre-set a distance Δd to define the narrow band. The front can move inside the narrow band until it collides with the narrow-band frontiers. Then, the function G should be reinitialized by treating the current zero set configuration as the initial one.

Also, this method can be made cheaper by observing that the grid points that do not belong to the narrow band can be treated as sign holders [8], following the same idea of the characteristic function defined in Equation (2). Thus, the result of steps (1)-(5) (Section 5) can be used to initialize the Level Sets model if the narrow-band extension technique is applied.

At first, the user interaction procedure can also be implemented by using the narrow-band approach. From the entropy condition, manually burnt nodes remain burnt and consequently the split components will not merge again. However, we should be careful to rebuild the narrow band consistently after the manual intervention. We believe that this is the main challenge with this direction.

Offsets can also be implemented through Level Sets in a manner that resembles the application of level sets for grid generation [36]. For example, in the case of convex initial shape, $F = -K$, where K is given in Eq. (15), is effective. For a non-convex initial body, points with high curvature can move against the front. A possible solution is to include a threshold value that ensures that the front always moves outward: $F = \min\left(-K, F_{threshold}\right)$. However, for highly non-convex bodies, like the ones generated by steps (1)–(5), the speed function is not simple. Then, sorting of domain decomposition would be required [36, 30]. These are further directions for our work, as dicussed next.

8. CONCLUSIONS AND FUTURE WORK

In the present work we generalize our previous works [16, 15]. We demonstrate that steps (1)–(6) can be applied without scale or topological restrictions. Besides, we present a general interactive procedure to change the topology of a surface.

The purpose of this work will be to extend the user interaction method by using a scalpel and allowing the user to drag the scalpel.

In addition, we aim to apply the gradient vector flow (GVF), described in Appendix A, to improve the precision of the final result. We expect that with the proposed modifications for the GVF we will get a method less sensitive to noise and artifacts.

Another interesting point is to implement our approach by Level Sets, instead of T-Surfaces, following the discussion in Section 7. Finally, we expect that surface offsets will be useful to automatically initialize dual approaches for deformable surfaces.

9. ACKNOWLEDGMENTS

We would like to acknowledge the Brazilian Agency for Scientific Development (CNPq) and PCI-LNCC for their financial support of this work.

10. REFERENCES

1. Kass M, Witkin A, Terzopoulos D. 1988. Snakes: active contour models. *Int J Comput Vision* **1**(4):321–331.
2. McInerney T, Terzopoulos D. 1996. Deformable models in medical image analysis: a survey. *Med Image Anal* **1**(2): 91–108.
3. Cohen LD, Cohen I. 1993. Finite-element methods for active contour models and balloons for 2D and 3D images. *IEEE Trans Pattern Anal Machine Intell* **15**(11): 1131–1147.
4. ter Haar Romery BM, Niessen WJ, Viergever MA. 1998. Geodesic deformable models for medical image analysis. *IEEE Trans Med Imaging* **17**(4):634–641.
5. Sapiro G. 1997. Color snakes. *Comput Vision Image Understand* **68**(2):247–253.
6. Black A, Yuille A, eds. 1993. *Active vision*. Cambridge: MIT Press.
7. Caselles V, Kimmel R, Sapiro G. 1997. Geodesic active contours. *Int J Comput Vision* **22**(1):61–79.
8. Malladi R, Sethian JA, Vemuri BC. 1995. Shape modeling with front propagation: a level set approach. *IEEE Trans Pattern Anal Machine Intell* **17**(2):158–175.
9. McInerney TJ. 1997. *Topologically adaptable deformable models for medical image analysis*. PhD dissertation. University of Toronto.
10. McInerney T, Terzopoulos D. 1999. Topology adaptive deformable surfaces for medical image volume segmentation. *IEEE Trans Med Imaging* **18**(10):840–850.
11. McInerney T, Terzopoulos D. 1995. Topologically adaptable snakes. In *Proceedings of the fifth international conference on computer vision (ICCV'95), Cambridge, MA, USA*, pp. 840–845.

12. Sutton P, Hansen C. 2000. Accelerated isosurface extraction in time-varying fields. *IEEE Trans Visualiz Comput Graphics* **6**(2):98–107.

13. Allgower EL, Georg K. 1990. *Numerical continuation methods: an introduction.* Berlin: Springer-Verlag.

14. Lorensen WE, Cline HE. 1987. Marching cubes: a high-resolution 3D surface construction algorithm. *Comput Graphics* **21**(4):163–169.

15. Strauss E, Jimenez W, Giraldi G, Silva R, Oliveira A. 2002. *A surface extraction approach based on multi-resolution methods and T-surfaces framework.* Technical report, National Laboratory for Scientific Computing, ftp://ftp.lncc.br/pub/report/rep02/rep1002.ps.Z.

16. Giraldi G, Strauss E, Apolinario A, Oliveira AF. 2001. An initialization method for deformable models. In *Fifth world multiconference on systemics, cybernetics and informatics (SCI).*

17. Strauss E, Jimenez W, Giraldi GA, Silva R, Oliveira AF. 2002. A semiautomatic surface reconstruction framework based on T-surfaces and isosurface extraction methods. In *Proceedings of the international symposium on computer graphics, image processing and vision (SIBGRAPI'2001), Florianópolis, Brazil, October 15–18.*

18. Giraldi GA, Strauss E, Oliveira AF. 2003. Dual-T-snakes model for medical imaging segmentation. *Pattern Recognit Lett* **24**(7):993–1003.

19. Xu C, Pham D, Rettmann M, Yu D, Prince J. 1999. Reconstruction of the human cerebral cortex from magnetic resonance images. *IEEE Trans Med Imaging* **18**(6):467–480.

20. Giraldi GA, Strauss E, Oliveira AF. 2000. An initialization method for active contour models. In *Proceedings of the 2000 international conference on imaging science, systems, and technology (CISST'2000).*

21. Pohle R, Behlau T, Toennies KD. 2003. Segmentation of 3D medical image data sets with a combination of region based initial segmentation and active surfaces. In *Progress in biomedical optics and imaging. Proc SPIE Med Imaging* **5203**:1225–1231.

22. Cohen LD. 1991. On active contour models and balloons. *Comput Vision Graphics Image Process: Image Understand* **53**(2):211–218.

23. Falcão AX, da Cunha BS, Lotufo RA. 2001. Design of connected operators using the image foresting transform. *Proc SPIE Med Imaging* **4322**:468–479.

24. Jolion JM, Montanvert A. 1992. The adaptive pyramid: a framework for 2D image analysis. *Comput Vision Graphics Image Process: Image Understand* **55**(3):339–348.

25. Xu C, Prince J. 1998. Snakes, shapes, and gradient vector flow. *IEEE Trans Image Process* **7**(3):359–369.

26. Giraldi GA, Oliveira AF. 1999. *Convexity analysis of snake models based on hamiltonian formulation.* Technical report, Universidade Federal do Rio de Janeiro, Departamento Engenharia de Sistemas e Computação, http://www.arxiv.org/abs/cs.CV/0504031.

27. Chiang Y-J, Silva C, Schroeder W. 1998. Interactive out-of-core isosurface extraction. In *IEEE Visualization '98*, pp. 167–174.

28. Carneiro BP, Silva CT, Kaufman AE. 1996. Tetra-cubes: An algorithm to generate 3D isosurfaces based upon tetrahedra. In *Proceedings of the international symposium on computer graphics, image processing and vision (SIBGRAPI'96).*

29. Berger MJ, Oliger J. 1984. Adaptive mesh refinement for hyperbolic partial differential equations. *J Comput Phys* **54**:484–512.

30. Sethian JA. 1996. *Level set methods: evolving interfaces in geometry, fluid mechanics, computer vision and materials sciences.* Cambridge: Cambridge UP.

31. Cohen J, Varshney A, Manocha D, Turk G, Weber H, Agarwal P, Brooks F, Wright W. 1996. Simplification envelopes. *Comput graphics* **30**:119–128.

32. Perona P, Malik J. 1990. Scale-space and edge detection using anisotropic diffusion. *IEEE Trans Pattern Anal Machine Intell* **12**(7):629–639.

33. Sarti A, Ortiz C, Lockett S, Malladi R. 1998. A unified geometric model for 3D confocal image analysis in cytology. In *Proceedings of the international symposium on computer graphics, image processing and vision (SIBGRAPI'98)*, pp. 69–76.

34. Giraldi GA, Strauss E, Oliveira AF. 2001. Dual and topologically adaptable snakes and initialization of deformable models. In *Proceedings of the International conference on imaging science, systems, and technology (CISST'2001)*.

35. Taubin G. 2001. *Linear anisotropic mesh filtering*. Technical report RC-22213, IBM T.J. Watson Research Center.

36. Sethian JA. 1994. Curvature flow and entropy conditions applied to grid generation. *J Comput Phys* 115:440–454.

37. Xu C, Prince JL. 2000. Global optimality of gradient vector flow. In *Proceedings of the conference on information sciences and systems, Princeton University*.

APPENDIX A: DIFFUSION METHODS

In Eq. (13), if the function F depends on the curvature, we may have a geometric flow in which high curvatures are diffused.

In image processing, diffusion schemes for scalar and vector fields have also been applied. Gaussian blurring is the most commonly known one. Other approaches include anisotropic diffusion and Gradient Vector Flow. We will summarize these methods and conjecture their unification.

Anisotropic diffusion is defined by the following general equation:

$$\frac{\partial I\left(x,y,t\right)}{\partial t} = div\left(c\left(x,y,t\right)\nabla I\right), \tag{16}$$

where I is a graylevel image [32].

In this method, the blurring on parts with high gradient can be made much smaller than in the rest of the image. To show this property, we follow Perona-Malik [32]. First, we suppose that the edge points are oriented in the x direction. Thus, Eq. (16) becomes:

$$\frac{\partial I\left(x,y,t\right)}{\partial t} = \frac{\partial}{\partial x}\left(c\left(x,y,t\right) I_x\left(x,y,t\right)\right). \tag{17}$$

If c is a function of the image gradient: $c\left(x,y,t\right) = g\left(I_x\left(x,y,t\right)\right)$, we can define $\phi\left(I_x\right) \equiv g\left(I_x\right) \cdot I_x$ and then write Eq. (16) as

$$I_t = \frac{\partial I}{\partial t} = \frac{\partial}{\partial x}\left(\phi\left(I_x\right)\right) = \phi'\left(I_x\right) \cdot I_{xx}. \tag{18}$$

We are interested in the time variation of the slope: $\frac{\partial I_x}{\partial t}$. If $c\left(x,y,t\right) > 0$, we can change the order of differentiation and with a simple algebra demonstrate that

$$\frac{\partial I_x}{\partial t} = \frac{\partial I_t}{\partial x} = \phi'' \cdot I_{xx}^2 + \phi' \cdot I_{xxx}.$$

At edge points we have $I_{xx} = 0$ and $I_{xxx} << 0$, as these points are local maxima of the image gradient intensity. Thus, there is a neighborhood of the edge point in which the derivative $\partial I_x / \partial t$ has a sign opposite to $\phi'(I_x)$. If $\phi'(I_x) > 0$, the slope of the edge point decreases with time. Otherwise, it increases, which means that the border becomes sharper. Thus, the diffusion scheme given by Eq. (16) allows to blur small discontinuities and to enhance stronger ones. In this work, we have used ϕ as follows:

$$\phi = \left(\frac{\nabla I}{\left(1 + [\|\nabla I\| / K]^2\right)} \right), \tag{19}$$

as can be observed from Eq. (8).

In the above scheme, I is a scalar field. For vector fields, a useful diffusion scheme is the Gradient Vector Flow (GVF). It was introduced in [25] and can be defined through the following equation [37]:

$$\frac{\partial u}{\partial t} = \nabla \cdot (g \nabla u) + h(u - \nabla f), \tag{20}$$
$$u(x, 0) = \nabla f,$$

where f is a function of the image gradient (for example, P in Eq. (5)), and $g(x), h(x)$ are nonnegative functions defined on the image domain.

The field obtained by solving the above equation is a smooth version of the original one, which tends to be extended very far away from the object boundaries. When used as an external force for deformable models, it makes the methods less sensitive to initialization [25].

As the result of steps (1)–(6) (Section 5) is in general close to the target, we could apply this method to push the model toward the boundary when the grid is turned off. However, for noisy images some kind of diffusion (smoothing) must be used before applying GVF. Gaussian diffusion has been used [25], but precision may be lost due to nonselective blurring [32].

The anisotropic diffusion scheme presented above is an alternative smoothing method that can be used. Such an observation points toward the possibility of integrating anisotropic diffusion and GVF within a unified framework. A straightforward way of doing this is allowing g and h to be dependent upon the vector field u. The key idea would be to combine the selective smoothing of anisotropic diffusion with diffusion of the initial field obtained by GVF. Besides, we expect to get a more stable numerical scheme for noisy images.

2

PARAMETRIC CONTOUR MODEL IN
MEDICAL IMAGE SEGMENTATION

Bipul Das

Imaging Technology Division, GE India
Technology Centre, Bangalore, India

Swapna Banerjee

Department of Electronics and ECE, Indian
Institute of Technology, Kharagpur India

The model-based technique offers a unique and efficient approach toward medical image segmentation and analysis due to its power to unify image information within a physical framework. Of the model-based techniques, the deformable model is most effectively used for its ability to unify image statistics — both local and global — in a geometrically constrained framework. The geometric constraint imparts a compact form of shape information. This chapter reviews one of the most promising and highly used deformable approaches: the active contour model in medical image analysis. The active contour model is one of the most effective approaches due to its flexibility to adapt to various anatomical shapes while constraining the local geometric shape constraint. Within the geometric paradigm, local image statistics and regional information has been effectively used in segmentation purposes. In addition, various forms of a-priori information can be incorporated into this model. Active contour models are capable of accommodating a wide range of shape variability over time and space. The active contour also has to overcome the limitation of topological adaptibility by introducing a topology adaptive model. This chapter details the development and evolution of the active contour model with the growing sophistication of medical images.

Address all correspondence to: Bipul Das, Imaging Technology Division, John F. Welch Technology Centre, GE India Technology Centre, Plot #122, Export Promotion Industrial Park, Phase 2, Hoodi Village, Whitefield Road, Bangalore 560066, India. Phone: +91 (80) 2503 3225; Fax: +91 (80) 2525 5492. bipul.das@ge.com.

1. INTRODUCTION

The rapid development and proliferation of medical imaging technologies is revolutionizing medicine. Physicians and scientists noninvasively gather potentially life-saving anatomical information using the images obtained from these imaging devices. The need for identification and interaction with anatomical tissues by physiologists has led to an immense research effort into a wide range of medical imaging modalities. The intent of medical image analysis is manifold, ranging from interpretation, analysis, and visualization to a means for surgical planning and simulation, postoperative progression of the disease, and intraoperative navigation. For example, ascertaining the detailed shape and organization of the aortic arch in the abdomen for an aneurysm operation enables a surgeon preoperatively to plan an optimal stent design and other characteristics for the aorta.

Each of the imaging modalities captures a unique tissue property. Magnetic resonance imaging (MRI) uses the heterogeneous magnetic property of tissue to generate the image [1]. The response to an applied magnetic field is distinctive for each tissue and is reflected in the image. Doppler ultrasound, on the other hand, relies on the acoustic scattering property of each tissue [2]. X-ray and computed tomography (CT) imaging [3] are based on absorption. Functional imaging modalities like positron emission tomography (PET) and fMRI (functional MRI) highlight metabolic activities in the region of interest [4–6].

Although modern imaging devices provide exceptional views of internal anatomy as well as functional images, accurate quantification and analysis of the region of interest still remains a major challenge. Physicians manually segment and analyze the images, which is highly time consuming and prone to inter-observer variability. Accurate, reproducible quantification of medical images is required in order to support biomedical investigations and clinical activities. As imaging devices are moving toward higher-resolution images and the field of view (FOV) is increasing, the size of datasets is exploding. Manual analysis is becoming more challenging and nearly impossible. Thus, the need for computer-aided automated and semi-automated algorithms for segmenting and analyzing medical data is gaining importance.

The variability of anatomic shapes makes it difficult to construct a unique and compact geometric model for representation of an anatomic region. Furthermore, many factors contribute to degradation of image quality, which makes the process of segmentation even more challenging. Although the nature of artifacts may vary with imaging modality and the tissue concerned, their effect on image quality is nevertheless detrimental. Figures 1 and 2 the illustrate effects of two different types of artifacts in the process of image acquisition. In Figure 1 the inhomogeneity factor makes the middle region of the image darker compared to the top and lower side. In this case the inhomogeneity factor is a slowly varying intensity gradient

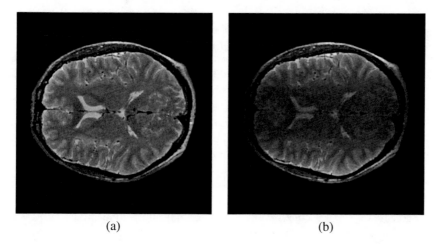

Figure 1. Effects of inhomogeneity in MRI images of brain: (a) images without inhomogeneity; (b) with inhomogeneity effects.

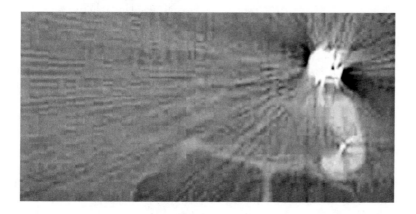

Figure 2. Illustration of streak artifacts in CT images.

from the middle to the outer sides. Figure 2 shows the effect of metal in CT, where radial streaks are observed from the metal sites (right region in the image).

The resolution of the imaging device also determines image quality. A low-resolution device suffers from problems of fuzzification and occlusion of boundaries, giving rise to blurred and disconnected anatomical edges. But an increase in image resolution is limited by factors like a low signal-to-noise ratio, exposure to more radiation, extended imaging time, and increasing contrast dosages. With all these factors affecting image quality, the challenge for the image analysis community is to find suitable algorithms to accurately and reproducibly segment anatomical structures for clinical studies.

Traditional low-level image processing techniques perform operations using local image statistics, producing localized patterns that need unification to form a meaningful segmentation. However, in most cases it leads to incorrect connected boundaries due to a lack of sufficient statistics in most regions. Moreover, the above-mentioned artifacts immensely bias the local statistics, making it impossible to generate anatomically correct structures. As a result, these techniques require a considerable amount of manual intervention to generate a meaningful structure, making it a tedious process, and one prone to operator subjectivity.

On the other hand, the use of global properties like intensity values or compact geometric models is also not always possible since these properties themselves do not necessarily have a one-on-one mapping with an anatomical structure or a desired region of interest. A methodology that can encapsulate local statistics in a global framework might prove to be a better alternative in this respect. Deformable models [7–11] comprise a step in that direction. The main idea of these models is that of using local statistics to deform a global geometric model. Through the last two decades, deformable models have been a promising and vigorously researched approach to computer-assisted medical image analysis. The source of the immense potential for the use of deformable models in segmentation, matching, and tracking of anatomic structures in medical images lies in its bottom–up approach, which exploits features derived from local image statistics along with a priori knowledge about the location, size, and shape of these structures [12]. This allows a high range of variability of these models to accommodate significant variation in biological structures.

The active contour model, commonly known as the snakes model, proposed by Kass et al. [10], defines a parametric framework for a curve that deforms under the action of local image statistics to conform into the perceived boundary of the structure in an image. For the last two decades, the active contour model has found widespread application in many fields of medical image segmentation and has undergone immense development in terms of its theoretical insight, as well as making itself more flexible and adaptable. This chapter tries to capture the evolution of this model and its use in medical image segmentation. Organization of the chapter is as follows: Section 2 provides the basic theory of an active contour and explains the underlying physics. The confluence of geometry and image properties is also explained in this section and the effects of each of the properties are explored. Section 3 describes the evolution of the snake model to address the requirements of medical image analysis applications. Section 4 describes the inclusion of a-priori information within the snake framework. Section 5 deals with the topological adaptability of the snake. We conclude with some discussion in Section 6.

2. ACTIVE CONTOUR MODEL: THEORY

This section will elaborate the theory of the active contour model. For easy reference, the definitions and notations used here are defined in the next subsection.

2.1. Definitions and Notations

We use $\Re$ is to denote a real number line, and $\Re^2$ will denote the Euclidean plane. An *image* is considered to be embedded on a rectangular subspace $R \subset \Re^2$. Over R, intensity values are acquired at every point with integral coordinates commonly referred to as *pixels*. A point in R will be represented as a two-dimensional position vector $\mathbf{u} = (x, y)$, where x, y denote the x- and y-coordinate values of $\mathbf{u}$. Let $f : R \rightarrow [0, 1, 2, 3, ..., \text{MaxIntensity}]$ denote the *intensity function* for a given image.

A *parametric curve* or *spline* is represented as a function $\tau : [0, 1] \rightarrow \Re^2$. A curve is closed if the initial and terminal points are identical, i.e., $\tau(0) = \tau(1)$. A point on the curve will be denoted by $\tau(s) = (x(s), y(s))$, where $s \in [0, 1]$ denotes the arc-length parameter, and $x(s)$ and $y(s)$ refer to its location in the xy-plane. Although in a continuous space any real value in $[0, 1]$ may be assigned to the parameter s, in the digital world only discrete values can be used. The snake is an ordered sequence of discrete points on a curve at a regular interval $\delta < 1.0$, where δ is a finitely small positive number. The points $..., \tau(-2\delta), \tau(-\delta), \tau(0), \tau(\delta), \tau(2\delta), ...$ on a snake τ at an interval of δ will be referred to as *control points*.

Let a contiguous set of pixels belonging to the structure of interest, sharing some similar attributes, be called the *foreground* and be denoted as $O \subset R$, where R is the image space. Any pixel $c \in O$ is called an object pixel. On the other hand, any pixel $c \in R - O$, i.e., belonging to the image space R but not belonging to the object space O, is a *background* pixel. The task of image segmentation is to identify the foreground O from the image space R. This requires representation of the foreground region into a compact geometric form.

2.2. Basic Snake Theory

Snakes are planar deformable contours that are useful in several image analysis tasks. In many images, the boundaries are not well delineated due to degradation by regional blurring, noise, and other artifacts. Despite these difficulties, human vision and perception interpolate between missing boundary segments. An active contour model is intended at inculcating this property of the human vision system. So the snake framework is formulated such that it approximates the locations and shapes of object boundaries in images based on the assumption that boundaries are piecewise continuous or smooth.

The mathematical basis for active contour models owes its foundation to the principle of unification of physics and optimization theory [12]. The laws of physics define the underlying principle of how a geometrical shape can vary over space and time. An active contour model permits an arbitrary shape to evolve to a meaningful shape guided by the image properties and constrained by the physical laws. The physical laws provide the desired intuitive nature to the evolving shape. In particular, for the snake, the points does not evolve independently but are constrained by the motion of the two nearest points on either side, thus confining its degrees of freedom, bringing an elastic model into the structure. Thus, it evolves from the elastic theory paradigm, generally in a Lagrangian dynamics setting. It stems from the theory of an elastic string deforming naturally to applied forces and constraints defined by various sources.

Guided by the physical laws, the model is driven to deform toward a lower-energy or equilibrium state monotonically. The local image statistics should be formulated within the deformable paradigm in such a way that the model is guided to delineate the desired anatomic structure. The optimization theory blends these two different forms of constraints within the same framework. The local image statistics-based features thus need to be defined within the framework of this physics-based geometric model, such that the "equilibrium state" is achieved only when the anatomic structure is delineated.

Definition of this physics-based model that governs the deformation property of the string is the main essence that makes the deformable model an attractive proposition to capture the local statistics of the image globally. A deformable model, and in particular an active contour model, by definition optimally integrates similar salient features within the geometric model.

The active contour model, or snake, proposed by Kass et al. [10] is an elastic contour that deforms under the guidance of attributed geometric and image properties. This phenomenon of deformation, as guided by physical laws, is defined in terms of an energy minimization framework. By definition, it is minimization of the total energy over the entire shape, defined by

$$E_{\text{snake}}(\tau) = E_{\text{int}}(\tau) + E_{\text{ext}}(\tau) \tag{1}$$

where $E_{\text{snake}}(\tau)$ is the total energy of the contour τ, composed of the internal energy $E_{\text{int}}(\tau)$ and external energy $E_{\text{ext}}(\tau)$. Internal energy is defined by the physical constraints that describe the degrees of freedom of the contour $\tau(s)$, and the external energy is defined by the image properties and other user constraints (e.g., landmark).

As defined previously, the physical constraints of the active contour model have their origin in the physics of an elastic body, which is described in the first term of the functional in Eq. (1). The internal energy term can be expressed as

$$E_{\text{int}}(\tau) = \int\limits_{0}^{1} \left[\alpha(s) \left| \frac{\partial \tau(s)}{\partial s} \right|^2 + \beta(s) \left| \frac{\partial^2 \tau(s)}{\partial s^2} \right|^2 \right] ds, \tag{2}$$

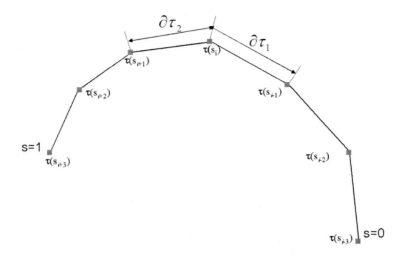

Figure 3. Illustration of computation of the surface tension and rigidity energies in the parametric snake framework. See attached CD for color version.

where the first term simulates the tension of the contour and the second, which is in essence the acceleration term, simulates the rigidity of the contour $\tau(s)$. $\alpha(s)$ and $\beta(s)$ $(\alpha(s), \beta(s) \in [0, 1])$ are the controlling strengths associated with the surface tension and rigidity terms. Although the strength factors are expressed as functions of the parameter s, in most cases they remain constant throughout the contour length. Thus, the term s will be dropped in future references to these factors for simplification.

Let us see how these terms control the contour behavior as the total energy functional tries to minimize itself. The first order derivative term in Eq. (2) can be minimized by reducing the value of the numerator. Thus, the difference between the two points $\partial \tau$ needs to be reduced (see Figure 3), which leads to shrinking the length of the contour $\tau(s)$. On the other hand, the second term in the expression is by definition the curvature term. Reduction of that term means the difference between $\partial \tau_1$ and $\partial \tau_2$ in Figure 3 needs to be minimized. Thus, minimizing this term leads to resistance to any bending and eventually straightening the contour $\tau(s)$, leading to a smooth contour. In case the contour is a closed one, the effect of these two terms will lead to a shrinking circle, in the absence of any other force.

Once the physical constraints are defined, the behavior of the contour is well set in terms of its geometric properties. However, its behavior on the image domain needs to be controlled by the image statistics-driven factors, such that the local minima coincide with the image feature of interest. For example, when the snake needs to converge onto image edges, then the external energy function needs to be defined as $-\gamma |\nabla G_\sigma * I(x,y)|^2$, where γ controls the magnitude of the potential, ∇ is the gradient operator, and $G_\sigma * I(x,y)$ denotes the image intensity $I(x,y)$ convolved with a (Gaussian) smoothing filter whose characteristic width σ controls the spatial extent of the local minima of the convolution kernel. Note here that the expression for the edge operator has a negative sign associated with it. The reason for this is that the local minima of the contour need to coincide with the maxima of the gradient functional. Also, note that the squared magnitude has been used for the edge functional computation. A different approach is also used, where the vector form of the gradient is used instead of the scalar information. However, in the Lagrangian setting an energy expression is required for solving the minimization problem. Thus, for the vector-based approach the dot product of the contour normal with the gradient is used for defining the energy functional and is expressed as $(\nabla G_\sigma * I(x,y)) \cdot \mathbf{N}(\tau(x(s), y(s)))$, where $\mathbf{N}(\tau(x(s), y(s)))$ is the normal to the contour $\tau(s)$ at location $x(s), y(s)$. Similarly, image intensity has been widely used along with edge information to formulate the external energy functional. The total external energy of the contour can be defined as

$$E_{\text{ext}}(\tau) = \int_0^1 \mathbf{E}_{\text{ext}}(\tau(s))ds, \tag{3}$$

where $\mathbf{E}_{\text{ext}}(\tau(s))$ denotes the energy functional given by the image properties at the point $\tau(s)$.

In summary, the basic definition of deformable parametric curve contains two terms: (a) internal energy, which defines the geometric properties of the curve; and (b) external energy, which combines all other forces that guide the curve to delineate the desired structure. Once the basic energy formulation is done, the idea is to find a methodology for energy minimization. A number of approaches have been proposed so far for energy minimization of the contour. The most well known is by solving the partial differential equation (PDE) for force (defined through an Euler-Lagrangian) using a finite-difference [10] or finite-element method [13]. A dynamic programming-based approach [14] and greedy snakes [15] are also used in many applications. The next subsection will briefly touch upon these approaches. Since these are quite standard ways of solving minimization problems, this chapter gives only the basic idea behind each of the methodologies. The pseudocode for the Euler-Lagrangian and greedy snakes are provided in Appendix 1.

2.3. Energy Minimization

According to the calculus of variations, the contour that minimizes the energy $E_{\text{snake}}(\tau)$ must satisfy the Euler-Lagrange equation [10]

$$\frac{\partial}{\partial s}\left(\alpha \frac{\partial \tau(s)}{\partial s}\right) - \frac{\partial^2}{\partial s^2}\left(\beta \frac{\partial^2 \tau(s)}{\partial s^2}\right) - \nabla \mathbf{E}_{\text{ext}}(\tau(s)) = 0. \tag{4}$$

This can be viewed as a vector-valued partial differential equation balancing internal and external forces at equilibrium given by

$$\mathbf{F}_{int} + \mathbf{F}_{ext} = 0, \tag{5}$$

where $\mathbf{F}_{int}$ represents the internal force due to stretching and bending factors, given by

$$\mathbf{F}_{int} = \frac{\partial}{\partial s}\left(\alpha\frac{\partial\tau(s)}{\partial s}\right) - \frac{\partial^2}{\partial s^2}\left(\beta\frac{\partial^2\tau(s)}{\partial s^2}\right). \tag{6}$$

The first term in Eq. (6) is the stretching force derived from the surface tension, while the second term represents the bending force. The external forces couple the contour to the image information in a way that equilibrium is accomplished when it balances with the physical constraints on the contour. Thus, $\mathbf{F}_{ext}$ is expressed as

$$\mathbf{F}_{ext} = -\nabla\mathbf{E}_{ext}(\tau(s)), \tag{7}$$

which pulls the contour toward the salient image features of interest. Other forces can be added to impose constraints defined by the user. We will make use of additional forces.

To solve the energy minimization problem, it is customary to construct the snake as a dynamical system that is governed by the functional to evolve the system toward equilibrium. The snake is made dynamic by treating the evolving contour τ as a function of both time t and arc-length s. This unifies the description of shape and motion within the same framework of Lagrangian mechanics. Thus, this formulation not only captures the shape of the contour but also quantifies its evolution over time. The Lagrange equations of motion for a snake is given by

$$\mu\frac{\partial^2\tau(s)}{\partial t^2} + \nu\frac{\partial\tau(s)}{\partial t} + \frac{\partial}{\partial s}\left(\alpha\frac{\partial\tau(s)}{\partial s}\right) - \frac{\partial^2}{\partial s^2}\left(\beta\frac{\partial^2\tau(s)}{\partial s^2}\right) = \nabla E_{ext}(\tau(s)), \tag{8}$$

where μ is the mass constant and ν the damping density following Newton's laws of motion. The system achieves equilibrium when the internal stretching and bending forces balance with the external forces and the contour ceases to move, i.e., both the acceleration and velocity terms vanish; in other words, $\frac{\partial^2\tau}{\partial t^2} = \frac{\partial\tau}{\partial t} = 0$.

For numerical solution of the equation, discretization of the equation is required. This is in general accomplished using a finite difference for solving the partial differential equation. In the discrete domain the energy equation can be expressed as

$$E(\mathbf{v}) = \frac{1}{2}\mathbf{v}\mathbf{A}\mathbf{v} + E_{ext}(\mathbf{v}), \tag{9}$$

where $\mathbf{v}$ is the discretized version of the contour $\tau(s)$, and $\mathbf{A}$ is the stiffness matrix. For all practical purposes, in this text we will use the symbol $\tau(\delta)$ for discrete representation of the contour. Minimum energy estimation is equivalent to setting the gradient of Eq. (10) to 0, which results in the following linear equation:

$$\mathbf{A}\tau = \mathbf{F}, \tag{10}$$

where $\mathbf{A}$ is the penta-diagonal stiffness matrix, and τ and $\mathbf{F}$ represent the position vectors $\tau_i = \tau(i\delta)$ and the corresponding force at these points $\mathbf{F}(\tau_i)$, respectively.

As the energy-space cannot be ascertained to be convex, so there is a high probability of getting local minima in the energy surface. In fact, finding the global minimum of the energy is not necessarily meaningful. Indeed, the main interest is finding a good contour that optimally fits to delineate the anatomic structure of interest in the best possible manner.

A neighborhood around each control point is considered and the total energy of the contour is computed for each neighborhood. Energy minimization continues until the energy between two consecutive iterations changes. This dynamic programming approach [14] searches for global minima in the image space. Greedy snakes [15], on the other hand, searches for local minima for each of the control points. The local motion of the points is considered in the neighborhood for energy minimization. In contrast to dynamic programming [14], greedy snakes [15] minimizes the energy of each local control point. Figure 4 illustrates the neighborhood search around a control point for dynamic programming and the greedy snakes algorithm.

3. ACTIVE CONTOUR EVOLUTION

The image processing task can be broadly classified into two categories: region-based and boundary based operations. Image processing techniques like mathematical morphological operations, region growing, and other region-based operations use regional homogeneity statistics to drive the task of image processing. Boundary-based operations (e.g., edge detection, gradient computation) use the statistics of variation in a local neighborhood. Low-level image processing techniques, if used independently for the purpose of segmentation, require a high level of manual intervention, rendering the result prone to inter- and intra-operator variability.

This chapter will focus on gradient-based approaches that rely mostly on image edges for convergence. Subsequent modifications for the gradient-based approaches and challenges faced at various levels of medical image segmentation will be discussed. Eventually, incorporation of region-based forces within the snake model help in providing a more compact model for the segmentation process. Region-based information can be incorporated in many ways into the energy minimization equation.

The active contour model allows user interaction at various stages. The main intention of the active contour is to reduce the amount of user intervention in the

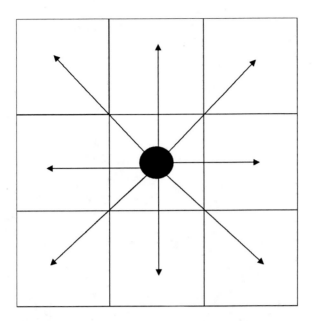

Figure 4. Neighborhood search for the minimum energy configuration.

process of segmentation. In particular, ideally, the user has to provide an initial contour near the desired edge. The snake deforms under the action of the local image forces and geometric constraints until it conforms to the final edges of the image.

The deformable model is in itself not free from limitations. In the original proposition, the user needs to provide the initial contour very near the desired edges; otherwise, the snake will not be able to deform to capture the desired anatomical structure. At the initial stage a number of solutions [17, 18] were provided in different forms to allow the snake more evolution. Cohen et al. [13] proposed a solution to propagate the contour faster toward the desired image edges. An internal pressure force was introduced by regarding the curve or surface as an inflating *balloon*. This pressure pushes the contour boundary toward the edges, and thus makes initialization of the snake a simpler process. However, the associated limitation of the snake remains in its ability to balance the strength of the balloon force with edge strength. As the balloon force is increased, there is a chance of leakage at weak edges. The addition of balloon pressure, though, adds to the propagation strength; however, this increases the instability of the snake framework. Berger et al. [18] proposed a "snake-growing" algorithm, where the snake grows based on the local contour information. Figure 6 shows the comparative result of a snake-growing compared to a conventional snake.

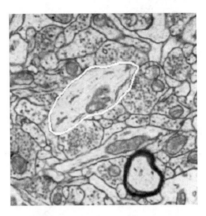

Figure 5. Illustration of segmentation of cellular structure in an EM photomicrograph. Reprinted with permission from [16]. Copyright ©1994, IEEE.

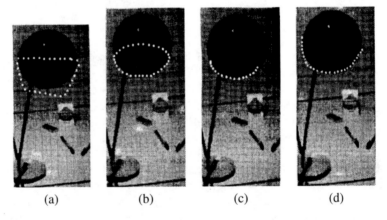

    (a)   (b)   (c)   (d)

Figure 6. Illustration of snake-growing algorithm in comparison to conventional snake. (a) Initial contour shown in white dots. (b) Result of conventional snake. (c–e) Performance of snake-growing algorithm. Reprinted with permission from [18]. Copyright ©1990, IEEE.

Leymarie and Levine [19] utilized a distance transform metric from the gradient information within the active contour framework to define a *grassfire transform*. The main motivation of the work was to define shape through skeletonization. In particular, an object's boundary is taken as the initial firefront that propagates within the interior of the object defined by the closed boundaries of the object. Points where the firefronts meet are considered the skeleton points of the representative object. The firefront propagation is accomplished using the active contour framework guiding the propagation using the distance transform from the boundaries. This work tries to bring in the gradient-based and regional informa-

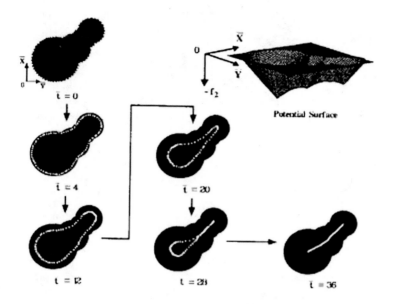

Figure 7. Example of grassfire propagation using an active contour model. The potential surface shows the valley in the distance transform function. Other images show the evolution of the snake toward the skeleton of the object. Reprinted with permission from [19]. Copyright ©1992, IEEE.

tion within the same framework to define the skeleton. However, this application has the probability of suffering from situations where noise plays a dominant role in determining the image gradient quality. Figure 7 depicts examples of skeletonization using this technique. Clearly, this formulation requires well-defined boundaries, which are absent in most medical images.

Lobregt et al. [20] tried to implicitly address the challenge due to fuzzy boundaries in medical images by controlling the local curvature of the contour in a local coordinate system. In this work, a local coordinate system was defined with respect to the vertex of the contour, and the change of curvatures in local and global coordinate system was taken into account. Thus, instead of global curvature variation, the contour deforms based on the variation in local and global curvature. This in turn retains the length of the contour, which otherwise has a shrinking property. It is important to mention that the curvature in this approach has been attributed to a direction both globally and locally. The approach intends that internal forces that act on the vertices should have the same (radial) direction as the curvature vectors. This means that internal forces can be derived from the curvature vectors by modifying only their lengths. Second, in order to reduce local curvature without affecting areas of constant curvature, the lengths of the internal force vectors

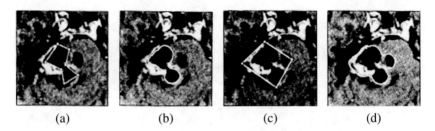

(a)   (b)   (c)   (d)

Figure 8. Illustration of dynamic discrete contour evolution on a cropped region from an MR image of brain. (a,c) Initial contour drawn manually. (b,d) Segmentation result from the contours of (a) and (c), respectively. Reprinted with permission from [20]. Copyright ©1995, IEEE.

should be zero for parts of the contour with constant curvature. To accomplish this, the dot product of the local r_i and global radial vectors c_i at point i is computed and convolved with a discrete filter f. The idea here is to reduce the high-frequency component and rather retain only the DC component. Thus, the choice of filter needs to be such that the result of convolution is zero. This approach results in a smoother contour and also allows an open contour to evolve within the snake framework. Figure 8 shows the results of deformation using the dynamic discrete contour.

3.1. Gradient Orientation

A different problem arises when two strong disconnected edges come close to each other. In these cases, the strong gradient acts independently to attract the contour. The final result thus becomes dependent on a number of factors like the contour's relative location with respect to the participating edges, their strengths, and possibly on all other force factors in the neighborhood. In many cases, the resulting contour alternates between the two strong edges. Falcaõ et al. [21, 22] addressed this problem in their proposed "live-wire" framework. The "live-wire" uses the gradient orientation information to detect the "true" boundary and avoids the possibility of getting trapped by strong edges. Similarly, the gradient orientation can be used in the snake framework [23]. Instead of using the gradient force without any reference to the contour, the external energy due to the gradient can be defined by the contour orientation and gradient direction. The idea is to make the "false" boundary invisible to the contour, so that it does not snap onto the "false" edge. Here, the direction of gradient is defined as whether it is a step-down or a step-up gradient. Now, this direction depends on the point from which we are looking at the gradient and the orientation of the contour. For example, in Figure 9, if we observe the edge marked green from the blue point, it seems to be a step-down gradient, while if it is observed from the red point, the gradient is a step-up gradient.

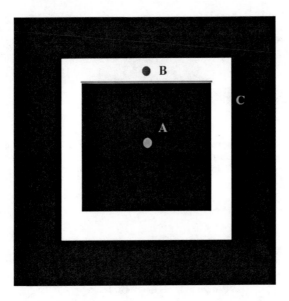

Figure 9. Illustration showing step-up and step-down edges from the observer's point of view. See attached CD for color version..

Now, if the contour approaches from the region marked A, then to track the interface between regions A and B it should latch onto a step-up edge along its outer normal. On the other hand, if it approaches from region B to the same interface, the contour point needs to snap at a step-down gradient inside the enclosed region of the contour. In other words, in the latter case the inward normal should see a step-down gradient. If the orientation of the contour is taken into account, then the desired edge would either be on the right- or left-hand side of the contour depending on whether it is considered in a clockwise or anticlockwise sense. Falcão et al. [21, 22] proposed a solution using the concept of contour orientation that relates gradient direction with the unit vector orthogonal to the local contour segment and directed from the "exterior" to the "interior".

Let $\theta_G(\tau(s_i)) = \tan^{-1} \nabla_y f(\tau(s_i)) / \nabla_x f(\tau(s_i))$ be the direction of the intensity gradient at the point $\tau(s_i)$, where s_i indicates the ith control point on contour τ. $\nabla_y f(\tau(s_i))$ and $\nabla_x f(\tau(s_i))$ are the gradients along the y- and x-directions, respectively, at the point $\tau(s_i)$. As previously mentioned, $f(x,y)$ denotes the image intensity at the location (x,y). If $\theta_N(\tau(s_i))$ is the normal to the contour at $\tau(s_i)$, then the energy due to the gradient field is defined as

$$
E_{\text{gradient}}(\tau(s_i)) = \begin{cases} -\mathbf{F}_{\text{gradient}}(\tau(s_i)) \bullet \mathbf{N} & \text{if } |\theta_G(\tau(s_i)) - \theta_N(\tau(s_i))| \leq \frac{\pi}{2} \\ 0 & \text{otherwise} \end{cases}
$$

$$(11)$$

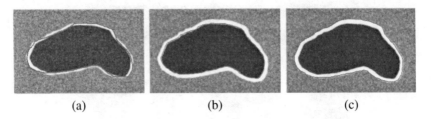

(a)   (b)   (c)

Figure 10. Illustration of gradient orientation on snake deformation: (a) contour deformation without gradient orientation information; (b) segmentation of region when foreground intensity is less than background and (c) when foreground intensity is greater than background intensity. In both (b) and (c) the contour has properly latched onto the desired boundary. See attached CD for color version. Reprinted with permission from [24]. Copyright ©2004, SPIE.

The normal $\theta_N(\tau(s_i))$ at a point $\tau(s_i)$ on the contour τ at s_i is defined as

$$\theta_N(\tau(s_i)) = \theta_C(\tau(s_i)) + \lambda\frac{\pi}{2}, \tag{12}$$

where $\theta_C(\tau(s_i))$ is the tangent at the point $\tau(s_i)$. The value of λ can be +1 or −1 depending on the desired direction of the normal. If the object intensity is greater than the background, then for contour in the counterclockwise direction the value of lambda should be 1, indicating an inward normal. This ensures that the contour will only be able to see the gradient, which is in the direction of the inward normal. But if it encounters a step-up gradient, then the difference between the two gradient angles and the growing normal will be more than $\frac{\pi}{2}$, so that the step-up gradient will be invisible to the growing contour. The reverse is the case if the contrast is changed. The effect of using the gradient orientation information within the snake framework is shown in Figure 10b,c. Snake deformation without the orientation information is illustrated in Figure 10a, which shows the final contour alternating between the two disconnected strong edges [24].

3.2. Convergence to Concavities

One of the major challenges faced in the initial phases of snake formulation was its inability to converge into concavities. Xu and Prince [25] designed a new external static force field vector $\mathbf{F}_{\text{ext}}(x, y) = \mathbf{v}(x, y)$, called the gradient vector flow field. This field originates from the edges and makes the snake converge to the gradient concavities. The gradient vector flow field is the vector field $\mathbf{v}(x, y) = [u(x, y), v(x, y)]$, which minimizes the energy functional

$$E = \iint \mu(u_x^2 + u_y^2 + v_x^2 + v_y^2) + |\nabla g|^2 |\mathbf{v} - \nabla g|^2 dxdy, \tag{13}$$

where g is the intensity gradient.

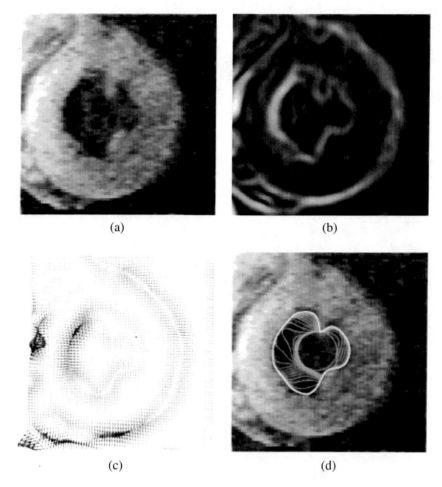

Figure 11. Illustration for performance of gradient vector flow (GVF) snake in segmentation of left ventricle from an MR image of heart: (a) original MR image showing left ventricle; (b) gradient map derived from (a); (c) vector flow field of the gradient map; (d) segmentation result using GVF snake. Reprinted with permission from [25]. Copyright ©1998, IEEE.

The basic nature of this force field is such that deformation near the nonhomogeneous regions of the image is governed by the gradient function, while in the homogeneous region the first term dominates. This results in a flow vector that converges into the edges of the image. Figure 11 illustrates the performance of gradient vector flow-based active contour model in segmentation of the left ventricle from MR images of the heart.

Anatomical structures vary widely in shape, size, and geometry. Segmentation of this wide range of anatomical structures requires highly deformable models to

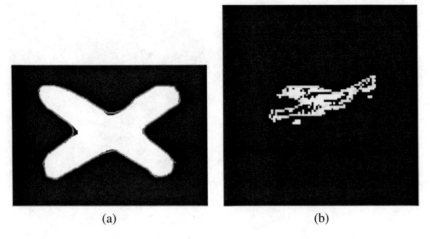

Figure 12. Images showing the performance of the inertial snake on (a) computer-generated phantom image and (b) ultrasound image of an artery of the lower limb [26]. See attached CD for color version.

fit into the process. As the contour itself is evolving under the effect of geometric physical constraints, the framework in its very definition imposes a geometric smoothness into it. Although this is effective in many situations, many other cases require relaxation of the physical constraints for appropriate segmentation. While in tracking geometric deformation in smooth structures the curvature is helpful, in segmentation of structures like white matter or convex structures the effect of curvature needs to be reduced. A study on the discrete computation and effect of curvature is presented in [15].

A potential way of controlling snake movement to conform into image boundaries and to avoid leaking is by incorporating an adaptable propagation force that modifies itself as it moves from a homogeneous to a nonhomogeneous region [26]. At this point, this is done by using an inertial snake, where the propagation term of active contour deformation is controlled by its distance from the initial contour. In that approach, the balloon force modifies itself and slows down at a rate directly proportional to the deformation rate between the successive iterations. Thus, in homogeneous region the force is higher, supporting faster propagation. But as the contour approaches the high-gradient region, the force reduces itself, thus discouraging propagation. The uncontrolled motion of the balloon force is thus controlled by the homogeneity and gradient information. Figure 12 illustrates the result of the inertial snake on computer-generated phantoms and ultrasound images.

Other significant attempts to improve the snake model using gradient-based information and internal energy has been pursued by other researchers [27, 28]. However, the main limitation remained its dependence on local image statistics, which is not reliable in many situations. Mostly for medical image analysis and

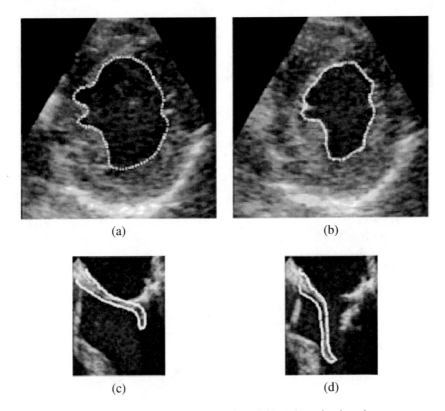

(a)   (b)

(c)   (d)

Figure 13. Images showing tracking of (a,b) endocardial boundary using the active contour model and (c,d) the mitral valve leaflet boundary. Reprinted with permission from [28]. Copyright © 1998, IEEE.

segmentation problem, one of the major challenges lies in the occurrence of fuzzy boundaries, as previously mentioned. Thus, transition from one region to another remains occluded by a lack of strong edges. Visually the transition can be observed by a change in other features and from the global information. Thus, where local statistics proved to have limitations in making a clear distinction between two regions, utilization of global statistics within the snake framework was found to be helpful.

3.3. Regional Information

Deformable models attracted the attention of the medical image analysis community for its ability to conform to the same framework constraints for a geometric shape and image information. In particular, after the introduction of regional energy that controls the propagation term, this model became more popular. The main motivation was to use global features and reduce reliance on local features. The rationale behind this approach was the fact that the features derived from local statistics are prone to errors due to noise and other artifacts that arise during the imaging process. Thus, a more global statistics would be helpful in detecting the region of interest. In fact, the basic definition of a structure can be stated as the region with similar attributes. If the features of interest can be isolated, the region connected by the similar features can be defined as the same structure. This gives rise to an entirely new approach toward the deformable model and has been studied in various forms by different researchers [29–32].

Region-based information is in general incorporated into the snake structure through a probabilistic model. As mentioned earlier, regional information attempts to capture the likelihood of a pixel (or point) belonging to any specified region. In general, the "region" is defined using some feature parameter, namely intensity, texture, etc. Based on the feature value, a pixel has a finite probability of belonging to a region defined in the feature space. The most widely used measures for feature space definition in snake-based segmentation is intensity. In some approaches, spatial intensity correlation and connectivity are used. The homogeneity of a space is normally defined as the cost function for traveling from a seed pixel to another location in the spatial domain based on a feature value.

Poon et al. [29] introduced the concept of region-based energy, where the homogeneity of a region is computed based on the intensity of a scalar image. For a vector image like that obtained with multispectral MRI (i.e., homogeneity, T1, T2, PD images), vector information from all the channels has been used for computing regional features. Figure 14 shows the results at different stages of snake deformation in delineation of the left ventricle from an MR image sequence using regional information. Other researchers [33–37] have also integrated region-based information into deformable contour models.

Region-based information is integrated along with the gradient into the snake model using a probabilistic approach [35]. A parametric curve is defined using a Fourier-based approach, where the idea is to use the number of harmonics depending on the required smoothness of the resulting contour. Thus, if the desired shape has more convexities, then higher Fourier harmonics are used, since the high frequency is encouraged by the geometry. Thus, the contour is expressed as

$$v(t) = \begin{pmatrix} x(t) \\ y(t) \end{pmatrix} = \begin{bmatrix} a_0 \\ c_0 \end{bmatrix} + \sum_{k=1}^{\infty} \begin{bmatrix} a_k & b_k \\ c_k & d_k \end{bmatrix} \begin{bmatrix} \cos(kt) \\ \sin(kt) \end{bmatrix}, \quad (14)$$

where $v(t)$ is the contour and a_k, b_k, c_k, and d_k are the Fourier coefficients, with k ranging from 1 to ∞. The smoothness of the desired contour determines the number of harmonics to be used to define the geometry of the contour.

The contour can be deformed by changing the coefficients in the Fourier expression in Eq. (15). This is analogous to the internal energy of conventional snakes. The external features that guide the final destiny of the contour are defined

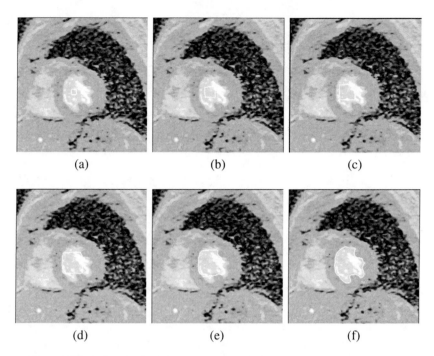

Figure 14. Evolution of region information-based snake for left ventricle segmentation from MR images. The homogeneity parameter is used in conjunction with the other standard energy functions, like geometric and edge functional, to evolve to the final contour, as shown by the white line in (g) from the initial contour in (a).   See attached CD for color version.. Reprinted with permission from [29]. Copyright ©1997, Institute of Physics.

by maximizing the probability that the contour traverses through a high-gradient region and encloses a region having similar regional features. The regional feature can be defined in terms of the homogeneity of intensity or any other desired attribute. The intensity feature was used in the work reported by Chakraborty and colleagues [35], Thus, mathematically the work contour searches for minimizing the entropy or maximizing the likelihood function, defined by

$$\max_{p}\{P(p|\,I_g, I_s)\} = \max_{p}[\ln P(p) + \ln P(I_g\,|p) + \ln P(\,I_s\,|p)], \qquad (15)$$

where the first term on the right-hand side (RHS) defines the geometric shape parameter, and the second term is defined by the gradient along the contour. This term can be defined by computing the gradient, using the derivative of the Gaussian convolved with the intensity. The integral is taken over the entire curve. Thus, maximizing this function represents that for a given pattern of geometric shape the maximum possible need of the contour to cover the high-gradient region. In most medical images, due to the previously mentioned causes, the gradients in many

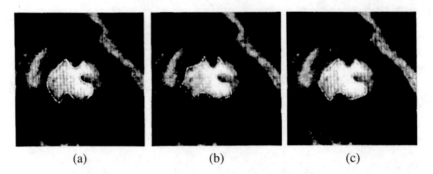

Figure 15. Illustration delineation of endocardium of heart using different methodologies: (a) manual segmentation by an expert; (b) semi-automated segmentation using only the gradient information into the deformable model; (c) same as (b) but with the regional information integrated along with geometric and gradient information. Reprinted with permission from [35]. Copyright ©1994, IEEE.

regions are very weak. Thus, with relaxation in geometric shape the contour tends to leak into other structures. Once the contour leaks, there is no force to stop this leakage, and return the contour to the desired structure. The regional features come to play in these regions of the image. The regional features are intended to prevent leakage through fuzzy and weak boundaries, since they use attributes other than simple local statistics. In a different form, these region-based approaches try to use global information derived in some form or other. The contour tries to maximize the homogeneous region enclosed by it. The region-based energy is thus defined as [35]

$$\ln P(I_s|p) = \iint\limits_{A} I_s(x,y)dA, \qquad (16)$$

where $I_s(x,y)$ is the intensity at the pixel location (x,y) in the image, and the integral gives the total area A enclosed by the curve p.

The result of using regional information within a deformable model framework as described in Eqs. (12) and (13) is shown in Figure 15 for segmentation of the endocardium. As is evident, the region-based information visually improved the segmentation quality compared to the one using only gradient information.

The homogeneity feature has also been used for segmentation of an ultrasound image (see [32]). The external energy is defined using the homogeneity of the region through which a control point is moving. As the curve moves from one position to another while deforming, the position of the point also changes, and thus the associated intensity value (provided it is not moving through a homogeneous surface). Both the edge- and region-based energies have their own advantages and disadvantages. Edge-based energy can give good localization of the contour near the boundaries. Unfortunately, it has a small realm of attraction, thus requiring good initialization or a balloon force [13]. On the other hand, the region-based energy has a large realm of attraction and can converge even if explicit edges are not present. However, it does not as give good localization as the edge-based energy at image boundaries. The region-based energy defined in [32] attempts to ensure that in the region having maximum inhomogeneity the region-based force factor approaches zero to complement the gradient force. Also, the region-based energy is designed with the property that any control point will want to preserve the "nearness" to the initial intensity value from where it started. Thus, the defined force field has two factors — intensity difference from the initial location and local edge strength — and is equated as follows:

$$\gamma(\tau(s_i^t)) = \left(1.0 - \left\|\psi(f(\tau(s_i^t))) - \psi(f(\tau(s_i^0)))\right\|\right) * \left(1.0 - \psi\left(|\nabla G_\sigma \otimes f|\right)\right).$$

(17)

In Eq. (18) the term $\left\|\psi(f(\tau(s_i^t))) - \psi(f(\tau(s_i^0)))\right\|$ gives the difference of the normalized feature image between the points $\tau(s_i^t)$ and $\tau(s_i^0)$, where $\tau(s_i^t)$ and $\tau(s_i^0)$ represent the ith point on the contour at the tth and 0th iterations, respectively. f represents the feature image, which in this case is intensity. ψ represents a normalized feature. The first term in Eq. (18) tends to reduce the force, while the difference between the two feature values increases, i.e., tends to 1.0. On the other hand, the second term vanishes as the point approaches a high-gradient region. This force field thus tends to balance between the region-based homogeneity information and the local edge information [32]. Figure 16 illustrates the use of the above-mentioned region-based force field for segmenting ultrasound images. In both the cases the contour has been initiated outside the region of interest. It is to be noted that the active contour models that have been discussed so far are unidirectional in nature. Thus, they have the ability to either expand or contract depending on how they are set. Thus, the major challenge of this framework is that once the contour leaks through a boundary to the background, there is no force to bring it back to the object region. This limitation is due to the fact that the active contour does not have the knowledge of which region it belongs to. If this information can be imparted a priori to the snake process, then the deformation could be more controlled.

4. A-PRIORI INFORMATION

Use of factors like homogeneity provides better segmentation results compared to the local statistics-based approach; however, as discussed previously, they are limited by their inability to undertake bidirectional motion. The active contour model has unidirectional motion because of its lack of knowledge about object and background in any form of statistical information. If the snake can distinguish between object class and background class, then once it leaks from one structure to the other, the snake could go back to the desired interface. Thus, the active contour needs to be intelligent enough to distinguish between object

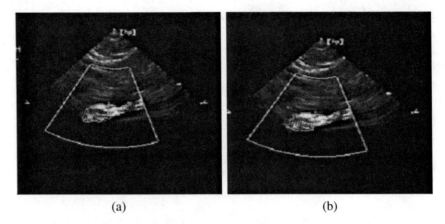

(a)   (b)

Figure 16. Illustration of homogeneity-induced inertial snake [32] in segmentation of Doppler ultrasound images. See attached CD for color version.

and background. This can be accomplished if only some form of information that discriminates between object and background is known a priori.

4.1. Shape A Priori

Among other features, shape can be used to discriminate object from background. This is applicable where the target object has a well-defined shape, distinct from most other structures in the image. Some work has been reported using shape [38, 39] to identify object from background. If the shape pattern is known a priori from a set of statistical distributions of object shapes, then a shape model can be defined based on those available shapes. These shape models are usually defined as probabilistic distributions, where a Gaussian distribution is defined for each of the "modes" of the shape about a mean model. This "mode" can be represented in any form, like a Fourier [38] or point-wise representation [40, 41], or some other form of expression. In each case, the underlying theory is to define a symmetric model that captures the statistical variation of the a-priori shapes from a mean shape defined as

$$\bar{\mathbf{x}} = \frac{1}{N} \sum_{i=0}^{N-1} \mathbf{x}_i, \tag{18}$$

where $\bar{\mathbf{x}}$ is the mean shape, and $\mathbf{x}_i$ is the ith shape vector defined by some form of shape descriptor. N is the total number of shapes known a priori. The main motivation is to represent a curve in using a shape descriptor and associate a probability distribution on the parameters based a-priori knowledge about the shape. The prior information available is a flexible bias toward more likely shapes. The parameterization itself should be expressive enough to represent any potential shape of a given geometric type, and the associated probability distribution will introduce a bias toward an expected range of shapes. The spread in distributions is due to the variability among instances of the object. If a particular distribution is known to govern the parameters, it can be used as prior probability. On the other hand, if the mean and standard deviation of the distribution is known, an independent multivariate Gaussian can be used for all parameters:

$$P(\mathbf{p}) = \prod_{i=0}^{N} P(p_i) = \prod_{i=0}^{N} \frac{1}{\sigma_i \sqrt{2\pi}} e^{-\frac{(p_i - m_i)^2}{2\sigma_i}}, \tag{19}$$

where N is the number of parameters, p_i is the ith parameter value, and m_i and σ_i are the mean and standard deviation.

It is important to mention at this stage that a Gaussian distribution has certain beautiful properties that make it the choice for most probabilistic distributions. Among the probability densities with a given variance, the Gaussian is the one with maximum entropy [38]. Moreover, the Gaussian is a symmetric distribution about its mean. Thus, the Gaussian density follows directly from knowing no information other than mean and variance. Since for most of the distribution any bias is not desirable, the Gaussian distribution is the most effective choice in approximating a probability density function.

Once the probabilistic model has been designed, to apply this a-priori knowledge to the problem of boundary determination, a maximum a-posteriori criterion has been formulated. Let $I(x, y)$ be the image data and $t_\mathbf{p}(x, y)$ an image template corresponding to a particular value of the parameter vector. In terms of probability, to decide which template $t_\mathbf{p}$ and image I correspond with the probability of the template, given the image given by $P(t_\mathbf{p}|I)$, the maximum over $\mathbf{p}$ needs to be determined, which can be mathematically expressed as [38]

$$P(t_{\max}|I) = \max_{\mathbf{p}} P(t_\mathbf{p}|I) = \max_{\mathbf{p}} \frac{P(t_\mathbf{p}|I)P(t_\mathbf{p})}{P(I)}. \tag{20}$$

Maximizing a-posteriori probability gives the desired template fit in an image. Figure 17 illustrates segmentation of synthetic images using a-priori shape information within the deformable model framework.

4.1.1. Application and Discussion

Shape a priori was used within the snake framework for detection of brain cortex in [39]. A cross-section of brain cortex is modeled as a ribbon, and a constant speed mapping of its spine is sought. A variational formulation and associated force balance conditions are used for convergence of the snake. The model uses only elastic forces, and the curvature term is dropped from the force balance equation. The external force is tailored for application into structures like

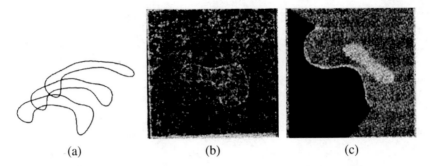

(a)   (b)   (c)

Figure 17. Illustration of using shape-based prior in the deformable model framework:
(a) shape priors with the mean shape and with a standard deviation around one parameter;
(b,c) results of [38] on synthetic images. Reprinted with permission from [38]. Copyright
©1992, IEEE.

the cortex, which has a nearly constant width throughout its extent. The force field
is defined such that if a small disk centered at a point on the active contour rests
entirely within the ribbon, it experiences no external force; if, on the other hand, a
portion of the disk intersects adjacent tissue, the disk experiences a force drawing
it back toward the cortex.

These approaches showed some promise in the particular cases where the
shape distributions are known a priori or the solution was tailored for the specific
application and shape [39]. However, the main limitations of incorporating this
information into the active contour model is a loss of its generality and deforma-
bility within a geometric paradigm, which is probably the most attractive feature
of an active contour model. Unifying the a-priori shape information with image
data in an active contour model has been proposed by many researchers [42–46].
A separate class of compact representations of shape and image data within the
deformable model framework inspired the active shape model [40] and the active
appearance model [41].

4.2. Feature Space

The purpose of incorporating a-priori features is principally to balance the
force equation in such a way that the contour will converge from both the object and
background toward the interface. To strike this balance it is required to optimally
use information about object and background so that the regional features will
drive the snake from any image location toward the object–background interface.
Therefore, the image surface needs to be defined in such a manner that when the
contour lies within object class (defined in some form), the force field acts in such
a way that the energy minimization criteria are reached if and only if the contour
expands to propagate toward the interface. On the other hand, if a contour point

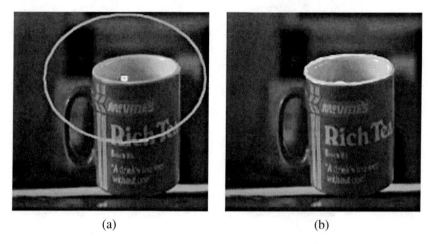

(a)   (b)

Figure 18. Illustration of the result of dual active contour model (a) initialization of the two contours (shown in white); (b) result after convergence. Reprinted with permission from [47]. Copyright ©1997, IEEE.

lies in the background region, it should experience a contracting force. In this particular situation, it is assumed that the object is entirely contained within the background. Figure 18 illustrates some results using the dual active contour model, where two contours attempt to integrate the information from a contour expanding within a feature to a contour contracting from outside the feature [47]. Though conceptually this is something the a-priori information is designed to accomplish, this method in principle does not use any explicit form of prior statistical image information to drive the snake. Object feature information can be used analogous to how shape information has been incorporated within the snake framework. The idea is to define the statistical distribution of the feature space from prior-known segmented object–background data and define a regional force field using this information.

The statistical snake proposed by Ivins and Porill [31] addressed this feature by incorporating an energy term that generates a bidirectional pressure force depending on a-priori information of the image data. A regional feature defines the modified external energy over the area as follows:

$$E_{\text{region}} = -\iint\limits_{R} G(f(x,y))dxdy, \tag{21}$$

where G is the function that measures the nature of the image data. For a unidirectional snake with a balloon or like forces the value of $G(f(x,y))$ is set to +1 or −1 depending on whether the snake is expanding or contracting. In a statistical snake, this measure will change the direction depending on the nature of $f(x,y)$

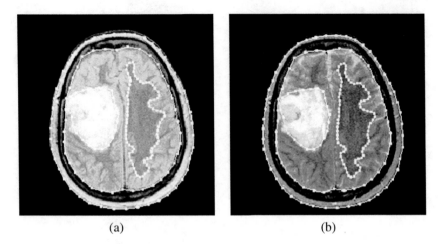

(a)   (b)

Figure 19. Segmentation results in sections of NMR images of brain using statistical snake. Reprinted with permission from [31]. Copyright ©1994, British Machine Vision Association Press.

and is defined as

$$G(f(x,y)) = \begin{cases} +1 & \text{if } |f(x,y) - \mu| \le k\sigma, \\ -1 & \text{if } |f(x,y) - \mu| > k\sigma, \end{cases} \quad (22)$$

where μ defines the mean, and σ is the standard deviation of the intensity distribution in the object region. Thus, the force field exerts a unit outward pressure when the contour is inside the object region and an inward pressure when the contour lies outside the object region. This is attributable to the bidirectional nature of the active contour model. The force can be modeled to vary with the distance from the mean of the object intensity, i.e., when the control point of the snake is near a mean object feature, the propagation force is high, and as it moves away from the mean the force decreases, until it starts reversing direction as it crosses the entire object feature distribution zone. A linear model and a model based on Mahalanobis distance are also computed in [31].

These approaches are essentially a probabilistic approach with a pixel having a certain confidence level belonging to some a-priori distribution. Suppose the image has two main regions, with different probability distributions. A simple example is the case where we have to segment a white object from a dark background; the regions will have different means and possibly different variances. Jacob et al. [48] used a region likelihood function defined as follows:

$$E_{\text{region}} = -\int_S \log(P(f(s)|s \in R_1))ds - \int_{S'} \log P(f(s)|s \in R_2))ds, \quad (23)$$

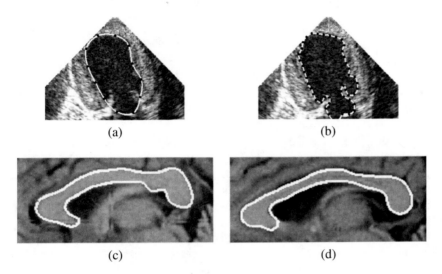

Figure 20. Segmentation results using the probabilistic model proposed in [48]: (a) initial contour drawn on an ultrasound image of dog heart; (b) final segmentation result; (c,d) segmentation of corpus callosum from MR images. Reprinted with permission from [48]. Copyright ©2004, IEEE.

where R_1 and R_2 are two regions in the image and the entire image domain $R = R_1 \cup R_2$. S and S' are the regions inside and outside the curve, respectively. Thus, the optimal segmentation is obtained when $S = R_1$ and $S = R_2$. It can be shown that Eq. (23) can be rewritten as [48]

$$E_{\text{region}} = \int_S - \left(\frac{\log(P(f(s)|s \in R_1))}{\log(P(f(s)|s \in R_2))} \right) ds. \qquad (24)$$

Figure 20 illustrates segmentation results using the probabilistic model in [48]. Evaluation of the energy minimization equation for the snake using this kind of probability density function requires estimation of these functions. As previously mentioned, the probability is estimated from the a-priori information and approximated as a Gaussian distribution with a certain mean and standard deviation. In situations where the a-priori distributions are not known, they can be estimated dynamically [48]. However, there is risk involved with this dynamic approach of incorporating more uncertainty into the system. Nevertheless, the probabilistic approach has proved to be a better solution for snake decomposition compared to the one without any a-priori information. It is important to note that Eqs. (24) and (25) balance the force from both the object and background feature space in contrast to Eq. (23), which uses information about only the object feature. Since by principle the requirement is to optimally use the information from the two regions, so it is recommended that both feature spaces be used for definition of the force equation.

Many other investigators have used the a-priori Gaussian distribution model (see, e.g., [24, 49–51]). With all these approaches, the main intention is to capture the confidence level of a pixel belonging to some region. Das et al. [24] developed an active contour model using the a-priori information within a class uncertainty [52] framework.

Given a priori knowledge of object/background intensity probability distributions, the object/background class of any location can be determined based on its intensity value and establish the confidence level of the classification [52]. The pixels with a higher confidence of belonging to the object class exert a high expanding force on the contour, while those with a high confidence of belonging to the background generate a high contracting force. It can be conjectured that the pixels near the object–background interface will have the lowest confidence of belonging to either of the classes and will represent the region of highest uncertainty. This is based on the assumption that there is a certain amount of mixing between the two intensities at the interface, which is true for most practical images due to effects like blurring, partial voluming effect, etc.

Given the probabilities for any pixel with intensity f belonging to object and background as $p_O(f)$ and $p_B(f)$, respectively, and $p(f)$ being the total probability given by $p(f) = p_O(f) + p_B(f)$, the class uncertainty of a pixel with intensity f is expressed as

$$h(f) = -\frac{p_O(f)}{2p(f)} \log \frac{p_O(f)}{2p(f)} - \frac{p_B(f)}{2p(f)} \log \frac{p_B(f)}{2p(f)}. \tag{25}$$

The class uncertainty is highest at the object–background interface, where the pixel intensities are in the most un-deterministic state. The force field is defined as follows:

$$\mathbf{F}_{\text{region}}(\tau(s_i)) = \begin{cases} 1 - h(f(\tau(s_i))) & \text{if } f(\tau(s_i)) \in \text{object}, \\ -(1 - h(f(\tau(s_i)))) & \text{if } f(\tau(s_i)) \in \text{background}. \end{cases} \tag{26}$$

Thus, the force field will assist faster movement of the contour in the homogeneous region and will slow down as it approaches the boundary. Other conventional force fields have been used with this contour model [49]. The performance of a class uncertainty-induced snake on medical phantoms and MR images of carotid artery is depicted in Figure 21.

Other deformable model classes like the level sets also use a-priori classification information. Many significant works have been published using this technique [53–57]. However, active shape models and level sets are not within the purview of this chapter, and so interested readers are encouraged to refer to the above-mentioned references.

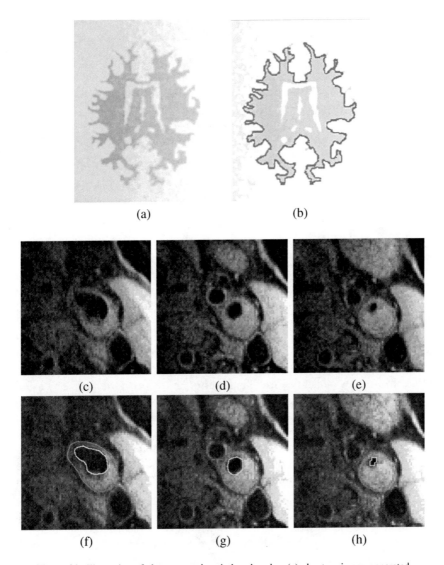

(a)   (b)

(c)   (d)   (e)

(f)   (g)   (h)

Figure 21. Illustration of class uncertainty-induced snake: (a) phantom image generated from segmented mask of brain with noise and inhomogeneity added; (b) segmentation using class uncertainty-induced active contour [49]; (c–e) cropped region showing carotid artery in MR images (courtesy Hospital of the University of Pennsylvania); (f–h) segmentation of lumen (green) and outer vessel wall (red) using the class uncertainty based snake. See attached CD for color version.

One of the major advantages of the level set approach is its adaptability to topological changes. Traditional snakes, on the other hand, are restricted by their inability to respond to topological variations. The topology of the structure of interest must be known a priori since traditional snakes models being parametric representations are incapable of topological transformations without additional intervention. Samadani [58] used a heuristic technique based on deformation energies to split and merge active contours. More recently, Malladi et al. [54] and Caselles et al. [51] independently developed a topology-independent active contour scheme based on the modeling of propagating fronts with curvature-dependent speeds, where the propagating front is viewed as an evolving level set of some implicitly defined function.

5. TOPOLOGICAL SNAKE

Topological adaptivity requires the multiple instances of the model to be dynamically created or destroyed, or can seamlessly split or merge as the object to be segmented changes its topology. Much research has been dedicated to this area [59–61]. The main principle behind each of these approaches involves using the grid information to establish a relation between the parametric curve and the pixel domain. Conversion to and from the traditional snakes model formulation requires the ability to discard or impose the grid within the framework at any time. The grid needs to provide a simple and effective means to extend the geometric and topological adaptability of snakes. McInerney and Terzopoulos [59] developed a parametric snakes model that has the power of an implicit formulation by using a superposed simplicial grid to reparameterize the model during the deformation process. Of all the approaches, we will detail this approach since it is the one most widely used. As previously mentioned, the idea is to incorporate the traditional snakes model within the framework of simplicial domain decomposition.

The grid of discrete cells used to approximate the snake model is an example of space partitioning by simplicial decomposition. There are two main types of domain decomposition methods: non-simplicial and simplicial. Most non-simplicial methods employ a regular tessellation of space. The marching cubes algorithm is an example of this type of method. These methods are fast and easy to implement, but they cannot be used to represent surfaces or contours unambiguously without the use of a disambiguation scheme.

Simplicial methods, on the other hand, are theoretically sound because they rely on classical results from algebraic topology. In simplicial decomposition, space is partitioned into cells defined by open simplices, where an n-simplex is the simplest geometrical object of dimension n. A simplicial cell decomposition is also called a *triangulation*.

The simplest triangulation of Euclidean space R^n is a Coxeter-Freudenthal triangulation (Figure 22a). It is constructed by subdividing space using a uniform cubic grid, and the triangulation is obtained by subdividing each cube into $n!$ simplices. Simplicial decompositions provide an unambiguous framework for

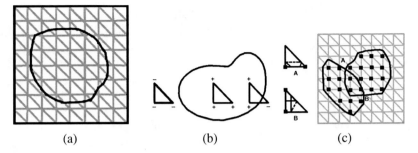

Figure 22. (a) Simplicial approximation of contour model using a Freudenthal triangulation [59]. (b) Cell classification. (c) Intersection of two snakes with "inside" grid cell vertices marked. Snake nodes in triangles A and B are reconnected. Reprinted with permission from [59]. Copyright ©1995, IEEE.

the creation of local polygonal approximations of a contour or surface model. In an n-simplex, the negative vertices can always be separated from the positive vertices by a single plane; thus, an unambiguous polygonalization of the simplex always exists, and as long as neighboring cubes are decomposed so that they share common edges (or faces in 3D) at their boundaries, a consistent polygonization will result. The set of simplices (or triangles in 2D) of the grid that intersect the surface or contour (the boundary triangles) form a two-dimensional combinatorial manifold that has as its dual a one-dimensional manifold that approximates the contour. The one-dimensional manifold is constructed from the intersection of the true contour with the edges of each boundary triangle, resulting in one line segment that approximates the contour inside this triangle (Figure 22a). The contour intersects each triangle in two distinct points, each located on a different edge. The set of all these line segments constitutes the combinatorial manifold that approximates the true contour.

The cells of the triangulation can be classified in relation to the partitioning of space by a closed contour model by testing the "sign" of the cell vertices during each time step. If the signs are the same for all vertices, the cell must be totally inside or outside the contour. If the signs are different, the cell must intersect the contour (Figure 22b).

The simplicial decomposition of the image domain also provides a framework for efficient boundary traversal or contour tracing. This property is useful when models intersect and topological changes must take place. Each node stores the edge and cell number it intersects, and, in a complementary fashion, each boundary cell keeps track of the two nodes that form the line segment cutting the cell. Any node of the model can be picked at random to determine its associated edge and cell number. The model can then be traced by following the neighboring cells indicated by the edge number of the connected nodes.

When a snake collides with itself or with another snake, or when a snake breaks into two or more parts, a topological transformation must take place. In order to effect consistent topological changes, consistent decisions must be made about disconnecting and reconnecting snake nodes. The simplicial grid provides us with an unambiguous framework from which to make these decisions. Each boundary triangle can contain only one line segment to approximate a closed snake in that triangle. This line segment must intersect the triangle on two distinct edges. Furthermore, each vertex of a boundary triangle can be unambiguously classified as inside or outside the snake. When a snake collides with itself, or when two or more snakes collide, there are some boundary triangles that will contain two or more line segments. We then choose two line segment endpoints on different edges of these boundary triangles and connect them to form a new line segment. The two endpoints are chosen such that they are the closest endpoints to the outside vertices of the triangle and such that the line segment joining them separates the inside and outside vertices (Figure 22c). Any unused node points are discarded.

Once the topological transformations have taken place, the list of nodes generated can be visited and contour tracings perform via the grid cells, marking off all nodes visited during the tracings. All new snakes generated are determined by the topological transformation phase and assign each a unique identifier.

Topological adaptive snakes are widely used [59,60,63] for their ability to handle complex structures which are so often encountered in medical imaging. Figure 23 illustrates some of the implementation results for tracking blood vessels in a retinal angiogram, on the cerebral vasculature surface (3D), and in different regions of brain. It is important to notice that topological adaptability has allowed an immense amount of flexibility in the snake framework, and thus enabled it to segment geometrically and topologically complex structures.

6. DISCUSSION AND CONCLUSIONS

The basic snake algorithm thus developed originally for computer vision applications has found widespread application in medical image analysis for its ability to capture local image statistics within a global geometric framework. This framework is widely appreciated in segmenting anatomical structures and quantifying various features in images of different modalities, including MR, x-ray, CT, and ultrasound. The task of segmentation using an active contour model ranges throughout the anatomical atlas, covering areas, like spine, heart, brain, cerebrum, kidney, lungs, and liver, and various artery segmentation, like the carotid and the aorta. An extensive amount of work has been done in delineating and quantifying the growth of objects like tumors, multiple sclerosis lesions, a fetus, micro-calcifications in breast from mammography images, etc. Thus, applications range from identifying white matter in the brain to quantifying diseases through imaging. Also, application of the active contour model has gone a step further in

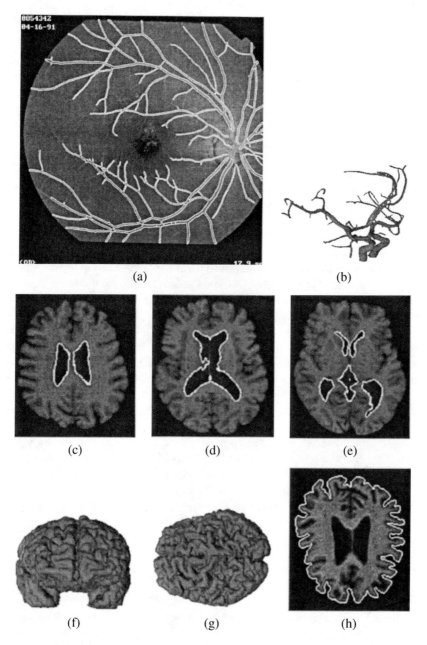

(a)   (b)

(c)   (d)   (e)

(f)   (g)   (h)

Figure 23. Illustration of results of segmentation using topology-adaptive active contour model on 2D images and 3D volumes [60]. (a) Segmentation of blood vessels in retinal angiography. T-surface segmentation of (b) cerebral vasculature from MR image volume; (c–e) ventricles from MR image volume of the brain; (f–h) different view of cerebral cortex segmentation using T-surface. Reprinted with permission from [60]. Copyright ©1999, IEEE.

identifying cellular structures and cell motion. This wide range of applications essentially covers both the 2D and 3D image domain for signifying both volume and temporal data. Motion tracking using 3D temporal data has also been widely studied for cardiac, pulmonary, and arterial motion in 4D MR, CT, etc., and even to the level of cellular motion from molecular imaging devices. At the present time, the deformable model-based segmentation algorithm has become a vital part of the most advanced image processing toolbox associated with medical imaging devices.

Most clinical applications presently use manual segmentation of the region of interest, that is, a domain expert goes through each of the image slices over the entire volume, or temporal data, and manually identifies and delineates the region of interest by using a mouse-guided framework. This has several disadvantages: the manual segmentation process is extremely tedious and time consuming. Furthermore, the image segmentation is nonreproducible and prone to operator bias. Thus, computer-assisted methodologies with minimal user intervention need to replace the manual segmentation process to obtain accurately reproducible segmentation.

This chapter has attempted to focus on the development of the active contour model to meet the various requirements in medical image segmentation and analysis. Segmentation of medical images is required for accurate and reproducible analysis of data for a huge range of applications, including diagnosis, postoperative study, and interactive surgical procedures. Manual segmentation is the most common technique used by physicians to process data. However, with the amount of data exploding and due to the nonreproducibility of the results, there is an inherent need for automated or semi-automated computerized algorithms that can generate segmentation results accurately and reproducibly. Segmentation processes that use low-level image processing have not been sufficient to segment complex structures from images and provide an accurate continuous boundary due to their dependence on local statistics, which in turn are corrupted by noise and other artifacts. The deformable model has been found to be quite efficient in this context, since it uses physics-based constraints along with local image statistics in a very natural way. The initial design of the active contour itself generated a lot of interest. With the complexity of the task increasing, the requirements are becoming more demanding, and subsequent improvements have followed. Efforts are being made to make the deformation less sensitive to initialization [13, 26]. Dependence on the gradient force alone for growth and termination of the active contour forces the snake to fail in images with weak and fuzzy boundaries, since the edge functional is not well defined in those regions. Regional information, like homogeneity and contrast, improved the active contour model. The snake evolution using regional information and local statistics, like gradient, captured the object effectively as the propagation was controlled by the regional force rather than a blind force. A-priori information even made the snake bidirectional, thus helping it to prevent leakage. Performance was thus enhanced with incorporation of this form of energy. Another major advancement of the active contour model came in the form of inclusion of topological adaptability, where the snake can merge and split to capture complex geometries and topologies.

The equations in this chapter mostly deal with a 2D space. However, they are extendable to 3D in all cases [25, 60]. The basic energy equation remains the same for all dimensionalities. Only the computation of geometric properties and image forces is changed. The geometric properties then need to be evaluated for a surface rather than a line segment. This makes the estimation computationally expensive, but the main essence is retained. The snake framework can be utilized in a different form often to segment 3D volumes. Rather than using the surface, the 3D volume can be broken down into an array of 2D slices (which comes naturally in medical images). Each of the 2D slices can be separately segmented and stacked up to form a 3D volume. However, in this approach the 3D information of the medical data is not utilized optimally.

A similar approach has also been used for motion tracking in various medical applications like tracking heart motion [64] and cell deformation [28, 65–69]. Deformable models have been used to track nonrigid microscopic and macroscopic structures in motion, such as blood cells [65] and neurite growth cones [70] in cine-microscopy, as well as coronary arteries in cine-angiography [71]. However, the primary use of deformable models for tracking in medical image analysis is to measure the dynamic behavior of the human heart, especially the left ventricle. Regional characterization of heart wall motion is necessary to isolate the severity and extent of diseases such as ischemia. The most conventional approach is to track the 2D contour in an image frame and propagate the contour to the temporally next frame for deformation. Some approaches have utilized motion vectors and Kalman filtering approaches [66] to boost snake performance in tracking motions of this kind.

The increasingly important role of medical imaging in the diagnosis and treatment of disease and the rapid advancement in imaging devices have opened up challenging problems for the medical image analysis community. Deformable models offer an attractive solution to situations where we intend to capture complex shapes and wide shape variability of anatomical structures. Deformable models overcome many of the limitations of traditional low-level image processing techniques by providing compact and analytical representations of object shape, by incorporating anatomic knowledge, and by providing interactive capabilities.

APPENDIX A

Energy minimization of the snake is accomplished within an Euler-Lagrangian framework of solving PDEs or a dynamic programming approach that uses neighborhood information on an energy surface. Note that the energy-based approach of dynamic programming and the greedy snake does not optimally use the image vector information. Pseudocode for the PDE-based and the greedy snake methods are provided in this appendix:

A. Pseudocode for Snake Computation Using the PDE Approach

1. **Input image** $I(x, y)$

2. **Preprocessing**

   (a) **Compute feature map (Input Image I)**

       i. **Compute gradient map G = $\nabla G_\sigma \oplus$ I**

          A. **Normalize G**

       ii. **Compute regional information-based normalized feature map F**

3. **Input discrete points**

4. **Define a contour through the sample points on the curve**

5. **Input parameter values for snake computation:** α = strength of elasticity; β = rigidity strength; γ = gradient strength; η = other factor (**might be regional or user-defined constraints). The number of parameters introduced will be equal to the number of force fields used.**

6. **Define stiffness matrix**

$$K = \begin{bmatrix} c_1 & b_1 & a_1 & \ldots & \ldots & \ldots & \ldots & \ldots & a_{N-1} & b_N \\ b_1 & c_2 & b_2 & a_2 & \ldots & \ldots & \ldots & \ldots & 0 & a_N \\ a_1 & b_2 & c_3 & b_3 & a_3 & \ldots & \ldots & \ldots & 0 & 0 \\ 0 & a_2 & b_3 & c_4 & b_4 & a_4 & \ldots & \ldots & \ldots & \ldots \\ \ldots & \ldots & \ldots & \ldots & \ldots & \ldots & \ldots & \ldots & \ldots & \ldots \\ \ldots & \ldots & \ldots & \ldots & \ldots & \ldots & \ldots & \ldots & \ldots & \ldots \\ \ldots & \ldots & \ldots & \ldots & \ldots & \ldots & \ldots & \ldots & \ldots & \ldots \\ 0 & 0 & \ldots & \ldots & \ldots & a_{N-4} & b_{N-3} & c_{N-2} & b_{N-2} & a_{N-2} \\ a_{N-1} & 0 & \ldots & \ldots & \ldots & 0 & a_{N-3} & b_{N-2} & c_{N-1} & b_{N-1} \\ b_N & a_N & \ldots & \ldots & \ldots & 0 & 0 & a_{N-2} & b_{N-1} & c_N \end{bmatrix},$$

$$h^4 a_i = \beta_{i+1},$$
$$h^4 b_i = -2\beta_i - 2\beta_{i+1} - h^2 \alpha_{i+1},$$
$$h^4 c_i = \beta_{i-1} + 4\beta_i + \beta_{i+1} + h^2 \alpha_i + h^2 \alpha_{i+1},$$

where α, β are the coefficient values.

1. **While (Iterations $\neq$ Maximum Iterations)**

(a) **Construct the coordinate matrix:** $\mathbf{X} = \{x(0), x(1), x(2), ..., x(N\text{-}1)\}^T$
$\mathbf{Y} = \{y(0), y(1), y(2), ..., y(N\text{-}1)\}^T$

(b) **Construct matrix from external energy and information:** $\mathbf{B}_x(\bullet, t - \Delta t, t - 2\Delta t), \mathbf{B}_y(\bullet, t - \Delta t, t - 2\Delta t)$**, where** $\mathbf{B}_x$ **denotes the** x**-derivative values of the external energy** $\left(\frac{\partial}{\partial x} E_{\text{ext}}\right)$ **and** $\mathbf{B}_y = \frac{\partial}{\partial y} E_{\text{ext}}$**.** t **represents the iteration index with separation** $\Delta t = 1$ **for most cases.**

(c) **Solve** $\mathbf{X} = \mathbf{K}^{-1}\mathbf{B}_x$ **and** $\mathbf{Y} = \mathbf{K}^{-1}\mathbf{B}_y$

(d) **iterations++**

(e) **ReSample Curve**

2. **End and fit spline to the final contour.**

B. Pseudocode for Snake Computation Using Local Neighborhood Energy-Based Approach

1. **Input image** $I(x, y)$

2. **Preprocessing**

   (a) **Compute feature map (Input Image** I**)**

      i. **Compute gradient map** $\mathbf{G} = \nabla G_\sigma \oplus \mathbf{I}$

         A. **Normalize G**

      ii. **Compute regional information-based normalized feature map F**

3. **Input discrete points**

4. **Define a contour through the sample points on the curve**

5. **Input parameter values for snake computation:** α = strength of elasticity; β = rigidity strength; γ = gradient strength; η = other factor (**might be regional or user-defined constraints**). **The number of parameters introduced will be equal to the number of force fields used.**

6. **While (Iterations != Maximum Iterations)**

   (a) **For (i=0; i<N; i++) /* N = Number Of Control Points */**

      i. **Search the** 3×3 **neighborhood (for 2D)**

         A. **Compute Energy due to all the factors at each neighborhood**

         B. **Find the lowest energy neighborhood pixel**

         C. **Assign the point to this lowest energy neighborhood**

      ii. **Update the contour information**

  (b) **Iterations++;**

7. **End and fit spline to the final contour.**

Note that in both cases it important to ensure that any movement of the contour that violates the topological circle configuration of the curve is avoided, that is, there cannot be any self-intersecting lines in the contour.

APPENDIX B

Incorporation of a priori information in the form of some probabilistic approach is detailed in this appendix. Specifically, the pseudocode for defining intensity-based object background confidence classification is provided.

Pseudocode for Object–Background Classification Based on Intensity

1. **Input Image** $I(x, y)$

2. **Input object distribution information (object mean, object std deviation)**

3. **Input background intensity distribution (background mean, background std. deviation)**

4. **Construct One-Sided Gaussian Probability Density Function:**

  (a) **If (Object mean > Background mean)**

      i. **For (intensity = Minimum Intensity; intensity < =Maximum Intensity, intensity++)**

        A. **if (intensity < =Object Mean)**

        B. **Object Probability (intensity) = exp(–(intensity – Object Mean)^2/(2*(Object Std Deviation)^2);**

        C. **else**

        D. **Object Probability (intensity) = 1.0;**

        E. **if (intensity<=background mean)**

        F. **Background Probability (intensity) =1.0;**

        G. **else**

        H. **Background Probability (intensity) = exp(–(intensity – Background Mean)^2/(2*(Background Std Deviation)^2);**

  (b) **else**

      i. **For (intensity = Minimum Intensity; intensity < =Maximum Intensity, intensity++)**

A. **if (intensity < = Object Mean)**

B. **Object Probability (intensity) = exp(–(intensity – Object Mean)^2/(2*(Object Std Deviation)^2);**

C. **else**

D. **Object Probability (intensity) = 1.0;**

E. **if((intensity<=background mean)**

F. **Background Probability (intensity) =1 .0;**

G. **else**

H. **Background Probability (intensity) = exp(–(intensity – Background Mean)^2/(2*(Background Std Deviation)^2);**

(c) **For the entire image compute the probability map at each pixel.**

7. REFERENCES

1. Haacke EM, Brown RW, Thompson MR, Venkatesan R. 1999. *Magnetic resonance imaging: physical principles and sequence design.* New York: Wiley-Liss.

2. Kurut EK, McIlwain EF, Plotnick GD. 2004. *Handbook of echo-doppler doppler interpretation,* 2d ed. Boston: Blackwell Futura.

3. Calender WA. 2000. *Computed tomography: fundamentals, system technology, image quality, applications.* Weinheim: Wiley-VCH.

4. Wahl RL. 2002. *Principles and practice of positron emission tomography.* Philadelphia: Lippincott Williams & Wilkins.

5. Huettel SA, Song AW, McCarthy MC. 2004. *Functional magnetic resonance imaging.* Sunderland, MA: Sinauer Associates.

6. Wernick MN, Aarsvold JN. 2004. *Emission tomography: the fundamentals of PET and SPECT.* New York: Academic Press.

7. Fischler M, Elschlager R. 1973. The representation and matching of pictorial structures. *IEEE Trans Comput* **22**(1):67–92.

8. Widrow B. 1973. The rubber mask technique, part I. *Pattern Recognit* **5**(3):175–211.

9. Terzopoulos D. 1986. Regularization of inverse visual problems involving discontinuities. *IEEE Trans Pattern Anal Machine Intell* **8**(4):413–424.

10. Kass M, Witkin A, Terzopoulos D. 1988. Snakes: active contour models. *Int J Comput Vision* **1**:321–331.

11. Terzopoulos D, Fleischer K. 1988. Deformable models. *Visual Comput* **4**(6):306–331.

12. McInerney T, Terzopoulos D. 1996. Deformable models in medical image analysis: a survey. *Med Image Anal* **1**(2):91–108.

13. Cohen LD, Cohen I. 1993. Finite-element methods for active contour models and balloons for 2-d and 3-d images. *IEEE Trans Pattern Anal Machine Intell* **15**(11):1131–1147.

14. Amini AA, Weymouth TE, Jain RC. 1990. Using Dynamic programming for solving variational problems in vision. *IEEE Trans Pattern Anal Machine Intell* **12**:855–867.

15. Williams DJ, Shah MA. 1992. Fast algorithm for active contours and curvature estimation. *Comput Vision Graphics Image Process: Image Understand* **55**:14–26.

16. Carlbom I, Terzopoulos D, Harris K. 1994. Computer-assisted registration, segmentation, and 3D reconstruction from images of neuronal tissue sections. *IEEE Trans Med Imaging* **13**(2):351–362.

17. Cohen I, Cohen LD, Ayache N. 1992. Using deformable surfaces to segment 3D images and infer differential structures. *Comput Vision Graphics Image Process: Image Understand* **56**(2):242–263.

18. Berger M-O, Mohr R. 1990. Towards autonomy in active contour models. In *Proceedings of the 19th international conference on pattern recognition*, Vol. 1, pp. 847–857. Washington, DC: IEEE.

19. Leymarie F, Levine MD. 1992. Simulating the grassfire transform using an active contour model. *IEEE Trans Pattern Anal Machine Intell* **14**:56–75.

20. Lobregt S, Viergever MA. 1995. A discrete dynamic contour model. *IEEE Trans Med Imaging* **14**:12–24.

21. Falcao AX, Udupa JK, Samarasekera S, Hirsch BE. 1996. User-steered image boundary segmentation. *Proc SPIE* **2710**:278–288.

22. Falcao A, Udupa JK. 1997. Segmentation of 3D objects using live wire. *Proc SPIE* **3034**:228–235.

23. Park HW, Schoepflin T, Kim Y. 2001. Active contour model with gradient directional information: directional snake. *IEEE Trans Circ Syst Video Technol* **11**:252–256.

24. Das B, Saha PK, Wehrli FW. 2004. Object class uncertainty induced snake with application to medical image segmentation. *Proc SPIE* **5370**:369–380.

25. Xu C, Prince J. 1998. Snakes, shapes, and gradient vector flow. *IEEE Trans Image Process* **7**:359–369.

26. Das B, Banerjee S. 2004. Inertial snake for contour detection in ultrasonography images. *IEEE Proc Image Signal Process* **151**:235–240.

27. Paragios N, Deriche R. 2000. Geodesic active contours and level sets for the detection and tracking of moving objects. *IEEE Trans Pattern Anal Machine Intell* **22**:266–280.

28. Ma T, Tagare HD. 1999. Consistency and stability of active contours with euclidean and non-Euclidean arc lengths. *IEEE Trans Image Process* **8**:1549–1560.

29. Poon CS, Braun M. 1997. Image segmentation by a deformable contour model incorporating region analysis. *Phys Med Biol* **42**:1833–1841.

30. Amini AA, Duncan JS. 1992. Bending and stretching models for lv wall motion analysis from curves and surfaces. *Image Vision Comput* **10**:418–430.

31. Ivins J, Porill J. 1994. Statistical snakes: active region models. In *Proceedings of the fifth British machine vision conference (BMVC'94)*, pp. 377–386. Washington, DC: IEEE.

32. Das B, Banerjee S. 2004. Homogeneity induced inertial snake with applications to medical image segmentation. In *Proceedings of the IEEE Symposium on computer-based medical systems*, pp. 304–309. Washington, DC: IEEE Computer Society.

33. Rougon N, Prêteux F. 1991. Deformable markers: mathematical morphology for active contour models control. *Proc. SPIE* **1568**:78–89.

34. Chakraborty A, Staib LH, Duncan JS. 1994. Deformable boundary finding influenced by region homogeneity. In *Proceedings of the fourth international conference on computer vision (ICCV'94)*, pp. 624–627. Washington, DC: IEEE Computer Society.

35. Chakraborty A, Duncan JS. 1995. Integration of boundary finding and region-based segmentation using game theory. In *Fourteenth international conference on information processing in medical imaging*, pp. 189–200. New York: Kluwer.

36. Herlin IL, Ayache N. 1992. Features extraction and analysis methods for sequences of ultrasound images. *Image Vision Comput* **10**:673–682.

37. Gauch JM, Pien HH, Shah J. 1994. Hybrid boundary-based and region-based deformable models for biomedical image segmentation. *Proc SPIE* **2299**: pp. 72–83.

38. Staib LH, Duncan JS. 1992. Boundary finding with parametrically deformable models. *IEEE Trans Pattern Anal Machine Intell* **14**:1061–1075.

39. Davatzikos CA, Prince JL. 1995. An active contour model for mapping the cortex. *IEEE Trans Med Imaging* **14**:65–81.

40. Cootes TF, Taylor CJ, Cooper D, Graham J. 1995. Active shape models: their training and application. *Comput Vision Image Understand* **61**:38–59.

41. Cootes TF, Edwards GJ, Taylor CJ. 1998. Active appearance models. In *Proceedings of the European conference on computer vision*, Vol. 2, pp. 484–498. New York: Springer.

42. Storvik G. 1994. A Bayesian approach to dynamic contours through stochastic sampling and simulated annealing. *IEEE Trans Pattern Anal Machine Intell* **16**:976–986.

43. Lai KF, Chin RT. 1995. Deformable contours: modeling and extraction. *IEEE Trans Pattern Anal Machine Intell* **17**:1084–1090.

44. Liu L, Sclaroff S. 2001. Medical image segmentation and retrieval via deformable models. In *Proceedings of the international conference on image processing (ICIP'2001)*, Vol. 3, pp. 3–7. Washington, DC: IEEE Computer Society.

45. Olstad B, Torp AH. 1996. Encoding of a priori information in active contour models. *IEEE Trans Pattern Anal Machine Intell* **18**:863–872.

46. Gastaud M, Barlaud M, Aubert G. 2004. Combining shape prior and statistical features for active contour segmentation. *IEEE Trans Circ Syst Video Technol* **14**:726–734.

47. Gunn SR, Nixon MS. 1997. A robust snake implementation: a dual active contour. *IEEE Trans Pattern Anal Machine Intelll* **19**:63–68.

48. Jacob M, Blu T, Unser M. 2004. Efficient energies and algorithms for parametric snakes. *IEEE Transactions on Image Processing* **13**:1231–1244.

49. Das B, Saha PK, Wolf R, Song HK, Wright AC, Wehrli FW. 2005. Cerebrovascular plaque segmentation by using object class uncertainty snake in mr images. *Proc. SPIE* **5747**:1720–1731.

50. Yushkevich PA, Piven J, Cody H, Ho S, Gee JC, Gerig G. 2005. User-guided level set segmentation of anatomical structures with ITK-SNAP. *Insight J* **1** (Special Issue on ISC/NA-MIC/MICCAI Workshop on Open-Source Software, November).

51. Caselles V, Kimmel R, Sapiro G. 1995. Geodesic active contours. In *Proceedings of the fifth international conference on computer vision (ICCV'95)*, pp. 694–699. Washington, DC: IEEE Computer Society.

52. Saha PK, Udupa JK. 2001. Optimum threshold selection using class uncertainty and region homogeneity. *IEEE Trans Pattern Anal Machine Intell* **23**:689–706.

53. Osher S, Sethian JA. 1988. Fronts propagating with curvature dependent speed: algorithms based on Hamilton-Jacobi formulation. *J Computat Phys* **79**:12–49.

54. Malladi R, Sethian J, Vemuri BC. 1995. Shape modeling with front propagation: A level set approach. *IEEE Trans Pattern Anal Machine Intell* **17**(2):158–175.

55. Chan TF, Vese LA. 2001. Active contours without edges. *IEEE Trans Image Process* **10**:266–277.

56. Paragios N, Deriche R. 2000. Geodesic active contours and level sets for the detection and tracking of moving objects. *IEEE Trans Pattern Anal Machine Intell* **22**:266–280.

57. Valdés-Cristerna R, Medina-Bañuelos V, Yáñez-Suárez O. 2004. Coupling of radial-basis network and active contour model for multispectral brain mri segmentation. *IEEE Trans Biomed Eng* **51**:459–470.

58. Samadani R. 1992. Changes in connectivity in active contour models. In *Proceedings of the Workshop on Visualization*, pp. 337–343. Washington, DC: IEEE Computer Society.

59. McInerney T, Terzopoulos D. 1995. Topologically Adaptable Snakes. In *Proceedings of the fifth international conference on computer vision (ICCV'95)*, pp. 840–845. Washington, DC: IEEE Computer Society.

60. McInerney T, Terzopoulos D. 1999. Topology adaptive deformable surfaces for medical image volume segmentation. *IEEE Trans Med Imaging* **18**:840–851.

61. Ji L, Yan H. 2001. Robust topology-adaptive snakes for image segmentation. In *Proceedings of the international conference on image processing (ICIP'2001)*, Vol. 2, pp. 797–800.

62. Lorenson WE, Cline HE. 1987. Marching cubes, a high resolution 3d surface construction algorithm. *Comput Graphics* **21**:163–169.

63. Giraldi GA, Strauss E, Oliveira AA. 2000. A boundary extraction method based on dual-t-snakes and dynamic programming. In *IEEE proceedings of computer vision and pattern recognition (CVPR'2000)*, Vol. 1, pp. 44–49. Washington, DC: IEEE Computer Society.

64. Mikić I, Krucinski S, Thomas JD. 1998. Segmentation and tracking in echocardiographic sequences: active contours guided by optical flow estimates. *IEEE Trans Med Imaging* **17**:274–285.

65. Leymarie F, Levine MD. 1993. Tracking deformable objects in the plane using an active contour model. *IEEE Trans Pattern Anal Machine Intell* **15**:617–634.

66. Curwen RW, Amini AA, Duncan JS, Lee F. 1994. Tracking vascular motion in x-ray image sequences with Kalman snakes. *Comput Cardiol*, **1**:109–112.

67. Freedman D, Zhang T. 2004. Active contours for tracking distributions. *IEEE Trans Image Process* **13**:518–526.

68. Ray N, Acton ST, Altes T, Lange EE, Brookeman JR. 2003. Merging parametric active contours within homogeneous image regions for mri-based lung segmentation. *IEEE Trans Med Imaging* **22**:189–200.

69. Ray N, Acton ST. 2004. Motion gradient vector flow: an external force for tracking rolling leukocytes with shape and size constrained active contours. *IEEE Trans Med Imaging* **23**:1466–1478.

70. Gwydir SH, Buettner HM, Dunn SM. 1994. Non-rigid motion analysis and feature labelling of the growth cone. In *Proceedings of the IEEE Workshop on biomedical image analysis*, pp. 80–87. Washington, DC: IEEE Computer Society.

71. Lengyel J, Greenberg DP, Popp R. 1995. Time-dependent three-dimensional intravascular ultrasound. *J Comput Graphics* **29**:457–464.

3

DEFORMABLE MODELS AND THEIR APPLICATION IN SEGMENTATION OF IMAGED PATHOLOGY SPECIMENS

Lin Yang

Department of Electrical and Computer Engineering
Rutgers University, Piscataway, New Jersey, USA

David J. Foran

Center for Biomedical Imaging,
UMDNJ-Robert Woods Johnson Medical School,
Piscataway, New Jersey, USA

Microsopic evaluation of peripheral blood smears and stained tissue analysis are performed routinely in pathology departments worldwide for cancer diagnosis and/or early detection. Recently, there has been an increase in the number of institutions using digital imaging and analysis to assist in assesment before a dignosis is rendered. Before the computer can be used to index, achive, analyze, or classify an imaged specimen, it must first be delineated into "homogeneous" regions based on the similarity of pixel attributes. Deformable models, or snakes, have gained significant attention and have become popular image segmentation methods since their first introduction by Kass, Witkin, and Terzopoulus in 1989. In this chapter, we will review recent advances and improvements on deformable models. We will focus primarily on the application and performance of different types of deformable models for analyzing microscopic pathology specimens.

1. INTRODUCTION

In many applications where computer-assisted analysis of pathology specimens is performed ([1, 2, 3]), one of the most difficult challenges is how to

---

Address all correspondence to: David Foran, Department of Biomedical Imaging, UMDNJ-Robert Woods Johnson Medical School, Piscataway, NJ 08854. Phone: (732) 235-4858; Fax: (732) 235-4825. djf@pleiad.umdnj.edu, foran@umdnj.edu.

accurately segment the objects of interest. Image segmentation is the process of delineating an image into several "homogeneous" regions based on the similarity of pixel attributes. If the segmentation is performed independently by the computer, the processing is referred to as *unsupervised*. This is in contrast to *supervised* image segmentation, which requires human input and intervention. Depending on whether or not prior knowledge has been used in the image segmentation, it can be classified as either "high-level" or "low-level" segmentation. Low-level image segmentation relies upon the pixel attributes of the image without consideration of prior knowledge. For many practical applications, however, it is often necessary to incorporate additional information into the analysis.

New segmentation methods have emerged that guide the partitioning process by utilizing cues based on shape, appearance, and/or contextual models. In early low-level segmentation pixels are clustered based on their similarity in spatial and feature space and the resulting subregions are then assigned object labels. In contrast, high-level approaches attempt to detect and extract objects from images using prior knowledge and establish models that allow the segmentation method to adapt to the object of interest. Deformable models belong to this family of high-level image segmentation approaches.

There are two general types of deformable models described in the literature: parametric deformable models [4] and geodesic or level set-based deformable models [5, 6]. Parametric deformable models have gained significant attention throughout the image-processing community since its first introduction by Kass, Witkin, and Terzopoulus [4]. Snakes are curves that are defined within the image domain and move under the influence of internal forces within the curve and external forces derived from the image data. All deformable model properties and behaviors are specified through a function called the *energy function* by analogy with physical systems. A partial differential equation controlling the deformable model causes it to evolve so as to reduce its energy, and the local minima of this energy then correspond to desired image properties. Parametric deformable models have been used in a range of applications, including edge detection [4], object recognition [7, 8], shape modeling [8, 9], and motion tracking [7, 10], to mention only a few. In an almost parallel effort, a variety of deformable models based on utilizing the image gradients as external forces have been proposed. Examples include the traditional deformable model [11, 12], the balloon-deformable model [13], the pressure forces model [14], and the more recently reported gradient vector flow (GVF) model [15, 16]. The GVF deformable model often outperforms other gradient-based models because it is insensitive to initialization values and can move into boundary concavities. It also has a much larger capture region than earlier approaches. However, the GVF deformable model was designed for binary or graylevel images, and it is not straightforward to adapt this approach to segment imaged pathology specimens. Simply transforming color images into graylevel images suffers from the fact that this process can often serve to eliminate potentially useful chromatic attributes, which may contain extremely valuable informational content especially where stained pathology specimens are concerned. In order to apply the GVF deformable model strategy to chromatic pathology images, a robust color GVF deformable model [17] based on Luv color gradients and L_2E robust estimation was proposed for segmenting stained blood smear specimens. Geometric deformable models, or level set-based deformable models, were almost simultaneously proposed by Caselles et al. [6] and by Malladi et al. [5] to address the fact that parametric active contour models could not resolve topological changes. Geodesic deformable models are based on the theory of curve evolution and are numerically implemented using level set methods. They can automatically handle topology changes in an image and allow for multiple simultaneous boundary estimations. Furthermore, they are not sensitive to initial starting positions as parametric deformable models are. Therefore, these groups of deformable models continue to gain increasing interests throughout the research community [18, 19, 20, 21]. However, due to their computational complexity, their speed of convergence is slower than parametric deformable models. In addition, because of the inaccuracy in the computation of the level set, this group of deformable models may sometimes need to be reinitialized several times throughout the whole iterative procedure.

1.1. A Quick Look at Deformable Model

Defined within an image domain, the traditional deformable model [4] is parametrically defined as $\mathbf{x}(s) = (x(s), y(s))$, where $x(s)$ and $y(s)$ are x and y coordinates along the contour and s represents the arc-length with value in $[0, 1]$, to minimize an energy function as follows:

$$E_{df} = \int_0^1 (E_{int}(\mathbf{x}(s)) + E_{ext}(\mathbf{x}(s)))ds, \tag{1}$$

where the first term represents the internal energy of deformable model, and the second term represents the external forces pushing the deformable model toward the desired objects' edges. The internal energy is defined as

$$E_{int}(\mathbf{x}(s)) = (\alpha |\mathbf{x}_s(s)|^2 + \beta |\mathbf{x}_{ss}(s)|^2)/2, \tag{2}$$

where $\mathbf{x}_s(s)$ is the first derivative of $\mathbf{x}(s)$ and $\mathbf{x}_{ss}(s)$ is the second derivative of $\mathbf{x}(s)$ with respect to s. The external energy is defined as the image energy, which is derived from the image data over the position that the deformable model lies. This energy function attracts deformable models to salient features in images such as lines and edges. The edges of the image is actually the boundary between color differences. Therefore, the external energy is usually defined as follows:

$$E_{ext}(\mathbf{x}(s)) = -\left|\nabla \left\{G_{\sigma(x,y)} * I(x,y)\right\}\right|, \tag{3}$$

where $I(x, y)$ is the image intensity at point (x, y), $G_{\sigma(x,y)}$ is the two-dimensional Gaussian kernel with σ as standard deviation. Therefore, the external energy in the traditional deformable model is defined as the minus value of the gradient of the Gaussian smoothing image.

The goal of the active contour models is to find the local minima of E_{df} defined in Eq. (1), based on the Euler-Lagrange principle. Equation (1) has a minimum only if the Euler-Lagrange differential equation is satisfied as

$$\alpha * \mathbf{x}_{ss}(s) - \beta * \mathbf{x}_{ssss}(s) - \gamma * \nabla E_{\text{ext}}(\mathbf{x}(s)) = 0, \tag{4}$$

where $\mathbf{x}_{ss}(s)$ and $\mathbf{x}_{ssss}(s)$ are the second and fourth derivatives of the curve with respect to the parameter s.

In order to find the solution for Eq. (4), the deformable model is made dynamic by defining $\mathbf{x}$ as the function of time t and s as follows:

$$\mathbf{x}_t(s, t) = \alpha * \mathbf{x}_{ss}(s, t) - \beta * \mathbf{x}_{ssss}(s, t) - \gamma * \nabla E_{\text{ext}}(\mathbf{x}(s, t)). \tag{5}$$

Then the partial derivative of $\mathbf{x}$ with respect to t is the same as the left side in Eq. (4). When $\mathbf{x}$ becomes a stable value, its partial derivative with respect to t will be 0 and we get the solution for Eq. (4). The solution to Eq. (5) can be achieved by solving the discrete equations iteratively.

The success of the deformable model depends greatly on the design of the external force. The external force of the traditional deformable model, defined as the gradient magnitude of the original image, suffers from the following weakness:

1. **Initialization problem**: Because the external force is only around the edges and the gradient magnitude of many other homogeneous places will be zero, the capture range of this kind of deformable model is quite limited. Therefore, the deformable model fails to capture the edges even if initialized even just a small distance from the edges.

2. **Boundary concavities**: Because the forces in concave regions act in opposite directions, they can become balanced in these areas and will therefore fail to enable the deformable model to detect the edges.

3. **Topological changes**: There is no way for this deformable model to handle topological changes in an image. Therefore, it is quite difficult to segment multiply objects in the image without conducting special procedures.

1.2. Introduction to Essential Tools and Methods

This chapter is written for the purpose of introducing readers to the essential elements, tools, and methods of deformable models and to provide a basic understanding as to when it is appropriate to utilize them in practical problems in which stained pathology specimens are to be segmented. With a limited set of mathematical jargon and symbols, the emphasis is weighted to inspire interest for the problems at hand. This has been done by selecting those methods that are best suited for conveying the fundamental characteristics of deformable models. Of course, our selection of the techniques and numerical examples are limited by the usual constraints: author bias and author limitations. Our goal is to provide a general framework for deformable models while providing references which will enable readers to pursue any remaining details.

In this chapter, we will review two deformable models: the parametric deformable model and the geodesic or level set-based deformable model. The chapter is organized as follows: the next section provides the essential mathematical background related to deformable models. It discusses some selected numerical methods for solving discretized optimization problems in deformable models. Emphasis is given to the well developed Finite Difference Method (FDM). Section 3 serves as a review of different types of parametric deformable models. We will also provide the numerical solution to the optimization problem. Stained pathology specimens will be used as the test set for evaluating the performance of the algorithms. Section 4 is devoted to illustrating how to use level set techniques to solve topological changes that include a description of the geodesic deformable models. This section also provides their applications in pathology image segmentation and the actual experimental results.

2. MATHEMATICAL BACKGROUND OF DEFORMABLE MODELS

In the present section we provide a brief overview of some of the requisite mathematics that are needed to understand deformable models. While detailed proofs are not included, we have provided citations for proof and additional detailed descriptions.

2.1. Calculus of Variations and Euler-Lagrange Differential Equation

Let's consider a real function $y = f(x)$ with both x and $y \in \mathbb{R}$. We claim that a necessary condition for y to have an extreme points is $f'(x_0) = 0$. Furthermore, if $f_J(x_0) \neq 0$, we can conclude that x_0 is the extreme point of y. Similarly a functional is defined as $f(G(x)) = y$ with $G(x)$ denoting a set of functions defined in $\mathbb{R}$ and $y \in \mathbb{R}$. Therefore, *the fundamental problem of calculus of variations* is: how to find the extreme function $G_0(x)$ that will minimize the value of y. This is also called a variational problem.

Theorem 1 (Euler-Lagrange principle) *For a functional defined as*

$$I(f(x)) = \int_a^b g(x, f(x), f'(x))dx \tag{6}$$

the variational problem for this type of function is solved by the following Euler-Lagrange differential equation:

$$\frac{\partial g}{\partial f} - \frac{d}{dx}\left(\frac{\partial g}{\partial f'}\right) = 0. \tag{7}$$

For a more general case with a functional defined as

$$I(f(x)) = \int_a^b g(x, f(x), f'(x), f''(x), ..., f^{(n)}(x))dx, \tag{8}$$

the variational problem is solved by the following Euler-Lagrange differential equation:

$$\frac{\partial g}{\partial f} - \frac{d}{dx}\left(\frac{\partial g}{\partial f'}\right) + \frac{d^2}{dx^2}\left(\frac{\partial g}{\partial f''}\right) - ... + (-1)^n \frac{d^n}{dx^n}\left(\frac{\partial g}{\partial f^{(n)}}\right) = 0. \tag{9}$$

The formal proof of the Euler-Lagrange equation is beyond the scope of this chapter. We refer the reader to [22] for further details.

2.2. Finite-Difference Method (FDM)

The-finite difference method (FDM) consists of two steps: (1) replacing the (partial) derivatives by some numerical differentiation formulas to get a difference equation, in other words, derivatives are discretized by using the "difference"; and (2) solving the derived difference equation by using either an iterative or a direct method.

We first partition the domain Ω by a mesh grid. For example, we use a uniform mesh grid with grid lines

$$x_j = x_0 + jh, \ j = 0, 1, ..., J,$$
$$y_l = y_0 + lk, \ l = 0, 1, ..., L,$$

where $h = x_{i+1} - x_i$, and $k = y_{i+1} - y_i$, are the mesh size in the x and y directions, respectively. For simplicity, we write $f_{j,l} = f(x_j, y_l)$, where the function values are the nodes of the mesh.

Using Taylor expansion and the intermediate value theorem, we can derive the following numerical differentiation formulas:

Forward difference formula:

$$u_x(x, y) \approx \frac{1}{h}(u_{i+1,j} - u_{i,j}), \tag{10}$$
$$u_y(x, y) \approx \frac{1}{k}(u_{i,j+1} - u_{i,j}).$$

Backward difference formula:

$$u_x(x,y) \approx \frac{1}{h}(u_{i,j} - u_{i-1,j}), \tag{11}$$

$$u_y(x,y) \approx \frac{1}{k}(u_{i,j} - u_{i,j+1}).$$

Centered-difference formula:

$$u_x(x,y) \approx \frac{1}{2h}(u_{i+1,j} - u_{i-1,j}), \tag{12}$$

$$u_y(x,y) \approx \frac{1}{2k}(u_{i,j+1} - u_{i,j-1}).$$

Similarly, the three second-order partial derivatives are given by

$$u_{xx}(x,y) \approx \frac{1}{hk}(u_{i+1,j} - 2u_{i,j} + u_{i-1,j}), \tag{13}$$

$$u_{yy}(x,y) \approx \frac{1}{hk}(u_{i,j+1} - 2u_{i,j} + u_{,j-1}),$$

$$u_{xy}(x,y) \approx \frac{1}{hk}(u_{i+1,j+1} - 2u_{i,j} + u_{i-1,j-1}).$$

For clarity, we now demonstrate the idea of FDM using the following examples.

Example 1 *As an example, we consider using FDM to solve the following differential equation:*

$$y'(x) = y(x) + 5.$$

Applying the finite-difference scheme, we know that

$$y\prime(x) = \lim_{h \to 0} \frac{y(x+h) - y(x)}{h} \approx \frac{y(x+h) - y(x)}{h} \text{ for } h \to 0. \tag{14}$$

Therefore, we get

$$y(x+h) = y(x) + hy(x) + 5h, \tag{15}$$

and the problem can be solved iteratively. The error between the approximate solution and the real solution is called the discretization error or truncate error, which will be bigger as h increases. In practical applications, h should be chosen to be small in order to avoid big discretization errors introduced by the approximation of derivatives in (14).

Again, we will not provide a comprehensive description of the FDM. We refer the readers to [23] for details.

3. PARAMETRIC DEFORMABLE MODELS

Recalling equation (1),

$$E_{df} = \int_0^1 (E_{int}(\mathbf{x}(s)) + E_{ext}(\mathbf{x}(s)))ds. \tag{16}$$

Depending on the specific definition of the external energy, E_{ext}, there are several kinds of parametric deformable models. In this section we will introduce the traditional deformable model, the balloon deformable model, the GVF deformable model, and the robust color GVF deformable model.

3.1. Traditional Deformable Model

In the traditional deformable model [4], the external energy E_{ext} is simply defined as the gradient of the graylevel image. As the gradient edge detector is sensitive to noise, the actual external energy is defined as the gradient of smoothed image using Gaussian filter, which is

$$E_{ext}(\mathbf{x}(s)) = - \left| \nabla \left\{ G_{\sigma(x,y)} * I(x,y) \right\} \right|, \tag{17}$$

where G_σ is the Gaussian filter with σ as the deviation, and I denotes the graylevel image.

Using the calculus of variants theory introduced in the previous section, it can be determined that in order to minimize the integral E_{df} in (17), it is necessary to solve the following partial differential equation:

$$\alpha * \mathbf{x}_{ss}(s) - \beta * \mathbf{x}_{ssss}(s) - \gamma * \nabla E_{ext}(\mathbf{x}(s)) = 0, \tag{18}$$

where $\mathbf{x}_{ss}(s)$ and $\mathbf{x}_{ssss}(s)$ are the second and fourth derivatives of the curve with respect to the parameter s, and $\nabla E_{ext}(\mathbf{x}(s))$ is the gradient. Notice that the signs before each term are not important because the parameters α, β, and γ are adjustable. In order to solve the PDE (partial differential equation), we can apply the FDM introduced in the previous section and define x as the function of time t and s as follows:

$$\mathbf{x}(s,t) = \alpha * \mathbf{x}_{ss}(s,t) - \beta * \mathbf{x}_{ssss}(s,t) - \gamma * \nabla E_{ext}(\mathbf{x}(s,t)). \tag{19}$$

After simple mathematical deduction, we are left with the following iterative equations:

$$\mathbf{A} \cdot \mathbf{x}(s,t) + \gamma * \frac{\partial E_{ext}}{\partial x} = -(\mathbf{x}(s,t) - \mathbf{x}(s,t-1)), \tag{20}$$

$$\mathbf{A} \cdot \mathbf{y}(s,t) + \gamma * \frac{\partial E_{ext}}{\partial y} = -(\mathbf{y}(s,t) - \mathbf{y}(s,t-1)), \tag{21}$$

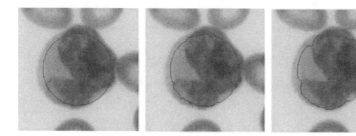

Figure 1. The image segmentation result of a Follicular Center Cell Lymphoma (FCC) applying traditional deformable model. The left panel shows the initial position, the center panel shows one snapshot of the evolving contours, and the right panel shows the final segmentation results after 150 iterations. See attached CD for color version.

and $\mathbf{A}$ and $\mathbf{x}$ spatially defined as

$$
\mathbf{A} = \begin{bmatrix} l & q & p & 0 & 0 \\ q & l & q & p & 0 \\ p & q & l & q & p \\ 0 & p & q & l & q \\ 0 & 0 & p & q & l \end{bmatrix}, \mathbf{x} = \begin{bmatrix} x_{i-2} \\ x_{i-1} \\ x_i \\ x_{i+1} \\ x_{i+2} \end{bmatrix}, \mathbf{y} = \begin{bmatrix} y_{i-2} \\ y_{i-1} \\ y_i \\ y_{i+1} \\ y_{i+2} \end{bmatrix},
$$

and $p = \beta$, $q = -\alpha - 4\beta$, and $l = 2\alpha + 6\beta$.

The limitations of the traditional deformable model are its small capture region and sensitivity to initial (starting) position. Figure 1 shows the performance of applying the traditional deformable model on segmenting a Follicular Center Cell Lymphoma (FCC). It can be seen that if the initial position is not sufficiently close to the object boundary, the traditional deformable model cannot segment the nuclei accurately. (Please note that all segmentation results are obtained after applying the color gradient described in [17], whereas using the traditional gradient[4] does not result in satisfactory convergence to the nuclear boundary.)

3.2. Balloon Deformable Model

In order to resolve the difficulties with the small capture region of the traditional deformable model, Cohen and Cohen [13] proposed a new external force that could enlarge the scope of the capture zone of the original model. Instead of defining E_{ext} as the negative gradient of the image, they define

$$
E_{\mathrm{ext}} = -\nabla P(\mathbf{x}), \tag{22}
$$

where $P(s)$ is the potential function calculated using a Euclidean (or Chamfer) distance map. Let $d(\mathbf{x})$ be the distance between a point x and the nearest edge

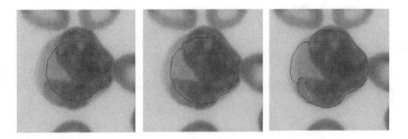

Figure 2. The image segmentation result of a Follicular Center Cell Lymphoma (FCC) applying the balloon deformable model. The left panel shows the initial position, the center panel shows one snapshot of the evolving contours, and the right panel shows the final segmentation results after 150 iterations. See attached CD for color version.

point; we have $P(x) = g(d(\mathbf{x}))$, and there are many ways to define the function P. For example,

$$P = -e^{-d(\mathbf{x})^2}. \tag{23}$$

Figure 2 shows the performance of applying the traditional deformable model on segmenting a Follicular Center Cell Lymphoma (FCC). Although it provides better performance compared to the traditional deformable model, it still fails to segment nuclei accurately. (Notice that all the segmentation results are obtained after applying the color gradients in [17]; otherwise, the result will not converge to the nuclei if applying the normal gradient used in [13].)

3.3. GVF Deformable Model

To effectively capture concave regions in graylevel images and enlarge the capture region of the traditional deformable model, Xu and Prince [15] proposed a new force field into the external force. The Helmholtz theorem [24] states that the most general static vector field can be decomposed into two components: an irrotational (curl-free) component and a solenoidal (divergence-free) component. The traditional force field is a static irrotational vector field. The GVF deformable model generates a more general field by combining these two components.

Rewriting (5) and replacing $-\nabla E_{\text{ext}}(\mathbf{x}(s))$ with Θ,

$$\mathbf{x}_t(s, t) = \alpha \mathbf{x}_{ss}(s, t) - \beta \mathbf{x}_{ssss}(s, t) + \Theta, \tag{24}$$

where Θ is the gradient vector flow defined as $\Theta(x, y) = [u(x, y), v(x, y)]$, that minimizes the energy functional

$$\begin{aligned}
\Psi \quad = \quad & \int\int \mu(u_x^2 + u_y^2 + v_x^2 + v_y^2)\, dx\, dy \\
& + (|\nabla\{G_{\sigma(x,y)} * f(x, y)\}|^2 \cdot \\
& |\Theta - \nabla\{G_{\sigma(x,y)} * f(x, y)\}|^2)\, dx\, dy,
\end{aligned} \tag{25}$$

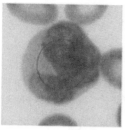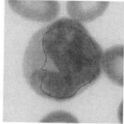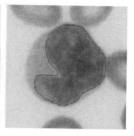

Figure 3. The image segmentation result of a Follicular Center Cell Lymphoma (FCC) applying the GVF deformable model. The left panel shows the initial position, the center panel shows one snapshot of the evolving contours, and the right panel shows the final segmentation results after 150 iterations. See attached CD for color version.

where $\nabla \{G_{\sigma(x,y)} * f(x,y)\}$ is the gradient of the input image $f(x,y)$ after Gaussian smoothing with variance σ and mean 0. Equation (25) is dominated by $u_x^2 + u_y^2 + v_x^2 + v_y^2$ when $|\nabla \{G_{\sigma(x,y)} * f(x,y)\}|$ is small. When $|\nabla \{G_{\sigma(x,y)} * f(x,y)\}|$ is large, the second term dominates the integrand and is minimized when $\Theta = \nabla \{G_{\sigma(x,y)} * f(x,y)\}$. This result keeps Θ nearly equal to the gradient of the edge when the deformable model is near the object, while enabling the deformable model to move toward the edges when it is far away from the object.

Figure 3 shows the performance using the GVF deformable model for segmenting a Follicular Center Cell Lymphoma (FCC). Based on the results of these experiments, we have demonstrated that the GVF deformable model provides large capture regions and at the same time the GVF vector flow enables the deformable model to enter into convex regions within the image. In fact, the GVF deformable model outperformed all the other gradient-based single-channel image segmentation algorithms that were tested. (Please note that all segmentation results were obtained after applying the color gradients in [17]; using the traditional gradient [15] does not result in accurate delineation of the boundaries.

3.4. Robust Color GVF Deformable Model

In graylevel images, the gradient is defined as the first derivative of the image luminance. It has a high value in those regions exhibiting high luminance contrast. However, this strategy is not suitable for color images. Simply transforming color images into graylevel images by averaging across the three channels and applying the graylevel image gradient operator does not provide satisfactory results for many pathology applications.

Imaged pathology specimens must be accurately segmented before any higher-level analysis can be performed. In order to apply the GVF deformable model to address the limitations of traditional approaches, Yang et al. [17] proposed a robust color GVF deformable model that integrated a color gradient and robust estimation in the original GVF deformable model. The definition of color gradients was first introduced in [25, 26, 27]. In contrast to previous approaches, the color gradient in [17] is defined in a Luv color space rather than an RGB color space because Euclidean metrics and distances are perceptually uniform in a Luv color space, which is not the case in an RGB color space [26].

Let $\Gamma(x, y) : \mathbb{R}^3$ be a color image; based on classical Riemannian geometry results [28], the L_2 norm can be written in matrix form:

$$d\Gamma^2 = \begin{bmatrix} dx \\ dy \end{bmatrix}^T \begin{bmatrix} g_{11} & g_{12} \\ g_{21} & g_{22} \end{bmatrix} \begin{bmatrix} dx \\ dy \end{bmatrix}, \tag{26}$$

where $g_{11} = [\frac{\partial \Gamma}{\partial x}]^2, g_{12} = g_{21} = \frac{\partial \Gamma}{\partial x} \frac{\partial \Gamma}{\partial y}, g_{22} = [\frac{\partial \Gamma}{\partial y}]^2$. The quadratic form (26) achieves its extrema changing rates in the directions of the eigenvectors of matrix $[g_{i,j}], i = 1, 2, j = 1, 2$ and the changing magnitude is decided by its eigenvalues λ_+ and λ_-. Define the color gradient as

$$\nabla\Theta = \sqrt{\lambda_+ - \lambda_-}, \tag{27}$$

where

$$g_{11} = \begin{bmatrix} |\frac{\partial L}{\partial x}|^2 \\ |\frac{\partial u}{\partial x}|^2 \\ |\frac{\partial v}{\partial x}|^2 \end{bmatrix} \quad g_{22} = \begin{bmatrix} |\frac{\partial L}{\partial y}|^2 \\ |\frac{\partial u}{\partial y}|^2 \\ |\frac{\partial v}{\partial y}|^2 \end{bmatrix}, \tag{28}$$

$$g_{12} = g_{21} = \begin{bmatrix} |\frac{\partial^2 L}{\partial x \partial y}| \\ |\frac{\partial^2 u}{\partial x \partial y}| \\ |\frac{\partial^2 v}{\partial x \partial y}| \end{bmatrix}, \tag{29}$$

where L, u, and v correspond to the three channels in the Luv color space. In the robust color GVF deformable model, the initial contour locations are obtained from L_2E robust estimation [17] to increase the converge speed. By applying the calculus of variations introduced in the previous section, it can be shown that minimizing the integral in Eq. (25) is equal to solving the following equation:

$$\mu\nabla^2 u - (u - f_x)(f_x^2 + f_y^2) = 0, \tag{30}$$

$$\mu\nabla^2 v - (v - f_y)(f_x^2 + f_y^2) = 0. \tag{31}$$

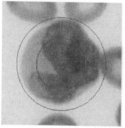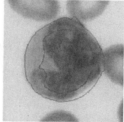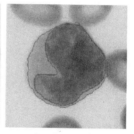

Figure 4. The image segmentation result of a Follicular Center Cell Lymphoma (FCC) applying robust color GVF deformable model. The left panel shows the two initial positions for the segmentation of both nuclei and cytoplasm, the center panel shows one snapshot of the evolving contours, and the right panel shows the final segmentation results after 125 iterations. See attached CD for color version.

The numerical solution to (30) and (31) can be solved by treating u and v as functions of time and solving

$$u_t(x,y,t) = \mu\nabla^2 u(x,y,t) -$$
$$(u(x,y,t) - f_x(x,y))(f_x^2(x,y) + f_y^2(x,y)), \quad (32)$$

$$v_t(x,y,t) = \mu\nabla^2 v(x,y,t) -$$
$$(v(x,y,t) - f_y(x,y))(f_x^2(x,y) + f_y^2(x,y)). \quad (33)$$

In order to set up an iterative solution, let the indices i, j and n correspond to x, y, and t will be derived from the iterative algorithm for (32) and (33).

Figure 4 shows the performance of applying double robust color GVF deformable models on segmenting both the nuclei and the cytoplasm of a Follicular Center Cell Lymphoma (FCC). Throughout our experiments, the robust color GVF deformable model provided accurate segmentation results while maintaining smooth boundaries.

4. GEODESIC OR LEVEL SET-BASED DEFORMABLE MODELS

As previously mentioned, parametric deformable models offer the advantages of fast converge speed and simple implementation. However, they are not able to address topological changes in the image, and they therefore cannot segment multiple objects simultaneously since the deformable models themselves cannot split or merge automatically. Furthermore, although the GVF deformable model enlarges the capture region significantly, it still requires the initial (starting) positions to cover at least the center of the object of interest. Otherwise, it may fail to find the whole object if the initial positions do not include the center [29]. Geodesic or level set-based deformable models offer a different approach than parametric deformable models. Instead of operating on the 2D contours directly, it embeds the contour into a 3D function set, called the level set function. The level set function evolved by solving a set of PDEs (partial differential equations), whereas the contour was modeled by the zero level set function:

$$C(s,t) = \{s, t | \Psi(s,t) = 0\}, \tag{34}$$

where $\Psi(s,t)$ is the 3D level set function and $C(s,t)$ denotes the contour of the object. The advantage of level set and geodesic deformable models are their powerful ability to handle arbitrary complex topological changes by merging or splitting of contours automatically. They are also quite insensitive to initial (starting) positions, which we will be shown in our examples. The disadvantages are their computational complexity and comparatively more difficult implementation. In addition, because of the inaccuracy of computing the level set function numerically, some algorithms may require reinitializations.

In this section, we will introduce the level set-based deformable models with front propagation and the geodesic deformable models. They have already been shown to be very similar [21].

4.1. Level Set-Based Deformable Models Using Front Propagation

This shape model with front propagation was proposed by Malladi et al. [5] and numerically implemented with the level set method. Let $\gamma(t)$ be the contour of the object modeled as the zero level set $\{\Psi = 0\}$ of a scalar Lipschitz function Ψ such that

$$\Psi(s, t = 0) > 0 \text{ on } \Omega_1, \Psi(s, t = 0) < 0 \text{ on } \Omega_2 \text{ and } \Psi(s, t = 0) = 0 \text{ on } C, \tag{35}$$

where Ω_1 is the region in which s locates inside the contour C, and Ω_2 is the region denoting those s outside the contour C. The evolution of the contour C is given by the zero-level set of the level set function $\{s, t | \Psi(s,t) = 0\}$. Assume the evolving speed function in the normal direction of contour C is defined as F; we then have [30]

$$\frac{\partial \Psi}{\partial t} = |\nabla \Psi| F, \Psi(s, 0) = \Psi_0(s), \tag{36}$$

where $\Psi_0(s)$ is the initial position of the contour C. For certain types of functions, F, we obtain the standard Hamilton-Jacobi equations.

Some approaches have different definitions of the speed function F. In [5], F is separated as F_A and F_G, where F_A is named as the advection term that is independent of the contour's geometry and F_G refers to the term that is related to the geometry of the contour. If we set $F_G = 0$ to denote the situation of moving the contour at a constant speed, then $F = F_A$. Let $F_A = \gamma$ be an adjustable parameter; we obtain

$$F = \gamma - \frac{\gamma}{M_1 - M_2} \left(|\nabla G_\sigma * I(x,y)| - M_2 \right), \tag{37}$$

where M_1 and M_2 are the maximum and minimum values of the magnitude of the image gradient $|\nabla G_\sigma * I(x,y)|$. When the Gaussian smoothed gradient reaches M_1, the value of the speed function will be 0 and the zero level set will provide the contour of the object.

By integrating (36) and (37) together, we have

$$\frac{\partial \Psi}{\partial t} = |\nabla \Psi| \left(\gamma - \frac{\gamma}{M_1 - M_2} \left(|\nabla G_\sigma * I(x,y)| - M_2 \right) \right), \Psi(s,0) = \Psi_0(s).$$
(38)

Applying the FDM, the numerical solution of (38) is given by the following iterative equation:

$$\Psi^{n+1} = \Psi^n + \Delta t \cdot \left[|\nabla \Psi| \left(\gamma - \frac{\gamma}{M_1 - M_2} \left(|\nabla G_\sigma * I(x,y)| - M_2 \right) \right) \right], \quad (39)$$

$$\Psi(s,0) = \Psi_0(s),$$

where Δt is the iteration step. Equation (39) can be implemented iteratively.

Figure 5 shows the experimental results applying the algorithm introduced in this section. From the experiments we conclude that level set-based deformable models are quite insensitive to initial positions and can handle topological changes successfully. (Similar as in the previous section, all the segmentation results are obtained after applying the color gradients in [17]; otherwise, the result will not converge to the nuclei if applying the normal gradient used in [5].)

4.2. Geodesic Deformable Models

In almost parallel efforts, the geodesic model was proposed by Caselles [6]. Equation (1) of the traditional deformable model can be rewritten in a more general form:

$$E(C) = \int_0^1 (E_{int}(C(s)) + E_{ext}(C(s))) \, ds, \quad (40)$$

where C is a specific allowed space of curves. By applying Fermat's principle, it is equivalent to solve the following intrinsic problem:

$$\arg \min_C \int_0^1 g(|\nabla I(C(s))| \cdot |C'(s)| \, ds), \quad (41)$$

where I is the image, and the function g is an edge detector defined as

$$g(|\nabla I(C(s))|) = \frac{1}{1 + |\nabla G_\sigma * I(x,y)|^p}, \quad (42)$$

where p is the rank with $p > 0$.

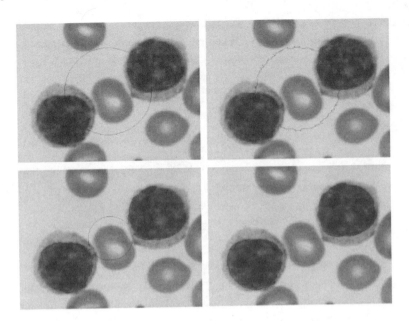

Figure 5. The image segmentation result of the nuclei of two Benign (BEN) cells simutaneously applying a level set-based deformable model. The top left panel shows the initial curve, the top right and bottom left panels show two snapshots of the evolving contours, and the bottom right panel shows the final segmentation results after 1000 iterations. See attached CD for color version.

Solving (41) is a problem of geodesic computation in a Riemannian space, according to a metric induced by the image I. It can be seen that when $|\nabla G_\sigma * I(x, y)|$ is large, the value of the edge detection function g will approach 0 and the energy term $E(C)$ is minimized and the evolution will stop at the boundary of the object.

The geodesic deformable model in [6] actually has a level set formulation, which established the relationship with these two apparently different approaches:

$$\frac{\partial \Psi}{\partial t} = |\nabla \Psi| \cdot g(|\nabla I(C(s))|) \cdot \varphi + \nabla g(|\nabla I(C(s))|) \cdot \nabla I, \ \Psi(s, 0) = \Psi_0(s), \ (43)$$

where

$$\varphi = div\left(\frac{\nabla I}{|\nabla I|}\right). \tag{44}$$

Applying the FDM, the numerical solution of (43) results in the following iterative equation:

$$\Psi^{n+1} = \Psi^n + \Delta t \cdot [|\nabla \Psi| \cdot g(|\nabla I(C(s))|) \cdot \varphi + \nabla g(|\nabla I(C(s))|) \cdot \nabla I],$$
$$\Psi(s, 0) = \Psi_0(s), \tag{45}$$

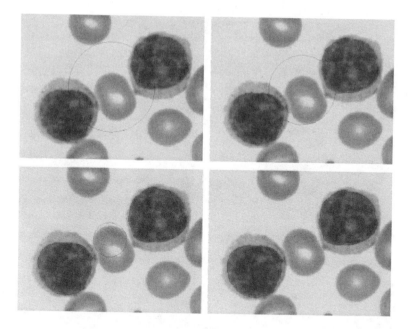

Figure 6. The image segmentation result of the nuclei of two Benign (BEN) cells being detected and delineated simultaneously by applying the geodesic deformable model. The top left panel shows the initial curve, the top right and bottom left panels show two snapshots of the evolving contours, and the bottom right panel shows the final segmentation results after 1000 iterations. See attached CD for color version.

where Δt is the iteration step. Equation (45) can be implemented iteratively, and the contour of the object is the zero level set of the functional Ψ.

Figures 6 and 7 show the experimental results applying the geodesic deformable model on the segmentation of two Benign (BEN) cells and an immunostained breast cancer tissue microarray disc. From these experiments we conclude that geodesic deformable models are also insensitive to initial positions and can automatically split or merge to address complex topological changes in the image. (As in the previous section, all the segmentation results are obtained after applying the color gradients in [17]; the result does not converge if applying the traditional gradient [6].)

5. CONCLUDING REMARKS

Medical imaging and computer-assisted diagnosis are extremely active fields of research with a wide range of application domains. In this chapter we have chosen to focus our emphasis on the use of deformable models in diagnostic pathology applications since this area has been relatively underrepresented in the literature.

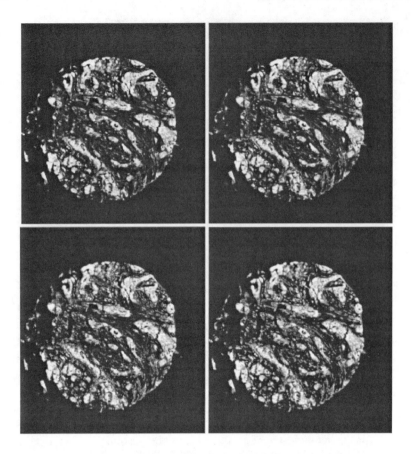

Figure 7. The image segmentation result with breast tissue applying the geodesic deformable model. The top left panel shows the initial curve, the top right and bottom left panels show two snapshots of the evolving contours, and the bottom right panel shows the final segmentation results after 8000 iterations. See attached CD for color version.

In addition to introducing the underlying logic and theory of deformable models, this chapter provides an overview of the requisite numerical techniques needed to implement the algorithms and analyze imaged pathology specimens. A range of different approaches were used to analyze identical image sets in order to illustrate the comparative performance among each of the various strategies. The segmentation results of actual imaged pathology specimens and stained tissue are also provided for different approaches introduced in the chapter. We expect that after reviewing this work, including the supporting mathematical background, that readers will have sufficient understanding to implement these methods for practical imaging applications. Given the brevity of the chapter, it was necessary to omit some related topics that are both important and exciting, but to mitigate this limitation we have made every attempt to include a comprehensive set of references for the interested reader to pursue.

6. ACKNOWLEDGMENTS

The research described in this chapter was funded, in part, by the National Institutes of Health under contract 5R01LM007455-03 from the National Library of Medicine and contract 1R01EB003587-01 from the National Institute of Biomedical Imaging and Bioengineering.

7. REFERENCES

1. Comaniciu D, Meer P, Foran DJ. 1999. Image-guided decision support system for pathology. *Machine Vision Appl* **11**:213–224.
2. Foran DJ, Comaniciu D, Meer P, Goodell LA. 2000. Computer-assisted discrimination among malignant lymphomas and leukemia using immunophentyping intelligent image repositories and telemicroscopy. *IEEE Trans Inform Technol Biomed* **4**(4):265–273.
3. Catalyurek U, Beynon MD, Chang C, Kurc T, Sussman A, Saltz J. 2003. The virtual microscope. *IEEE Trans Inform Technol Biomed* **7**(4):230–248.
4. Kass M, Witkin A, Terzopoulos D. 1987. Snakes: active contour models. *Int J Comput Vision* **1**:321–331.
5. Malladi R, Sethian JA, Vemuri BC. Shape modeling with front propagation: a level set approach. *IEEE Trans Pattern Anal Machine Intell* **17**(2):158–175.
6. Caselles V, Catte F, Coll T, Dibos F. 1993. A geometric model for active contours in image processing. *Num Math* **66**:1–32.
7. Leymarie F, Levine MD. 1993. Tracking deformable objects in the plane using an active contour model. *IEEE Trans Pattern Anal Machine Intell* **15**:617–634.
8. Durikovic R, Kaneda K, Yamashita H. 1995. Dynamic contour: a texture approach and contour operations. *Visual Comput* **11**:277–289.
9. Terzopoulos D. 1988. The computation of visible-surface representations. *IEEE Trans Pattern Anal Machine Intell* **10**(4):417–438.
10. Terzopoulos D, Szeliski R. 1992. Tracking with Kalman snakes. In *Active vision*, pp. 3–20. Ed A Blake, A Yuille. Cambridge: MIT Press.
11. Amini AA, Weymouth TE, Jain RC. 1990. Using dynamic programming for solving variational problems in vision. *IEEE Trans Pattern Anal Machine Intell* **12**(9):855–867.
12. Williams DJ, Shah M. 1992. A fast algorithm for active contours and curvature estimation. *Comput Vision Graphics Image Process: Image Understand* **55**(1):14–26.
13. Cohen LD. 1991. On active contour models and balloons. *Comput Vision Graphics Image Process: Image Understand* **53**(2):211–218.
14. Cohen LD, Cohen I. 1993. Finite-element methods for active contour models and balloons for 2d and 3d images. *IEEE Trans Pattern Anal Machine Intell* **15**(11):1131–1147.
15. Xu C, Prince JL. 1998. Snakes, shapes, and gradient vector flow. *IEEE Trans Image Process* **7**(3):359–369.
16. Xu C, Prince JL. 1998. Generalized gradient vector flow external forces for active contours. *Int J Signal Process* **71**(2):131–139.
17. Yang L, Meer P, Foran D. 2005. Unsupervised segmentation based on robust estimation and color active contour models. *IEEE Trans Inform Technol Biomed* **9**:475–486.

18. Jehan-Besson S, Gastaud M, Barlaud M, Aubert G. 2003. Region-based active contours using geometrical and statistical features for image segmentation. In *Proceedings of the IEEE international conference on image processing*, Vol. 2, pp. 643–646. Washington, DC: IEEE Computer Society.

19. Fedkiw RP, Sapiro G, Shu C. 2003. Shock capturing, level sets, and PDE-based methods in computer vision and image processing: a review of Osher's contributions. *J Comput Phys* **185**(2):309–341.

20. Chan TF, Vese LA. 2001. A level set algorithm for minimizing the Mumford-Shah functional in image processing. In *Proceedings of the IEEE Workshop on Variational and Level Set Methods*, pp. 161–171, Washington, DC: IEEE Computer Society.

21. Chan TF, Vese LA. Active contours withour edges. *IEEE Trans Image Process* **10**(2):266–277.

22. Arfken G. 1985. Calculus of variations. In *Mathematical Methods for Physicists*, 3rd ed, pp. 925–962 (chapter 17). Orlando, FL: Academic Press.

23. Smith GD. 1986. *Numerical solution of partial differential equations: finite-difference methods*, 3d ed. Oxford Applied Mathematics & Computing Science Series. Oxford: Oxford UP.

24. Gradshteyn IS, Ryzhik IM. 2000. *Tables of integrals series and products*, 6th ed. San Diego, CA: Academic Press.

25. Zenzo SD. 1986. A note on the gradient of a multi-image. *Comput Vision Graphics Image Process: Image Understand* **33**:116-125.

26. Sapiro G, Ringach DL. 1996. Anisotropic diffusion on multivalued images with applications to color filtering. *IEEE Trans Image Process* **5**(11):1582–1586.

27. Gevers T. 2002. Adaptive image segmentation by combining photometric invariant region and edge information. *IEEE Trans Pattern Anal Machine Intell* **24**(6):848–852.

28. Kreyszig E. 1991. *Differential geometry*. New York: Dover Publications.

29. Ray N, Acton ST, Altes T, de Lange EE. 2001. MRI ventilation analysis by merging parametric active contours. In *Proceedings of the 2001 international conference on image processing*, pp. 861–864. Washington, DC: IEEE Computer Society.

30. Osher S, Sethian JA. 1988. Fronts propagating with curvature-dependent speed: algorithms based on Hamilton-Jacobi fomulation. *J Comput Phys* **79**:12-49.

31. McInerney T, Terzopoulos D. 1995. A dymamic finite-element surface model for segmentation and tracking in multidimensional medical images with applications on cardiac 4d image analysis. *Comput Med Imaging Graphics* **19**:69–83.

4

IMAGE SEGMENTATION USING THE LEVEL SET METHOD

Yingge Qu, Pheng Ann Heng, and Tien-Tsin Wong

Department of Computer Science and Engineering
The Chinese University of Hong Kong

Construction of a speed function is crucial in applying the level set method to medical image segmentation. In this chapter we focus on the construction of the speed function. First of all, we have to investigate the curvature term in the speed function, and then show how to transform the image segmentation problem into an interface propagating problem. When segmenting medical images with classical level set methods, the propagating front may not be able to capture the real boundaries, although they are obvious to the human eye. We propose two formulations to enhance the speed function in level set methods, in order to tackle the segmentation problem of tagged MR images. First, a relaxation factor is introduced, aimed at relaxing the boundary condition when the boundary is unclear or blurry. Second, in order to incorporate human visual sensitive information from the image, a simple and general model is introduced to incorporate shape, texture, and color features. By further extending this model, we present a unified approach for segmenting and tracking of the high-resolution color anatomical Chinese Visible Human (CVH) data. The underlying relationship of these two applications relies on the proposed variational framework for the speed function. Our proposed method can be used to segment the first slice of the volume data. Then, based on the extracted boundary on the first slice, our method can also be adapted to track the boundary of the homogeneous organs among the subsequent serial images. In addition to the promising segmentation results, the tracking procedure requires only a small amount of user intervention.

Address all correspondence to: Pheng Ann Heng, Department of Computer Science and Engineering, The Chinese University of Hong Kong, Room 1028, Ho Sin-Hang Engineering Building, Shatin, N.T., Hong Kong. Phone: +852-2609 8424; Fax: +852-2603 5024. pheng@cse.cuhk.edu.hk; http://www.cse.cuhk.edu.hk/˜pheng/.

1. INTRODUCTION

As medical imaging plays an increasingly prominent role in the diagnosis and treatment of diseases, thousands of CT, MR, PET, and other images are acquired daily [1]. Their efficient and fast processing is challenging. Automatic or semiautomatic segmentation of different image components is useful for analyzing anatomical structures, the spatial distribution of their function or activity, and pathological regions. Segmentation is the basis for visualization and diagnosis.

Many segmentation methods have been proposed for medical image segmentation. Model-based methods utilize training in advance of obtaining sufficient prior knowledge, in order to get a fine parametric representation. However, these methods can only deal with one structure at a time. Although Snake-driven approaches [2, 3] have been successful in segmenting medical images that cannot be segmented well with traditional techniques, these approaches suffer from the strict requirement of initial contour and high computational load. In our work, we use level set methods as the tool, due to their strength in dealing with local deformations, multicomponent structures, and adaptability of topology. Such capabilities make these methods suitable for segmentation of medical images, which typically contain serial images of internal tissues with topological changes.

In the level set method, the construction of the speed function is vital with respect to the final result. The speed function is designed to control movement of the curve; and in different application problems, the key is to determine the appropriate stopping criteria for the evolution [4]. In our work, two improvements for enhancing the speed function of level set methods are presented, to tackle the segmentation of the left ventricle from tagged MR images. Both improvements are related to the construction of the speed function, which controls the propagating interfaces for the purpose of segmentation. Our method is especially efficient in segmenting the tagged MRI images with blurry boundaries and strong tag lines. Two ways to enhance the speed function for segmentation of images with blurry boundaries and strong tag lines are presented here. We first introduce the *relaxation factor*. It provides a way to stop the evolving curve at the ventricle boundary even when the boundary is blurry. In other words, the relaxation factor relaxes the bounding condition of the difference between the maximum and minimum gradient values of the image. This approach is described in detail in Section 4.1. This initial idea solves the leak problem at the blurry boundary by relaxing the bounding condition of the speed function. Second, *image content*-based items are incorporated in the speed function. The goal here is to take care of more image properties in order to control the front propagation instead of using the image gradient alone. We derive a simple and general model, through combining the image content items, to endow the speed function with more variability and better performance. By exploiting more image features than the image gradient, the constructed speed function can force the evolving boundary to stop at the object boundary, even if strong tag lines are close to the true boundary.

Based on the model described above, we further present a unified approach for semiautomatic segmenting and tracking of the high-resolution color anatomical Chinese Visible Human (CVH) data. A two-step scheme is proposed, starting with segmenting the first image slice. The user can initialize the first slice by clicking on the area of interest (AOI). The contours in the subsequent image slices are then automatically tracked. The underlying relationship of these two steps relies on the proposed variational framework for the speed function. Segmentation results are shown to be promising, while the tracking procedure demands very little user intervention.

The rest of this chapter is organized as follow. Section 2 discusses the related work. Section 3 covers the mathematical foundations of level set methods. We will discuss the fundamental formulation first. We will then look into why the curvature term is combined in the speed function, and how to adapt the speed function for image segmentation. The front propagation algorithm of the *narrow band* method and the numerical scheme are also mentioned in this section. In Section 4 we present the work on incorporating the speed function with the relaxation factor and the image content items to handle tagged cardiac MRI images. In Section 5 we present the semiautomatic segmentation and tracking of serial medical images. A two-step scheme is proposed to reduce the user intervention. A new scheme to construct the speed function for tracking is demonstrated with the high-resolution color anatomical images. Finally, we offer our conclusions in Section 6.

2. RELATED WORK

Medical image segmentation plays an important role in computer-aided diagnosis. Because of the complexity of organs and the structures and the limitation of different imaging modalities, medical images always show artifacts, including noises and weak boundaries. Such artifacts make medical image segmentation a difficult task. When applying classical segmentation techniques (such as thresholding, edge detection, and region growing), these artifacts may cause the boundaries to become indistinguishable and discontinuous. Figures 1a and 1b show typical tagged cardiac MRI and their corresponding edge image obtained using the Roberts operator. In Figure 1a, because of the blood flow, there is an artifact in the image of the left ventricle. In Figures 1a and 1b, the graylevel of boundaries varies from place to place, and these boundaries are not apparent, and hence cannot be detected by the Roberts operator. Examining Figures 1c and 1d, the segmentation results obtained using the Roberts operator, we can see that there are discontinuities on the boundaries, and they cannot be correctly segmented. As a result, these model-free techniques either fail completely or require a significant amount of expert intervention for such a segmentation problem.

To address these difficulties, *deformable models* have been proposed and are now widely used in medical image segmentation [5]. Deformable models are

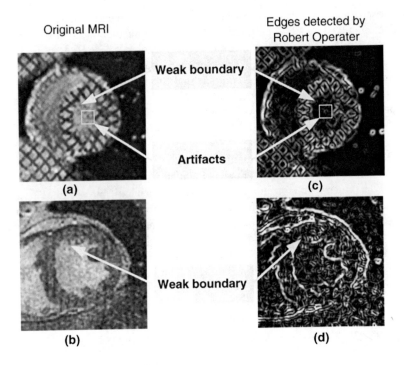

Figure 1. Cardiac MRI images (a,b) show the original MR images with weak boundary artifacts. (c,d) Results with the Roberts operator. See attached CD for color version.

physically motivated and model-based methods for describing region boundaries. They are described as closed parametric curves or surfaces that deform under the influence of internal and external forces. This term, "deformable model," first appeared in the work by Terzopoulos [6], where the generalized spline models with continuity constraints were applied. Similar work was proposed by Grenander et al. [7] and Miller et al. [8]. The most popular deformable model is the *snakes* model introduced by Kass et al. [2, 3]. Snake-driven approaches involve solving the energy-based active contours minimization problem by computing geodesics or minimal distance curves [9, 10, 11]. These approaches have been successfully applied to segment medical images that cannot be well segmented with other techniques. Along with the advances of front propagation modeling methods, a considerable number of specific modifications for various applications have been proposed. Various terms — such as snakes, active contours, balloons, and deformable contours — have been used in the literature to refer to this deformable model technique. Active contour models may incorporate a wide range of driving forces [12, 13]. Many of them are based on minimization of combined energy functions, which control the fairness of the resulting curve, on one hand, while attracting it to the object boundaries of the AOI.

However, two main limitations of deformable templates have been noted. First, snakes are quite sensitive to initial conditions. Deformable models may converge to a wrong boundary if the initial position is not close enough to the desired boundary. Second, its topological constraint is another disadvantage. Terzopoulos et al. [14] and Cohen [15] used balloon forces to free the deformable models from the initial conditions problem. The key is to introduce a constant force, which continuously expands or shrinks the initial contour. Caselles et al. [16] and Malladi et al. [9] tackled the variable topology problem by introducing the implicit snakes models. Many models have difficulties in progressing into boundary concavities. Addressing these problems, a new class of external forces has been proposed by deriving from the original image a gradient vector flow field in a variational framework [17]. Sensitivity to initialization has been drastically reduced, and contours have a more sensible behavior in the regions of concavities.

The level set technique, introduced by Osher and Sethian [4, 18, 19, 20], is an emerging method to represent shapes and track moving interfaces. Such techniques have been intensively studied in segmentation and tracking [9]. The ability of handling local deformations, multicomponent structures, and changes of topology are its major strengths. In this approach, the initial curve is interpreted as the zero level curve of a function $\Phi(t,0) : \Omega \rightarrow R$. The evolution of these curves is controlled by a Partial Differential Equation (PDE) [4]. The attempts to evolve interfaces with level set methods has received much attention in the last few years due to its ability in a boundary-driven approach for image segmentation [16, 10, 21, 22, 23].

Recently, a general variational framework for *Mumford-Shah* [24] and Geman [25]-type functionals has been introduced [26]. Edge boundaries are represented by a continuous function, yielded by minimizing an energy function. Caselles et al. [27], Kichenassamy et al. [11], and Paragios [28] developed another classical snake model, the *geodesic active contour*, as the geometric alternative to the original snake. Its implicit parametrization allows one to handle the topological changes naturally.

In the level set method, the construction of the speed function is vital to the final result. The speed function is designed to control the movement of the curve. In different applications, the key is to determine the appropriate stopping criteria for the evolution [4]. In case of segmentation, segmentation accuracy depends on the termination criteria of the evolving surface, which in turn depends on the speed term. When segmenting or localizing an anatomical structure, having prior information about the expected shape can significantly help in the segmentation process. This was recently addressed in various forms [29, 30, 31, 32]. Cootes et al. [33] and Wang et al. [34] found a set of corresponding points across a set of training images and constructed the statistical model of shape variation that is then used in the localization of the boundary. Staib and Duncan [13] incorporated the global shape information into segmentation by using an elliptic Fourier decomposition of the boundary and placing a Gaussian prior on the Fourier coefficient. Chan et al. [35] and Leventon et al. [29] introduced the shape priors into geodesic active models. To improve the robustness of level set-based methods to noisy and incomplete data, Rousson and Paragios combined a shape influence term [36].

3. LEVEL SET METHODS AND IMAGE SEGMENTATION

3.1. Formulations

The level set method, developed by Osher and Sethian, is a zero equivalent surface method [18]. Its basic idea is to change the movement track of a planar curve into the movement track of a three-dimensional surface. Though this conversion complicates the solution, it exhibits many other advantages: parameter-free representation, topological flexibility, and the ability to handle local deformations are its main strengths. These properties make the level set framework a suitable choice for describing cardiac structure.

The classical level set boundary is defined as a zero level set of an implicit representation Φ of the evolving curve. In detail, we now evolve the implicit level set function $\Phi(x, y, t)$, to denote the evolution of a curve $\Gamma(t)$ in its normal direction with a speed $F(x, y)$. At time t, the zero level set $(x, y)|\phi(x, y, t) = 0$ describes the evolved contour $\Gamma(t)$, namely,

$$\Phi(\Gamma(t), t) = 0 \ . \tag{1}$$

When we differentiate this equation with respect to t and use the chain rule, we have

$$\frac{\partial \phi}{\partial t} + \nabla \phi \cdot \frac{\partial \Gamma}{\partial t} \ . \tag{2}$$

Because F denotes the speed of the curve in its normal direction, it can be characterized as

$$\frac{\partial \Gamma}{\partial t} \cdot N = F \ , \tag{3}$$

where N represents the outwards normal, and can be obtained by

$$N = \frac{\nabla \phi}{|\nabla \phi|} \ . \tag{4}$$

Substitute Eqs. (3) and (4) into (2), and we can get the evolution equation for ϕ as

$$\Phi_t + F|\nabla \Phi| = 0 \ . \tag{5}$$

This is the basic equation of the level set [4], and the zero level set denotes the object contour curve:

$$\Gamma(t) = \{(x, y) | \Phi(x, y, t) = 0\} . \tag{6}$$

The function Φ is usually calculated based on the signed distance measure to the initial front. Applying to the image domain, it can be simply the Euclidean distance between the curve and one image point. That is,

$$\Phi(x, y) = \pm d(x, y) , \tag{7}$$

where $d(x, y)$ is the Euclidean distance from the point to the boundary, and the sign is chosen such that points inside the boundary have a negative sign and those outside have a positive sign.

Now the evolution of the boundary is defined via a partial differential equation on the zero level set of Φ:

$$\frac{\partial \Phi}{\partial t} = -F |\nabla \Phi| . \tag{8}$$

Here, F is a known function, and is determined by the local curvature κ at the zero level set, i.e.,

$$F = F(\kappa) , \tag{9}$$

where the curvature κ is given by

$$\kappa = \nabla \cdot \frac{\nabla \phi}{|\nabla \phi|} = \frac{\phi_{xx} \phi_y^2 - 2\phi_x \phi_y \phi_{xy} + \phi_{yy} \phi_x^2}{(\phi_x^2 + \phi_y^2)^{3/2}} , \tag{10}$$

3.2. Speed Function

Consider a boundary separating one region from another (either a curve in 2D or a surface in 3D), and imagine that this interface moves in a direction normal to itself with a known speed function F. The purpose is to track the motion of this interface as it evolves [4], as illustrated in Figure 2. Sethian [4, 20] represents the speed function F as

$$F = F(L, G, I) , \tag{11}$$

where L is the *local information*, which is determined by the local geometric properties, such as curvature and normal direction; G is the *global property* of the front that depends on the shape and position of the front; I represents the *independent properties* that are independent of the front, such as an underlying fluid velocity that passively transports the front.

It is difficult to design a generic model for the speed function F, because it is closely related to the applications. In this section, we give a brief view of two important terms in the speed function. First we examine the curvature term in Eq. (9), and then we look at the speed term introduced by Caselles et al. [16] and Malladi et al. [9] for image segmentation purposes.

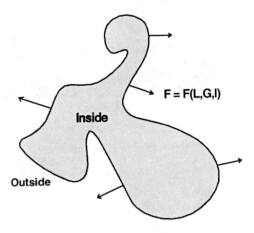

Figure 2. Interface propagation. See attached CD for color version.

3.2.1. Curvature Term In Speed Function

Suppose the speed function in Eq. (9) is $F = 1 - \epsilon\kappa$, where ϵ is a constant. Sethian [4] showed that the effects of the $\epsilon\kappa$ term on modifying the result are profound. It lays down the foundation for building accurate numerical schemes that follow the correct entropy condition.

Suppose we are propagating a cosine front $\gamma(0) = (1 - s, [1 + \cos 2\pi s]/2])$. The speed function is given by $F = 1 - \epsilon\kappa, \epsilon > 0$. With $\epsilon = 0.25$, Figure 3a shows the propagation result of the initial cosine curve. According to the action of the negative reaction term $-\epsilon\kappa$, we can note that, although the V-shape at $s = n + 1/2$

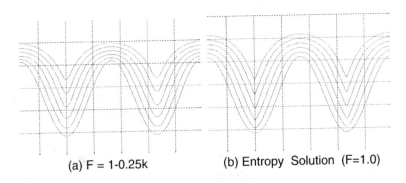

(a) F = 1-0.25k   (b) Entropy Solution (F=1.0)

Figure 3. The entropy solution is the limit of viscous solutions. See attached CD for color version.

is sharpened, the flow remains smooth and differentiable for all the time. A smaller ϵ will lead to sharper troughs. Until $-\epsilon = 0$, i.e. $F = 1$, to solve the propagation correctly, we must follow the entropy condition to avoid the "swallowtail." The weak solution following the entropy condition is shown in Figure 3b. Comparing Figure 3a with Figure 3b, Sethian [4] pointed out that at any time T,

$$\lim_{\epsilon \to 0} X^{\epsilon}_{curvature}(T) = X^{En}_{constant}(T) . \tag{12}$$

Here $X^{\epsilon}_{curvature}(t)$ is the solution obtained by evolving the curve with $F_{\kappa} = 1 - \epsilon\kappa$, and $X^{En}_{constant}(t)$ is the weak solution obtained with speed function $F = 1$ and the entropy condition. Equation (12) makes the point that the limit of motion under curvature, known as the "*viscosity solution*," is the entropy solution for the case of constant speed.

To examine the role of the curvature in the speed function, we now turn to a discussion of the relationship between propagating fronts and the hyperbolic conservation laws. For completeness, we present the basic idea below, and readers are referred to [4][37] for details.

We call the equation for $u_t(x, t)$ of the form

$$u_t + [G(u)]_x = 0 \tag{13}$$

the "hyperbolic conservation law." There is an example in [4] to demonstrate the relationship between the hyperbolic conservation law and the propagating front, given Burger's equation as the example, which follows the hyperbolic conservation law:

$$u_t + uu_x = 0. \tag{14}$$

Its physical meaning describes the motion of a compressible fluid in one dimension. Imagine there is a sudden expansion or compression of the fluid; then the solution will appear as discontinuities or "shocks." However if we change the right-hand side 0 with a second derivative,

$$u_t + uu_x = \varepsilon u_{xx}, \tag{15}$$

and then fluid viscosity will appear to retain the smoothness of the fluid, and such shocks are avoided.

Look at the propagating front again, which is given by ψ (Figure 4). Suppose the front propagates from time t to time $t + \Delta t$. The right-hand plot in Figure 4 shows the relation among speed F, tangent $(1, \psi_x)$, and change in height V, i.e.,

$$\frac{V}{F} = \frac{(1 + \psi_x^2)^{1/2}}{1}. \tag{16}$$

Rewriting it, we can obtain the motion equation as

$$\psi_t = F(1 + \psi_x^2)^{1/2}. \tag{17}$$

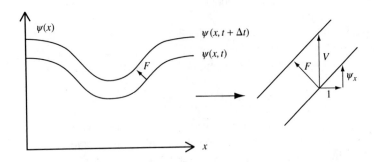

Figure 4. Variables for propagating graph.

Plugging the speed function $F(\kappa) = 1 - \epsilon\kappa$ and the formula $\kappa = -\psi_{xx}/(1 + \psi_x^2)^{3/2}$ into Eq. (17), we have

$$\psi_t - (1 + \psi_x^2)^{1/2} = \epsilon\frac{\psi_{xx}}{(1 + \psi_x^2)^{3/2}}. \tag{18}$$

Differentiating both side yields an evolution equation:

$$u_t + [-(1 + u^2)^{1/2}]_x = \epsilon[\frac{u_x}{1 + u^2}]_x, \tag{19}$$

where $u = d\psi/dx$.

Comparing this curvature-modified propagating equation with Eq. (15), it is analogous to a viscous hyperbolic conservation law. The linkage shows us that the role of curvature in a propagating front is analogous to the role of viscosity in this hyperbolic conservation law. It keeps the moving front smooth and differentiable during propagation.

3.2.2. Adapting Speed Function for Image Segmentation

After examining the curvature term in the speed function, we now return to the segmentation problem. Consider a medical image in which our goal is to isolate an organ from the background. Starting from an initial contour, we want the moving front to propagate inside the homogeneous region and stop at the boundaries.

Malladi, Sethian, and Vemuri [38, 39, 9] and Caselles et al. [16] [10, 40] first proposed to use the level set methods to solve the shape recovery problem. The propagating function is represented as

$$\frac{\partial\phi}{\partial t} = g_I(F_A + F_G)|\nabla\phi| . \tag{20}$$

Here the influence of the speed function F is split into two parts, F_A and F_G. The term F_A is the advection term, causing the front to uniformly expand or contract with a speed of F_A depending on its sign. The second term F_G is the part that depends on the geometry of the front, such as its local curvature. The affect of this curvature term was investigated in the previous section. An example is $\pm 1 - \epsilon\kappa$, where ϵ is a constant. The constant 1 or -1 acts as an advection term (F_A), to expand or contract the front. The diffusive term $\epsilon\kappa$ (F_G) keeps the propagating front smooth. The curve evolution is coupled with the image segmentation problem by multiplying $(F_A + F_G)$ by a stopping term:

$$g_I(x, y) = \frac{1}{1 + |\nabla(G_\sigma \otimes I(x, y))|}, \tag{21}$$

where the expression $G_\sigma \otimes I$ means that we convolute the image I with a Gaussian smoothing filter G_σ with characteristic width of σ. When in homogenous regions, $\nabla(G_\sigma \otimes I(x, y))$ will converge to zero, so that the affect of g_I on $F_A + F_G$ is minor. In the case when at the boundary the filter $g_I(x, y)$ drops to zero, it performs as a halting criteria for the speed function and stops the evolving front at the desired region.

An example of this speed function on a multi-object image is shown in Figure 5. The bottom images (Figure 5c,d) show topology adaptability during propagation.

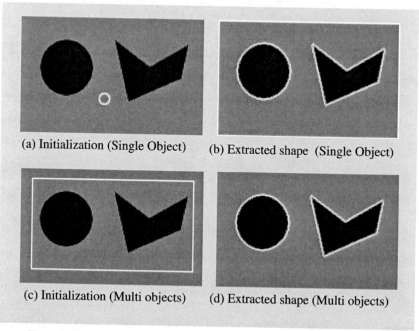

(a) Initialization (Single Object)   (b) Extracted shape (Single Object)

(c) Initialization (Multi objects)   (d) Extracted shape (Multi objects)

Figure 5. Shape extraction on multi-object image. See attached CD for color version.

3.3. Narrow-Band Algorithm and Implementation

Malladi et al. [9] implemented the level set approach using the *Narrow-Band Method*, which solves the initial value problem of level set methods. They then sped up the boundary-value problem by also employing a *Fast Marching Method* [41], which requires that the speed F should be strictly positive or negative. In this chapter, we focus on Narrow-Band methods with our particular application.

Instead of using all the grid points, the key idea of the Narrow-Band approach is to constrain the computation only to the pixels that are close to the zero level set. The pseudocode of this method is:

1. *Initialize* the signed distance function $\Phi(x, 0)$ of the initial contour Γ;

2. *Find* the narrow band points: determine those points X_i whose distance $|\Phi(x, t)|$ is less than the specified narrow bandwidth, and mark them as the narrow band points;

3. *Update*: resolve level set Eq. (20), and track the zero level set curve; update the level set function value $|\Phi(x, t + \Delta t)|$ in the narrow band;

4. *Reinitialize*: reinitialize the narrow band when the zero level set reaches the boundary of the narrow band. Repeat steps 3 and 4.

5. *Convergence test*: check whether the iteration converges or not. If so, stop; otherwise, enter the calculation of the next step, and go to step 3.

In step 1 the signed distance is always obtained by the closest distance from the narrow band points to the zero level set. The sign is chosen such that the inner part of the zero level set is negative, and the outer part is positive. In this way, the signed distance function can be seen as the projection of ϕ from the one-dimensional higher space to the image space.

In step 3, when solving propagation Eq. (20), the normal $\vec{n}$ and curvature $F(\kappa)$ terms actually are only defined on the zero level set. We need to extend the speed function to the whole narrow band area. A simple way to do this is to extrapolate the value on the zero level set to the nearby grid points. Many approaches for such extensions have been discussed in [4].

When the curve evolves to the boundary of the narrow band, the narrow band should be reinitialized. If the point difference between sequential time steps is smaller than the designed threshold in the narrow band, the propagating speed will be set to zero. When the narrow band is not reinitialized within a certain time, this means that curve evolvement has stopped. So the iteration ends, and the final zero level curve is the boundary of the desired object.

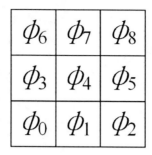

Figure 6. Numbering scheme for derivative computation.

3.4. Numerical Implementation

In image segmentation case, the previous discussion in Section 3.2.2 shows that the speed function usually includes: (1) a curvature-based speed term $F(\kappa)$; (2) a constant speed term (F_A), where the speed can be expressed as a function $F_A(x, y)$ of the location (x, y); (3) a stopping criterion g_I based on the image gradient to extract the boundary (Eq. (21)). The level set partial differential equation for this curve evolution is:

$$\frac{\partial \phi}{\partial t} = g_I(\alpha \kappa |\nabla \phi| + \beta F_A(x, y)|\nabla \phi|), \tag{22}$$

where α and β are constants; F_A is a constant speed term; g_I is also constant during the propagation.

Consider the implementation of this PDE within the image domain. First, define the function $\phi(t)$ in the narrow band area. We use the Euclidean distance from point (x, y) to the zero level set as the value of the signed distance. The sign is negative if the point is inside the curve, and positive if (x, y) is outside the curve. All the calculations are carried out only within the narrow band area.

The evolution equation can now be represented as

$$\phi(t + \Delta t) = \phi(t) + g_I(\alpha T_1 + \beta T_2)\Delta t. \tag{23}$$

First, we describe the finite-difference derivatives required for level set update and curvature computation in T_1 and T_2. For the convenience of representation of derivatives, the neighborhood of ϕ is specified with the numbering scheme shown in Figure 6.

The central point ϕ_4 denotes the current pixel. Using the central difference approximations, the derivatives of the level set function ϕ are defined as

$$
\begin{aligned}
D_x &= (\phi_5 - \phi_3)/2 & D_y &= (\phi_7 - \phi_1)/2 \\
D_{xx} &= (\phi_5 - 2\phi_4 + \phi_3)/2 & D_{yy} &= (\phi_7 - 2\phi_4 + \phi_1)/2 \\
D_{xy} &= (\phi_2 - \phi_8 - \phi_0 + \phi_6)/4 \\
D_x^+ &= \phi_5 - \phi_4 & D_y^+ &= \phi_7 - \phi_4 \\
D_x^- &= \phi_4 - \phi_3 & D_y^- &= \phi_4 - \phi_1 \\
D_x^{+y} &= (\phi_8 - \phi_6)/2 & D_x^{-y} &= (\phi_2 - \phi_0)/2 \\
D_y^{+x} &= (\phi_8 - \phi_2)/2 & D_y^{-x} &= (\phi_6 - \phi_0)/2
\end{aligned}
\tag{24}
$$

The stretch of $|\nabla\phi|$ is obtained by $[D_x^2 + D_y^2]^{1/2}$. The individual terms of T_1 and T_2 are then calculated as:

$$
T_1 = \kappa[D_x^2 + D_y^2]^{1/2},
\tag{25}
$$

where the curvature κ can be obtained by

$$
\kappa = \frac{D_{xx}(D_y)^2 - 2D_y D_x D_{xy} + D_{yy}(D_x)^2}{(D_x^2 + D_y^2)^{3/2}},
\tag{26}
$$

and T_2 can be calculated as

$$
T_2 = \max(F_{i,j}, 0)\nabla^+ + \min(F_{i,j}, 0)\nabla^-,
\tag{27}
$$

where

$$
\nabla^+ = [\max(D_x^-, 0)^2 + \min(D_x^+, 0)^2 + \max(D_y^-, 0)^2 + \min(D_y^+, 0)^2]^{1/2}
$$

$$
\nabla^- = [\max(D_x^+, 0)^2 + \min(D_x^-, 0)^2 + \max(D_y^+, 0)^2 + \min(D_y^-, 0)^2]^{1/2}
\tag{28}
$$

To certify the stability of the evolution, the size of the time step is restricted following the Courant Friedrich Levy (CFL) condition $\Delta t \leq 1/\max(g_I(\alpha T_1 + \beta T_2))$ (Section 4.3). This requires that the curve cannot move more than one grid point at each time step. Here the maximum is calculated in the whole image domain.

4. AUGMENTING THE SPEED FUNCTION

Many challenges in interface problems arise from the production of an appropriate model for the speed term [4]. As mentioned before, the construction of speed function is vital for final results. The speed function is designed to control the movement of the curve. In different problems, the key is to determine the appropriate stopping criteria for the evolution. In a segmentation case, the segmentation precision depends on when and where the evolving curved surface stops, and the stopping criteria of the evolving surface also depends on the speed term F. So the construction of F is critical. However, when segmenting the medical images with the classical speed function, especially when there are blurry boundaries and a strong tag line, the propagating front may not capture the true boundary, by either leaking through it, or stopping at the non-boundary area.

In this section, two improvements to augment the speed function are introduced to handle the tagged MRI. A relaxation factor is first introduced, followed by image content items.

4.1. Relaxation Factor

In [9], the construction of a speed term is described as $F = F_A + F_G$, where F_A is a constant. It does not depend on the geometry of the front, but its sign determines the direction of front movement. F_G depends on the geometry of the front. In [9], a negative speed term is constructed as in Eq. (29), and then the speed term is constructed as: $F = F_A + F_I$, where F_I is defined as

$$F_I(x, y) = \frac{-F_A}{M_1 - M_2} \{ |\nabla G_\sigma \cdot I(x, y)| - M_2 \} . \tag{29}$$

The expression $G_\sigma \cdot I(x, y)$ denotes the image convolved with a Gaussian smoothing filter whose characteristic width is σ. M_1 and M_2 are the maximum and minimum values of the magnitude of image gradient $|\nabla G_\sigma \cdot I(x, y)|$. So the speed term F tends to zero when the image gradient is large.

However, in practice, the gradient values on the object boundary seldom reach the maximum value (M_1). In other words, the evolvement cannot stop at the object boundary. Especially for MR images in which the boundaries are blurry, results are even worse. To solve this problem, a *relaxation factor* δ is introduced to relax the bounding of $M_1 - M_2$:

$$r' = \frac{|\nabla G_\sigma \cdot I(x, y)| - M_2}{M_1 - M_2 - \delta}, \tag{30}$$

where $\delta \in [0, M_1 - M_2]$. We trim r to 1:

$$r = \begin{cases} r' & \text{if } r < 1 \\ 1 & \text{if } r \geq 1 \end{cases},$$

and the reconstructed negative speed term will be $F_I'(x, y) = -r \cdot F_A$.

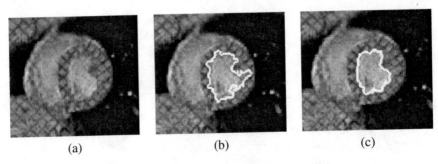

(a) (b) (c)

Figure 7. (a) Original MR image. The white line in (b) is the propagated front obtained by a classical level set speed term. It can easily leak beyond the true boundary due to the blurry boundary. (c) Result obtained by introducing the relaxation factor into the speed term.

By introducing this relaxation factor, when the front propagates to places where the gradient of the object boundary are close to M_1, but not exactly M_1, the speed F drops to zero and the evolving curve will be stopped appropriately. Figure 7c shows the result of solving this problem with $\delta = 0.23$.

4.2. Image Content Items

The visual content of an image includes the color, shape, texture, and spatial layout, reflecting the human visual response directly. The image/object feature extraction techniques have been fully developed based on these items. In typical level set methods, the construction of a speed function mainly uses the gradient information. However, as medical imaging techniques advance, complex content in the image imposes new challenges to level set-based segmentation methods. Various image content-based speed items have been introduced in order to tackle different application problems. Here we derive a simple yet general model to incorporate image features into the speed function, so as to endow the speed function with more variability and better performance.

The form of the speed function can be written as [9]: $F = F_A + F_G$. By adding the control items or another image force, it can be expressed in a general but simple form:

$$F = A(F_A + F_G) + B, \tag{31}$$

$$A = 1/(1 + \text{dist}(C_{\text{img}}, C_{\text{front}})), \tag{32}$$

$$B = \overrightarrow{\text{dist}}(C_{\text{img}}, C_{\text{front}}). \tag{33}$$

The dist() can be any appropriate distance function. Its purpose is to measure the difference of image features between the propagating front and the propagated areas. B stands for the additional forces that arise from the image content. C

stands for the image content model, including any of the color, shape, and texture features. A is used to balance the force from the front and the force from additional items, and $A \to 1$.

4.3. Courant Friedrich Levy Condition

To ensure the stability when employing the numerical schemes to solve the PDEs, the full matrix approach requires a time step that satisfies a Courant Friedrich Levy (CFL) condition with regard to the maximum velocity over the entire domain, not simply in response to the speed of the front itself. Analogous with the underlying wave equation, for an advective speed function F and the first-order space scheme, a CFL condition requires the front to cross no more than one grid cell in each time step. Thus, we require that

$$\max_{\Omega} F \Delta t \leq \Delta x \,, \tag{34}$$

where the maximum is taken over values for F at all possible grid points, not simply those corresponding to the zero level set. In practice, one can quickly scan the range of the values for the speed function F and choose an appropriate time step accordingly.

In a narrow-band implementation, the time step can be adaptively chosen according to the maximum velocity field achieved within the narrow band. This is advantageous when the front speed changes substantially as it moves (such as in curvature flow). In such problems, the CFL restriction for the velocity field for all the level sets may be much more stringent than the one for those sets within the narrow band.

4.4. Augmented Speed Function for Segmentation

Some researchers [9, 42] introduce the stop term based on the image gradient:

$$K_I(x, y) = \frac{1}{1 + |\nabla G_\sigma \cdot I(x, y)|}. \tag{35}$$

Here, the gradient can be treated as the difference measurement of gray/brightness values. To adjust the influence of the image gradient on the speed term, we can redefine it:

$$K_I'(x, y) = \frac{1}{1 + |\nabla G_\sigma \cdot I(x, y)|^p} = 1 - \frac{|\nabla G_\sigma \cdot I(x, y)|^p}{1 + |\nabla G_\sigma \cdot I(x, y)|^p} \,, \tag{36}$$

where the constant $p \geq 1$. When p is larger, K_I' will be smaller, so it will control the speed to decrease faster. Then the speed term can be written as

$$F = K_I'(k + F_A) \,, \tag{37}$$

where $k = \dfrac{\phi_{yy}\phi_x^2 - 2\phi_x\phi_y\phi_{xy} + \phi_{xx}\phi_y^2}{(\phi_x^2 + \phi_y^2)^{3/2}}$ is the curvature of the front at point (x,y).

To resolve the boundary-leaking problem, Kichenassamy et al. [43] and Yezzi et al. [23] introduced a pull-back term $(\nabla c \cdot \nabla \phi)$ due to the edge strength; here $c(x,y) = \frac{1}{1+|\nabla G_\sigma \cdot I(x,y)|}$. It is an additional force term based on the color feature. To provide an additional attraction force when the front was in the vicinity of an edge, Siddiqui et al. [44] introduced an extra term $\frac{1}{2} div \left[\begin{pmatrix} x \\ y \end{pmatrix} \phi \right]$ according to area minimization. It is an additional force term based on the shape feature.

In the case of tagged MR, new features can also be introduced along the same lines. The high clarity of tag lines makes segmentation more difficult than with an untagged image. According to human response, texture is the most distinguishable feature (Figure 8a). In this example, the tag lines are in the vertical direction; hence we design an additional term B based on texture feature BPV [45]:

$$BPV(x,y) = \frac{1}{N} \sum_{y-\lceil \frac{N-1}{2} \rceil}^{y+\lceil \frac{N-1}{2} \rceil} (I(x,i) - M)^2 ,$$

$$M = \frac{1}{N} \sum_{y-\lceil \frac{N-1}{2} \rceil}^{y+\lceil \frac{N-1}{2} \rceil} |I(x,i) - I(x,y)|. \tag{38}$$

Here, the distance is measured by the standard deviation. $BPV(x,y)$ is the BPV value of point (x,y), $1 \le x \le m$, $\frac{N-1}{2} \le y \le n - \frac{N-1}{2}$, m and n are the height and width of the image, and N is the width of the window, which is approximately 7 or 9 according to the width of the tag lines. $I(x,y)$ is the intensity value of the block center. The reasoning of the above equation is as follows. When the intensity value of some point is quite distinct compared to points that are on the same line and whose center is located at the point, the BPV value of this point is smaller, and vice versa. Now, the speed function has been augmented to

$$F = K'_I(\varepsilon k + F_A + F'_I) + \beta \frac{\nabla c \cdot \nabla \phi}{|\nabla \phi|} + \mu \, div \left[\begin{pmatrix} x \\ y \end{pmatrix} \phi \right] + \gamma(BPV), \tag{39}$$

where K'_I is the A item, used to control the balance between the original speed term and the additional speed term. Larger K'_I will speed up the decrease in value of the speed term. The coefficients β, μ, and γ are constants, which should be defined according to the contribution of their corresponding part. In Eq. (39), such image features as curvature, shape, and texture information have been combined into the speed term. An experiment based on this augmented speed item is carried out in the following section.

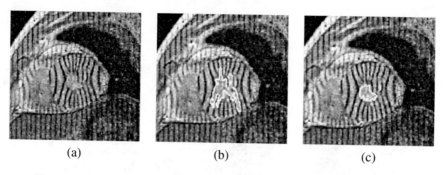

(a)   (b)   (c)

Figure 8. Segmentation of tagged MRI image: (a) strong tagged MR image; (b) result obtained using the standard level set method. This result has a serious leak phenomenon due to the strong tag lines. (c) Improved result obtained using the BPV feature to control propagation of the front.

4.5. Results and Discussion: Segmentation of tagged MRI Data

Segmentation experiments were performed on the 2D slices of MR images with weak boundaries and artifacts. For the following experiments, the training set consisted of 30 nearby slices of the left ventricle.

The first experiment was aimed to demonstrate the effect of the relaxation factor. Figure 9 shows the result of introducing this factor. By adjusting the value of the factor δ, its influence on stopping the propagating front can be seen clearly. The first one shows the original leaking problem. The following results were obtained by setting δ to 0.5 and 1.5.

Two other segmentation results from tagged MR and anatomical images are shown here to demonstrate the effectiveness of the image content, and using the augmented speed term described in the previous sections. In both examples, by defining the seed point inside the region of interest, initialization can be done simply by one mouse click. Then the narrow-band method, as described in Section 3.3, is employed to propagate the front.

The first experiment was carried out on a cardiac MRI and showed the left ventricle with tag lines. Because of the blood flow, tag lines within the left ventricle decrease rapidly in the last stage of the cardiac shrink, until they disappear. But tag lines in the myocardium decrease slowly, which can be seen from Figure 8a. Inside the left ventricle the intensity changes are smaller and the relative BPV value is larger. On the other hand, in the myocardium the intensity changes are larger and the relative BPV value is smaller. As for images like Figure 8a whose tag lines are very strong, the weight of the BPV feature should be greater in construction of the speed term.

In the above experiment, the spatial step length is 1, the temporal step length 0.001, $F_A = -20$, $\beta = 5$, $\mu = 0.0025$, $\gamma = 280$, and $\delta = 0.23$. The number of iterations is 150. As the tag lines in Figure 8 are strong, a large γ should be set, while in other cases it could be small. For MR images without tag lines, we

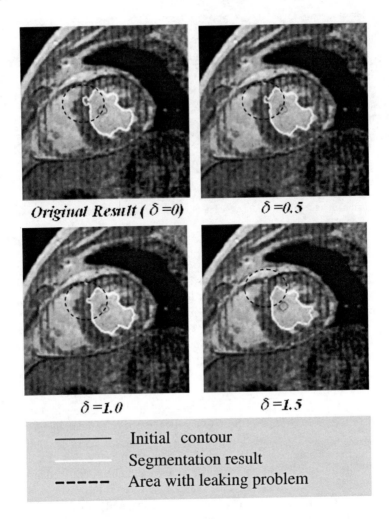

Figure 9. Introducing the relaxation factor into the front propagation to solve the leaking problem. See attached CD for color version.

do not have to impose the BPV term (namely, $\gamma = 0$). These parameters are fine tuned empirically and adjusted manually. An automatic process to estimate the parameters could be further studied in the future [46].

This model can be applied to various cases. Another experimental result can be seen in Figure 10. The original segmentation result is far from satisfactory (Figure 10b) because the stronger image details stop the propagation easily. In this case, the introduction of color and texture into the speed term makes the result closer to the user's expectation. We introduced a block color histogram and

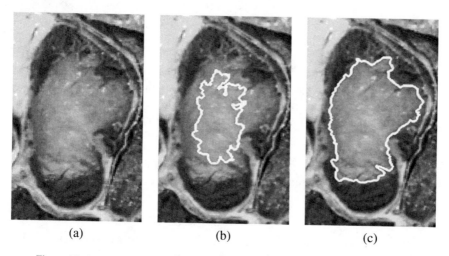

(a)   (b)   (c)

Figure 10. Segmentation of color slide image: (a) original color slide image; (b) propagation front stops in a non-boundary area; (c) result after incorporating color and texture features into the speed function. See attached CD for color version.

the BPV texture feature in our experiment. The distance measures are: histogram intersection, as a measure of the block-wise histogram, and the Euclidean distance, as a measure in the BPV item. The balancing items are: $F_A = -15$, $\beta = 5$, $\mu = 0.002$, $\gamma = 20$, and $\delta = 0.2$.

5. SEMIAUTOMATIC SEGMENTATION AND TRACKING OF SERIAL MEDICAL IMAGES

The Chinese Visible Human (CVH) data were acquired in 2002 (for males) and 2003 (for females). It is the first volumetric data representing a complete normal human of Asian extraction [47]. Higher resolution, distinguishable blood vessels, data completeness, and freedom from organic lesions are the main advantages of this dataset. It is useful in a variety of research and educational applications. At the same time, it brings a new challenges to the research of segmentation due to the high-resolution color details without obvious boundaries. Although the property of high resolution in details can present difficulties in segmenting the CVH data, it offers convenience for tracking-based serial image segmentation. When segmenting the serial dataset, a two-step scheme based on Level Set segmentation and tracking is proposed as follows:

1. *Segmentation Step:* This step segments the first slice of volumetric data (e.g., a stack of slices containing the target organ(s)). In this step, the speed function is designed for the purpose of segmentation (Section 4.4), which incorporates the gradient, texture, and color information. The user can set

the initial seed by simply clicking on the AOI, as shown in the leftmost image of Figure 11;

2. *Tracking Step:* For subsequent image slices, level set segmentation is performed with the initial curve (the same as the segmented result from the previous image). The front is propagated with a newly proposed speed function (Section 5.1), which is designed for tracking.

This segmentation process is demonstrated in Figure 11. The underlying relationship between the segmentation and tracking methods relies on the proposed variational framework (Section 4.2) for the speed function.

5.1. Speed Function for Tracking

The 0.1-mm inter-layer distance of the CVH data makes tracking easier and more reliable for the segmentation task. We also extended the speed model in Section 4 for the tracking problem. Due to the visual consistency constraint between two continuous layers, we can assume that the transformation of the edge between images I_n and I_{n+1} is between a narrow band with width δ. All the following calculations are done only within the narrow band.

We propose a new speed function for evolving the contour, from image I_n to the next slice I_{n+1}. Taking the segmentation result in I_n as the initial contour in I_{n+1}, the front propagates under the speed function (Eq. (40)), to attract the front moving to the new AOI boundary. Here, the curvature term κ is still adopted in order to avoid a "swallowtail" during the propagation. F_D is the cost function between the two images I_n and I_{n+1}. It can be measured by the sum of square differences between the image intensities in a window, as shown in Figure 12. Equation 41 tells us how to determine the magnitude and signal of F_D, where $+n$ and $-n$ indicate whether the pixels are outside or inside the zero level set, respectively, in I_n. C_+^n and C_-^n are the content models of these pixels in I_n. ID represents the overlapped non-homogenous areas (Figure 12):

$$F = KI_{n+1}(\epsilon\kappa + F_D) + \beta F_C, \tag{40}$$

$$F_D = S \cdot (I_n - I_{n+1})^2, F_C = S \cdot \text{dist}(C_n, C_{n+1}), \tag{41}$$

$$S = \text{Sign}(\text{dist}(C_{ID}, C_+^n) - \text{dist}(C_{ID}, C_-^n). \tag{42}$$

Note that F_D, convolved by KI_{n+1}, forces the front to move in the homogeneous area and to stop at the boundaries in I_{n+1}. The sign of F_D determines whether the curve will expand or shrink.

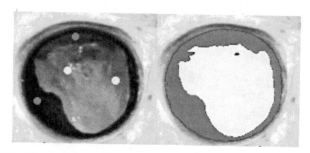

(a) Initial contour segmented in the first slice by level set

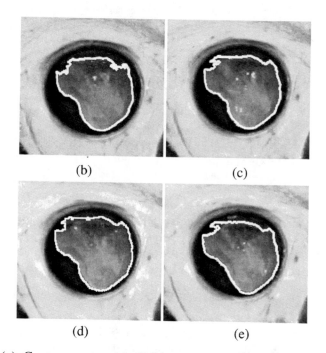

(b)-(e): Contours automatically detected in the subsequent slices

Figure 11. The user need only to click on the AOI to initialize the first slice. The contours in the subsequent image slices are then automatically tracked. See attached CD for color version.

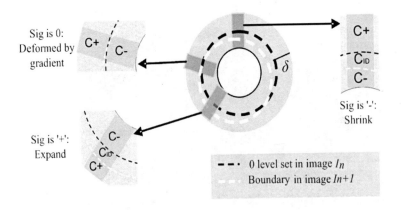

Figure 12. Design of the speed function for tracking: value and signal. See attached CD for color version.

5.2. Results and Discussion: Segmentation and Tracking of CVH Data

For the tracking task, experiments are carried out on the volumetric CVH data. Referring to the speed function (Eqs. (40–42)), in addition to the color information, which is introduced by the distance of $(I_n - I_{n+1})^2$ in Eq. (41), we still incorporate the BPV (Eq. (38)) texture feature as the image content item C term in Eqs. (41) and (42), because of its effectiveness as a texture measure and the convenience of calculation.

Satisfactory results have been obtained (Figure 11). The boundaries of the AOI are well tracked and delineated using the proposed speed function model. We tested it in a topology-coherent case (Figure 11) and a topology-changing case (Figure 13). Figure 13a shows the first slice of a section of CVH data containing the brain. The two white dots in Figure 13b depict initialization in the AOI. Figure 13c gives the boundaries in the subsequent image slices that are automatically tracked. We can notice the topology changing by comparing the top left and bottom right images in Figure 13c.

We should note that this method benefitted from the close inter-layer distance within the CVH data. If the object displacements between slices are so large that there are no overlapping regions, the model would fail.

6. CONCLUSION

To summarize, a variational framework for the speed function of level set methods has been proposed for segmentation and tracking of medical images. For segmenting the tagged MR images with blurry boundaries and strong tag lines,

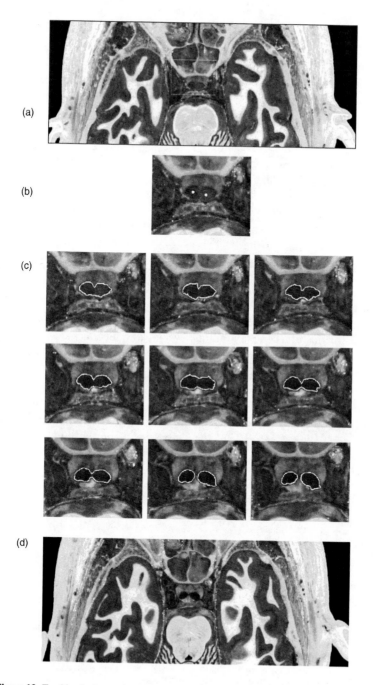

Figure 13. Tracking in the topology-changing case: (a) the first slice of serial CVH data; (b) initialization in the AOI; (c) boundaries in the subsequent image slices that are automatically tracked. See attached CD for color version.

two improvements are proposed to augment the speed function. The relaxation factor is first introduced. It provides a relaxing boundary condition, so as to stop the evolving curve at a blurred or unclear boundary. Second, the speed term is augmented by introducing visual content items. A simple and general model is proposed to incorporate image features into the speed item in order to improve the flexibility and performance of the speed function. Promising experimental results have demonstrated that incorporation of the distance measure and proper image features in the speed function can improve the segmentation result significantly.

As a further step, we present a unified approach for semiautomatic segmentation and tracking of the high-resolution color anatomical Chinese Visible Human (CVH) data. A two-step scheme is proposed, starting from segmenting the first image slice. The user need only to initialize on the first slice by clicking on the area of interest. The contours in subsequent image slices can then be automatically tracked. The advantage of this methods lies in two factors. The first is its ability to deal with non-rigid objects, using a simple model that does not require important prior knowledge. This makes it especially feasible in the context of general medical segmentation. Furthermore, the proposed two-step scheme for segmentation and tracking requires very little user intervention.

These advantages make it possible to employ this technique in future work on the reconstruction of a complex vascular system with topological changes.

7. ACKNOWLEDGMENTS

The work described in this chapter was supported by a grant from the Research Grants Council of the Hong Kong Special Administrative Region, China (Project No. CUHK4223/04E) and the CUHK Shun Hing Institute of Advanced Engineering.

8. REFERENCES

1. Bankman IN. 2000. *Handbook of medical imaging: processing and analysis.* New York: Academic Press.
2. Kass M, Witkin A, Terzopoulos D. 1987. Snakes: active contour models. In *Proceedings of the international conference on computer vision,* pp. 261–268. Washington, DC: IEEE Computer Society.
3. Kass M, Witkin A, Terzopoulos D. 1987. Snakes: active contour models. *Int J Comput Vision* 1:321–331.
4. Sethian J. 1999. *Level set methods and fast marching methods: evolving interfaces in computational geometry, fluid mechanics, computer vision, and materials science.* Cambridge: Cambridge UP.
5. Xu C, Pham DL, Prince JL. 2000. Medical image segmentation using deformable models. In *Handbook of medical imaging,* Vol. 2: *Medical image processing and analysis,* pp. 129–174. Ed M Sonka, JM Fitzpatrick. Bellingham, WA: SPIE Press.
6. Terzopoulos D. 1986. Regularization of inverse visual problems involving discontinuities. *IEEE Trans Pattern Anal Machine Intell* 8(4):413–424.

7. Grenander U, Chow Y, Keenan D. 1991. *A pattern theoretic study of biological shapes*. New York: Springer-Verlag.

8. Miller M, Christensen G, Amit Y, Grenander U. 1993. Mathematical textbook of deformable neuroanatomies. *Proc Natl Acad Sci USA* **24**:11944–11948.

9. Malladi R, Sethian J, Vemuri B. 1995. Shape modeling with front propagation: a level set approach. *IEEE Trans Pattern Anal Machine Intell* **17**:158–175.

10. Caselles V, Kimmel R, Sapiro G. 1997. Geodesic active contours. *Int J Comput Vision* **22**:61–79.

11. Kichenassamy S, Kumar A, Olver PJ, Tannenbaum A, Yezzi AJ. 1995. Gradient flows and geometric active contour models. In *Proceedings of the fifth international conference on computer vision (ICCV'95)*, pp. 810–815. Washington, DC: IEEE Computer Society.

12. Terzopoulos D, Metaxas D. 1991. Dynamic 3D models with local and global deformations: deformable superquadrics. *IEEE Trans Pattern Anal Machine Intell* **13**(7):703–714.

13. Staib L, Duncan J. 1992. Boundary finding with parametrically deformable models. *IEEE Trans Pattern Anal Machine Intell* **14**(11):1061–1075.

14. Terzopoulos D, Platt J, Barr A, Fleischer K. 1987. Elastically deformable models. *Comput Graphics* **21**(4):205–214.

15. Cohen LD. 1991. On active contour models and balloons. *Comput Vision Graphics Image Process: Image Understand* **53**(2):211–218.

16. Caselles V, Catte F, Coll T, Dibos F. 1993. A geometric model for active contours in image processing. *Num Math* **66**(1):1–31.

17. Xu C, Prince JL. 1998. Snakes, shapes, and gradient vector flow. *IEEE Trans Image Process* **7**(3):359–369.

18. Osher S, Sethian J. 1988. Fronts propagating with curvature-dependent speed: algorithms based on Hamilton-Jacobi formulations. *J Comput Phys* **79**(1):12–49.

19. Osher S, Fedkiw R. 2001. Level set methods: an overview and some recent results. *J Comput Phys* **169**:463–502.

20. Sethian J. 1996. *Level set methods*. Cambridge: Cambridge UP.

21. Lauziere Y, Siddiqi K, Tannenbaum A, Zucker S. 1998. Area and length minimizing flows for segmentation. *IEEE Trans Image Process* **7**:433–444.

22. Tek H, Kimia BB. 1995. Image segmentation by reaction-diffusion bubbles. In *Proceedings of the fifth international conference on computer vision (ICCV'95)*, pp. 156–162. Washington, DC: IEEE Computer Society.

23. Yezzi A, Kichenassamy S, Kumar A, Olver P, Tannenbaum A. 1997. A geometric snake model for segmentation of medical imagery. *IEEE Trans Med Imaging* **16**(2):199–209.

24. Tsai A, Yezzi AJ, Willsky AS. 2000. A curve evolution approach to smoothing and segmentation using the Mumford-Shah functional. In *Proceedings of the international conference on computer vision and pattern recognition (CVPR'2000)*, pp. 1119–1124. Washington, DC: IEEE Computer Society.

25. Geman D, Geman S, Gragne C, Dong P. 1990. Boundary detection by constrained optimization. *IEEE Trans Pattern Anal Machine Intell* **12**(7):609–628.

26. Hewer GA, Kenney C, Manjunathg BS. 1998. Variational image segmentation using boundary functions. *IEEE Trans Image Process* **7**(9):1269–1282.

27. Caselles V, Kimmel R, Sapiro G. 1995. Geodesic active contours. In *Proceedings of the fifth international conference on computer vision (ICCV'95)*, pp. 694–699. Washington, DC: IEEE Computer Society.

28. Paragios N, Deriche R. 2000. Geodesic active contours and level sets for the detection and tracking of moving objects. *IEEE Trans Pattern Anal Machine Intell* **22**:266–280.

29. Leventon M, Grimson E, Faugeras O. 2000. Statistical shape influence in geodesic active contours. In *Proceedings of the international conference on computer vision and pattern recognition*, Vol. 1, pp. 316–322. Washington, DC: IEEE Computer Society.

30. Chen Y, Thiruvenkadam H, Tagare H, Wilson D. 2002. Using prior shapes in geometric active contours in variational framework. *Int J Comput Vision* **50**:313–328.

31. Rousson M, Paragios N. 2002. Shape priors for level set representations. In *Proceedings of the European conference on computer vision*, Vol. 2, pp. 78–93. New York: Springer.

32. Paragios N. 2003. A level set approach for shape-driven segmentation and tracking of the left ventricle. *IEEE Trans Med Imaging* **22**(6):773–776.

33. Cootes T, Beeston C, Edwards G, Taylor C. 1999. A unified framework for atlas matching using active appearance models. In *Lecture notes in computer science*, Vol. 1613, pp. 311–333. New York: Springer.

34. Wang Y, Staib L. 1998. Elastic model based non-rigid registration incorporating statistical shape information. In *Proceedings of the conference on medical image computing and computer-assisted intervention*, Vol. 2, pp. 1162–1173. Washington, DC: IEEE Computer Society.

35. Chen Y, Thiruvenkadam S, Tagare H, Huang F, Wilson D, Geiser E. 2001. On the incorporation of shape priors into geometric active contours. In *IEEE workshop on variational and level set methods*, pp. 145–152. Washington, DC: IEEE Computer Society.

36. Rousson M, Paragios N. 2002. Shape priors for level set representations. In *Proceedings of the European conference on computer vision*, Vol. 2, pp. 78–92. New York: Springer.

37. Sethian J. 1985. Curvature and the evolution of fronts. *Commun Math Phys* **101**:487–499.

38. Malladi R, Sethian J, Vemuri B. 1993. A topology-independent shape modeling scheme. *Proc SPIE* **2031**:246–258.

39. Malladi R, Sethian J, Vemuri B. Evolutionary front for topology-independent shape modeling and recovery. In *Proceedings of the third European conference on computer vision*, Vol. 800, pp. 3–13. New York: Springer.

40. Dibos F, Caselles V, Coll T, Catte F. 1995. Automatic contours detection in image processing. In *Proceedings of the first world congress of nonlinear analysts*, pp. 1911–1921. Hawthorne, NJ: de Gruyter.

41. Malladi R, Sethian J, Hege H, Polthier K. 1997. Level set methods for curvature flow, image enhancement, and shape recovery in medical images. In *Proceedings of the first world congress of nonlinear analysts*, pp. 329–345. Hawthorne, NJ: de Gruyter.

42. Suri J, Liu K, Singh S, Laxminarayana S, Reden L. 2001. Shape recovery algorithms using level sets in 2-d/3-d medical imagery: a state-of-the-art review. *IEEE Trans Inform Technol Biomed* **6**(1):9–12.

43. Kichenassamy S, Kumar A, Olver P, Tannenbaum A, Yezzi A. 1996. Conformal curvature flows: from phase transitions to active vision. *Arch Rat Mech Anal* **134**(3):275–301.

44. Siddiqui K, Lauriere Y, Tannenbaum A, Zucker SW. 1998. Area and length minimizing flows for shape segmentation. *IEEE Trans Image Process* **7**(3):433–443.

45. Looney CG. 1997. *Pattern recognition using neural networks*. Oxford: Oxford UP.

46. Yezzi AJ, Tsai A, Willsky AS. 1999. Binary and ternary flows for image segmentation. In *Proceedings of the 1999 international conference on Image processing*, Vol. 2, pp. 1–5. Washington, DC: IEEE Computer Society.

47. Zhang S, Heng P, Liu Z, Tan L, Qiu M, Li Q, Liao R, Li K, Gy GC, Guo Y, Yang X, Liu G, Shan J, Liu J, Zhang W, Chen X, Chen J, Wang J, Chen W, Lu M, You J, Pang X, Xiao H, Xie Y, Cheng C. 2004. The Chinese visible human (CVH) datasets incorporate technical and imaging advances on earlier digital humans. *J Anat* **204**:165–173.

5

PARALLEL CO-VOLUME SUBJECTIVE SURFACE METHOD FOR 3D MEDICAL IMAGE SEGMENTATION

Karol Mikula

Department of Mathematics and Descriptive Geometry, Slovak University of Technology, Bratislava, Slovakia

Alessandro Sarti

Dipartmento di Elettronica, Informatica e Sistemistica, University of Bologna, Bologna, Italy

In this chapter we present a parallel computational method for 3D image segmentation. It is based on a three-dimensional semi-implicit complementary volume numerical scheme for solving the Riemannian mean curvature flow of graphs called the subjective surface method. The parallel method is introduced for massively parallel processor (MPP) architecture using the message passing interface (MPI) standard, so it is suitable, e.g., for clusters of Linux computers. The scheme is applied to segmentation of 3D echocardiographic images.

1. INTRODUCTION

The aim of segmentation is to find boundaries of an object in an image. In a generic situation these boundaries correspond to edges. In the presence of noise, which is intrinsically linked to modern noninvasive acquisition techniques (such as ultrasound), the object boundaries (image edges) can be very irregular or even interrupted. The same happens in images with occlusions, subjective contours (in

Address all correspondence to: Karol Mikula, Department of Mathematics and Descriptive Geometry, Slovak University of Technology, Radlinsk,ho 11, 813 68 Bratislava, Slovakia. Phone: 02 5292 5787; Fax: 02 5292 5787. mikula@vox.svf.stuba.sk some psychologically motivated examples), or in case of partly missing information (like in problems of inpainting). Then simple segmentation techniques fail and image analysis becomes a difficult task. In all these situations, the subjective surface method can help significantly. It is an evolutionary method based on numerical solution of time-dependent highly nonlinear partial differential equations (PDEs), solving a Riemannian mean curvature flow of a graph problem. The segmentation result is obtained as a "steady state" of this evolution. In case of a large dataset (3D images or image sequences), where the amount of processed information is huge, a discretization of the partial differential equation leads to systems of equations with a huge amount of unknowns. Then parallel implementation of the method is necessary, first, due to a large memory requirement, and second, due to a necessity for fast computing times. For both purposes, an implementation on the massively parallel processor (MPP) architecture using the message passing interface (MPI) standard is a favourable solution.

2. MATHEMATICAL MODELS IN IMAGE SEGMENTATION

Image segmentation based on the subjective surface method is related to geodesic (or conformal) mean curvature flow of level sets (level curves in case of 2D images and level surfaces in case of 3D images). Let us outline first the curve and surface evolution models and their level set formulations, preceding the subjective surface method.

A simple approach to image segmentation (similar to various discrete region-growing algorithms) is to place a small seed, e.g., a small circle in the 2D case, or a small ball in the 3D case, inside the object and then evolving this *segmentation curve* or *segmentation surface* to find automatically the object boundary (cf. [1]). Complex mathematical models as well as Lagrangean numerical schemes have been suggested and studied for evolving curves and surfaces over the last two decades (see, e.g., [2, 3, 4, 5, 6, 7, 8, 9, 10]). For moving curves and surfaces the robust level set models and methods were introduced (see, e.g., [11, 12, 13, 14, 15, 16, 17, 18]). A basic idea in the level set methods is that the moving curve or surface corresponds to the evolution of a particular level curve or level surface of the so-called level set function u that solves some form of the following general level set equation: $u_t = F|\nabla u|$, where F represents the normal component of the velocity of this motion.

The first segmentation level set model with the speed of the segmentation curve (surface) modulated by $F = g^0 \equiv g(|\nabla G_\sigma * I^0|)$, where G_σ is a smoothing kernel and g is a smooth edge detector function, e.g., $g(s) = 1/(1 + Ks^2)$, and was given in [19] and [20]. Due to the shape of the Perona-Malik function g, the moving curve is strongly slowed down in a neighbourhood of an edge, and a "steady state" of the segmentation curve is taken as the boundary of segmented object. However, if an edge is crossed during evolution (e.g., in a noisy image),

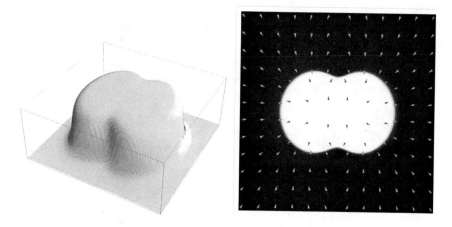

Figure 1. Left: A graph of the image intensity function $I^0(x)$. **Right**: Image given by the intensity $I^0(x)$ plotted together with arrows representing the vector field $-\nabla g(|\nabla I^0(x)|)$. See attached CD for color version.

there is no mechanism to reverse the motion since F is always positive. Moreover, if there is a missing part of the object boundary, such an algorithm, as with any other simple region-growing method, is completely useless.

Not only the segmentation models but also image smoothing (filtering) models and methods have been suggested either using the original Perona-Malik idea of nonlinear diffusion depending on an edge indicator (cf. [21, 22, 23, 24, 25, 26, 27, 28, 29, 30, 31, 32, 33, 34]) or using geometrical PDEs in the level set formulations (cf. [35, 36, 37, 38, 16, 39, 40, 41, 42]).

Later on, the level set models for image segmentation were significantly improved by introducing a driving force in the form $-\nabla g(|\nabla I^0(x)|)$ ([43, 44, 45, 46, 47]). The vector field $-\nabla g(|\nabla I^0(x)|)$ has an important geometric property: it points toward regions where the norm of the gradient ∇I^0 is large (see Figure 1, illustrating the 2D situation). If an initial segmentation curve or surface belongs to a neighborhood of an edge, it is driven automatically to this edge by the velocity field.

However, the situation is more complicated in the case of noisy images (see Figure 2). The advection is not sufficient, the evolving curve can be attracted to spurious edges, and no reasonably convergent process is observed. Adding a curvature dependence (regularization) to the normal velocity F, the sharp curve irregularities are smoothed, as presented in the right-hand part of Figure 2. It turns out that an appropriate regularization term is given by $g^0 k$, where the amount of curve intrinsic diffusion is small in the vicinity of an un-spurious edge. Following this 2D example, we can write the geometrical equation for the normal velocity v

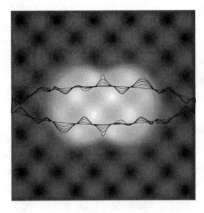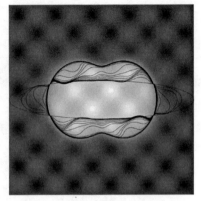

Figure 2. Evolution only by advection leads to attracting a curve (initial ellipse) to spurios edges, but adding a regularization term related to the curvature of evolving curve, the edge is found smoothly also in the case of a 2D noisy image (right).

as

$$v = g^0 k + \nabla g^0 \cdot \vec{N}$$

of the segmentation curve, where k is its curvature and $\vec{N}$ is its normal vector. Similarly, the geometrical equation for the moving segmentation surface has the form

$$v = g^0 H + \nabla g^0 \cdot \vec{N},$$

where H is its mean curvature and $\vec{N}$ is its normal vector. The level set formulation of either such curve or surface evolution is given by ([43, 44, 45, 46, 47])

$$u_t = g^0 |\nabla u| \nabla \cdot \left(\frac{\nabla u}{|\nabla u|} \right) + \nabla g^0 \cdot \nabla u = |\nabla u| \nabla \cdot \left(g^0 \frac{\nabla u}{|\nabla u|} \right), \qquad (1)$$

where the moving curve or surface is given by the same evolving level line and, respectively, level surface of the level set function u.

There is still a practical problem with the previous approach. It gives satisfactory results if the initial segmentation curve or surface belongs to the vicinity of an edge; otherwise, it is difficult to drive an arbitrary initial state there. An important observation, leading to the subjective surface method ([48, 49, 50]), is that Eq. (1) moves not only one particular level set, but all the level sets, by the above mentioned advection-diffusion mechanism. So we can consider the evolution of the whole (hyper)surface u, which we call the *segmentation function*, composed by those level sets. Moreover, we are a bit free in choosing the precise form of the diffusion term in the segmentation model. In fact,

$$u_t = \sqrt{\varepsilon^2 + |\nabla u|^2}\, \nabla \cdot \left(g(|\nabla G_\sigma * I^0|) \frac{\nabla u}{\sqrt{\varepsilon^2 + |\nabla u|^2}} \right), \tag{2}$$

where the Evans-Spruck regularization [51]

$$|\nabla u| \approx |\nabla u|_\varepsilon = \sqrt{\varepsilon^2 + |\nabla u|^2} \tag{3}$$

is used, gives the same advection term $-\nabla g^0 \cdot \nabla u$ as (1). The parameter ε shifts the model from the mean curvature motion of level sets ($\varepsilon = 0$) to the mean curvature flow of graphs ($\varepsilon = 1$). This means that either level sets of the segmentation function move in the normal direction proportionally to the (mean) curvature ($\varepsilon = 0$), or the graph of the segmentation function itself moves (as a 2D surface in 3D space in segmentation of 2D images, or a 3D hypersurface in 4D space in segmentation 3D images) in the normal direction proportionally to the mean curvature. In both cases large variations in the graph of the segmentation function outside edges are smoothed due to large mean curvature. On edges the advection dominates, so all the level sets that are close to the edge are attracted from both sides to this edge and a shock (steep gradient) is subsequently formed. For example, if the initial "point-of-view" surface, as plotted in the top right portion of Figure 3, illustrating the 2D situation, is evolved by Eq. (2), the so-called subjective surface is formed finally (see Figure 3, bottom right), and it is easy to use one of its level lines, e.g., $(\max(u) + \min(u))/2$, to get the boundary of the segmented object.

In the next example we illustrate the role of the regularization parameter ε. The choice of $\varepsilon = 1$ is not appropriate for segmentation of an image object with a gap, as seen in Figure 4 (top). However, decreasing ε, i.e., if we go closer to the level set flow Eq. (1), we get very good segmentation results for that image containing a circle with a large gap, as presented in Figure 4 (middle and bottom). If the image is noisy, the motion of the level sets to the shock is more irregular, but finally the segmentation function is smoothed and flattened as well. For a comprehensive overview of the role of all the model parameters, the reader is referred, e.g., to [52].

The subjective surface segmentation (2) is accompanied by Dirichlet boundary conditions:

$$u(t, x) = u^D \quad \text{in } [0, T] \times \partial\Omega, \tag{4}$$

where $\partial\Omega$ is a Lipschitz continuous boundary of a computational domain $\Omega \subset \mathbb{R}^d$, $d = 3$, and with initial condition

$$u(0, x) = u^0(x) \quad \text{in } \Omega. \tag{5}$$

We assume that the initial state of the segmentation function is bounded, i.e., $u^0 \in L_\infty(\Omega)$. The segmentation is an evolutionary process given by the solution

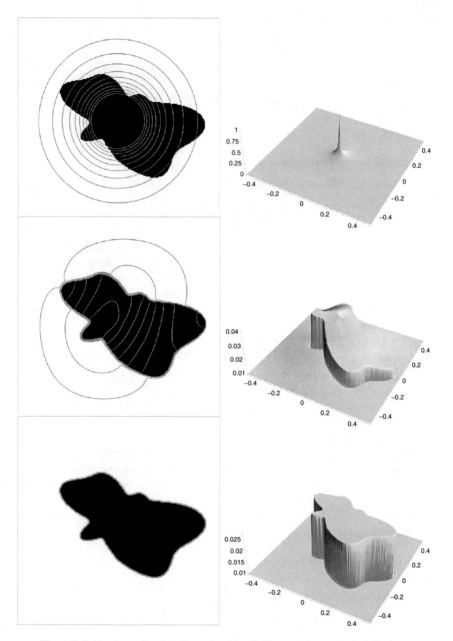

Figure 3. Subjective surface-based segmentation of a "batman" image. In the left column we plot the black-and-white image to be segmented together with isolines of the segmentation function. In the right column there is the shape of the segmentation function. The rows correspond to time steps 0, 1, and 10, which gives the final result. The regularization parameter $\varepsilon = 1$ is used in this example. See attached CD for color version.

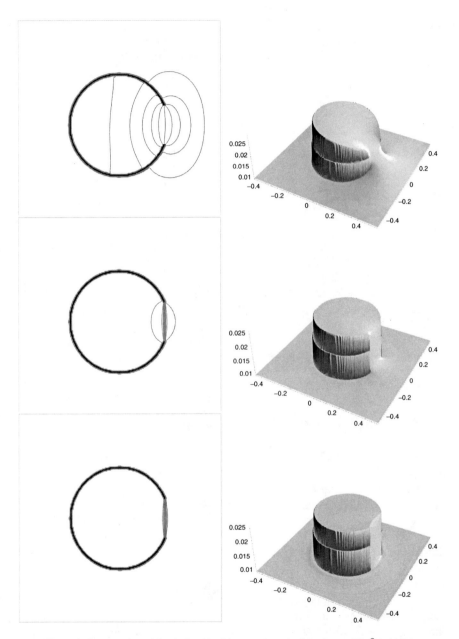

Figure 4. Segmentation of the circle with a big gap using $\varepsilon = 1$ (top), $\varepsilon = 10^{-2}$ (middle), and $\varepsilon = 10^{-5}$ (bottom). For a bigger missing part, a smaller ε is desirable. In the left column we see how closely to the edges the isolines are accumulating and closing the gap; on the right we see how steep the segmentation function is along the gap. See attached CD for color version.

of Eq. (2), where T represents a time when a segmentation result is achieved. The Perona-Malik function $g : \mathbb{R}_0^+ \rightarrow \mathbb{R}^+$ is nonincreasing, $g(0) = 1$, admitting $g(s) \rightarrow 0$ for $s \rightarrow \infty$ [21]. Usually we use the function $g(s) = 1/(1 + Ks^2)$, $K \geq 0$. $G_\sigma \in C^\infty(\mathbb{R}^d)$ is a smoothing kernel, e.g., the Gauss function

$$G_\sigma(x) = \frac{1}{(4\pi\sigma)^{d/2}} e^{-|x|^2/4\sigma}, \tag{6}$$

which is used in pre-smoothing of image gradients by the convolution

$$\nabla G_\sigma * I^0 = \int_{\mathbb{R}^d} \nabla G_\sigma(x - \xi) \tilde{I}^0(\xi) d\xi, \tag{7}$$

with $\tilde{I}^0$ the extension of I^0 to $\mathbb{R}^d$ given by periodic reflection through the boundary of the image domain. The computational domain Ω is usually a subdomain of the image domain, and it should include the segmented object. In fact, in most situations Ω corresponds to the image domain itself. Due to the properties of function g and the smoothing effect of convolution, we always have $1 \geq g^0 \geq \nu_\sigma > 0$ [22, 24]. In [51, 53], the existence of a viscosity solution [54] of the curvature driven level set equation [11], i.e., Eq. (1) with $g^0 \equiv 1$, was proven. For analytical results on Eqs. (1) and (2), respectively, we refer the reader to [47, 45] and [49, 55], respectively.

3. SEMI-IMPLICIT 3D CO-VOLUME SCHEME

Our computational method for solving the subjective surface segmentation equation (2) uses an efficient and unconditionally stable semi-implicit time discretization, first introduced for solving level set-like problems in [16], and a three-dimensional complementary volume spatial discretization introduced in [56] for image processing applications. In this section we present the serial algorithm of our method, and in the next section we introduce its parallel version suitable for a massively parallel computer architecture using the message passing interface standard.

For time discretization of nonlinear diffusion equations there are basically three possibilities: implicit, semi-implicit, or explicit schemes. For spatial discretization usually finite differences [13, 14], finite volumes [57, 58, 59, 26], or finite-element methods [60, 61, 62, 63, 64, 30, 24] are used. The co-volume technique (also called the complementary volume or finite volume-element method) is a combination of the finite-element and finite-volume methods. The discrete equations are derived using the *finite-volume methodology*, i.e., integrating an equation into the so-called control (complementary, finite) volume. Very often the control volumes are constructed as elements of a dual (complementary) grid to a *finite-element triangulation* (tetrahedral grid in the 3D case). Then the nonlinear quantities in PDEs, as an absolute value of the solution gradient in Eq. (2), are evaluated using piecewise linear representation of the solution on a tetrahedral grid thus employing the methodology of the linear finite-element method. The finite-volume methodology brings in the naturally discrete minimum–maximum principle. The piecewise linear representation (reconstruction) of the segmentation function on the finite-element grid yields a fast and simple evaluation of nonlinearities. Implicit, i.e., nonlinear time discretization and co-volume techniques, for solution of the level set equations were first introduced in [65]. The implicit time stepping as in [65], although unconditionally stable, leads to solution of a nonlinear system in every discrete time update. On the other hand, the semi-implicit scheme leads in every time step to solution of a linear algebraic system that is much more efficient. Using explicit time stepping, stability is often achieved only under severe time step restriction. Since in nonlinear diffusion problems (like the level set equations or the subjective surface method) the coefficients depend on the solution itself and thus must be recomputed in every discrete time update, an overall computational time for an explicit scheme can be tremendous. From such a point of view, the semi-implicit method seems to be optimal regarding stability and computational efficiency.

In the next subsections we discuss the semi-implicit 3D co-volume method. We present the method formally in discretization of Eq. (1), although we always use its ε-regularization (2) with a specific $\varepsilon > 0$. The notation is simpler in case of (1), and it will be clear where the ε-regularization appears in the numerical scheme.

3.1. Semi-Implicit Time Discretization

We first choose a uniform discrete time step τ and a variance σ of the smoothing kernel G_σ. We then replace the time derivative in (1) by backward difference. The nonlinear terms of the equation are treated from the previous time step while the linear ones are considered on the current time level, which means semi-implicitness of the time discretization. By such an approach we get our semi-discrete in a time scheme:

Let τ and σ be fixed numbers, I^0 be a given image, and u^0 a given initial segmentation function. Then, for every discrete time moment $t_n = n\tau$, $n = 1, \ldots N$, we look for a function u^n, the solution of the equation

$$\frac{1}{|\nabla u^{n-1}|} \frac{u^n - u^{n-1}}{\tau} = \nabla \cdot \left(g^0 \frac{\nabla u^n}{|\nabla u^{n-1}|} \right). \tag{8}$$

3.2. Co-Volume Spatial Discretization in 3D

A 3D digital image is given on a structure of voxels with a cubic shape, in general. Since discrete values of image intensity I^0 are given in voxels and they influence the model, we will relate spatially discrete approximations of the segmentation function u also to the voxel structure; more precisely, to voxel centers. In every discrete time step t_n of the method (8) we have to evaluate the gradient of the segmentation function at the previous step $|\nabla u^{n-1}|$. To that goal we put the 3D tetrahedral grid into the voxel structure and take a piecewise linear representation of the segmentation function on such a grid. Such an approach will give a constant value of the gradient in tetrahedra (which is the main feature of the co-volume [65, 16] and linear finite-element [62, 63, 64] methods in solving the mean curvature flow in the level set formulation), allowing simple, clear, and fast construction of a fully-discrete system of equations.

The formal construction of our co-volumes will be given in the next paragraph, and we will see that the co-volume mesh corresponds back to the image voxel structure, which is reasonable in image processing applications. On the other hand, the construction of the co-volume mesh has to use a 3D tetrahedral finite-element grid to which it is complementary. This will be possible using the following approach. First, every cubic voxel is split into 6 pyramids with a vertex given by the voxel center and base surfaces given by the voxel boundary faces. The neighbouring pyramids of the neighbouring voxels are joined together to form an octahedron that is then split into 4 tetrahedra using diagonals of the voxel boundary face (see Figure 5). In such way we get our *3D tetrahedral grid*. Two nodes of every tetrahedron correspond to the centers of neighbouring voxels, and the further two nodes correspond to the voxel boundary vertices; every tetrahedron intersects a common face of neighbouring voxels. In our method, only the centers of the voxels will represent degree-of-freedom nodes (DF nodes), i.e., solving the equation at a new time step, we update the segmentation function only in these DF nodes. Additional nodes of the tetrahedra will not represent degrees of freedom, and we will call them non-degree-of-freedom nodes (NDF nodes), and they will be used in piecewise linear representation of the segmentation function. Let a function u be given by discrete values in the voxel centers, i.e., in DF nodes. Then in the NDF nodes we take the average value of the neighbouring DF nodal values. By such defined values in the NDF nodes a piecewise linear approximation u_h of u on the tetrahedral grid is built.

For the tetrahedral grid $\mathcal{T}_h$, given by the previous construction, we construct a co-volume (dual) mesh. We modify the approach given in [65, 16] in such a way that our co-volume mesh will consist of cells p associated only with DF nodes p of $\mathcal{T}_h$, say $p = 1, \ldots, M$. Since there will be one-to-one correspondence between co-volumes and DF nodes, without any confusion, we use the same notation for them. For each DF node p of $\mathcal{T}_h$, let C_p denote the set of all DF nodes q connected to the node p by an edge. This edge will be denoted by σ_{pq} and its length by h_{pq}. Then

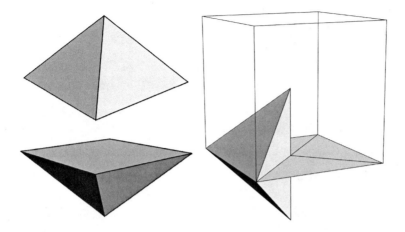

Figure 5. Neighbouring pyramids (left) that are joined together and which, after splitting into four parts, give tetrahedra of our 3D grid. We can the see intersection of one of these tetrahedra with the bottom face of the voxel co-volume (right). See attached CD for color version.

every *co-volume* p is bounded by the planes e_{pq} that bisect and are perpendicular to the edges $\sigma_{pq}, q \in C_p$. By this construction, if e_{pq} intersects σ_{pq} in its center, the co-volume mesh corresponds exactly to the voxel structure of the image inside the computational domain Ω where the segmentation is provided. Then the co-volume boundary faces do cross in NDF nodes. So we can also say that the NDF nodes correspond to zero-measure co-volumes and thus do not add additional equations to the discrete model (cf. (10)), and they do not represent degrees of freedom in the co-volume method. We denote by $\mathcal{E}_{pq}$ the set of tetrahedra having σ_{pq} as an edge. In our situation (see Figure 4), every $\mathcal{E}_{pq}$ consists of 4 tetrahedra. For each $T \in \mathcal{E}_{pq}$, let c_{pq}^T be the area of the portion of e_{pq} that is in T, i.e., $c_{pq}^T = m(e_{pq} \cap T)$, where m is a measure in $I\!\!R^{d-1}$. Let $\mathcal{N}_p$ be the set of all tetrahedra that have a DF node p as a vertex. Let u_h be a piecewise linear function on $\mathcal{T}_h$. We will denote a constant value of $|\nabla u_h|$ on $T \in \mathcal{T}_h$ by $|\nabla u_T|$ and define regularized gradients by

$$|\nabla u_T|_\varepsilon = \sqrt{\varepsilon^2 + |\nabla u_T|^2}. \qquad (9)$$

We will use the notation $u_p = u_h(x_p)$, where x_p is the coordinate of the DF node p of $\mathcal{T}_h$.

With these notations, we are ready to derive co-volume spatial discretization. As is usual in finite-volume methods [59, 58, 57], we integrate ((8)) over every co-volume $p, 1 = 1, \ldots, M$. We get

$$\int_p \frac{1}{|\nabla u^{n-1}|} \frac{u^n - u^{n-1}}{\tau} dx = \int_p \nabla \cdot \left(g^0 \frac{\nabla u^n}{|\nabla u^{n-1}|} \right) dx. \qquad (10)$$

For the right-hand side of (10) using the divergence theorem we get

$$
\int_p \nabla \cdot \left(g^0 \frac{\nabla u^n}{|\nabla u^{n-1}|} \right) dx \;=\; \int_{\partial p} \frac{g^0}{|\nabla u^{n-1}|} \frac{\partial u^n}{\partial \nu} ds
$$

$$
=\; \sum_{q \in C_p} \int_{e_{pq}} \frac{g^0}{|\nabla u^{n-1}|} \frac{\partial u^n}{\partial \nu} ds.
$$

So we have an integral formulation of (8):

$$
\int_p \frac{1}{|\nabla u^{n-1}|} \frac{u^n - u^{n-1}}{\tau} dx = \sum_{q \in C_p} \int_{e_{pq}} \frac{g^0}{|\nabla u^{n-1}|} \frac{\partial u^n}{\partial \nu} ds, \tag{11}
$$

expressing a "local mass balance" in the scheme. Now the exact "fluxes" $\int_{e_{pq}}$ $\frac{g^0}{|\nabla u^{n-1}|} \frac{\partial u^n}{\partial \nu} ds$ on the right-hand side and the "capacity function" $\frac{1}{|\nabla u^{n-1}|}$ on the left-hand side (see, e.g., [59]) will be approximated numerically using piecewise linear reconstruction of u^{n-1} on the tetrahedral grid $\mathcal{T}_h$. If we denote by g_T^0 the approximation of g^0 on a tetrahedron $T \in \mathcal{T}_h$, then for the approximation of the right-hand side of (11) we get

$$
\sum_{q \in C_p} \left(\sum_{T \in \mathcal{E}_{pq}} c_{pq}^T \frac{g_T^0}{|\nabla u_T^{n-1}|} \right) \frac{u_q^n - u_p^n}{h_{pq}}, \tag{12}
$$

and the left-hand side of (11) is approximated by

$$
M_p m(p) \frac{u_p^n - u_p^{n-1}}{\tau}, \tag{13}
$$

where $m(p)$ is a measure in $\mathbb{R}^d$ of co-volume p and M_p is an approximation of the capacity function inside the finite volume p. For that goal we use the averaging of the gradients in tetraherda crossing co-volume p, i.e.,

$$
M_p = \frac{1}{|\nabla u_p^{n-1}|}, \quad |\nabla u_p^{n-1}| = \sum_{T \in \mathcal{N}_p} \frac{m(T \cap p)}{m(p)} |\nabla u_T^{n-1}|. \tag{14}
$$

Then the regularization of the capacity function is given by

$$
M_p^\varepsilon = \frac{1}{|\nabla u_p^{n-1}|_\varepsilon}, \tag{15}
$$

and if we define coefficients (where the ε-regularization is taken into account),

$$
d_p^{n-1} = M_p^\varepsilon m(p), \tag{16}
$$

$$
a_{pq}^{n-1} = \frac{1}{h_{pq}} \sum_{T \in \mathcal{E}_{pq}} c_{pq}^T \frac{g_T^0}{|\nabla u_T^{n-1}|_\varepsilon}, \tag{17}
$$

we get from (12)–(13) our **3D fully-discrete semi-implicit co-volume scheme**:

Let u_p^0, $p = 1, \ldots, M$ be given discrete initial values of the segmentation function. Then, for $n = 1, \ldots, N$ we look for $u_p^n, p = 1, \ldots, M$, satisfying

$$d_p^{n-1} u_p^n + \tau \sum_{q \in C_p} a_{pq}^{n-1} (u_p^n - u_q^n) = d_p^{n-1} u_p^{n-1}. \tag{18}$$

The system (18) can be rewritten into the form

$$\left(d_p^{n-1} + \tau \sum_{q \in C_p} a_{pq}^{n-1} \right) u_p^n - \tau \sum_{q \in C_p} a_{pq}^{n-1} u_q^n = d_p^{n-1} u_p^{n-1}, \tag{19}$$

and, applying the Dirichlet boundary conditions (which contribute to the right-hand side), it gives a system of linear equations with a matrix $\mathbf{A}_{M \times M}$, the off-diagonal elements of which are symmetric and nonpositive, namely $\mathbf{A}_{pq} = -\tau a_{pq}^{n-1}$, $q \in C_p$, $\mathbf{A}_{pq} = 0$, otherwise. Diagonal elements are positive, namely, $\mathbf{A}_{pp} = d_p^{n-1} + \tau \sum_{q \in C_p} a_{pq}^{n-1}$, and dominate the sum of the absolute values of the nondiagonal elements in every row. Thus, the matrix of the system is symmetric and a diagonally dominant M-matrix, which implies that it always has a unique solution for any $\tau > 0$, $\varepsilon > 0$, and for every $n = 1, \ldots, N$. The M-matrix property gives us the minimum–maximum principle:

$$\min_p u_p^0 \leq \min_p u_p^n \leq \max_p u_p^n \leq \max_p u_p^0, \ 1 \leq n \leq N, \tag{20}$$

which can be seen by the following simple trick. We may temporary rewrite (18) into the equivalent form:

$$u_p^n + \frac{\tau}{d_p^{n-1}} \sum_{q \in C_p} a_{pq}^{n-1} (u_p^n - u_q^n) = u_p^{n-1}, \tag{21}$$

and let $\max(u_1^n, \ldots, u_M^n)$ be achieved in the node p. Then the whole second term on the left-hand side is nonnegative, and thus $\max(u_1^n, \ldots, u_M^n) = u_p^n \leq u_p^{n-1} \leq \max(u_1^{n-1}, \ldots, u_M^{n-1})$. In the same way, we can prove the relation for the minimum, and together we have

$$\min_p u_p^{n-1} \leq \min_p u_p^n \leq \max_p u_p^n \leq \max_p u_p^{n-1}, \ 1 \leq n \leq N, \tag{22}$$

which by recursion implies the L_∞ stability estimate (20).

The evaluation of g_T^0 included in coefficients (17) can be done in several ways. First, we may replace the convolution by the weighted average to get $I_\sigma^0 := G_\sigma * I^0$ (see, e.g., [26]), and then relate discrete values of I_σ^0 to voxel centers. Then, as above, we may construct its piecewise linear representation on the grid and get a constant value of $g_T^0 \equiv g(|\nabla I_\sigma^0|)$ on every tetrahedron $T \in \mathcal{T}_h$. Another possibility is to solve numerically the linear heat equation for time t corresponding to variance σ with the initial datum given by I^0 (see, e.g., [30]) by the same method as above. The convolution represents a preliminary smoothing of the data. It is also a theoretical tool to have bounded gradients and thus a strictly positive weighting coefficient g^0. In practice, the evaluation of gradients on a fixed discrete grid (e.g., described above) always gives bounded values. So, working on a fixed grid, one can also avoid the convolution, especially if preliminary denoising is not needed or not desirable. Then it is possible to work directly with gradients of the piecewise linear representation of I^0 in evaluation of g_T^0.

A change in the L_2 norm of numerical solutions in subsequent time steps is used to stop the segmentation process. We check whether

$$\sqrt{\sum_p m(p)\,(u_p^n - u_p^{n-1})^2} < \delta, \tag{23}$$

with a prescribed threshold δ. For our semi-implicit scheme and small ε, a good choice of threshold is $\delta = 10^{-5}$.

We start all computations with an initial function given as a peak centered in a "focus point" inside the segmented object. Such a function can be described at a sphere with center s and radius R by $u^0(x) = \frac{1}{|x-s|+v}$, where s is the focus point and $\frac{1}{v}$ gives a maximum of u^0. Outside the sphere we take the value u^0 equal to $\frac{1}{R+v}$. R usually corresponds to the halved inner diameter of the image domain. For small objects, a smaller R can be used to speed up computations. Usually we put the focus point s inside a small neighborhood of a center of the mass of the segmented object.

3.3. Semi-Implicit 3D Co-Volume Scheme in Finite-Difference Notation

The presented co-volume scheme is designed for the specific mesh given by the cubic voxel structure of a 3D image. For simplicity of implementation, reader convenience, and due to the relation to the next section devoted to parallelization, we will write the co-volume scheme (18) in a "finite-difference notation." As is usual for 3D rectangular grids, we associate co-volume p and its center (DF node) with a triple (i, j, k), i representing the index in the x-direction, j in the y-direction, and k in the z-direction (see Figure 7 for our convention of coordinate notation). The unknown value u_p^n then can be denoted by $u_{i,j,k}^n$. If Ω is a rectangular subdomain of the image domain (usually Ω is the image domain itself) and $N_1 + 1$, $N_2 + 1$, $N_3 + 1$ are the numbers of voxels of Ω in the x, y, z-directions, and if we consider Dirichlet boundary conditions (i.e., the values u_p^n in boundary voxels are not considered as unknown), then $i = i_l, \ldots, i_r$, $j = j_l, \ldots, j_r$, $k = k_l, \ldots, k_r$, where $i_r - i_l \leq N_1 - 2$, $j_r - j_l \leq N_2 - 2$, $k_r - k_l \leq N_3 - 2$. We define the space discretization step $h = \frac{1}{N_1}$, and for simplicity we assume that voxels have cubic shape. For every co-volume p, the set $C_p = \{w, e, s, n, b, t\}$ consists of 6 neighbours, west $u_{i-1,j,k}$, east $u_{i+1,j,k}$, south $u_{i,j-1,k}$, north $u_{i,j+1,k}$, bottom $u_{i,j,k-1}$, and top $u_{i,j,k+1}$, and the set $\mathcal{N}_p$ consists of 24 tetrahedra.

In every discrete time step $n = 1, \ldots, N$ and for every i, j, k, we compute the absolute value of gradient $|\nabla u_T^{n-1}|$ on these 24 tetrahedra. We denote by $G_{i,j,k}^{z,l}, l = 1, \ldots, 4, z \in C_p$ the square of the gradient on the tetrahedra crossing the west, east, south, north, bottom, and top co-volume faces. If we define (omitting upper index $n - 1$)

$$s_{i,j,k} = (u_{i,j,k} + u_{i-1,j,k} + u_{i,j-1,k} + u_{i-1,j-1,k} +$$
$$+ \ u_{i,j,k-1} + u_{i-1,j,k-1} + u_{i,j-1,k-1} + u_{i-1,j-1,k-1})/8,$$

the value at the left-south-bottom NDF node of the co-volume, then for the west face we get

$$G_{i,j,k}^{w,1} = \left(\frac{u_{i,j,k} - u_{i-1,j,k}}{h}\right)^2 + \left(\frac{s_{i,j,k+1} - s_{i,j,k}}{h}\right)^2 +$$
$$\left(\frac{u_{i,j,k} + u_{i-1,j,k} - s_{i,j,k+1} - s_{i,j,k}}{h}\right)^2,$$

$$G_{i,j,k}^{w,2} = \left(\frac{u_{i,j,k} - u_{i-1,j,k}}{h}\right)^2 + \left(\frac{s_{i,j+1,k+1} - s_{i,j,k+1}}{h}\right)^2 +$$
$$\left(\frac{s_{i,j+1,k+1} + s_{i,j,k+1} - u_{i,j,k} - u_{i-1,j,k}}{h}\right)^2, \tag{24}$$

$$G_{i,j,k}^{w,3} = \left(\frac{u_{i,j,k} - u_{i-1,j,k}}{h}\right)^2 + \left(\frac{s_{i,j+1,k+1} - s_{i,j+1,k}}{h}\right)^2 +$$
$$\left(\frac{s_{i,j+1,k+1} + s_{i,j+1,k} - u_{i,j,k} - u_{i-1,j,k}}{h}\right)^2,$$

$$G_{i,j,k}^{w,4} = \left(\frac{u_{i,j,k} - u_{i-1,j,k}}{h}\right)^2 + \left(\frac{s_{i,j+1,k} - s_{i,j,k}}{h}\right)^2 +$$
$$\left(\frac{u_{i,j,k} + u_{i-1,j,k} - s_{i,j+1,k} - s_{i,j,k}}{h}\right)^2,$$

and correspondingly we get all $G_{i,j,k}^{z,l}$ for the further co-volume faces.

In the same way, but only once at the beginning of the algorithm, we compute values $G_{i,j,k}^{\sigma,z,l}, l = 1, \ldots, 4, z \in C_p$, changing u by I_σ^0 in the previous expressions, and we apply function g to all these values to get discrete values of g_T^0.

Then in every discrete time step and for every i, j, k we construct (west, east, south, north, bottom and top) coefficients

$$a_{i,j,k}^{w} = \tau \frac{1}{4} \sum_{l=1}^{4} \frac{g(\sqrt{G_{i,j,k}^{\sigma,w,l}})}{\sqrt{\varepsilon^2 + G_{i,j,k}^{w,l}}}, \quad a_{i,j,k}^{e} = \tau \frac{1}{4} \sum_{l=1}^{4} \frac{g(\sqrt{G_{i,j,k}^{\sigma,e,l}})}{\sqrt{\varepsilon^2 + G_{i,j,k}^{e,l}}},$$

$$a_{i,j,k}^{s} = \tau \frac{1}{4} \sum_{l=1}^{4} \frac{g(\sqrt{G_{i,j,k}^{\sigma,s,l}})}{\sqrt{\varepsilon^2 + G_{i,j,k}^{s,l}}}, \quad a_{i,j,k}^{n} = \tau \frac{1}{4} \sum_{l=1}^{4} \frac{g(\sqrt{G_{i,j,k}^{\sigma,n,l}})}{\sqrt{\varepsilon^2 + G_{i,j,k}^{n,l}}}, \quad (25)$$

$$a_{i,j,k}^{b} = \tau \frac{1}{4} \sum_{l=1}^{4} \frac{g(\sqrt{G_{i,j,k}^{\sigma,b,l}})}{\sqrt{\varepsilon^2 + G_{i,j,k}^{b,l}}}, \quad a_{i,j,k}^{t} = \tau \frac{1}{4} \sum_{l=1}^{4} \frac{g(\sqrt{G_{i,j,k}^{\sigma,t,l}})}{\sqrt{\varepsilon^2 + G_{i,j,k}^{t,l}}},$$

and we use, cf. (14),

$$m_{i,j,k} = \frac{1}{\sqrt{\varepsilon^2 + \left(\frac{1}{24} \sum_{z \in C_p} \sum_{l=1}^{4} \sqrt{G_{i,j,k}^{z,l}}\right)^2}}$$

to define diagonal coefficients

$$a_{i,j,k}^{p} = a_{i,j,k}^{w} + a_{i,j,k}^{e} + a_{i,j,k}^{s} + a_{i,j,k}^{n} + a_{i,j,k}^{b} + a_{i,j,k}^{t} + m_{i,j,k} h^2.$$

If we define the right-hand sides at the nth discrete time step by

$$b_{i,j,k} = m_{i,j,k} h^2 u_{i,j,k}^{n-1},$$

then for the DF node corresponding to triple (i, j, k) we get the equation

$$a_{i,j,k}^{p} u_{i,j,k}^{n} - a_{i,j,k}^{w} u_{i-1,j,k}^{n} - a_{i,j,k}^{e} u_{i+1,j,k}^{n} - a_{i,j,k}^{s} u_{i,j-1,k}^{n} - \qquad (26)$$
$$a_{i,j,k}^{n} u_{i,j+1,k}^{n} - a_{i,j,k}^{b} u_{i,j,k-1}^{n} - a_{i,j,k}^{t} u_{i,j,k+1}^{n} = b_{i,j,k}.$$

Collecting these equations for all DF nodes and taking into account Dirichlet boundary conditions we get the linear system to be solved.

3.4. Solution of Linear Systems

We can solve system (26) by any efficient preconditioned linear iterative solver suitable for sparse, symmetric, diagonally dominant M-matrices [66]. For example, the so-called SOR (Successive Over Relaxation) method can be used. Then, at the nth discrete time step we start the iterations by setting $u_{i,j,k}^{n(0)} = u_{i,j,k}^{n-1}$, $i = i_l, \ldots, i_r$, $j = j_l, \ldots, j_r$, $k = k_l, \ldots, k_r$, and in every iteration $l = 1, \ldots$ and for every $i = i_l, \ldots, i_r$, $j = j_l, \ldots, j_r$, $k = k_l, \ldots, k_r$ the following two-step procedure is used:

$$
Y = (a_{i,j,k}^{w} u_{i-1,j,k}^{n(l)} + a_{i,j,k}^{e} u_{i+1,j,k}^{n(l-1)} + a_{i,j,k}^{s} u_{i,j-1,k}^{n(l)} +
$$
$$
a_{i,j,k}^{n} u_{i,j+1,k}^{n(l-1)} + a_{i,j,k}^{b} u_{i,j,k-1}^{n(l)} + a_{i,j,k}^{t} u_{i,j,k+1}^{n(l-1)} + b_{i,j,k})/a_{i,j,k}^{p} \quad (27)
$$

$$
u_{i,j,k}^{n(l)} = u_{i,j,k}^{n(l-1)} + \omega(Y - u_{i,j,k}^{n(l-1)}).
$$

We define the squared L_2-norm of the residuum after the lth SOR iteration by

$$
R^{(l)} = \sum_{i,j,k} (a_{i,j,k}^{p} u_{i,j,k}^{n(l)} - a_{i,j,k}^{w} u_{i-1,j,k}^{n(l)} - a_{i,j,k}^{e} u_{i+1,j,k}^{n(l)} -
$$
$$
a_{i,j,k}^{s} u_{i,j-1,k}^{n(l)} - a_{i,j,k}^{n} u_{i,j+1,k}^{n(l)} a_{i,j,k}^{b} u_{i,j,k-1}^{n(l)} - a_{i,j,k}^{t} u_{i,j,k+1}^{n(l)} - b_{i,j,k})^2.
$$

The iterative process is stopped if $R^{(l)} < \text{TOL } R^{(0)}$. The relaxation parameter ω is chosen by the user to improve the convergence rate of the method.

4. BUILDING UP THE PARALLEL ALGORITHM

4.1. MPI Programming

A parallel computer architecture (cf. [67]) is usually categorized by two aspects: whether the memory is physically centralized or distributed, and whether or not the address space is shared. On one hand there is so-called SMP (symmetric multi-processor) architecture that uses shared system resources, e.g., memory and an input/output subsystem, equally accessible from all processors. On the other hand, there is the MPP (massively parallel processors) architecture, where the so-called nodes are connected by a high-speed network. Each node has its own processor, memory, and input/output subsystem, and the operating system is running on each node. Massively does not necessarily mean a large number of nodes, so one can consider, e.g., a cluster of Linux system computers of a reasonable size (and price) to solve a particular scientific or engineering problem. But, of course, parallel computers with a huge number (hundreds) of nodes are used at large computer centers.

The main goal of parallel programming is to utilize all available processors and minimize the elapsed time of the program. In SMP architecture one can assign the parallelization job to a compiler, which usually parallelizes some DO loops (for image processing applications based on such an approach we refer the reader to, e.g., [68]). This is a simple approach but is restricted to having such memory resources with a shared address space at one's disposal. In MPP architecture, where the address space is not shared among the nodes, parallel processes must transmit data over a network to access data that other processes update. To that goal, message-passing is employed.

In parallel execution, several programs can cooperate in providing computations and handling data. But our parallel implementation of the co-volume subjective surface algorithm uses so-called the SPMD (single program multiple data) model. In the SPMD model, there is only one program built, and each parallel process uses the same executable working on different sets of data. Since all the processes execute the same program, it is necessary to distinguish between them. To that goal, each process has its own *rank*, and we can let processes behave differently, although executing one program, using the value of *rank*. In our case, we split the huge amount of voxels into several parts, proportional to the number of processors, and then we have to rewrite the serial program in such a way that each parallel process handles the correct part of the data and transmits the necessary information to other processes.

Parallelization should reduce the time spent on computation. If there are p processes involved in parallel execution, ideally, the parallel program could be executed p times faster than a sequential one. However, this is not true in practice because of the necessity for data transmission due to data splitting. This drawback of parallelization can be overcome in an efficient and reliable way by so-called message-passing, which is used to consolidate what has been separated by parallelization.

The Message Passing Interface (MPI) is a standard specifying a portable interface for writing parallel programs that have to utilize the message-passing. It aims at practicality, efficiency, and flexibility at the same time. The MPI subroutines solve the problems of environment management, point-to-point and collective communication among processes, construction of derived data types, input/output operations, etc.

The environment managment subroutines, MPI_Init and MPI_Finalize, initiate and finalize an MPI environment. Using subroutine MPI_Comm_size, one can get a number of processes involved in parallel execution belonging to a *communicator*– identifier associated with a group of processes participating in the parallel job, e.g., MPI_COMM_WORLD. Subroutine MPI_Comm_rank gives a *rank* to a process belonging to communicator. The MPI parallel program should include the file mpi.h, which defines all MPI-related parameters (cf. Figure 6).

Collective communication subroutines allow one to exchange data among a group of processes specified by the communicator, e.g., MPI_Bcast sends data from a specific process called the *root* to all the other processes in the communicator. Or, subroutine MPI_Allreduce does reduction operations such as summation of data distributed over all processes in the communicator and places the result on all of the processes.

```
#include <mpi.h>
int main(int argc, char *arvg[])
{
 MPI_Init(&argc, &argv);
 MPI_Comm_size(MPI_COMM_WORLD, &nprocs);
 MPI_Comm_rank(MPI_COMM_WORLD, &myid);
  .
  .
  .
 MPI_Finalize():
}
```

Figure 6. Typical structure of an MPI parallel program.

Using point-to-point communication subroutines, a message is sent by one process and received by another. We distinguish between unidirectional and bidirectional communications. At the sending process, the data are first collected into the *user sendbuffer* (scalar variables or arrays used in the program), and then one of the MPI send subroutines is called, the system copies the data from the user sendbuffer to *system buffer*, and finally the system sends the data from the system buffer to the destination process. During the receiving process, one of the MPI receive subroutines is called, the system receives the data from the source process, and copies it to the *system buffer*, and then the system copies the data from the system buffer to the *user recvbuffer*, and finally the data can be used by the receiving process. In MPI, there are two modes of communication: blocking and non-blocking. Using blocking communication subroutines, the program will not return from the subroutine call until the copy to/from the system buffer has finished. Using non-blocking communication subroutines such as MPI_Isend and MPI_Irecv, the program immediately returns from the subroutine call. This indicates that the copy to/from the system buffer is only initiated, so one has to assure that it is also completed by using the MPI_Wait subroutine. In other cases, incorrect data could be copied to the system buffer. In spite of the higher complexity of non-blocking subroutines, we generally prefer them, because their usage is more safe from *deadlock* in bidirectional communication. Deadlocks can take place either due to the incorrect order of blocking send and receive subroutines or due to the limited size of the system buffer, and when a deadlock occurs, the involved processes will not proceed any further.

In the next subsection we show how the message-passing subroutines mentioned above are employed to parallelize the 3D semi-implicit co-volume subjective surface segmentation method.

4.2. Parallelization of the Co-Volume Algorithm Using MPI

There are two main goals for parallelization of a program: to handle huge amounts of data that cannot be placed into the memory of one single serial computer, and to run the program faster. Let us suppose that in terms of running time, a fraction p of a program can be parallelized. In an ideal situation, executing the parallelized program on n processors, the running time will be $1 - p + \frac{p}{n}$. We can see that, if, e.g., only 80% of the program can be parallelized, i.e., $p = 0.8$, the maximal speed-up (estimated from above by $\frac{1}{1-p}$) cannot exceed 5, although with infinitely many processors. This illustrative example shows that it is very important to identify the fraction of the program that can be parallelized and maximize it. Fortunately, every time-consuming part of our algorithm can be efficiently parallelized either directly (reading and writing data, computing coefficients of the linear system), or it is possible to change the serial linear solver (SOR method) to the parallel solver (e.g., RED-BLACK SOR method), which can be parallelized efficiently. The next important issue in parallelization is to balance the workload of the parallel processes. This problem can be addressed by as uniform as possible splitting of the data so that every process provides approximately the same number of operations. The final and very important step is to minimize the time spent for communication. This leads, e.g., to a requirement that the data transmitted (e.g., multidimensional arrays) be contiguous in memory, so that one can exchange it among processors directly in one message using only one call of MPI send and receive subroutines. For parallel algorithms implemented in C language this means that multidimensional arrays should be distributed in row-wise blocks, or, better, say we have to split the multidimensional array like $u[i][j][k]$ in the first index i (cf. Figure 7).

In Figure 8 we can see the main structure of our parallel program. First, the MPI environment is initiated, and every process involved in parallel execution gets its rank stored in variable $\text{myid} = 0, \ldots, n_{\text{procs}} - 1$, where 0 represents the root process and n_{procs} is the number of parallel processes. Then by the root process we read the time step τ and the upper estimate of the number of time steps nts. These parameters are sent to all processes by the MPI_Bcast subroutine. In the beginning of the algorithm we also read the image, compute the discrete values of g_T^0 in function Coefficients0, and construct the initial segmentation function. All these procedures work independently on their own (overlapping) subsets of data, and no exchange of information between processes is necessary in this part of the program. Then in the cycle we call procedure EllipticStep, which in every time step contains computing of coefficients (25) and solving the linear system (26). In the iterative solution of the linear system we will need to exchange overlapping data between neighbouring processes. The cycle is finished when condition ((23)) is fulfilled, and finally the MPI environment is finalized.

Figure 9 shows our distribution of data among the processes. Both the 3D image and the discrete values of the segmentation function are represented by a

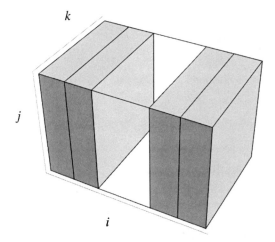

Figure 7. Splitting of a 3D image to n_{procs} 3D rectangular subareas, where n_{procs} corresponds to the number of processes involved in parallel execution. See attached CD for color version.

```
#include <mpi.h>

int main(int argc, char &argv[])
{
 MPI_Init(&argc, &argv);
 MPI_Comm_rank(MPI_COMM_WORLD, &myid);
 if (myid==0)
    {
    printf("tau, number of time steps:\n");
    scanf("%if %d",&tau,&nts);
    }
 MPI_Bcast(&tau, 1, MPI_DOUBLE,0,MPI_COMM_WORLD);
 MPI_Bcast(&nts, 1, MPI_INT,0,MPI_COMM_WORLD);
 ReadingImage();
 Coefficients0();
 InitialSegmentationFunction();
 for (k=1;k<=nts;k++)
    {
     change=EllipticStep();
     if (change < delta)
        {
         WritingSegmentationResult();
         break;
        }
    }
 MPI_Finalize();
 }
```

Figure 8. Main structure of our MPI parallel program for the 3D semi-implicit co-volume subjective surface segmentation method.

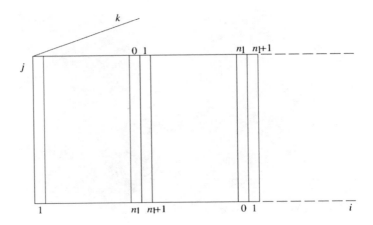

Figure 9. Data distribution and its overlap over parallel processes.

three-dimensional array indexed by i, j, k. The 3D image is given in index ranges $i = 1, \ldots, N_1 + 1, j = 1, \ldots, N_2 + 1, k = 1, \ldots, N_1 + 3$. Let us suppose that our computational domain, i.e., the domain where we update the segmentation function, is equal to the image domain. Then the boundary positions with $i = 1$, $i = N_1 + 1, j = 1, j = N_2 + 1, k = 1, k = N_3 + 1$ are reserved for Dirichlet boundary conditions and all the inner voxel positions correspond to DF nodes of the 3D co-volume algorithm. In order to distribute the data (3D image as well as the segmentation function), we define $n_1 = \frac{N_1}{n_{\text{procs}}} + 1, n_1^{\text{last}} = N_1 - (n_{\text{procs}} - 1)n_1$, and we set $n_2 = N_2, n_3 = N_3$. Then on the root process with rank 0 we store the first part of the 3D image as well as the first part of the discrete segmentation function, namely, the array with indices $i = 1, \ldots, n_1 + 1, j = 1, \ldots, n_2 + 1$, $k = 1, \ldots, n_3 + 1$ (cf. Figure 9). The next process with rank 1 handles the next part of the image and the segmentation function, namely, all 2D slices $j = 1, \ldots, n_2 + 1$, $k = 1, \ldots, n_3 + 1$ locally indexed by i in the range $i = 0, \ldots, n_1 + 1$, where the 2D slice with index $i = 0$ corresponds to the slice with index $i = n_1$ in the root process (cf. Figure 9). This is similar for further processes, with the only difference that on the last process with rank $n_{\text{procs}} - 1$ the index i of the last 2D slice is n_1^{last} instead of n_1. The merging of all 2D slices for $i = 1, \ldots, n_1$ (n_1^{last} on the last process) from all the subsequent processes gives the non-distributed complete 3D image as well as the complete segmentation function. In order to solve iteratively the linear system and to compute its coefficients, we need the overlap. The overlap in which it is necessary to exchange information between neighbouring processes is given by the slices $n_1, n_1 + 1$ and slices $0, 1$ of subsequent processes (cf. Figure 9).

As a first example showing how the data distribution is realized, we present the procedure for the parallel reading of the 3D image in Figure 10. In all subsequent figures the value of parameter $p = 1$. Depending on the rank of the process, we

```
void ReadingImage()
{
 input=fopen("3Dimage.dat","r");

 for (n=0;n<nprocs;n++)
   {
     if (myid==n)
       {
        if(myid==0)
          {
            fseek(input,0,SEEK_SET);
            for(i=p;i<=n1+p;i++)
            for(j=p;j<=n2+p;j++)
            for(k=p;k<=n3+p;k++)
            {
              ll=getc(input); u[i][j][k]=ll/255.;
            }
          }
        if((myid>0)&&(myid<nprocs-1))
          {
            fseek(input,(n1*myid-1)*(n2+1)*(n3+1),SEEK_SET);
            for(i=p-1;i<=n1+p;i++)
            for(j=p;j<=n2+p;j++)
            for(k=p;k<=n3+p;k++)
            {
              ll=getc(input); u[i][j][k]=ll/255.;
            }
          }
        if (myid==nprocs-1)
          {
            fseek(input,(n1*myid-1)*(n2+1)*(n3+1),SEEK_SET);
            for(i=p-1;i<=nllast+p;i++)
            for(j=p;j<=n2+p;j++)
            for(k=p;k<=n3+p;k++)
            {
              ll=getc(input); u[i][j][k]=ll/255.;
            }
          }
       }
   }
 fclose(input);
}
```

Figure 10. Parallel reading of a 3D image.

start the reading of the input file at the desired position and put the graylevel image intensity to the array $0 \le u[i][j][k] \le 1$.

After reading of the image, the discrete values of g_T^0 are computed in the procedure Coefficients0 (cf. the paragraph following (24)). Then we do not need an image anymore in the program, so the discrete initial segmentation function is

```
for (i=p+1;i<=N1+p-1;i++)
for (j=p+1;j<=N2+p-1;j++)
for (k=p+1;k<=N3+p-1;k++)
  {
  z=(b[i][j][k]+aw[i][j][k]*u[i-1][j][k]+
     ae[i][j][k]*u[i+1][j][k]+as[i][j][k]*u[i][j-1][k]+
     an[i][j][k]*u[i][j+1][k]+ab[i][j][k]*u[i][j][k-1]+
     at[i][j][k]*u[i][j][k+1])/ap[i][j][k];
  u[i][j][k]=u[i][j][k]+omega*(z-u[i][j][k]);
  }
```

Figure 11. One iteration of the standard serial SOR method.

built and stored in the same array $u[i][j][k]$ by the procedure InitialSegmentation-Function.

In every time step, the values of the discrete segmentation function are updated in the DF nodes, solving iteratively the linear system with coefficients given by (25). Figure 11 shows one iteration of the serial SOR method described in (25). We can see the dependence of the currently updated value $u[i][j][k]$ on its six neighbours (the west, east, south, north, bottom, and top DF nodes). In every iteration three of them should already be known (cf. (27)), so in parallel run every consecutive process should wait until its preceding process is finished in order to get the west values updated. Such dependence is not well suited for parallelization. But there exists an elegant way to change the standard SOR method to be efficiently parallelized (see, e.g., [67]). It is possible to split all voxels to RED elements, given by the condition that the sum of its indices is an even number, and to BLACK elements, given by the condition that sum of its indices is an odd number. Then the six neighbours of RED elements are BLACK elements (cf. Figure 12), and the value of RED elements depends only on those of the BLACK elements, and vice versa. Due to this fact, we can split one SOR iteration into two steps. First we update RED elements and then BLACK elements, and this splitting is perfectly parallelizable. Figure 13 shows one iteration of the so-called RED-BLACK SOR method operating on RED elements.

After computing one RED-BLACK SOR iteration for the RED elements on every parallel process, we have to exchange RED updated values in overlapping regions, and then we can compute one iteration for BLACK elements. The data exchange is implemented as shown in Figure 14 using non-blocking MPI_Isend and MPI_Irecv subroutines. This iterative process is stopped using the condition for a relative residual stated at the end of Section 3.4. Computing the initial residual $R^{(0)}$ as well as all further residuals $R^{(l)}$, we have to collect partial information from all the processes and send the collected value to all processes to check the stopping criterion by every process. Figure 15 shows how the MPI_Allreduce subroutine is used toward that end in computing $R^{(0)}$. In fact, we compute by the

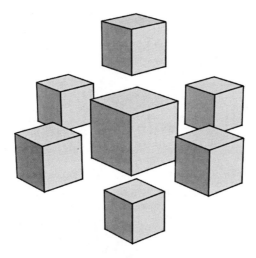

Figure 12. The RED element is in the middle, and its 6 neighbors (west, east, south, north, bottom, and top) have the sum of indices different by 1 from the middle one, so they are all BLACK elements. See attached CD for color version.

same strategy the residuals $R^{(l)}$ not after every RED-BLACK iteration, since it is time consuming in itself, but after every ten RED-BLACK iterations. Fulfiling the stopping criterion for the SOR iterations, we get an approximate solution in the new time step. In checking the stopping condition (23) of the overall segmentation process, we have to employ in a similar way the procedure MPI_Allreduce in evaluation of the L_2 norm of difference of subsequent time step solutions.

Using the PARAVER software, in Figures 16–19 we visualize the run of our parallel program, computing just one time step of the method on four processors. In Figure 16 we can see in green color the time spent for the MPI_Init and MPI_Finalize functions. In blue color we can see the running time of the program outside the MPI subroutines. First there is the parallel reading of the image, computing g_T^0 coefficients and construction of the initial segmentation function, and then we can see 50 iterations of the RED-BLACK SOR method, indicated by yellow lines corresponding to data exchanges. Figure 17 shows the zoom of the previous visualization at the start of the iteration process. The time spent in the MPI_Allreduce subroutine by every process is visualized in orange. This corresponds to a synchronization of all processes at the first computation of initial residual before starting iterations of the RED-BLACK SOR method. Next, MPI_Allreduce we can see almost on the right end of the picture, when the residual after ten RED and ten BLACK iterations is computed. Figure 18 zooms in on this part of the parallel run. Together with MPI_Allreduce in orange, we can see the MPI_Wait procedure in red, the data exchanges expressed by the yellow lines, and

```
if (myid==0)
{
  for (i=p+1;i<=n1+p-1;i++)
  for (j=p+1;j<=n2+p-1;j++)
  for (k=p+1;k<=n3+p-1;k++)
   {if ((i+j+k) % 2 ==0)
    {z=(b[i][j][k]+aw[i][j][k]*u[i-1][j][k]+
        ae[i][j][k]*u[i+1][j][k]+as[i][j][k]*u[i][j-1][k]+
        an[i][j][k]*u[i][j+1][k]+ab[i][j][k]*u[i][j][k-1]+
        at[i][j][k]*u[i][j][k+1])/ap[i][j][k];
     u[i][j][k]=u[i][j][k]+omega*(z-u[i][j][k]);}}
}
if ((myid>0)&&(myid<nprocs-1))
{
  for (i=p;i<=n1+p-1;i++)
  for (j=p+1;j<=n2+p-1;j++)
  for (k=p+1;k<=n3+p-1;k++)
   {if ((i+j+k) % 2 ==0)
    {z=(b[i][j][k]+aw[i][j][k]*u[i-1][j][k]+
        ae[i][j][k]*u[i+1][j][k]+as[i][j][k]*u[i][j-1][k]+
        an[i][j][k]*u[i][j+1][k]+ab[i][j][k]*u[i][j][k-1]+
        at[i][j][k]*u[i][j][k+1])/ap[i][j][k];
     u[i][j][k]=u[i][j][k]+omega*(z-u[i][j][k]);}}
}
if (myid==nprocs-1)
{
  for (i=p;i<=n1last+p-1;i++)
  for (j=p+1;j<=n2+p-1;j++)
  for (k=p+1;k<=n3+p-1;k++)
   {if ((i+j+k) % 2 ==0)
    {z=(b[i][j][k]+aw[i][j][k]*u[i-1][j][k]+
        ae[i][j][k]*u[i+1][j][k]+as[i][j][k]*u[i][j-1][k]+
        an[i][j][k]*u[i][j+1][k]+ab[i][j][k]*u[i][j][k-1]+
        at[i][j][k]*u[i][j][k+1])/ap[i][j][k];
     u[i][j][k]=u[i][j][k]+omega*(z-u[i][j][k]);}}
}
```

Figure 13. One iteration for RED elements in the parallel RED-BLACK SOR method. One iteration for BLACK elements differs only in the Boolean condition of the **if** command, which has the form $(i + j + k) \% 2 == 1$.

of course in blue we can see the running of the program in updating the values of $u[i][j][k]$, either for all RED elements or for all BLACK elements by every process. Figure 19 gives insight into the MPI data transmission process. The time spent in MPI_Isend is shown in violet, MPI_Irecv in gray, and we can see again MPI_Wait in red, which controls so that the desired data are completely transfered from one process to another.

```
if (myid==0)
{
 MPI_Isend(&(u[n1][p+1][p+1]),(n2-1)*(n3-1),MPI_DOUBLE,
           myid+1,7,MPI_COMM_WORLD,&req1);
 MPI_Irecv(&(u[n1+p][p+1][p+1]),(n2-1)*(n3-1),MPI_DOUBLE,
           myid+1,7,MPI_COMM_WORLD,&req2);
}
if ((myid>0)&&(myid<nprocs-1))
{
 MPI_Isend(&(u[n1][p+1][p+1]),(n2-1)*(n3-1),MPI_DOUBLE,
           myid+1,7,MPI_COMM_WORLD,&req1);
 MPI_Isend(&(u[p][p+1][p+1]),(n2-1)*(n3-1),MPI_DOUBLE,
           myid-1,7,MPI_COMM_WORLD,&req2);
 MPI_Irecv(&(u[n1+p][p+1][p+1]),(n2-1)*(n3-1),MPI_DOUBLE,
           myid+1,7,MPI_COMM_WORLD,&req3);
 MPI_Irecv(&(u[0][p+1][p+1]),(n2-1)*(n3-1),MPI_DOUBLE,
           myid-1,7,MPI_COMM_WORLD,&req4);
}
if (myid==nprocs-1)
{
 MPI_Isend(&(u[p][p+1][p+1]),(n2-1)*(n3-1),MPI_DOUBLE,
           myid-1,7,MPI_COMM_WORLD,&req1);
 MPI_Irecv(&(u[0][p+1][p+1]),(n2-1)*(n3-1),MPI_DOUBLE,
           myid-1,7,MPI_COMM_WORLD,&req2);
}
MPI_Wait(&req1, &status);
MPI_Wait(&req2, &status);
if (myid > 0 && myid < nprocs-1)
{
 MPI_Wait(&req3, &status);
 MPI_Wait(&req4, &status);
}
```

Figure 14. Point-to-point communication after one RED-BLACK SOR iteration for RED elements. The same exchange of data is done also after one iteration for BLACK elements.

5. DISCUSSION OF COMPUTATIONAL RESULTS

In this section we discuss the numerical examples computed using scheme (18) and by its parallel implementation as presented in the previous section.

In [56] we have shown, using comparisons of our numerical solutions with known nontrivial exact solutions, that the 3D semi-implicit co-volume method (18) is second-order accurate for smooth (or mildly singular) solutions and first-order accurate for highly singular solutions (when the gradient is vanishing on a large subset of a domain and a discontinuity set of the gradient field is nontrivial). This means that the method is experimentally convergent and reliable for computing graph evolutions forming the flat regions as arising in the subjective surface segmentation method.

```
deltain=0;
if (myid==0)
  {
    for (i=p+1;i<=n1+p-1;i++)
    for (j=p+1;j<=n2+p-1;j++)
    for (k=p+1;k<=n3+p-1;k++)
    {
     deltain+=sqr(-aw[i][j][k]*u[i-1][j][k]-ae[i][j][k]*u[i+1][j][k]
               -as[i][j][k]*u[i][j-1][k]-an[i][j][k]*u[i][j+1][k]
               -ab[i][j][k]*u[i][j][k-1]-at[i][j][k]*u[i][j][k+1]
               +ap[i][j][k]*u[i][j][k]-b[i][j][k]);
    }
  }
if ((myid>0)&&(myid<nprocs-1))
  {
    for (i=p;i<=n1+p-1;i++)
    for (j=p+1;j<=n2+p-1;j++)
    for (k=p+1;k<=n3+p-1;k++)
    {
     deltain+=sqr(-aw[i][j][k]*u[i-1][j][k]-ae[i][j][k]*u[i+1][j][k]
               -as[i][j][k]*u[i][j-1][k]-an[i][j][k]*u[i][j+1][k]
               -ab[i][j][k]*u[i][j][k-1]-at[i][j][k]*u[i][j][k+1]
               +ap[i][j][k]*u[i][j][k]-b[i][j][k]);
    }
  }
if (myid==nprocs-1)
  {
    for (i=p;i<=n1last+p-1;i++)
    for (j=p+1;j<=n2+p-1;j++)
    for (k=p+1;k<=n3+p-1;k++)
    {
     deltain+=sqr(-aw[i][j][k]*u[i-1][j][k]-ae[i][j][k]*u[i+1][j][k]
               -as[i][j][k]*u[i][j-1][k]-an[i][j][k]*u[i][j+1][k]
               -ab[i][j][k]*u[i][j][k-1]-at[i][j][k]*u[i][j][k+1]
               +ap[i][j][k]*u[i][j][k]-b[i][j][k]);
    }
  }
MPI_Allreduce(&deltain,&tmp,1,MPI_DOUBLE,MPI_SUM,MPI_COMM_WORLD);
deltain=tmp;
```

Figure 15. Computing the initial residual in parallel.

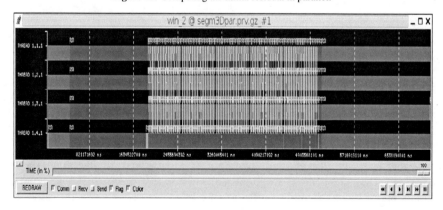

Figure 16. Visualization of the parallel run on 4 processors. See attached CD for color version.

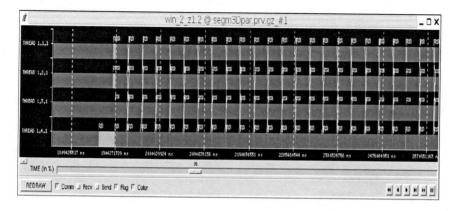

Figure 17. Zoom of the parallel run. See attached CD for color version.

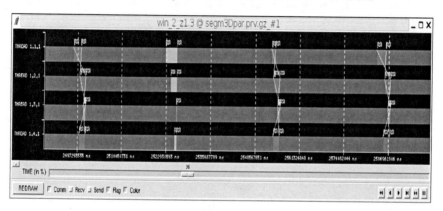

Figure 18. Further zoom of the parallel run. See attached CD for color version.

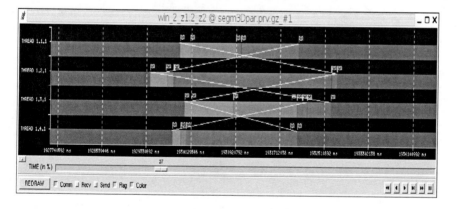

Figure 19. Final zoom of the parallel run. See attached CD for color version.

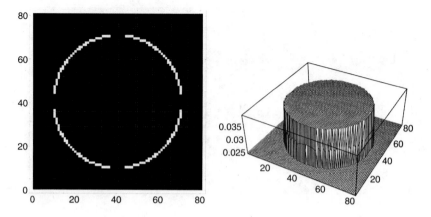

Figure 20. Subjective surface segmentation of 3D sphere with four holes. See attached CD for color version.

As a first example, we segment a 3D image with 81^3 voxels containing a white sphere with four holes on a black background. One 2D slice along the equator is presented in Figure 20 (left). On the right-hand side of Figure 20 we can see a 2D cut of the segmentation function in the same 2D slice after 28 steps of the semi-implicit scheme using $\tau = 0.002$, $\varepsilon = 10^{-3}$, $K = 1$, $TOL = 0.001$ and $\delta = 10^{-5}$. This state of the segmentation function with a shock profile along the edges continuing also into gaps can be successively used to segment the sphere with completion of the holes. The result, where we visualize level surface 0.03, is plotted in Figure 21.

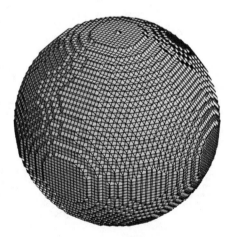

Figure 21. Result of subjective surface segmentation of a 3D sphere with four holes. See attached CD for color version.

Table 1. Computing times and speed-up of parallel program
running on 2 to 32 processors.

# processors	2	4	8	16	32
time(secs)	373.4	198.15	112.5	62.85	38.5
speed-up	2	3.77	6.64	11.88	19.4
rel. speed-up	1	0.94	0.83	0.74	0.61

In the next example, we solve the same problem but with an image resolution given by 128^3 voxels. This 3D example we solved on an MPP cluster at CINECA in Bologna. Since due to the huge amount of unknowns we cannot solve the problem on a single processor, we started the report on the results with computation on two processors. Table 1 shows the computing times in seconds for 34 time steps when the segmentation was achieved using the same parameters as above. As we can see, the computation times are well scaled using a larger number of processors. As expected, due to the increasing complexity of communication using a large number of processors, the relative speed-up (i.e., speed-up over a number of processors) is decreasing.

Next, we present an example of subjective surface segmentation of a 3D echocardiographic image of size $81 \times 87 \times 166$ voxels. We use $\tau = 0.001$, $K = 1, TOL = 0.001$, and $\delta = 10^{-5}$. As one can see from the volume rendering visualization in Figure 22, the 3D image is very noisy; however, the surface of the left ventricle is observable. How noisy is the image intensity can be seen also from Figure 23, where we plot intensity and its graph in one 2D slice. Due to the high complexity of this image, we start the segmentation process with an initial function with maxima in several "points of view" inside the desired object. We again evolve the segmentation function until the L_2 norm of the difference of the two subsequent time steps is less than the prescribed threshold δ. We then check a 2D slice with relatively good ventricular boundary edges (Figure 24), where we can see an accumulation of level sets along the inner boundary of the ventricle (Figure 24, left). The largest gap in the histogram (Figure 24, right) indicates the shock in the segmentation function, which can be used for segmentation. We choose one level inside the gap, and plot it inside the slice (Figure 25, left). We can check what this level set looks like in other noisy slices (Figure 25, right, Figure 27), and then we visualize the corresponding 3D isosurface (Figure 28), which gives a realistic representation of the left ventricle.

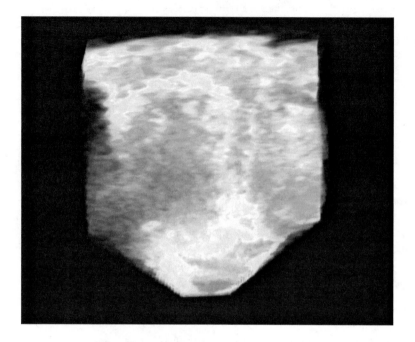

Figure 22. Volume rendering of the original 3D data set.   See attached CD for color version.

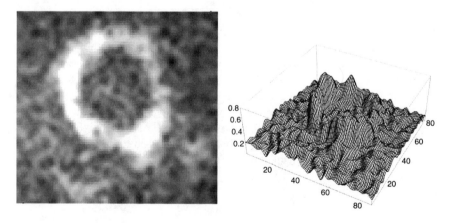

Figure 23. Plot of image intensity in slice $k = 130$ (left), and its 3D graphical view (right). See attached CD for color version.

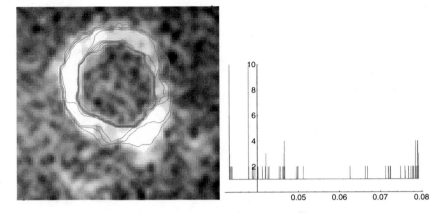

Figure 24. Plot of accumulated level sets in slice $k = 130$ (left); the histogram of the segmentation function in this slice (right). See attached CD for color version.

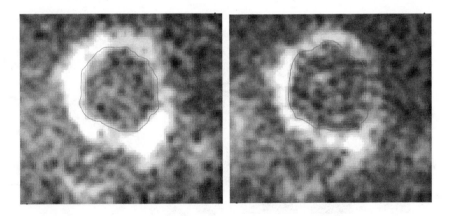

Figure 25. Plot of image intensity together with level line 0.052 in slices $k = 130$ (left) and $k = 125$ (right). Visualization of 3D surface in Figure 22 is done with the same level set. See attached CD for color version.

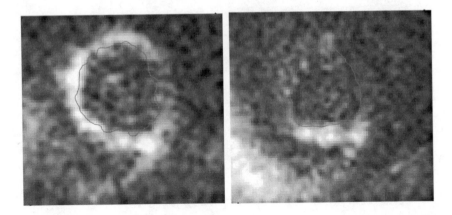

Figure 26. Plot of image intensity together with level line 0.052 in slices $k = 115$ (left) and $k = 100$ (right). Visualization of 3D surface in Figure 22 is done with the same level set. See attached CD for color version.

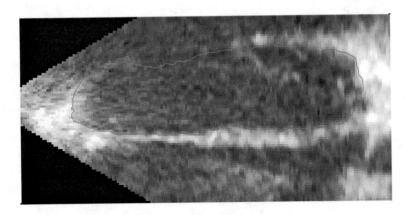

Figure 27. Plot of image intensity together with level line 0.052 in two other slices, $j = 40$. Visualization of 3D surface in Figure 22 is done with the same level set. See attached CD for color version.

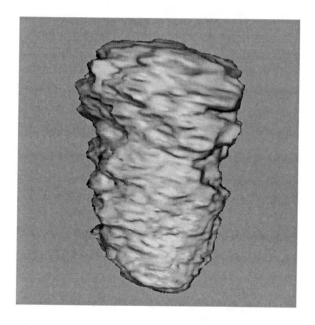

Figure 28. Isosurface visualization of the segmentation result for the left ventricle. See attached CD for color version.

6. ACKNOWLEDGMENTS

This work was supported by Project HPC-EUROPA at the CINECA Super-Computing Center, Bologna, by EU projects Embryomics, and BioEmergences and by grants VEGA 1/3321/06 and APVT-20-040902. We thank to G. Ballabio, C. Calonaci, and R. Gori from CINECA for an introduction to MPI parallel programming and for 3D visualizations.

7. REFERENCES

1. Kass M, Witkin A, Terzopulos D. 1987. Snakes: active contour models. *Int J Comput Vision* **1**:321–331.

2. Gage M, Hamilton RS. 1986. The heat equation shrinking convex plane curves. *J Diff Geom* **23**:69–96.

3. Grayson M. 1987. The heat equation shrinks embedded plane curves to round points. *J Diff Geom* **26**:285–314.

4. Dziuk G. 1991. Algorithm for evolutionary surfaces. *Numer Math* **58**:603–611.

5. Dziuk G. 1994. Convergence of a semi-discrete scheme for the curve shortening flow. *Math Models Methods Appl Sci* **4**:589–606.

6. Dziuk G. 1999. Discrete anisotropic curve shortening flow. *SIAM J Numer Anal* **36**:1808–1830.

7. Mikula K, Ševčovič D. 2001. Evolution of plane curves driven by a nonlinear function of curvature and anisotropy. *SIAM J Numer Anal* **61**:1473–1501.

8. Mikula K, Ševčovič D. 2004. Computational and qualitative aspects of evolution of curves driven by curvature and external force. *Comput Visualiz Sci*, **6**(4):211–225.

9. Mikula K, Ševčovič D. 2004. A direct method for solving an anisotropic mean curvature flow of planar curve with an external force. *Math Methods Appl Sci* **27**(13):1545–1565.

10. K. Mikula, Ševčovič D. 2006. Evolution of curves on a surface driven by a geodesic curvature and external force. *Applic Anal* **85**(4):345–362.

11. Osher S, Sethian JA. 1988. Front propagating with curvature dependent speed: algorithms based on the Hamilton-Jacobi formulation. *J Comput Phys* **79**:12–49.

12. Sethian JA. 1990. Numerical algorithm for propagating interfaces: Hamilton–Jacobi equations and conservation laws. *J Diff Geom* **31**:131–161.

13. Sethian JA. 1999. Level set methods and fast marching methods. In *Evolving interfaces in computational geometry, fluid mechanics, computer vision, and material science*. Cambridge: Cambridge UP.

14. Osher S, Fedkiw R. 2003. *Level set methods and dynamic implicit surfaces*. New York: Springer.

15. Sapiro G. 2001. *Geometric partial differential equations and image analysis*. Cambridge: Cambridge UP.

16. Handlovičová A, Mikula K, Sgallari F. 2003. Semi-implicit complementary volume scheme for solving level set-like equations in image processing and curve evolution. *Numer Math* **93**:675–695.

17. Frolkovič P, Mikula K. 2003. *Flux-based level set method: a finite volume method for evolving interfaces*. Preprint IWR/SFB 2003-15, Interdisciplinary Center for Scientific Computing, University of Heidelberg.

18. Frolkovič P, Mikula K. 2005. *High resolution flux-based level set method*. Preprint 2005-12, Department of Mathematics and Descriptive Geometry, Slovak University of Technology, Bratislava.

19. Caselles V, Catté F, Coll T, Dibos F. 1993. A geometric model for active contours in image processing. *Numer Math* **66**:1–31.

20. Malladi R, Sethian JA, Vemuri B. 1995. Shape modeling with front propagation: a level set approach. *IEEE Trans Pattern Anal Machine Intell* **17**:158–174.

21. Perona P, Malik J. 1990. Scale space and edge detection using anisotropic diffusion. *IEEE Trans Pattern Anal Machine Intell* **12**(7):629–639.

22. Catté F, Lions PL, Morel JM, Coll T. 1992. Image selective smoothing and edge detection by nonlinear diffusion. *SIAM J Numer Anal*, **29**:182–193.

23. Weickert J, Romeny BMtH, Viergever MA. 1998. Efficient and reliable schemes for nonlinear diffusion filtering. *IEEE Trans Image Processing* **7**:398–410.

24. Kačur J, Mikula K. 1995. Solution of nonlinear diffusion in image smoothing and edge detection. *Appl Numer Math* **17**:47–59.

25. Kačur J, Mikula K. 2001. Slow and fast diffusion effects in image processing. *Comput Visualiz Sci* **3**(4):185–195.

26. Mikula K, Ramarosy N. 2001. Semi-implicit finite volume scheme for solving nonlinear diffusion equations in image processing. *Numer Math* **89**(3):561–590.

27. Mikula K, Sgallari F. 2003. Semi-implicit finite volume scheme for image processing in 3D cylindrical geometry. *J Comput Appl Math* **161**(1):119–132.

28. Mikula K. 2002. Image processing with partial diferential equations. In *Modern methods in scientific computing and applications*, pp. 283–321. Eds A Bourlioux, MJ Gander. NATO Science Ser. II, Vol. 75. Dodrecht: Kluwer Academic.

29. Krivá Z, Mikula K. 2002. An adaptive finite volume scheme for solving nonlinear diffusion equations in image processing. *J Vis Commun Image Represent* **13**:22–35.

30. E. Bänsch, Mikula K. 1997. A coarsening finite element strategy in image selective smoothing. *Comput Visualiz Sci* **1**(1):53–61.

31. E. Bänsch, Mikula K. 2001. Adaptivity in 3D image processing. *Comput Visualiz Sci* **4**(1):21–30.
32. Sarti A, Mikula K, Sgallari F. 1999. Nonlinear multiscale analysis of three-dimensional echocardiographic sequences. *IEEE Trans Med Imaging* **18**:453–466.
33. Sarti A, Mikula K, Sgallari F, Lamberti C. 2002. Nonlinear multiscale analysis models for filtering of 3D + time biomedical images. In *Geometric methods in biomedical image processing*, pp. 107–128. Ed R Malladi. New York: Springer.
34. Sarti A, Mikula K, Sgallari F, Lamberti C. 2002. Evolutionary partial differential equations for biomedical image processing. *J Biomed Inform* **35**:77–91.
35. Alvarez L, Lions PL, Morel JM. 1992. Image selective smoothing and edge detection by nonlinear diffusion, II. *SIAM J Numer Anal* **29**:845–866.
36. L Alvarez, Guichard F, Lions PL, Morel JM. 1993. Axioms and fundamental equations of image processing. *Arch Rat Mech Anal* **123**:200–257.
37. Mikula K, Sarti A, Lamberti C. 1997. Geometrical diffusion in 3D-echocardiography. In *Proceedings of ALGORITMY'97, a conference on scientific computing*, pp. 167–181. http://www.math.sk/mikula/msl_alg97.pdf
38. Handlovičová A, Mikula K, Sarti A. 1999. Numerical solution of parabolic equations related to level set formulation of mean curvature flow. *Comput Visualiz Sci* **1**.(2):179–182.
39. Handlovičová A, Mikula K, Sgallari F. 2002. Variational numerical methods for solving nonlinear diffusion equations arising in image processing. *J Vis Commun Image Represent* **13**:217–237.
40. Mikula K. 2001. Solution and applications of the curvature driven evolution of curves and surfaces. In *Numerical methods for viscosity solutions and applications*, pp. 173–196. Eds M Falcone, Ch Makridakis. Advances in Mathematics for Applied Sciences, Vol. 59. Singapore: World Scientific.
41. Mikula K, Preusser T, Rumpf M, Sgallari F. 2002. On anisotropic geometric diffusion in 3D image processing and image sequence analysis. In *Trends in nonlinear analysis*, pp. 307–322. Ed M Kirkilionis, et al. New York: Springer.
42. Mikula K, Preusser T, Rumpf M. 2004. Morphological image sequence analysis. *Comput Visualiz Sci* **6**(4):197–209.
43. Caselles V, Kimmel R, Sapiro G. 1995. Geodesic active contours. In *Proceedings of the fifth international conference on computer vision (ICCV'95)*, pp. 694–699. Washington, DC: IEEE Computer Society.
44. Caselles V, Kimmel R, Sapiro G. 1997. Geodesic active contours. *Int J Comput Vision* **22**:61–79.
45. Caselles V, Kimmel R, Sapiro G, Sbert C. 1997. Minimal surfaces: a geometric three dimensional segmentation approach. *Numer Math* **77**:423–451.
46. Kichenassamy S, Kumar A, Olver P, Tannenbaum A, Yezzi A. 1995. Gradient flows and geometric active contours models. In *Proceedings of the fifth international conference on computer vision (ICCV'95)*, pp. 810–815. Washington, DC: IEEE Computer Society.
47. Kichenassamy S, Kumar A, Olver P, Tannenbaum A, Yezzi A. 1996. Conformal curvature flows: from phase transitions to active vision. *Arch Rat Mech Anal* **134**:275–301.
48. Sarti A, Malladi R, Sethian JA. 2000. Subjective surfaces: a method for completing missing boundaries. *Proc Natl Acad Sci USA* **Vol. 12**(97):6258–6263.
49. Sarti A, Citti G. 2001. Subjective surfaces and riemannian mean curvature flow graphs. *Acta Math Univ Comenianae* **70**(1):85–104.
50. Sarti A, Malladi R, Sethian JA. 2002. Subjective surfaces: a geometric model for boundary completion. *Int J Comput Vision* **46**(3):201–221.
51. Evans LC, Spruck J. 1991. Motion of level sets by mean curvature, I. *J Diff Geom* **33**:635–681.
52. Mikula K, Sarti A, Sgallari F. 2005. Semi-implicit co-volume level set method in medical image segmentation. In *Handbook of biomedical image analysis: segmentation and registration models*, pp. 583–626. Ed JS Suri, D Wilson, S Laxminarayan. New York: Springer.

53. Chen Y-G, Giga Y, Goto S. 1991. Uniqueness and existence of viscosity solutions of generalized mean curvature flow equation. *J Diff Geom* **33**:749–786.

54. Crandall MG, Ishii H, Lions PL. 1992. User's guide to viscosity solutions of second order partial differential equations. *Bull Amer Math Soc* **27**:1–67.

55. Citti G, Manfredini M. 2002. Long time behavior of Riemannian mean curvature flow of graphs. *J Math Anal Appl* **273**(2):353–369.

56. Corsaro S, Mikula K, Sarti A, Sgallari F. 2004. *Semi-implicit co-volume method in 3D image segmentation*. Preprint 2004-12, Department of Mathematics and Descriptive Geometry, Slovak University of Technology, Bratislava.

57. Patankar S. 1980. *Numerical heat transfer and fluid flow*. New York: Hemisphere Publishing.

58. Eymard R, Gallouet T, Herbin R. 2000. The finite volume method. In *Handbook for numerical analysis*, Vol. 7, pp. 715–1022. Ed Ph Ciarlet, JL Lions. New York: Elsevier.

59. Le Veque R. 2002. *Finite volume methods for hyperbolic problems*. Cambridge Texts in Applied Mathematics, Cambridge: Cambridge UP.

60. Brenner SC, Scott LR. 2002. *The mathematical theory of the finite element method*. New York: Springer.

61. Thomée V. 1997. *Galerkin finite element methods for parabolic problems*. Berlin: Springer.

62. Deckelnick K, Dziuk G. 1995. Convergence of a finite element method for non-parametric mean curvature flow. *Numer Math* **72**:197-222.

63. Deckelnick K, Dziuk G. 2000. Error estimates for a semi-implicit fully discrete finite element scheme for the mean curvature flow of graphs. *Interfaces Free Bound* **2**(4):341–359.

64. Deckelnick K, Dziuk G. 2003. Numerical approximation of mean curvature flow of graphs and level sets. In *Mathematical aspects of evolving interfaces*, pp. 53–87. Ed L Ambrosio, K Deckelnick, G Dziuk, M Mimura, VA Solonnikov, HM Soner. New York: Springer.

65. Walkington NJ. 1996. Algorithms for computing motion by mean curvature. *SIAM J Numer Anal*, **33**(6):2215–2238.

66. Saad Y. 1996. *Iterative methods for sparse linear systems*. Spanish Fork, UT: PWS Publishing.

67. Aoyama Y, Nakano J. 1999. *RS/6000 SP: Practical MPI Programming, IBM* www.redbooks.ibm.com.

68. Mikula K. 2001. Parallel filtering of three dimensional image sequences. In *Science and supercomputing at CINECA*, pp. 674–677. Ed F Garofalo, M Moretti, M Voli. Bologna: CINECA.

69. Kanizsa G. 1979. *Organization in vision*. New York: Praeger.

70. Mikula K, Sarti A, Sgallari F. 2006. Co-volume method for Riemannian mean curvature flow in subjective surfaces multiscale segmentation. *Comput Visualiz Sci* **9**(1):23–31.

6

VOLUMETRIC SEGMENTATION USING SHAPE MODELS IN THE LEVEL SET FRAMEWORK

Fuxing Yang and Milan Sonka

Department of Electrical and Computer Engineering
The University of Iowa, Iowa City, Iowa, USA

Jasjit S. Suri

Biomedical Research Institute, Idaho
State University, Pocatello, Idaho, USA

It is an arduous task to extract the structural detail in medical images because of noisy or partial volume effects, or incomplete information. However, expert-identified segmentation results are often available, and most of the structures to be extracted have a similar shape from one subject to another. Then to model the family of shapes and restricting the new structure to be extracted within the class is of particular interest. Generally, active shape models are used to implement this framework. However, the definition of the image term is the most challenging factor in such an approach. The level set methods define a powerful optimization framework via an implicit description of different shapes in various dimensional spaces. This advantage can help recover objects of interest by the propagation of curves or surfaces. The properties of the level set methods support complex topologies, considered in higher dimensions, are implicit, intrinsic, and parameter free. In this chapter, we give a review of the level set method and show the usage of the shape models for segmentation of objects in 2D and 3D in a level set framework via regional information.

1. INTRODUCTION

The level set method is a numerical technique for tracking interfaces and shapes. Level set methods are nowadays widely used in medical image processing. This chapter is an attempt to survey the latest techniques in 2D and 3D for fast shape recovery based on the class of deformable models in level set frameworks and to emphasize a state-of-the-art family of the model using shape and regional information.

Aside from medical imagery, the diversity of applications of level sets has reached into several fields. These applications and their relevant works include [1]: geometry (Angenent et al. [2], Chopp et al. [3], and Sethian et al. [4]); grid generation (Sethian and Malladi [5]); fluid mechanics (Sethian et al. [6] and Sussman et al. [7]); combustion (Rhee et al. [8]); solidification (Sethian and Strain [9]); device fabrication (Adalsteinsson and Sethian [10]); morphing (Breen and Whitaker [11]); object tracking/image sequence analysis in images (Mansouri and Konrad [12], Paragios and Deriche [13] and Kornprobst et al. [14]); stereo vision (Faugeras and Keriven from INRIA [15]); shape from shading (Kimmel et al. [16, 17]); mathematical morphology (Sapiro et al. [18] and Sochen et al. [19]); color image segmentation (Sapiro et al. [20]); 3D reconstruction and modeling (Caselles et al. [21]); surfaces and level sets (Chopp [3] and Kimmel et al. [22]); topological evaluations (DeCarlo and Gallier [23]); inpainting (Telea [24]); 2D and 3D medical image segmentation (which will be discussed in more detail in the following).

Segmentation has always been a critical component in two-dimensional (2D) and three-dimensional (3D) medical imagery since it greatly assists in the process of medical therapy [1]. The applications of shape recovery have been increasing as scanning methods have become faster, more accurate, and less artifacted [25]. The recovery of the shapes of the human body is more difficult compared to other imaging fields. This is primarily due to the great shape variability involved, the complexity of medical structures, several kinds of artifacts, and restrictive body scanning methods.

Since the introduction of the level set method, the concept of deformable models for image segmentation defined in a level set framework has motivated the development of geometric active contours. Much work on 2D and 3D segmentation has been done around this method. For example, Malladi and Sethian [26] proposed a real-time algorithm for medical shape recovery using the level set method. Application of level sets for cortex unfolding was studied Faugeras and coworkers from INRIA [27]. Application of the level set technique in cell segmentation was introduced by Sarti et al. [28]. Niessen et al. [29] worked on application of geodesic active contours for cardiac image analysis. There are also many applications in brain imaging, like the work on gray matter/white matter (GM/WM) boundary estimation by Gomes and Faugeras [30], GM/WM boundary estimation with fuzzy models by Suri [31], and GM/WM thickness estimation by Zeng et al. [32]. Angelini et al. [33] and Lin et al. [34] worked on 3D ultrasound image analysis using a three-dimensional level set.

As applications are becoming more and more widely used in medical image segmentation and relative analysis, the challenges facing researchers are becoming more difficult and complex. Initially, a level set without complicated regularizers was utilized to solve the simple case where medical images had good contrast, less noise, and simple shape. However, the recovery of shapes of the human body is more difficult compared to other imaging fields, and the original level set-based method was not capable of solving the more complicated medical imaging tasks. Thus, the segmentation methods in the level set framework were embedded with many different powerful regularizers or propagating forces to improve robustness. These methods can be classified in four categories: clustering-based [31], Bayesian bidirectional classifier-based [35], shape-based [36], and coupled constrained-based [32]. All these features did improve the robustness and accuracy in specific applications. However, these methods did not make full use of the regional information combined with statistic shape information.

Motivated by combining regional and statistic shape information, many attempts have been made in order to make good use of the global shape and regional information, including work by Tsai et al. [37] and Rousson et al. [38]. In this chapter, we will introduce this family of state-of-the-art medical image segmentation methods within a level set framework. The reader will gain an understanding of what is the regional-based active contour in the level set framework, how it solves the segmentation problem without using image gradient information, which is a major control factor for other approaches, and how it could be implemented via the level set method. In addition, the reader will be shown how statistical shape information can be extracted from a training procedure and combined with regional information for segmentation.

The layout of the remainder of this chapter is as follows In the Section 2, a short introduction to the level set method and the theoretical background appears. Section 3 describes a typical application using the level set method. Section 4 deals with the relationship between active methods and level set methods. Additionally, active contours using the level set framework will be discussed in more detail, including the mathematical background and applications in image processing. Section 5 discusses a segmentation method in the level set framework using regional information and prior shape knowledge in greater detail. Relative applications are also introduced. Finally, Section 6 offers a brief conclusion of to the chapter and discusses the pros and cons of this method.

2. BRIEF MATHEMATICAL FORMULATION OF LEVEL SETS

2.1. Front Evolution

Front evolution is a useful technique in image analysis for object extraction, object tracking, etc. The basic idea behind the method is to evolve a curve toward the lowest potential of a cost function, where its definition reflects the task to be addressed and imposes certain smoothness constraints. Propagating interfaces occur in a wide variety of settings, and include ocean waves, flames, and material boundaries. Less obvious boundaries are equally important and include shapes against backgrounds, handwritten characters, and iso-intensity contours in images. Furthermore, there are applications not commonly thought of as moving interface problems, like optimal path planning and construction of the shortest geodesic paths on surfaces, which can be recast as front propagation problems with significant advantages [39].

Consider a boundary, either a curve in 2D or a surface in 3D, separating one region from another. Assume that this curve/surface moves in a direction normal to itself with a known speed function F. The goal is to track the motion of this interface as it evolves. Here, the motions of the interface in its tangential directions are ignored. At a specific moment, the speed function $F(L, G, I)$ describes the motion of the interface in the normal direction.

1. Speed factor L depends on local geometric information (e.g., curvature and normal direction).

2. Speed factor G depends on the shape and position of the front (e.g., integrals along the front, heat diffusion).

3. Speed factor I does not depend on the shape of the front (e.g., an underlying fluid velocity that passively transports the front).

Langragian techniques are based on parameterizing the contour according to some sampling strategy and then evolving each element according to the speed function. While such a technique can be very efficient, it suffers from various limitations, like deciding on the sampling strategy, estimating the internal geometric properties of the curve, and changing its topology, addressing problems in higher dimensions [40].

The level set method was initially proposed to track a moving front by Osher and Sethian in 1988 [41] and was widely applied across various imaging domains in the late 1990s. They can be used to efficiently address the problem of curve or surface propagation in an implicit manner. The central idea is represent the evolving contour using a signed function, which is in a higher-dimensional space, where its zero level corresponds to the actual contour. Then, according to the motion equation of the contour, one can easily derive a similar flow for the implicit surface such that when applied to the zero level it will reflect the propagation of the contour. Basically, there are two kinds of formulations regarding the level set method: boundary value formulation and initial value formulation.

2.2. Boundary Value Formulation

Assume for the moment that $F > 0$, and the front is moving all the way outward. We can define the arrival time $T(x, y)$ of the front as it crosses each (x, y). Based on the fact that distance = rate × time, we have the following expression in the 1D situation:

$$1 = F\frac{dT}{dx}. \tag{1}$$

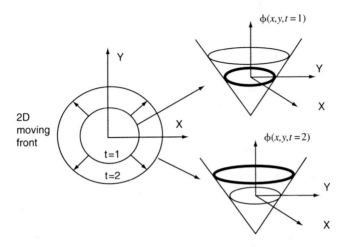

Figure 1. The level set function.

∇T is orthogonal to the level sets of T, and its magnitude is inversely proportional to the speed. So

$$|\nabla T|F = 1, \quad T = 0 \quad \text{on} \quad \Gamma, \tag{2}$$

where Γ is the initial location of the interface. Then, the front motion is characterized as the solution of a boundary value problem. If the speed F depends only on position, then the equation reduces to what is known as the *Eikonal* equation.

The most efficient way to solve the Eikonal equation is by employing the fast marching method. For readers who are interested in the details of this method, please refer to [5].

2.3. Initial Value Formulation

Assume that the front moves with a speed that is neither strictly positive nor negative, so the front can move inward and outward and a point (x, y), and can be crossed several times. $T(x, y)$ is not a single-value function. The solution is to treat the initial position of the front as the zero level set of a higher-dimensional function Φ (Figure 1). Evolution of this function will give the propagation of the front through a time-dependent initial value problem, and at any time the front is given by the zero level set of the time-dependent level set function Φ. Taking the one-dimensional situation as an example and $x(t)$ as the front, we have the following definition of the zero level set:

$$\Phi(x(t), t) = 0. \tag{3}$$

Taking the partial differential of the above equation, we have the following equations system:

$$\Phi_t + \nabla\Phi(x(t), t).x'(t) = 0, \tag{4}$$

$$F = x'(t) \cdot n, \qquad \text{where} \qquad n = \frac{\nabla\Phi}{|\nabla\Phi|}, \tag{5}$$

$$\Phi_t + F|\nabla\Phi| = 0, \qquad \text{given} \qquad \Phi(x, t = 0). \tag{6}$$

From these equations, the time evolution of the level set function Φ can be described, and the zero level set of this evolving function is always identified with the propagating interface.

There is also an efficient way to solve the initial value problem as just introduced: the narrow band method. For readers who are interested in the details of this method, please refer to [42].

3. BASIC APPLICATION OF LEVEL SET METHODS

The level set method includes numerous advantages: it is implicit, parameter free, allows easy estimation of the geometric properties of the evolving front or surface, can change the topology, and is intrinsic. Therefore, one can conclude that it is a very convenient framework for addressing numerous applications of computer vision and image processing.

In this section we provide some typical examples of applications in image processing, without complicated controlling or regularizers.

3.1. Curvature-Based Applications

In differential geometry, any simple closed curve moving under its curvature collapses nicely to a circle and then disappears. The wider applications include the study of the surface tension of an interface, the evolution of boundaries between fluids, and image noise removal. In order to prove this theorem and apply it to further applications, we chose the level set method to track the propagation of the front. The only factor affecting front propagation is the curvature. The speed F is defined as below. We only need to update the level set value in the whole domain and choose the positions of the zero crossing pixels as the locations of the new zero level set:

$$F = f(F_{\text{curv}}), \tag{7}$$

where $f()$ is a function defined on the curvature. In the following example, two different definitions are used. One is the signed curvature itself, and the other is the negative curvature only. Based on the different definition of the function, the movement of the front or surface is showing a different pattern. For the first case, all the parts of the contour are moving, while the parts with positive curvature are moving inward and the parts with negative curvature are moving outward. For the second case, only the concave parts (parts with negative curvature) are moving outward.

Figure 4 depicts propagation of the closed curve in 4 steps, which proves the theorem. At the same time, it also proves the ability of the level set method to deal with curvature-related problems. It is straightforward for higher-dimensional applications around curvature. In the following images, propagation of a closed 3D surface is also shown. An important application could be to help unwrap the fold parts of the original 3D image.

The level set methods exploit the fact that curves moving under their curvature smooth out and disappear. If we take pixel values as a topographic map from an image, the graylevel value is the height of the surface at that point. Let each closed curve move under the curvature. Then very small ones, like spikes of noise, will disappear quickly. The real boundaries still remain sharp, and they will not blur. They just move according to their curvature (Figure 3).

The extension of this noise removal application is valuable for image segmentation. By leaving the longer edges with smaller curvatures, the regions of interests are highly enhanced.

3.2. Image Segmentation Using the Fast Marching Method

The Narrow-Band Method is able to combine the relative geometric factors onto the front propagation. Thus, more complex speed functions F could be used and the front line could be moving more accurately. Positive speed functions F that depend on position and vary widely from point to point are best framed as boundary value problems and approximated through the use of Fast Marching Methods. With the help of the min heap method, Fast Marching Methods are extremely more computationally efficient than the level set method. The boundary value formulation does not need a time step and its approximation is not subject to CFL conditions, so the implementation is simpler. Note that the domain of dependence of a hyperbolic partial differential equation (PDE) for a given point in the problem domain is that portion of the problem domain that influences the value of the solution at the given point. Similarly, the domain of dependence of an explicit finite-difference scheme for a given mesh point is the set of mesh points that affect the value of the approximate solution at the given mesh point. The CFL condition, named for its originators — Courant, Friedrichs, and Lewy — requires that the domain of dependence of the PDE must lie within the domain of dependence of the finite-difference scheme for each mesh point of an explicit finite-difference scheme for a hyperbolic PDE. Any explicit finite-difference scheme that violates

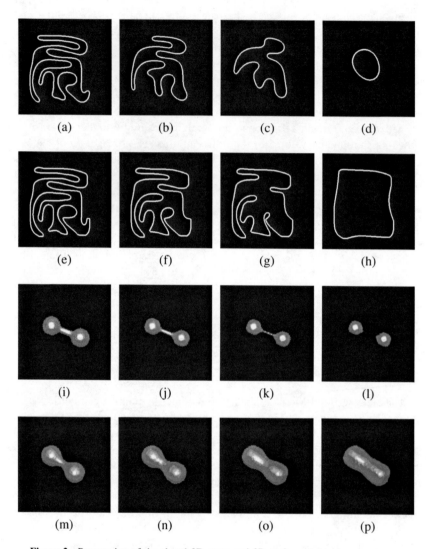

Figure 2. Propagation of the closed 2D curve and 3D surface: (a) under curvature at iteration 100; (b) under curvature at iteration 2000; (c) under curvature at iteration 4000; (d) under curvature at iteration 17000; (e) under negative curvature at iteration 100; (f) under negative curvature at iteration 2000; (g) under negative curvature at iteration 4000; (h) under negative curvature at iteration 17000; (i) under curvature at iteration 100; (j) under curvature at iteration 2000; (k) under curvature at iteration 4000; (l) under curvature at iteration 17000; (m) under negative curvature at iteration 100; (n) under negative curvature at iteration 2000; (o) under negative curvature at iteration 4000; (p) under negative curvature at iteration 17000. See attached CD for color version.

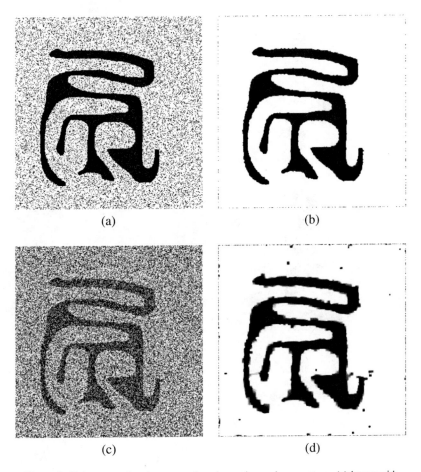

Figure 3. Noise removal and segmentation via moving under curvature: (a) image with mild noise; (b) after removing the noise; (c) image with strong noise; (d) after removing the noise.

the CFL condition is necessarily unstable, but satisfying the CFL condition does not necessarily guarantee stability.

In the cases where the gradient information is strong enough, the fast marching method can be directly used for segmentation. An extra stopping criterion has to be defined. A widely used definition of the gradient-based speed is $e^{-\alpha|\nabla I|}$, where α is a constant. A simple threshold value could be defined on the gradient. The speed factor could also be defined based on intensity itself. When the front touches the pixel with a gradient value above the threshold, the front point is frozen. If all the candidate pixels on the front are frozen, the Fast Marching Methods stop. In the following, several segmentation examples using this method are illustrated.

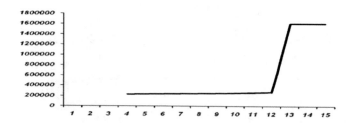

Figure 4. Number of voxels visited by the front using different threshold values.

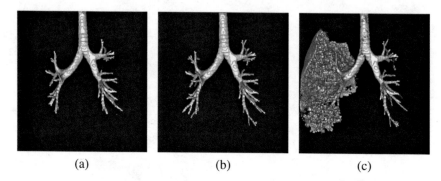

(a)   (b)   (c)

Figure 5. Pulmonary airway tree segmentation using 3D Fast Marching Methods: (a) result using stopping criterion as 6 in gray value; (b) result using stopping criterion as 11 in gray value; (c) result using stopping criterion as 13 in gray value.

The first is pulmonary airway tree segmentation from volumetric CT data. The definition of F is simply 1/Intensity. The stopping criterion is defined as if the gradient at the current pixel is smaller than threshold T_g and the intensity is smaller than threshold T_i. Since the percentage of airway or vessel volume to the volume of the whole dataset is small, it can be regarded as important a priori knowledge. So the optimal threshold could be found via the method developed by Mori et al. The method proposed in [43] can be applied to make control flooding of the Fast Marching into the parenchyma. If we choose the gray value from Figure 4, we can find that a value around 12 is optimal. Whenever a higher value is used, an obvious leakage is detected by looking at the number of traveled voxels (Figure 4c). Based on the requirement of the application, there is no need to use the Narrow-Band Method to execute segmentation, which will greatly increase the computational cost. More examples using this approach are shown in Figure 6.

We used a similar procedure for coronary artery segmentation of mouse hearts from Micro CT datasets. A Sigma filter for edge enhancement and noise removal was first applied to the datasets. Then we define the speed factor as $F = \text{sigma}(I)/\text{Max}(\text{sigma}(I)) + \text{const}$. The intensity threshold is also used

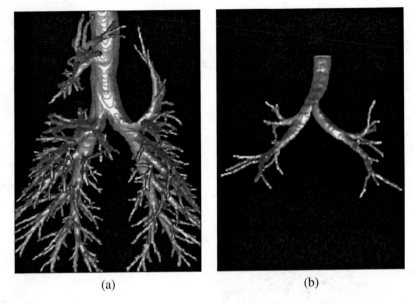

(a)   (b)

Figure 6. Results of pulmonary airway tree segmentation using 3D Fast Marching Methods from 3D CT image data: (a) pulmonary airway tree of a sheep lung from 3D CT data; (b) pulmonary airway tree of a human lung from low-dose 3D CT data.

as a tool to prevent leakage. An example is shown in Figure 7a,b. The size of this dataset is $319 \times 400 \times 382$. The processing time using the Fast Marching Methods is less than 20 seconds. The high proceeding speed due to the Fast Marching Method is very valuable in clinical usage. A modified version of this method was applied to measurement of coronary vasoreactivity in sheep using 64-slice multidetector computed tomography and 3d segmentation [44]. Some results are shown in Figure 7c,d.

One similarity of the above examples is that the boundary of the object to be segmented is easy to find. That is why the simple speed factor is defined based on intensity or as a function of intensity. However, in most cases, especially in medical image processing, medical image segmentation often faces difficult challenges, including poor image contrast, noise, and missing or diffuse boundaries.

3.3. Other Applications

To determine the minimum cost path after the endpoint is reached, a backpropagation from the endpoint to the starting point is carried out [45]. In the isotropic marching case, the fastest traveling is always along the direction perpendicular to the wave front, i.e., the iso-curve of the arrival time. Therefore, the minimum cost path can be found by a gradient descent in the arrival time function. A simple

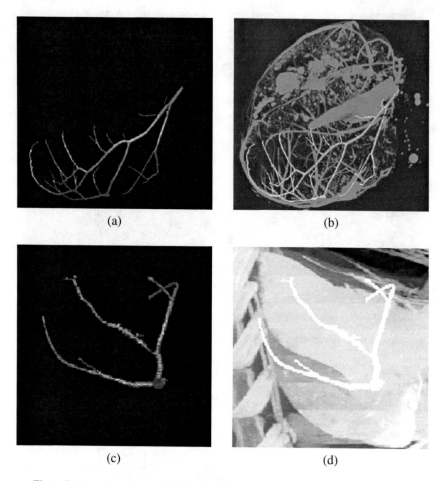

(a)   (b)

(c)   (d)

Figure 7. Comparison between 3D Fast Marching Methods for coronary artery segmentation and Maximum Intensity Projection: (a) segmentation result for the coronary artery tree of a mouse heart from 3D micro CT data; (b) Maximum Intensity Projection of the original data with skeleton; (c) segmentation result for the coronary artery tree of a sheep heart from 3D CT data; (d) Maximum Intensity Projection of the original data with segmentation.

descent can be implemented by point-by-point stepping to the neighbor with the smallest T-value. The smoothness of the path extracted this way is restricted by the pixel resolution and might be zigzagged [46]. By using distance information, the centerline could be easily extracted in binary images, which provides the skeleton for the segmentation result. By using a special function of image intensity as the cost, the method will help to find the path of the vessel in an angiographic image directly.

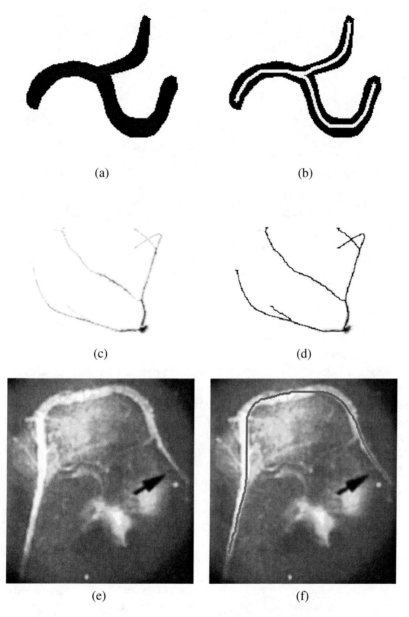

Figure 8. Centerline extraction and optimal path finding; (a) original 2D binary image; (b) centerline extracted using distance information; (c) inverse of 3D distance map corresponding to the segmented coronary artery from sheep heart in Figure 7c; (d) 3D centerline extracted from the inverted distance map; (e) original angiographic image; (f) path found by using gray value as cost. See attached CD for color version.

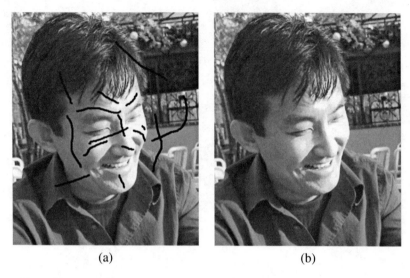

(a)   (b)

Figure 9. Image inpainting using level set methods: (a) corrupted image; (b) restored image after the fast marching-based inpainting. See attached CD for color version.

Front movement provides distance information and the normal direction, which can be effectively used as a reference for image inpainting [24]. An example is shown in Figure 9.

The signed distance is important information that could control front movement to the goal shape. This would help make the Level Set Metamorphosis a simple procedure. Since the front is not moving in only one direction, the narrow-band method has to be used. An example is shown in Figure 10, where (a) is the initial shape and (f) is the given goal state. Using the signed distance map of (f), the initial shape in (a) is driven to the final shape (f). The interim steps of the shape changing procedure are shown in (b)–(e). More details about these methods and more interesting examples can be found in [11].

4. ACTIVE CONTOURS IN THE LEVEL SET FRAMEWORK

From the previous section, the reader may find that the level set method can be applied directly to image processing tasks. The method is closely connected with the active contour or deformable model method, which has been employed as a powerful tool for image analysis. Active contours are object-delineating curves or surfaces that move within two- or three-dimensional digital images under the influence of internal and external forces and user-defined constraints. Since their introduction by Kass et al. [47], these algorithms have been at the core of one of the most active and successful research areas in edge detection, image segmentation,

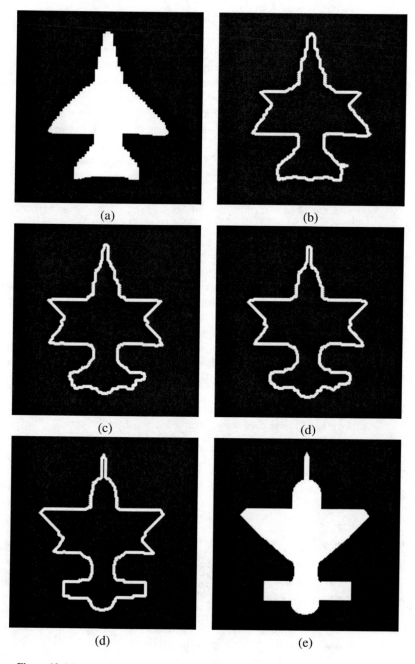

Figure 10. Metamorphosis using level set methods: (a) original shape; (b) interim step 1; (c) interim step 2; (d) interim step 3; (e) interim step 4; (f) final target shape.

shape modeling, and visual tracking. The first kind of active contour models are represented explicitly as parameterized contours (i.e., curves or surfaces) in a Lagrangian framework, which are called parametric active contours. Due to the special properties of the level set method, active contours can be represented implicitly as level sets function that evolve according to an Eulerian formulation, which are called geometric active contours. Although it involves only a simple difference in the representation for an active contour, the level set method-based geometric active contours have many advantages over parametric active contours.

1. They are completely intrinsic and therefore are independent of the parameterization of the evolving contour. In fact, the model is generally not parameterized until evolution of the level set function is complete. Thus, there is no need to add or remove nodes from an initial parameterization or adjust the spacing of the nodes as in parametric models.

2. The intrinsic geometric properties of the contour such as the unit normal vector and the curvature can be easily computed from the level set function, in contrast to the parametric case, where inaccuracies in the calculations of normals and curvature result from the discrete nature of the contour parameterization.

3. The propagating contour can automatically change topology in geometric models (e.g., merge or split) without requiring an elaborate mechanism to handle such changes, as in parametric models.

4. The resulting contours do not contain self-intersections, which are computationally costly to prevent in parametric deformable models.

Since its introduction, the concept of active contour for image segmentation defined in a level set framework has motivated the development of several families of methods, which include: the front-evolving geometric model, geodesic active contours, and region-based level set active contours.

4.1. Front-Evolving Geometric Models of Active Contours

Front-evolving geometric models of active contours (Caselles et al. [48] and Malladi et al. [49]) are based on the theory of curve evolution, implemented via level set algorithms. They can automatically handle changes in topology. Hence, without resorting to dedicated contour tracking, unknown numbers of multiple objects can be detected simultaneously. Evolving the curve C in the normal direction with speed F amounts to solving the following differential equation:

$$\frac{\partial \Phi}{\partial t} = |\nabla \Phi| g(|\nabla u_0|)(div(\frac{\nabla \Phi}{|\nabla \Phi|}) + \gamma), \tag{8}$$

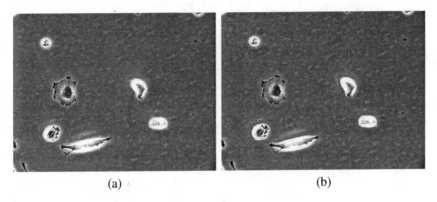

(a)   (b)

Figure 11. Using the front-evolving geometric model for segmentation of living tumor cells in the LSDCAS system: (a) original image; (b) result. See attached CD for color version.

where Φ is the level set function corresponding to the current curve C, $g()$ is the gradient function on the image, and γ is a constant to regulate the evolving speed.

The following is an example using the front-moving geometric model for image segmentation in a living tumor cell analyzed using the LSDCAS system [50]. The result is shown in Figure 11. The border of the image was chosen as the initial location of the contour, and the moving direction was initialized as inward.

The special property of the microscopic image is that at some points of the cell boundary the contrast is very low and the gradient from the original image data is not strong enough for accurate segmentation. In order to solve this problem, a preprocessing is applied for image boundary enhancement to prevent the moving front from evolving into the internal portion of the cells, which have weak boundary areas. The method is adopted from [20]. The original method is for color images with multiple bands, but the microscopic imaging here is gray-valued. So, let $\theta(x, y) : R^2 \to R$, and the arc is defined as

$$d\theta = \frac{\partial\theta}{\partial x}dx + \frac{\partial\theta}{\partial y}dy. \tag{9}$$

The norm is defined as:

$$d\theta^2 = \frac{\partial\theta^2}{\partial x^2}dxdx + \frac{\partial\theta^2}{\partial y^2}dydy + 2\frac{\partial\theta^2}{\partial x\partial y}dxdy. \tag{10}$$

$$d\theta^2 = \begin{bmatrix} dx \\ dy \end{bmatrix}^T \begin{bmatrix} s_{xx} & s_{xy} \\ s_{xy} & s_{yy} \end{bmatrix} \begin{bmatrix} dx \\ dy \end{bmatrix}, \tag{11}$$

where the second-order derivatives $s_{xx} = (\frac{\partial\theta}{\partial x}).(\frac{\partial\theta}{\partial x})$, $s_{yy} = (\frac{\partial\theta}{\partial y}).(\frac{\partial\theta}{\partial y})$, $s_{xy} = s_{yx} = (\frac{\partial\theta}{\partial x}).(\frac{\partial\theta}{\partial y})$.

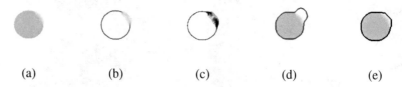

(a)   (b)   (c)   (d)   (e)

Figure 12. Weak boundary enhancement: (a) original image with partial weak edge; (b) gradient of original image; (c) new image after enhancement; (d) segmentation result using a front-evolving model on original image; (e) segmentation result using a front-evolving model on the enhanced image.

The extrema of the above form are in the directions of the eigenvectors of the metric tensor, with corresponding eigenvalues

$$\lambda_\pm = \frac{s_{xx} + s_{yy} \pm \sqrt{(s_{xx} - s_{yy})^2 + 4s_{xy}}}{2}. \tag{12}$$

In the image, the maximal and minimal changes at a specific location are provided by the eigenvalues $\lambda_\pm$. Different functions of $\lambda_\pm$ could be used to define the edges. In our approach, we define the following equation:

$$F = e^{-\rho*(\lambda_+ - \lambda_-)}, \tag{13}$$

where ρ is a constant. When we place this speed factor into the Eikonal equation, $|\nabla T|F = 1$, the moving front will stop at the location where F is small enough—in another words, where the difference between λ_+ and λ_- is large enough.

In order to prove the proposed edge enhancement, consider the example depicted in Figure 12. From this image, a big difference can be observed. Without using the weak boundary enhancement, the evolving front will move out of the dark region from the weak edge; after applying the enhancement, the moving front is stopped by the enhancement and it successfully accomplishes the segmentation without leakage.

From this microscopic imaging segmentation, the reader may find difficulty in using the edge-based method in some special cases where the objects have a very weak boundary. The method used in the above cell segmentation is only one example. Many attempts have been made to enhance image contrast so that the boundary information will be strong enough to stop the moving front, as with Lee's sigma filter [51], nonlinear anisotropic diffusion [52], the heat and shock filter [53], among others. These methods have to provide the intra-regional smoothing while enhance the inter-regional contrast, so that the moving front is able to move over small speckles of the noise and stop at the boundary of the big region.

4.2. Geodesic Active Contour Models

The geodesic model was proposed in 1997 by Caselles et al. [54]. This involves a problem of geodesic computation in a Riemannian space, according to a metric induced by the image. Solving the minimization problem consists in finding the path of minimal new length in that metric:

$$J(C) = 2 \int_0^1 |C'(s)| . g(|\nabla u_0(C(s))|) ds, \qquad (14)$$

where the minimizer C will be obtained when $g(|\nabla u_0(C(s))|)$ vanishes, i.e., when the curve is on the boundary of the object. The geodesic active contour model also has a level set formulation as follows:

$$\frac{\partial \Phi}{\partial t} = |\nabla \Phi| (div(g(|\nabla u_0|) \frac{\nabla \Phi}{|\nabla \Phi|}) + \nu g(|\nabla u_0|)). \qquad (15)$$

The geodesic active contour model is based on the relation between active contours and the computation of geodesics or minimal distance curves. The minimal distance curve lies within a Riemannian space whose metric is defined by the image content. This geodesic approach for object segmentation allows connecting classical "snakes" based on energy minimization and geometric active contours based on the theory of curve evolution. Previous models of geometric active contours are improved, allowing stable boundary detection when their gradients suffer from large variations.

4.3. Tuning Geometric Active Contour with Regularizers

The main problem of boundary-based level set segmentation methods is related to contour leakage at locations of weak or missing boundary data information. One approach can be followed to solve these limitations: to fuse regularizer terms in the speed function.

Suri et al. review in [1] recent works on the fusion of classical geometric and geodesic deformable models speed terms with regularizers, i.e., regional statistics information from the image. Regularization of the level set speed term is desirable to add prior information on the object to segment and prevent segmentation errors when using only gradient-based information in definition of the speed. Four main kinds of regularizers were identified by the review authors:

1. clustering-based regularizers;

2. Bayesian-based regularizers;

3. Shape-based regularizers;

4. Coupling-surfaces regularizers.

We will now give a brief overview of each method.

4.3.1. Clustering-Based Regularizers

Clustering-based regularizers: Suri [31] has proposed the following energy functional for level set segmentation:

$$\frac{\partial \Phi}{\partial t} = (\varepsilon k + F_p)|\nabla \Phi| - F_{ext}\nabla \Phi, \tag{16}$$

where F_p is a regional force term expressed as a combination of the inside and outside regional area of the propagating curve. The term is proportional to a region indicator taking a value between 0 and 1, derived from a fuzzy membership measure. The second part of the classical energy model constituted the external force given by F_{ext}. This external energy term depends upon image forces that are a function of the image gradient.

4.3.2. Bayesian-based regularizers

Baillard et al. [35] proposed an approach similar to the previous one where the level set energy functional is expressed as

$$\frac{\partial \Phi}{\partial t} = g(|\nabla I|)(k + F_0)|\nabla \Phi|. \tag{17}$$

It employs a modified propagation term F_0 as a local force term. This term was derived from the probability density functions inside and outside the structure to be segmented.

4.3.3. Shape-based regularizers

Another application of the fusion of Bayesian statistics with the geometric boundary/surface to model the shape within the level set framework was done by Leventon et al. [36]. The authors introduced shape-based regularizers where curvature profiles act as boundary regularization terms more specific to the shape in order to extract more than standard curvature terms. A shape model is built from a set of segmented exemplars using principal component analysis applied to the signed-distance level set functions derived from the training shapes (analogous to Cootes et al.'s [55] technique). The principal modes of variation around a mean shape are computed. Projection coefficients of a shape on the identified principal vectors are referred to as shape parameters. Rigid transformation parameters aligning the evolving curve and the shape model are referred to as pose parameters. To be able to include a global shape constraint in the level set speed term, shape and pose parameters of the final curve $\Phi^*(t)$ are estimated using the maximum a posteriori estimation. The new functional is the solution for the evolving surface, expressed as

$$\Phi(t+1) = \Phi(t) + \lambda_1(g(|\nabla I|)(k+c)|\nabla \Phi| + \nabla g(|\nabla I|).\nabla \Phi) + \lambda_2(\Phi^*(t) - \Phi(t)), \tag{18}$$

where λ_1 and λ_2 are two parameters that balance the influence of the gradient-curvature term and the shape-model term.

In [56], Leventon et al. proposed further refinements of their method by introducing prior intensity and curvature models using statistical image–surface relationships in the regularizer terms. Some clinical validation has reported showing efficient and robust performance of the method.

4.3.4. Coupling-surfaces regularizers

This kind of regularizer was motivated by segmentation of embedded organs such as the brain cortical gray matter. The application is to attempt to employ a level set segmentation framework to perform simultaneous segmentation of the inner and outer organ surfaces with coupled level set functions. This method was proposed by Zeng et al. [32]. In this framework, segmentation is performed with the following system of equations:

$$\begin{cases} \Phi_{\text{in}} + F_{\text{in}}|\nabla\Phi_{\text{in}}| = 0, \\ \Phi_{\text{out}} + F_{\text{out}}|\nabla\Phi_{\text{out}}| = 0. \end{cases} \tag{19}$$

where the terms F_{in} and F_{out} are functions of the surface normal direction (e.g., curvature), image-derived information and the distance between the two surfaces. When this distance is within the desired range, the two surfaces propagate according to the first two terms of the speed term. When the distance is outside the desired range, the speed term based on the distance controls the deformation so as to correct for the surface positions.

4.4. Region-Based Active Contour Models

These classical snakes and active contour models rely on the edge function, depending on the image gradient, to stop curve evolution, and these models can detect only objects with edges defined by the gradient. Some of the typical edge functions are illustrated in Figure 13. In practice, the discrete gradients are bounded, and then the stopping function is never zero on the edges, and the curve may pass through the boundary. If the image is very noisy, the isotropic smoothing Gaussian has to be strong, which will smooth the edges as well. This region-based active contour method is a different active contour model, without a stopping edge-function, i.e., a model that is not based on the gradient of the image for the stopping process.

4.4.1. Mumford-Shah (MS) function

One kind of stopping term is based on the Mumford-Shah [57] segmentation techniques. In this way, the model can detect contours with or without gradient, for instance, objects with very smooth boundaries or even with discontinuous

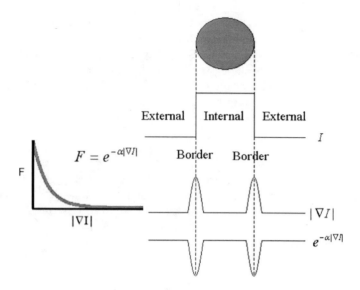

Figure 13. Typical definition of the edge functions to control propagation of the moving front.

boundaries. In addition, the model has a level set formulation, interior contours are automatically detected, and the initial curve can be anywhere within the image.

The original MS function is defined as follows:

$$F^{MS}(u, C) = \mu Length(C) \quad + \quad \lambda \int_{\Omega} |u_0(x, y) - u(x, y)|^2 \, dxdy$$

$$+ \quad \lambda \int_{\Omega \backslash C} |\nabla u(x, y)|^2 \, dxdy, \qquad (20)$$

where u_0 approximates original image u, u_o does not vary too much on each segmented region, and the boundary C is becoming as short as possible. In fact, u_0 is simply a cartoon version of the original image u. Basically, u_0 is a new image with edges drawn sharply. The objects are drawn smoothly without texture. Such cartoons are perceived correctly as representing the same scene as a simplification of the scene containing most of its essential features. In Chan and Vese's approach [58], a level set approach is proposed to solve the modified Mumford-Shah functional.

4.4.2. The level set approach to solve the Mumford-Shah function

In order to explain this model clearly, let us first define the evolving curve C in Ω as the boundary of an open subset w of Ω (i.e., $w \subset \Omega$, and $C = \partial w$). In what follows, inside(C) denotes the region w, and outside(C) denotes the region $\Omega \backslash \bar{w}$. The method is the minimization of an energy based-segmentation. Assume that the image u_0 is formed by two regions of approximatively piecewise-constant intensities, of distinct values u_0^i and u_0^o. Assume further that the object to be detected is represented by the region with the value u_0^i. Denote its boundary by C_0. Then we have $u_0 \approx u_0^i$ inside the object [or inside (C_0)], and $u_0 \approx u_0^o$ outside the object [or outside (C_0)]. The following fitting term is defined as:

$$F_1(C) + F_2(C) = \int_{\text{inside}(C)} |u_0(x,y) - c_1|^2 \, dx dy$$
$$+ \int_{\text{outside}(C)} |u_0(x,y) - c_2|^2 \, dx dy, \tag{21}$$

where C is any other variable curve, and the constants c_1, c_2, depending on C, are the averages of u_0 inside C and, respectively, outside C. In this simple case, it is obvious that C_0, the boundary of the object, is the minimizer of the fitting term:

$$\inf_C \{F_1(C) + F_2(C)\} \approx 0 \approx F_1(C_0) + F_2(C_0). \tag{22}$$

If the curve C is outside the object, then $F_1(C) > 0$ and $F_2(C) \approx 0$. If the curve C is inside the object, then $F_1(C) \approx 0$ and $F_2(C) > 0$. If the curve C is both inside and outside the object, then $F_1(C) > 0$ and $F_2(C) > 0$. The fitting term is minimized when $C = C_0$, i.e., the curve C is on the boundary of the object (Figure 14).

In order to solve more complicated segmentation, we require regularizing terms, like the length of the curve C, or the area of the region inside C. A new energy functional $F(c_1, c_2, C)$ is defined as

$$F(c_1, c_2, C) = \mu \cdot \text{Length}(C) + \nu \cdot \text{Area}(\text{inside}(C)) +$$
$$\lambda_1 \int_{\text{inside}(C)} |u_0(x,y) - c_1|^2 \, dx dy +$$
$$\lambda_2 \int_{\text{outside}(C)} |u_0(x,y) - c_2|^2 \, dx dy, \tag{23}$$

where $\mu \geq 0$, $\nu \geq 0$, $\lambda_1, \lambda_2 \geq 0$. (In Chan-Vese's approach, $\lambda_1 = \lambda_2 = 1$ and $\nu = 0$). Correspondingly, the level set based on C is defined as

$$\left\{ \begin{array}{c} C = \partial w = \{(x,y) \in \Omega : \Phi(x,y) = 0\} \\ \text{inside}(C) = w = \{(x,y) \in \Omega : \Phi(x,y) > 0\} \\ \text{outside}(C) = \Omega \backslash \bar{w} = \{(x,y) \in \Omega : \Phi(x,y) < 0\} \end{array} \right\}. \tag{24}$$

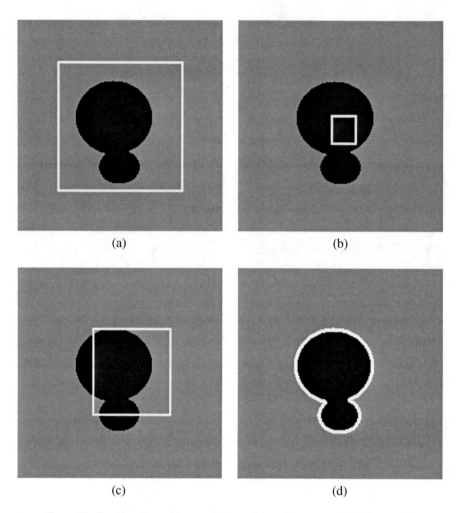

Figure 14. Consider all possible cases in the position of the curve. The fitting term is minimized only in the case when the curve is on the boundary of the object. (a) The curve C is outside the object, and $F_1(C) > 0$ and $F_2(C) \approx 0$. (b) The curve C is inside the object; then $F_1(C) \approx 0$ and $F_2(C) > 0$. (c) The curve C is both inside and outside the object; then $F_1(C) > 0$ and $F_2(C) > 0$. (d) The fitting term is minimized when the curve C is on the boundary of the object.

So, the unknown C could be replaced by Φ. Using Heaviside function H and Dirac measure Δ_0, which are defined by

$$H(z) = \begin{cases} 1, & (z \geq 0) \\ 0, & (z < 0) \end{cases}, \delta_0 = \frac{dH(z)}{dz}, \tag{25}$$

the energy function $F(c_1, c_2, C)$ can be rewritten as

$$F(c_1, c_2, \Phi) = \mu \int_\Omega \delta(\Phi(x,y))|\nabla\Phi(x,y)| \, dxdy + \nu \int_\Omega H(\Phi(x,y)) \, dxdy$$
$$+\lambda_1 \int_{inside(C)} |u_0(x,y) - c_1|^2 H(\Phi(x,y)) \, dxdy$$
$$+\lambda_2 \int_{outside(C)} |u_0(x,y) - c_2|^2 (1 - H(\Phi(x,y))) \, dxdy$$

$$(26)$$

where $c_1(\Phi)$ and $c_2(\Phi)$ are defined as

$$c_1(\Phi) = \frac{\int_\Omega u_0(x,y) H(\Phi(x,y)) \, dxdy}{\int_\Omega H(\Phi(x,y)) \, dxdy},$$

$$c_2(\Phi) = \frac{\int_\Omega u_0(x,y)(1 - H(\Phi(x,y))) \, dxdy}{\int_\Omega (1 - H(\Phi(x,y))) \, dxdy}.$$

$$(27)$$

Finally, the corresponding level set equation that is minimizing the energy can be solved by the following equation:

$$\frac{\partial \Phi}{\partial t} = \delta(\Phi)[\mu div(\frac{\nabla\Phi}{|\nabla\Phi|}) - \nu - \lambda_1(u_0 - c_1)^2 + \lambda_2(u_0 - c_2)^2].$$

$$(28)$$

The level set equation could be solved iteratively using time step Δt. However, there are inherent time step requirements to ensure the stability of the numerical scheme via the CFL condition. In Chan and Vese's approach, the time step can be set based on the following equation:

$$\Delta t \leq \frac{min(\Delta x, \Delta y, \Delta z)}{(|\mu| + |\nu| + |\lambda_0 + \lambda_1|)}.$$

$$(29)$$

4.4.3. Applications of the region-based active contour

One example using the region-based active contour proposed by Chan and Vese in 2001 is demonstrated Figure 15. The original image to be segmented was badly noised, with the initial contour labeled in red and the final segmentation based on Eq. (23). In this example, the initial contour was not strictly placed inside or outside the object to be segmented. What is more, the 2D curvature was taken as the approximation for $div(\frac{\nabla\Phi}{|\nabla\Phi|})$.

The authors of [59] presented an implementation and validation of a 3D deformable model method based on Chan and Vese's energy functional for segmentation of 3D real-time ultrasound. The clinical study showed superior performance of the deformable model in assessing ejection fraction (EF) when compared to MRI measures. It also showed that the three-dimensional deformable model improved EF measures, which is explained by a more accurate segmentation of small

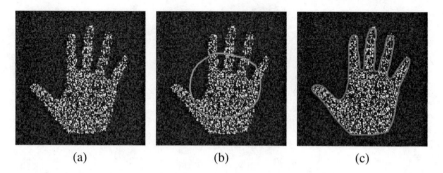

Figure 15. Segmentation using a region-based active contour: (a) original image; (b) image with initial contour; (c) image with segmentation result. See attached CD for color version.

and convoluted ventricular shapes when integrating the third spatial dimension. From this work the reader will also find out how to assign parameters for specific situations.

5. IMAGE SEGMENTATION USING SHAPE PRIOR

Missing or diffuse boundaries can be a very challenging problem in medical image processing, which may be due to patient movement, a low signal-to-noise (SNR) ratio of the acquisition apparatus, or blending with similar surrounding tissues. Under such conditions, without an a prior model to constrain the segmentation, most algorithms (including intensity- and curve-based techniques) fail— mostly due to the underdetermined nature of the segmentation process. Similar problems arise in other imaging applications as well, and they also hinder segmentation of an image. These image segmentation problems demand the incorporation of as much prior information as possible to help the segmentation algorithms extract the tissue of interest.

A number of model-based image segmentation algorithms in the literature were used to deal with cases when boundaries in medical images are smeared or missing. In 1995, Cootes et al. [55] developed a parametric point distribution model (PDM) for describing the segmenting curve by using linear combinations of the eigenvectors that reflect variations from the mean shape. The shape and pose parameters of this point distribution model were determined to match the points to strong image gradients. Wang and Staib [60] developed a statistical point model in 1998 for the segmenting curve by applying principal component analysis (PCA) to the covariance matrices that capture the statistical variations of the landmark points. They formulated their edge-detection and correspondence-determination problem in a maximum a posteriori Bayesian framework. The image gradient was used within that framework to calculate the pose and shape parameters that describe their segmenting curve. Leventon et al. [56] proposed a less restrictive model-based segmenter. They incorporated shape information as a prior model to restrict the flow of the geodesic active contour. Their prior parametric shape model was derived by performing PCA on a collection of signed distance maps of the training shape. The segmenting curve then evolves according to the gradient force of the image and the force exerted by the estimated shape. In 2002, Mitchell et al. [61] developed a model-based method for three-dimensional image segmentation. Comprehensive design of a three-dimensional (3D) active appearance model (AAM) was reported for the first time as an involved extension of the AAM framework introduced by Cootes et al. [62]. The model's behavior is learned from manually traced segmentation examples during an automated training stage. Information about shape and image appearance of the cardiac structures is contained in a single model. The clinical potential of the 3D AAM is demonstrated in short-axis cardiac MR images and four-chamber echocardiographic sequences. The AAM method showed good agreement with an independent standard using quantitative indices of border positioning errors, endocardial and epicardial volumes, and left-ventricular mass. The AAM method shows high promise for successful application to MR and echocardiographic image analysis in a clinical setting. The reported method combined the appearance feature with the shape knowledge, and it provided robust matching criteria for segmentation. However, this method needs to set up point correspondence, and it makes the procedure complicated.

The authors of [37] adopted implicit representation of the segmenting curve proposed in [36] and calculated the parameters of the implicit model to minimize the region-based energy based on a Mumford-Shah functional for image segmentation [58]. The proposed method gives a new and efficient framework for segmenting an image contaminated with heavy noise and delineating structures complicated by missing or diffuse boundaries. In the next section we will give a detailed description of this framework in a 2D space. The flowchart of the method is depicted in Figure 16.

5.1. Shape Model Training

Given is a set of binary images $\{B_1, B_2, \ldots, B_n\}$, each of which with 1 as object and 0 as background. In order to extract the accurate shape information, alignment has to be applied. Alignment is a task to calculate the following pose parameters $p = [a \ b \ h \ \theta]^T$, and correspondingly, these four parameters are for translation in x, y, scale, and rotation:

$$T(p) = \begin{bmatrix} 1 & 0 & a \\ 0 & 1 & b \\ 0 & 0 & 1 \end{bmatrix} \begin{bmatrix} h & 0 & 0 \\ 0 & h & 0 \\ 0 & 0 & h \end{bmatrix} \begin{bmatrix} \cos(\theta) & -\sin(\theta) & 0 \\ \sin(\theta) & \cos(\theta) & 0 \\ 0 & 0 & 1 \end{bmatrix}. \tag{30}$$

The strategy for computing the pose parameters for n binary images is to use the gradient descent method to minimize the special designed energy functional

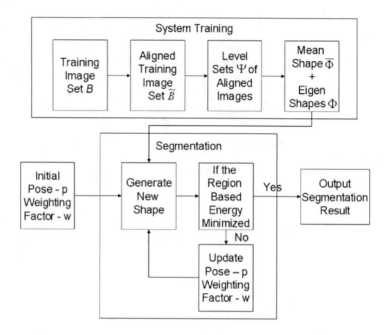

Figure 16. Flowchart of the algorithm presented in [37]. Basically, there are two stages. The first stage is system training to extract shape model, and the second is to segment the image using the shape model.

E^j_{align} for each binary image corresponding to the fixed one, say the first binary image B_1, and the energy is defined as follows:

$$E^j_{align} = \frac{\int \int_\Omega (\tilde{B}_j - B_1)^2 dA}{\int \int_\Omega (\tilde{B}_j + B_1)^2 dA}, \tag{31}$$

where Ω denotes the image domain, and $\tilde{B}_j$ denotes the transformed image of B_j based on the pose parameters p. Minimizing this energy is equivalent to minimizing the difference between the current binary image and the fixed image in the training database. The normalization term in the denominator is employed to prevent the images from shrinking to improve the cost function. Hill climbing or the Rprop method could be applied for the gradient descent.

An example is depicted in Figures 17 and 18 regarding the alignment procedure. There are in total 15 binary images about different plane shapes.

The popular and natural approach to represent shapes is by employing point models where a set of marker points is often used to describe the boundaries of the shape. This approach suffers from problems such as numerical instability, inability

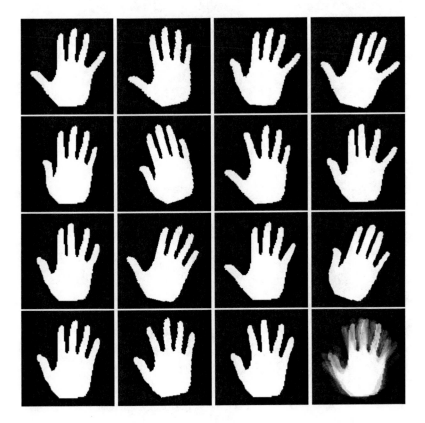

Figure 17. Binary images for training before alignment. The last image is the overlapping image before alignment.

to accurately capture high-curvature locations, difficulty in handling topological changes, and the need for point correspondences. In order to overcome these problems, an Eulerian approach to shape representation based on the level set methods of Osher and Sethian [41] can be utilized.

The signed distance function is chosen as the representation for shape. In particular, the boundaries of each of the aligned shapes are embedded as the zero level set of separate signed distance functions $\{\Psi_1, \Psi_2, \ldots, \Psi_n\}$, with negative distances assigned to the inside and positive distances assigned to the outside of the object. The mean level set function of the shape database as the average of these signed distance functions can be computed as $\bar{\Phi} = \frac{1}{n} \sum_{i=1}^{n} \Psi_i$. Figure 19 illustrates the implicit level set representation of the average shape and the zero level set represents the boundary of the average model.

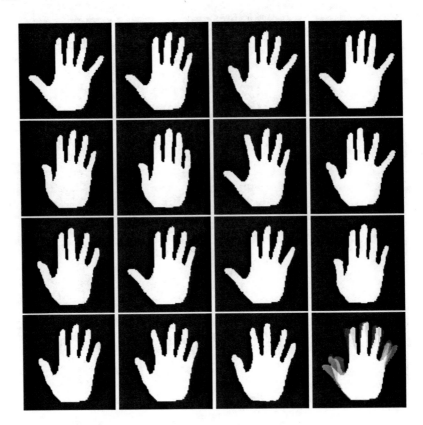

Figure 18. Binary image after alignment. The last image is the overlapping image after alignment.

To extract the shape variabilities, $\bar{\Phi}$ is subtracted from each of the n signed distance functions to create n mean-offset functions $\{\tilde{\Psi}_1, \tilde{\Psi}_2, \ldots, \tilde{\Psi}_n\}$. These mean-offset functions are analyzed and then used to capture the variabilities of the training shapes.

Specifically, n column vectors are created, $\tilde{\psi}_i$, from each $\tilde{\Psi}_1$. A natural strategy is to utilize the $N_1 \times N_2$ rectangular grid of the training images to generate $N = N_1 \times N_2$ lexicographically ordered samples (where the columns of the image grid are sequentially stacked on top of one another to form one large column). Next, we define the shape-variability matrix S as $S = [\tilde{\psi}_1, \tilde{\psi}_2, \ldots, \tilde{\psi}_n]$. The procedure for creation of the matrix S is shown in Figure 20.

An eigenvalue decomposition is employed to such that

$$\frac{1}{n}SS^T = U\Sigma U^T, \tag{32}$$

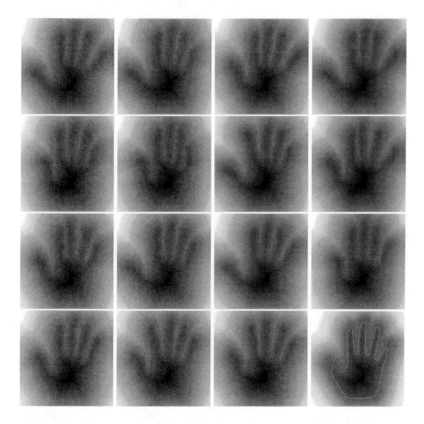

Figure 19. The level set for each image after alignment. The last image is the average level set, overlapped with the average shape after training. See attached CD for color version.

where U is an $N = N \times n$ matrix whose columns represent the orthogonal modes of variation in the shape, and Σ is an $n \times n$ diagonal matrix whose diagonal elements represent the corresponding nonzero eigenvalues. The N elements of the ith column of U, denoted by U_i, are arranged back into the structure of the $N = N_1 \times N_2$ rectangular image grid (by undoing the earlier lexicographical concatenation of the grid columns) to yield Φ_i, the ith principal mode or eigenshape. Based on this approach, a maximum of n different eigenshapes $\{\Phi_1, \Phi_2, \ldots, \Phi_n\}$ are generated. In most cases, the dimension of the matrix $\frac{1}{n}SS^T$ is large so that the calculation of the eigenvectors and eigenvalues of this matrix is computationally expensive. In practice, the eigenvectors and eigenvalues of $\frac{1}{n}SS^T$ can be efficiently computed from a much smaller $n \times n$ matrix W given by $\frac{1}{n}S^TS$. It is straightforward to show that if d is an eigenvector of W with corresponding eigenvalue λ, then Sd is an eigenvector of $\frac{1}{n}SS^T$ with eigenvalue λ.

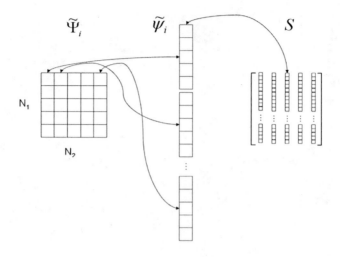

Figure 20. Creating the shape-variability matrix S.

For segmentation, it is not necessary to use all the shape variabilities after the above procedure. Let $k \leq n$, which is selected prior to segmentation, be the number of modes to consider. In general, k should be chosen large enough to be able to capture the main shape variations present in the training set. One way to choose the value of k is by examining the eigenvalues of the corresponding eigenvectors. In some sense, the size of each eigenvalue indicates the amount of influence or importance its corresponding eigenvector has in determining the shape. By looking at a histogram of the eigenvalues, one can estimate the threshold for determining the value of k. However, an automated algorithm is hard to implement as the threshold value for k varies for each different application. It is hard to define a universal k that can be set. The histogram of the eigenvalues for the above examples are listed in the Figure 21.

The eigenshapes are listed in Figure 22. In total there are 15 eigenshapes, corresponding to the 15 eigenvalues. Only the 12 2D eigenshapes of the first 12 eigenvalues are listed in the figure.

A new level set function,

$$\Phi[w] = \bar{\Phi} + \sum_{i=1}^{k} w_i \Phi_i, \tag{33}$$

where $w = \{w_1, w_2, \ldots, w_k\}$ are the weights for the k eigenshapes with the variances of these weights $\{\sigma_1^2, \sigma_2^2, \ldots, \sigma_k^2\}$ given by the eigenvalues calculated earlier. Now we can use this newly constructed level set function Φ as the implicit representation of shape. Specifically, the zero level set of Φ describes the shape,

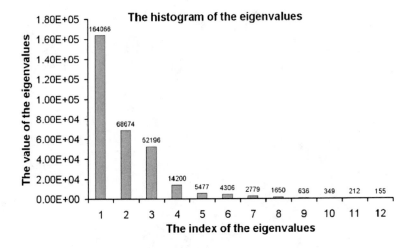

Figure 21. Histogram of the first 12 eigenvalues after PCA analysis on the 12 hand images.

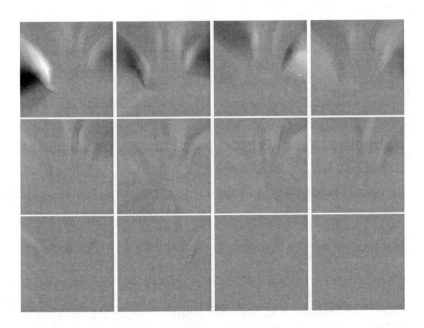

Figure 22. Output eigenshapes that have been scaled into the 0–255 range for illustration. Correspondingly, the largest 12 eigenvalues are 164066, 68674, 52196, 14200, 5477, 4306, 2779, 1650, 636, 349, 212, and 155. The smaller the value of the eignvalues, the smaller roles the eigenshapes will play in shape variation.

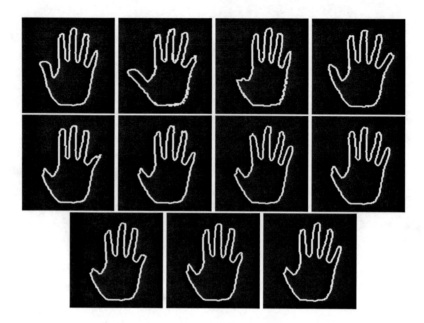

Figure 23. The first row is the shape after using the weight factor only from the first eigenshape. From left to right, the values of w are -0.3 and 0.3. The second row is the shape after using the weight factor only from the second eigenshape, and the same for other rows. The only image in the second column is the average shape without any shape variations.

with the shape's variability directly linked to the variability of the level set function. Therefore, by varying w, Φ will be changed, which indirectly varies the shape. However, the shape variability allowed in this representation is restricted to the variability given by the eigenshapes. Several examples are illustrated in Figure 23 using different w to control the shape. From this example, the reader will find it is very powerful to use different w for different eigenshapes to control shape variations.

5.2. Model for Segmentation

As of now, the training procedure is concluded, and we can make full use of the information after shape analysis. However, the implicit representation of shape cannot accommodate shape variabilities due to a differences in pose. To have the flexibility of handling pose variations, p is added as another parameter to the level set function:

$$\Phi[w, p](x, y) = \bar{\Phi}(\tilde{x}, \tilde{y}) + \sum_{i=1}^{n} w_i \Phi_i(\tilde{x}, \tilde{y}), \tag{34}$$

where

$$
\begin{bmatrix} x \\ y \\ 1 \end{bmatrix} = T(p) \begin{bmatrix} \tilde{x} \\ \tilde{y} \\ 1 \end{bmatrix}. \tag{35}
$$

As a segmentation using shape knowledge, the task is to calculate w and pose parameters p. The strategy for this calculation is quite similar to the image alignment for training. The only difference is the specially defined energy function for minimization.

Energy minimization is based on Chan and Vese's active model as defined by Eq. (23), which is equivalent (up to a term that does not depend upon the evolving curve), to the energy functional below:

$$
E_{cv} = -(\mu^2 A_u + \nu^2 A_v) = - \left(\frac{S_u^2}{A_u} + \frac{S_v^2}{A_v} \right). \tag{36}
$$

Before explaining the special features of the above equation, additional terms are defined. The regions inside and outside the zero level set are denoted as R^u and R^v:

$$
R^u = \{(x,y) \in R^2 : \Phi(x,y) < 0\}, \quad R^v = \{(x,y) \in R^2 : \Phi(x,y) > 0\}. \tag{37}
$$

The area in R^u is A_u, the area in R^v is A_v, the sum intensity in R^u is S_u, the sum intensity in R^v is S_v, the average intensity in R^u is $\mu = \frac{S_u}{A_u}$, and the average intensity in R^v is $\nu = \frac{S_v}{A_v}$. The Chan-Vese energy functional can be viewed as a piecewise constant generalization of the Mumford-Shah functional. Based on this energy definition and the corresponding solution, the next step is to find the corresponding w and p to implicitly determine the segmenting curve. The gradients of the energy F are taken with respect to w and p. The gradient descent scheme like Hill climbing or Rprop [63], can be utilized to finally find the value of w and p.

In addition to the energy function introduced above, several other similar region-based energy functions are defined in [37]. The reader may refer to Tsai's work for more details.

In the following, we applied the hand shape into a segmentation procedure (see Figure 24).

We now present another example using the shape prior active contour based on level set methods, which involves mitotic cell segmentation. The first step is to align all the training images until the overlapping error is minimized. Then principal components analysis (PCA) is then utilized to extract the eigenvalues and eigenvectors for the shape variance. Next, the mean shape is computed. With all this information, a target image is tested. The initial contour is the mean shape. After using the Rprop method, the program yields the final segmentation

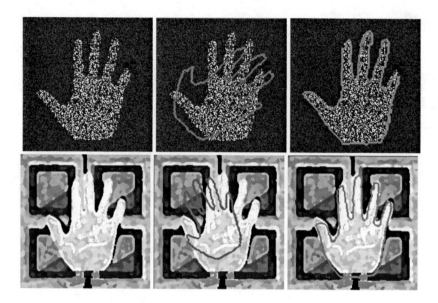

Figure 24. Segmentation using shape prior active contour. The first column includes the original noisy images for segmentation. The second column shows the images overlapped with initial average shape. The third column are the images with the final segmentation results. See attached CD for color version.

(see Figure 25). This method will automatically deal with the topological changes during training and segmentation that is due to the level set representation method.

There are many methods that can be utilized to adjust parameters for the model-based segmentation. Artificial neural networks, like Multi-Layer Perceptrons (MLPs), have become standard tools for regression. In general, an MLP with fixed structure defines a differentiable mapping from a parameter space to the space of functions. In the case where an MLP is with a fixed structure, a regression problem enters into the adaptation of parameters: the weights of the network given the sample data. This procedure is often referred to as learning. Because MLPs are differentiable, gradient-based adaptation techniques are typically applied to determine the weights. The earliest and most straightforward adaptation rule, ordinary gradient descent, adapts weights proportional to the partial derivatives of the error functional. Several improvements on this basic adaptation rule have been proposed, some based on elaborated heuristics, others on theoretical reconsideration of gradient-based learning. Resilient backpropagation (Rprop) is a well-established modification of the ordinary gradient descent. The basic idea is to adjust individual step size for each parameter to be optimized. These step sizes are not proportional to the partial derivatives but are themselves adapted based on

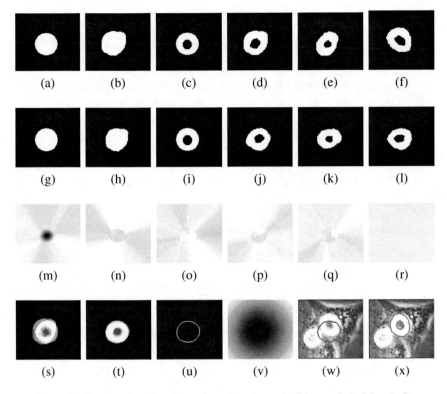

Figure 25. Segmentation using shape prior active contour: (a–f) images for training; (g–l) aligned training images; (m–r) eigenvectors after principal components analysis; (s) overlap before aligning; (t) overlap after aligning; (u) zero level set of the mean shape; (v) level set of mean shape; (w) target image to be segmented with initial contour; (x) segmentation result. See attached CD for color version.

some heuristics. Ordinary gradient descent computes the direction of the steepest descent by implicitly assuming a Euclidean metric on the weight space.

The Rprop algorithms are among the best performing first-order batch learning methods. There are many advantages for Rprop methods:

1. Speed and accuracy.

2. Robustness.

3. First-order methods; therefore, time and space complexity scales linearly with the number of parameters to be optimized.

4. Only dependent on the sign of the partial derivatives of the objective function and not on their amount; therefore, they are suitable for applications

where the gradient is numerically estimated or the objective function is noisy.

5. Easy to implement and not very sensitive to numerical problems.

The Rprop algorithms are iterative optimization methods. Let t denote the current iteration (epoch). In epoch t, each weight is changed according to

$$w^i(t+1) = w^i(t) - \text{sign}\left(\frac{\partial E(t)}{\partial w^i}\right) . \Delta^i(t). \tag{38}$$

The direction of the change depends on the sign of the partial derivative, but is independent of its amount. The individual step sizes $\Delta^i(t)$ are adapted based on changes of sign of the partial derivatives of $E(w)$ w.r.t. the corresponding weight:

- if $\frac{\partial E(t-1)}{\partial w^i} \cdot \frac{\partial E(t)}{\partial w^i} > 0$, then $\Delta^i(t)$ is increased by a factor $\eta^+ > 1$.

- if $\frac{\partial E(t-1)}{\partial w^i} \cdot \frac{\partial E(t)}{\partial w^i} \leq 0$, then $\Delta^i(t)$ is decreased by a factor $\eta^- \in [0, 1]$.

Additionally, some Rprop methods implement weight-backtracking, that is, they partially retract "unfavorable" previous steps. Whether a weight change was "unfavorable" is decided by a heuristic. In the following an improved version [64] of the original algorithm is described in pseudo-code. The difference compared to the original Rprop method is that the weight-backtracking heuristic considers both the evolution of the partial derivatives and the overall error:

1. Step 1. Enter the iteration n.

2. Step 2. For each weighting factor w^i, if $\frac{\partial E(t-1)}{\partial w^i} \cdot \frac{\partial E(t)}{\partial w^i} > 0$, then:

$$\begin{aligned} &\min(\Delta^i(t-1) \cdot \eta^+, \Delta_{\max}), \\ &w^i(t+1) = w^i(t) - \text{sign}\left(\frac{\partial E(t)}{\partial w^i}\right) . \Delta^i(t), \end{aligned} \tag{39}$$

3. Step 3. Elseif $\frac{\partial E(t-1)}{\partial w^i} \cdot \frac{\partial E(t)}{\partial w^i} < 0$, then: $\min(\Delta^i(t-1) \cdot \eta^-, \Delta_{\min})$ if $E(t) > E(t-1)$, then $w^i(t+1) = w^i(t-1)$, $\frac{\partial E(t)}{\partial w^i} = 0$.

4. Step 4. Elseif $\frac{\partial E(t-1)}{\partial w^i} \cdot \frac{\partial E(t)}{\partial w^i} = 0$, and then

$$w^i(t+1) = w^i(t) - \text{sign}\left(\frac{\partial E(t)}{\partial w^i}\right) \cdot \Delta^i(t). \tag{40}$$

5. Step 5. If there is still w^i to be updated, go to step 2; otherwise go to Step 6.

6. Step 6. If no more iteration is needed, exit. Otherwise, $n = n + 1$ go to Step 2.

In the following, the energy change though the first segmentation example in Figure 23 is plotted in Figure 26.

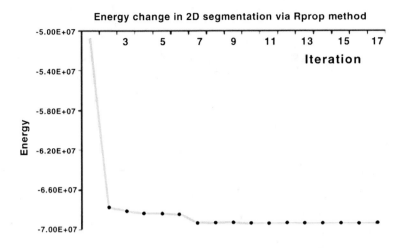

Figure 26. The region-based energy is decreasing as the Rprop method is applied for the 2D model-based segmentation.

5.3. Extend to Higher-Dimensional Problems

From the previous section, solution for the 2D segmentation using a shape model was introduced. As the imaging technology is becoming more and more powerful in clinical usage and medical research, 3D volumetric datasets or even 4D image datasets are used more often in diagnosis. Higher-dimensional imaging has multiple advantages over 2D imaging in many aspects. It can provide accurate quantification of the volumes and shape for the organ under observation without the need for geometric assumptions. It may also improve visualization of spatial relations between structures at different phases that are not readily obtained from conventional 2D images.

It is not a complicated task to extend the 2D version of the shape-based segmentation using level set methods to a higher-dimensional space. In the following, a 3D example is illustrated that is from synthesized 3D images. In Figure 27, five 3D images are listed that are used for training. The size of the image is 100 × 100 × 100 voxels. In Figure 28, six new shapes are generated by using the 3D eigenvalues after PCA in the training stage.

After 3D training, we applied the shape information to 3D segmentation. In Figure 29 the reader will find an extremely noised 3D image where a dumbbell-like shape is on the inside. Initially, the average shape is placed in the center of the 3D image. Then 3D model-based segmentation is applied. Three key steps illustrated in Figure 29. The red contours in the left column correspond to the current segmentation. The left column is the surface rendering of the current

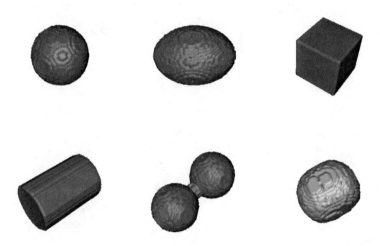

Figure 27. 3D images for training before alignment. The last image is the average 3D shape after training. See attached CD for color version.

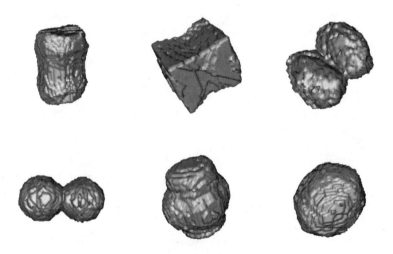

Figure 28. The first column are the two new shapes using the weight factor only from the first eigenshape, +1 and −1; correspondingly, the second column are the new shapes using the weight factor only from the second eigenshape, and the third column are from the third. See attached CD for color version.

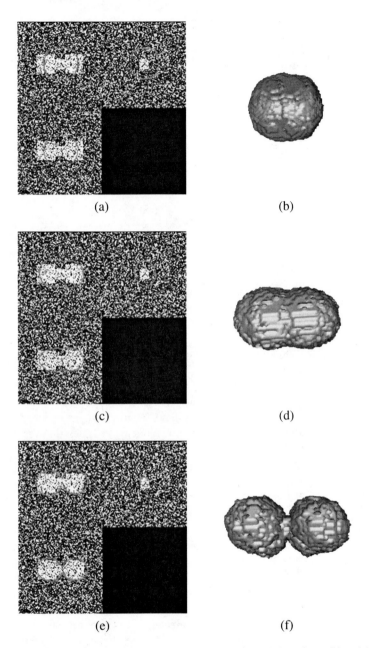

Figure 29. Example of 3D shape model-based segmentation: (a) three views of the original image to be segmented and the initial 3D average shape overlaid inside; (b) average 3D shape after surface rendering; (c) 3D surface at an interim step of the segmentation overlaid inside the original image; (d) surface rendering of the current 3D shape; (e) three views of the final segmentation; (f) surface rendering of the final segmentation. See attached CD for color version.

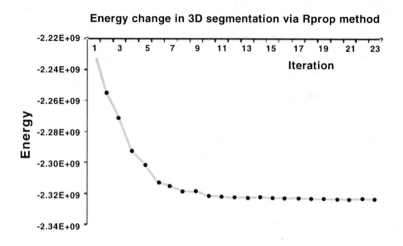

Figure 30. The region-based energy is decreasing as the Rprop method is applied for the 3D model-based segmentation.

segmentation. Correspondingly, the change in energy as the Rprop method was applied is plotted in Figure 30.

Practical medical imaging applications have been widely reported the literature. In [37], a 3D application was introduced that involves automated segmentation of the prostate from pelvic MRI, taken in conjunction with an endorectal coil (ERC) using T_1 and T_2 weighting. This imaging modality provides high-resolution images of the prostate with a smaller field of view and a thinner slice thickness than previously attainable. For assignment of appropriate radiation therapy after cancer detection, segmentation of the prostate gland from these pelvic MRI images is required. The authors employed a 3D version of the shape-based curve evolution technique to segment the prostate. By utilizing a 3D surface (instead of a 2D curve), the segmentation algorithm is able to utilize the full 3D spatial information to extract the boundaries of the prostate. A modified method was proposed in [65] that is for a similar application but from a different imaging modality: 3D CT scanning.

In the work of Rousson et al. [38], an example of similar analysis was introduced for 3D modeling of lateral brain ventricles. The model was built using a number of 3D surfaces from different subjects. This application showed the advantage of using the level set method to deal with topologies within the training set, like the separation between left and right ventricles. This 3D method can deal with noisy, incomplete, and occluded data because of its active shape nature. It is an intrinsic, implicit parameter and topology free, a natural property of the level set space. The brain ventricle extraction demonstrated the potential of the method in a higher-dimensional space.

Freedman et al. [65] presented an algorithm that uses learned models for both the shape and appearance of objects to achieve segmentation, which involves learning both types of information. The authors the application of the algorithm to segmentation of the prostate, as well as adjacent radiation-sensitive organs (e.g., bladder and rectum) from 3D computed tomography (CT) imagery, for the purpose of improving radiation therapy. The main innovation of this method over similar approaches is that there is no need to compute a pixel-wise correspondence between the model and the image; however, appearance information could be fully utilized.

6. CONCLUSIONS

Segmentation of deformable objects from medical images is an important and challenging problem. In the context of medical imagery, the main challenges include the following: (1) the edge information of the objects is too weak, (2) many objects have similar intensity profiles or appearance, and (3) a lot of the objects have a similar shape. Existing algorithms that use both shape and appearance models require a pixel-wise correspondence between the model and the image; this correspondence problem can sometimes be difficult to solve efficiently.

One type of segmentation algorithm incorporates learned shape models for the objects of interest using level set methods. One advantage with this method is that there is no need to compute a pixel-wise correspondence between the model and the image. The algorithm allows the shape to evolve until the optimal segmentation is found by minimizing a region-based energy factor.

In this chapter, this type of segmentation method was introduced in detail and practical applications were demonstrated. The applications not only proved that the method is an efficient and accurate solution in medical image analysis, but new attempts were also made to improve the original algorithm.

Although there are many advantages using the above methods within a level set framework, the computational cost is still a large barrier. The level set method is famous for speed due to heap sorting and signed distance transformation, but there are still many problems for advanced application in level set frameworks. For one thing, the Mumford-Shah model is fast without using the level set method, but, using the level set method, the iterative update of the level set brings a huge burden in terms of computation. From the segmentation results in [58], the reader will find that the approach is way too slow. (Like Figure 10 in [58], small images (e.g., 100×100) took more than 144 seconds to obtain the final segmentation.)

One important reason is solution of the PDEs involved in the frameworks. Efforts have been made to speed up the computation, e.g., estimation of the PDE [66], a multi-resolution approach [37], etc. However, it is limited to one aspect of the problem. Convergence of the gradient decent method is also playing a key role in the shape-based method. Therefore, processing speed is a big drawback of this method. Besides, for image segmentation, the initial position of the average shape is of great importance to the final segmentation. For complicated medical images, if the surrounding context around the object to be segmented has occupied a very large portion of the whole image, and similar structures are present in the images, the gradient descent method is not able to move the initial average shape to the place where the object is located, because the energy minimization method scheme makes the segmentation become stuck in a non-object position due to the local minimum. So, preprocessing has to be performed to restrict the segmentation to a smaller region. Or, statistic parameters can be assigned to the pose factors. For example, the largest size of the object (scaling), the largest tilting of the object (rotation), etc. However, this extra preprocessing will make the system more complex, with an unwieldy number of new parameters for controlling segmentation. Therefore, there is yet much work to be done to make the shape-based segmentation method more efficient in level set frameworks.

7. ACKNOWLEDGMENTS

The research presented in this chapter was supported, in part, by the following NIH grants: R01-HL63373, R01-HL071809, R01-HL075446, R33-CA94801, and R01-HL64368.

8. REFERENCES

1. Suri JS, Liu K, Singh S, Laxminarayan S, Zeng X, Reden L. 2002. Shape recovery algorithms using level sets in 2-d/3-d medical imagery: a state-of-the-art review. *IEEE Trans Inform Technol Biomed* **6**:8–28.

2. Angenent S, Chopp D, Ilmanen T. 1995. On the singularities of cones evolving by mean curvature. *Commun Partial Differ Eq* **20**:1937–1958.

3. Chopp DL. 1993. Computing minimal surfaces via level set curvature flow. *J Comput Phys* **106**:77–91.

4. Sethian JA. 1990. Numerical algorithms for propagating interfaces: Hamilton-Jacobi equations and conservation laws. *J Differ Geom* **31**:131–161.

5. Sethian JA, Malladi R. 1996. An $O(N \log N)$ algorithm for shape modeling. *Proc Natl Acad Sci USA* **93**:9389–9392.

6. Sethian JA. 1995. Algorithms for tracking interfaces in CFD and material science. *Annu Rev Comput Fluid Mech* **12**:125–138.

7. Sussman M, Smereka P, Osher SJ. 1994. A level set method for computing solutions to incompressible two-phase flow. *J Comput Phys* **114**:146–159.

8. Rhee C, Talbot L, Sethian JA. 1995. Dynamical study of a premixed V-flame. *J Fluid Mech* **300**:87–115.

9. Sethian JA, Strain JD. 1992. Crystal growth and dentritic solidification. *J Comput Phys* **98**:231–253.

10. Adalsteinsson D, Sethian JA. 1995. A unified level set approach to etching, deposition and lithography, I: algorithms and two-dimensional simulations. *J Comput Phys* **120**:128–144.

11. Breen DE, Whitaker RT. 2001. A level-set approach for the metamorphosis of solid models. *IEEE Trans Visualiz Comput Graphics* **7**:173–192.

12. Mansouri AR, Konrad J. 1999. Motion segmentation with level sets. *IEEE Trans Image Process* **12**(2):201–220.

13. Paragios N, Deriche R. 2000. Geodesic active contours and level sets for the detection and tracking of moving objects. *IEEE Trans Pattern Anal Machine Intell* **22**(3):266–280.

14. Kornprobst P, Deriche R, Aubert G. 1999. Image sequence analysis via partial differential equations. *J Math Imaging Vision* **11**:5–26.

15. Faugeras O, Keriven R. 1998. Variational principles, surface evolution, PDEs, level set methods and the stereo problem. *IEEE Trans Image Process* **7**:336–344.

16. Kimmel R. 1995. Tracking level sets by level sets: a method for solving the shape from shading problem. *Comput Vision Image Understand* **62**:47–58.

17. Kimmel R, Bruckstein AM. 1995. Global shape from shading. *Comput Vision Image Understand* **62**:360–369.

18. Sapiro G, Kimmel R, Shaked D, Kimia BB, Bruckstein AM. 1997. Implementing continuous-scale morphology via curve evolution. *Pattern Recognit* **26**:1363–1372.

19. Sochen N, Kimmel R, Malladi R. 1998. A geometrical framework for low level vision. *IEEE Trans Image Process* **7**:310–318.

20. Sapiro G, 1997. Color snakes. *Comput Vision Image Understand* **68**:247–253.

21. Caselles V, Kimmel R, Sapiro G, Sbert C. 1996. Three dimensional object modeling via minimal surfaces. In *Proceedings of the European conference on computer vision (ECCV)*, pp. 97–106. New York: Springer.

22. Kimmel R, Amir A, Bruckstein AM. 1995. Finding shortest paths on surfaces using level sets propagation. *IEEE Trans Pattern Anal Machine Intell* **17**:635–640.

23. DeCarlo D, Gallier J. 1996. Topological evolution of surfaces. In *Proceedings of the graphics interface 1996 conference*, pp. 194–203. Ed WA Davis, RM Bartels. Mississauga, Ontario: Canadian Human-Computer Communications Society.

24. Telea A. 2004. An image inpainting technique based on the fast marching method. *Graphics Tools* **9**:23–24.

25. Suri JS. 2001. Two dimensional fast mr brain segmentation using a region-based level set approach. *Int J Eng Med Biol* **20**(4):84–95.

26. Malladi R, Sethian JA. 1998. A real-time algorithm for medical shape recovery. In *Proceedings of the international conference on computer vision (ICCV'98)*, pp. 304–310. Washington, DC: IEEE Computer Society.

27. Hermosillo G, Faugeras O, Gomes J. 1999. Unfolding the cerebral cortex using level set methods. In *Proceedings of the second international conference on scale-space theories in computer vision. Lecture notes in computer science*, Vol. 1682, pp. 58–69. New York: Springer.

28. Sarti A, Ortiz C, Lockett S, Malladi R. 1996. A unified geometric model for 3d confocal image analysis in cytology. In *Proceedings of the international symposium on computer graphics, image processing, and vision (SIBGRAPI'98)*, pp. 69–76. Washington, DC: IEEE Computer Society.

29. Niessen WJ, ter Haar Romeny BM, Viergever MA. 1998. Geodesic deformable models for medical image analysis. *IEEE Trans Med Imaging* **17**:634–641.

30. Gomes J, Faugeras O. 2000. Level sets and distance functions. In *Proceedings of the European conference on computer vision (ECCV)*, pp. 588–602. New York: Springer.

31. Suri JS. 2000. Leaking prevention in fast level sets using fuzzy models: an application in MR brain. In *Proceedings of the International Conference on information technology applications in biomedicine*, pp. 220–226. Washington, DC: IEEE Computer Society.

32. Zeng X, Staib LH, Schultz RT, Duncan JS. 1999. Segmentation and measurement of the cortex from 3d mr images using coupledsurfaces propagation. *IEEE Trans Med Imaging* **18**:927–937.

33. Angelini E, Otsuka R, Homma S, Laine A. 2004. Comparison of ventricular geometry for two real time 3D ultrasound machines with a three dimensional level set. In *Proceedings of the IEEE international symposium on biomedical imaging (ISBI)*, Vol. 1, pp. 1323–1326. Washington, DC: IEEE Computer Society.

34. Lin N, Yu W, Duncan JS. 2003. Combinative multi-scale level set framework for echocardiographic image segmentation. *Med Image Anal* 7:529–537.

35. Baillard C, Hellier P, Barillot C. 2000. *Segmentation of 3-d brain structures using level sets*. Internal Publication of IRISA, Rennes Cedex, France.

36. Leventon ME, Grimson WL, Faugeras O. 2000. Statistical shape influence in geodesic active contours. In *Proceedings of the IEEE conference on computer vision and pattern recognition*, Vol. 1, pp. 316–323. Washington, DC: IEEE Computer Society.

37. Tsai A, Yezzi A, Wells W, Tempany C, Tucker D, Fan A, Grimson WE, Willsky A. 2003. A shape-based approach to the segmentation of medical imagery using level sets. *IEEE Trans Med Imaging* 22:137–154.

38. Rousson M, Paragios N, Deriche R. 2004. Implicit active shape models for 3d segmentation in MRI imaging. In *Proceedings of the international conference on medical image computing and computer-assisted intervention (MICCAI)*, pp. 209–216. New York: Springer.

39. Sethian JA. 1999. *Level set methods and fast marching methods evolving interfaces in computational geometry, fluid mechanics, computer vision, and materials science*. Cambridge: Cambridge UP.

40. Osher S, Paragios N. 2003. *Geometric level set methods in imaging vision and graphics*. New York: Springer.

41. Osher S, Sethian JA. 1988. Fronts propagating with curvature-dependent speed: algorithms based on Hamilton-Jacobi formulation. *Comput Phys* 79:12–49.

42. Adalsteinsson D, Sethian JA. 1995. A fast level set method for propagating interfaces. *J Comput Phys* 118:269–277.

43. Mori K, Hasegawa J, Toriwaki J, Anno H, Katada K. 1996. Recognition of Bronchus in three dimensional x-ray ct images with applications to virtualized bronchoscopy system. In *Proceedings of the IEEE international conference on pattern recognition (ICPR'96)*, pp. 528–532. Washington, DC: IEEE Computer Society.

44. Walker NE, Olszewski ME, Wahle A, Nixon E, Sieren JP, Yang F, Hoffman EA, Rossen JD, Sonka M. 2005. Measurement of coronary vasoreactivity in sheep using 64-slice multidetector computed tomography and 3-d segmentation. *Computer-assisted radiology and surgery (CARS 2005): proceedings of the 19th international congress and exhibition*. Amsterdam: Elsevier.

45. Cohen LD, Cohen RK. 1997. Global minimum for active contour models: a minimal path approach. *Comput Vision* 24:57–78.

46. Lin Q. 2003. *Enhancement, extraction, and visualization of 3d volume data*. PhD dissertation, Department of Electrical Engineering, Linkoping University, Sweden.

47. Kass M, Witkin A, Terzopoulos D. 1988. Snakes: active contour models. *Int J Comput Vision* 1:321–331.

48. Caselles V, Catte F, Coll T, Dibos F. 1993. A geometric model for active contours in image processing. *Numer Math* 66:1–31.

49. Malladi R, Sethian JA, Vemuri BC. 1994. Evolutionary fronts for topology-independent shape modeling and recovery. In *Proceedings of the third European conference on computer vision (ECCV'1994). Lecture notes in computer science*, Vol. 800, pp. 3–13.

50. Yang F, Mackey MA, Ianzini F, Gallardo G, Sonka M. 2005. Cell segmentation, tracking, and mitosis detection using temporal context. in *Proceedings of the international conference on medical image computing and computer-assisted intervention (MICCAI)*. New York: Springer. In press.

51. Lee J. 1983. Digital image noise smoothing and the sigma filter. *Comput Vision Graphics Image Process* 24:255–269.

52. Perona P, Malik J. 1990. Scale-space and edge detection using anisotropic diffusion. *IEEE Trans Pattern Anal Machine Intell* **12**(7):629–639.

53. Osher S, Rudin L. 1990. Feature-oriented image enhancement using shock filters. *SIAM J Numer Anal* **27**:919–940.

54. Caselles V, Kimmel R, Sapiro G. 1997. Geodesic active contours. *Int J Comput Vision* **22**:61–79.

55. Cootes TF, Taylor CJ, Cooper DH, Graham J. 1995. Active shape models—their training and application. *Comput Vision Image Understand* **61**:38–59.

56. Leventon ME, Grimson WL, Faugeras O, Wells III WM. 2000. Level set based segmentation with intensity and curvature priors. In *Proceedings of the IEEE workshop on mathematical methods in biomedical image analysis*, pp. 1121–1124. Washington, DC: IEEE Computer Society.

57. Mumford D, Shah J. 1989. Optimal approximations by piecewise smooth functions and associated variational problems. *Commun Pure Appl Math* **42**:577–685.

58. Chan TF, Vese LA. 2001. Active contours without edges. *IEEE Trans Image Process* **10**:266–277.

59. Angelini ED, Holmes J, Laine A, Homma S. 2003. Segmentation of RT3D ultrasound with implicit deformable models without gradients. In *Proceedings of the third international symposium on image and signal processing and analysis*, Vol. 2, pp. 711–716. Washington, DC: IEEE Computer Society.

60. Wang Y, Staib LH. 1998. Boundary finding with correspondence using statistical shape models. *Comput Vision Pattern Recognit* **22**(7):338–345.

61. Mitchell SC, Bosch JG, Lelieveldt BPF, van der Geest RJ, Reiber JHC, Sonka M. 2002. 3-d active appearance models: segmentation of cardiac mr and ultrasound images. *IEEE Trans Med Imaging* **21**(9):1167–1178.

62. Cootes TF, Edwards GJ, Taylor CJ. 2000. Active appearance models. *IEEE Trans Pattern Anal Machine Intell* **23**:681–685.

63. Riedmiller M, Braun H. 1993. A direct adaptive method for faster backpropagation learning: the rprop algorithm. In *Proceedings of the of the IEEE international conference on neural networks*, pp. 586–591. Washington, DC: IEEE Computer Society.

64. Igel C, Toussaint M, Weishui W. 2004. Rprop using the natural gradient compared to Levenberg-Marquardt optimization. In *Trends and applications in constructive approximation*. International Series of Numerical Mathematics, Vol. 151, 259–272. Heidelberg: Birkh,,user, Springer-Verlag.

65. Freedman D, Radke R, Zhang T, Jeong Y, Lovelock D, Chen G. 2005. Model-based segmentation of medical imagery by matching distributions. *IEEE Trans Med Imaging* **24**(3):281–292.

66. Tsai A, Yezzi A, Willsky AS. 2001. Curve evolution implementation of the Mumford-Shah functional for image segmentation, denoising, interpolation, and magnification. *IEEE Trans Image Process* **10**:1169–1186.

7

MEDICAL IMAGE SEGMENTATION BASED ON DEFORMABLE MODELS AND ITS APPLICATIONS

Yonggang Wang, Yun Zhu, and Qiang Guo

Institute of Image Processing and Pattern Recognition
Shanghai Jiaotong University, Shanghai, China

Deformable models, including parametric deformable models and geometric deformable models, have been widely used for segmenting and identifying anatomic structures in medical image analysis. This chapter discusses medical image segmentation based on deformable models and its applications. We first study several issues and methods related to medical image segmentation and then review deformable models in detail. Three applications in different medical fields are introduced: tongue image segmentation in Chinese medicine, cerebral cortex segmentation in MR images, and cardiac valve segmentation in echocardiographic sequences.

1. MEDICAL IMAGE SEGMENTATION

1.1. Background

Image segmentation plays a crucial role in image analysis. Its goal is to partition an image into non-overlapping and meaningful regions that are uniform with respect to certain characteristics, such as graylevel, color, and texture.

Medical image segmentation is becoming an increasingly indispensable step in image processing for identifying tissue organization from the human body in numerous medical imaging modalities, including X-ray Computed Tomography (CT), Magnetic Resonance (MR), Positron Emission Tomography (PET), and

---

Address all correspondence to: Yonggang Wang, Ju-Kong Apt. 848/704, YeongTong-Dong, YeongTong-Gu, Suwon-City, Gyeonggi-Do, South Korea 443-725. Phone: +82-31-890-8388. yonggangwang@sjtu.edu.cn. wygang@gmail.com.

mammography [1]. The segmentation of anatomic structures — the partitioning of the original set of image points into subsets corresponding to structures —
may at least make contributions in the following applications:

1. Preprocessing for multimodality image registration, labeling, and motion
   tracking. These tasks require anatomic structures in the original image to
   be reduced to a compact, analytic representation of their shapes.

2. Finding anatomic structures of interest or foci for diagnosis and treatment
   planning. A typical example is segmentation of the heart, especially the left
   ventricle (LV), from cardiac imagery. Segmentation of the left ventricle
   is a prerequisite for retrieving diagnostic information such as the ejection-
   fraction ratio, the ventricular volume ratio, and heart output, and for wall
   motion analysis, which provides information on wall thickening, etc. [2].
   Another example is tumor segmentation.

3. Providing quantification of outlined structures and 3D visualization of
   relevant image data.

Over the previous two decades, a number of researchers have devoted themselves to the development of eligible segmentation methods. Before analyzing
the state of the art of these methods, we first discuss several important issues in
medical image segmentation.

1.1.1. Complexity

Medical image segmentation is never a trivial task. Many factors should be
considered in the segmentation process. For instance, an obvious challenge is that
objects may be arbitrarily complex in terms of shape.

At present, various imaging modalities are in widespread clinical use for
anatomical and physiological imaging. A major hurdle in the effective use of these
imaging techniques, however, is reliable acquisition of anatomical structures. Ideally, the image obtained should be sufficiently clear and free of artifacts to facilitate
diagnosis of pathologies. However, this requirement is never realized in practice.
Some effects often occur during the final images, including significant signal loss,
noise artifacts, object occlusion, partial-volume effects, and nonuniformity of regional intensities. As mentioned below, these problems are readily present in
images acquired by brain MRI and cardiac ultrasound, where the boundary detection problem is further complicated by the presence of confusing anatomical
structures. Occluded objects are often contained in ultrasound datasets. Partial-
volume effects are common in medical images, particularly with CT and MRI data,
which derive from multiple tissue type location within a single pixel (voxel), and
lead to blurring of intensity across boundaries. To compensate for these artifacts,
there has been a recent growing interest in soft segmentation methods [3–5]. Soft

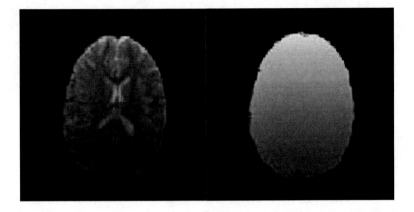

Figure 1. Intensity inhomogeneities in brain MR imaging.

segmentations allow for uncertainty in the location of object boundaries, where voxels may be classified into multiple classes with a varying degree of membership. The membership thus gives an indication of where partial-volume effects have occurred in the image.

Nonuniformity of regional intensities is a major difficulty that is specific to the segmentation of MR images [6,7]. It results in slow intensity variations of the same tissue over the image domain. The sources for this include poor radio-frequency (RF) coil uniformity, static field inhomogeneity, RF penetration, gradient-driven eddy currents, and overall patient anatomy and position [6]. This variability of tissue intensity values with respect to image location can significantly affect visual evaluation and degrade the performance of methods which assume that the intensity value of a tissue class is constant over the image. Recently, a number of image processing solutions [8–11] have been proposed as well as extended to simultaneously correct for the bias field and segment MR brain images in [12]. Figure 1 gives an example of intensity inhomogeneities in brain MRI.

1.1.2. Priors

In many applications, computer processing and analysis of medical images is limited due to low contrast of anatomical structures, variability of tissue features, fuzziness of boundaries between different tissues, and distributional complexities of tiny structures such as veins and nerves. In an effort to overcome these difficulties, various techniques have been developed to incorporate prior information into the segmentation process. When segmenting or locating an object, prior information — such as the general shape, size, location, and orientation of an object — can be quite helpful in improving the efficiency and accuracy of segmentation. Prior-based image segmentation that incorporates prior information of a certain object into the segmenting process makes the ambiguous, noise-stained, or occluded contour clear, and the final result becomes more robust, accurate, and efficient. The deformable models to be described below make it easy to incorporate prior knowledge to segment certain objects, where prior knowledge may be incorporated into models in the form of initial conditions, data constraints, or constraints on the model shape parameters [13].

Initially, deformable templates were used to embody a priori knowledge of the expected shape and shape variation of the structures. The idea can be traced back to the early work on spring-loaded templates by Fischler and Elshlager [14]. An example in medical image analysis is the work of Lipson et al. [15], who extracted vertebral contours using a deformable ellipsoidal template. Since then, more and more researchers have incorporated shape priors into their models to segment medical images. Staib and Duncan [16] applied a probabilistic deformable model on 2D echocardiograms and MR images to extract the LV of the heart and the corpus callosum of the brain, respectively. Probability distributions on the parameters of the representation bias the model toward a particular overall shape while allowing for deformations. Later, Staib and Duncan extended the model to 3D [17].

1.1.3. Interaction

A wide variety of approaches have been proposed for medical image segmentation. These approaches can be considered as three broad classes: manual, semiautomatic, and automatic. Currently, in most clinical segmentation, a skilled operator, using a computer mouse or trackball, manually traces the structure of interest on each slice of an image volume. Performing this segmentation manually is extremely labor intensive and time consuming, which is not even feasible for some applications with the increasing size of datasets. There are additional drawbacks in terms of achieving reproducible results due to operator bias and fatigue.

On the other hand, automatic segmentation of medical images can relieve clinicians from the laborious and tedious aspects of their work while increasing the consistency and reproducibility of segmentation. Although efficient, an automatic segmentation still aims at excellent performance. From this viewpoint, semiautomatic segmentation provides a good tradeoff between the precision of manual segmentation and the efficiency of automatic segmentation. Semiautomatic methods require user interaction to set algorithm parameters, to perform initial segmentation, or to select critical features. Many existing segmentation methods fall into this class. For example, when segmenting bony structures in CT images, a commonly used method is histogram thresholding, where one or more thresholds are selected from the histogram to group the pixels into several different clusters. In region-growing algorithms, seeds are generally chosen by the user, from which the final regions are formed. (Note that most of the deformable models used in this chapter are semiautomatic methods.) The user is required to set an initial contour for the object, and it will be driven to converge to the true boundary.

Most problems of segmentation inaccuracy can be overcome by human interaction. Even a correct automatic segmentation could not be obtained without relying on prior knowledge about images. Promising segmentation methods for complex images are therefore user guided and thus semiautomatic. An elegant semiautomatic should find an appropriate compromise between manual interaction and performance. In recent years, several effective interactive segmentation tools have been developed for delineating the boundaries of objects, which require manual intervention and guidance and consist of fast and accurate refinement techniques to assist the human operator. These tools include intelligent scissors [18], live wire/lane [19], graph-cut [20], and grab-cut [21]. It would will be meaningful to apply them to medical image segmentation.

1.2. Segmentation Methods

Many segmentation methods proposed for medical-image data are either direct applications or extensions of approaches from computer vision. Several general surveys on image segmentation can be found in the literature [22, 23]. Several surveys have targeted segmentation of MR images in particular [3, 24–26]. According to four time frames, Duncan and Ayache [1] critiqued the research efforts that have been put forth in the area of medical image analysis, including segmentation, over the past 20 years or so. Pham et al. [7] presented a critical appraisal of the current status of semiautomatic and automatic methods for the segmentation of anatomical medical images. In their work, the current segmentation approaches are subdivided into eight categories: (a) thresholding approaches, (b) region-growing approaches, (c) classifiers, (d) clustering approaches, (e) Markov random field (MRF) models, (f) artificial neural networks, (g) deformable models, and (h) atlas-guided approaches. Suetens et al. [27] reviewed different classes of image segmentation methods in diagnostic radiology and nuclear medicine. Based on the level of implemented model knowledge, they classified these methods into (a) manual delineation, (b) low-level segmentation, and (c) model-based segmentation.

Most of these methods are based on two basic properties of the pixels in relation to their local neighborhood: discontinuity and similarity. From this logic, in this chapter we coarsely classify the methods of medical image segmentation into three subcategories: region-based methods, boundary-based methods, and their combination. We will present brief overview of other notable methods that do not belong to these categories at the end of this section.

1.2.1. Region-based methods

Region-based methods are techniques that segment the image/volume into regions/sub-volumes. Several commonly used techniques belong to this class:

thresholding-, clustering-, and region-growing-based segmentation, and MRF models.

Thresholding is the most intuitive approach to segmentation [28]. It maps and clusters pixels in a feature space called a histogram. Thresholds are chosen at valleys between pixel clusters so that each pair represents a region of similar pixels in the image. Interactive selection of thresholds for the intracranial region has been reported [29]. This works well if the target object has distinct and homogeneous pixel values. On the other hand, spatial information is lost in the transformation, which may produce disjoint regions [30].

The difference between regions can be not only characterized by graylevel values, but also represented in other derived statistical parameters. Therefore, we can integrate various features — including intensity, and texture — into multidimensional cluster vectors in order to distinguish different regions. A commonly used example of clustering in medical image segmentation is the fuzzy c-means (FCM) algorithm [5], where fuzzy memberships are constructed to segment MR images that have been corrupted by intensity inhomogeneities. Problems similar to histogram thresholding are anticipated, and in practice only well-defined regions can be robustly identified.

Region growing [31, 32] is a classical segmentation technique extensively used in computer vision. Starting with selection of a seed region, the region-growing approach tends to group all similar neighbors according to a predefined homogeneity measure. Some early work on seed growing has been described by Cline et al. [33], who used seed growing to extract the brain surface. Region growing is seldom used alone, but is followed by a split-and-merge operation during the entire process of image segmentation. In this scenario, a threshold is required to decide whether to merge or split. The main disadvantage of region growing lies in selection of the seed. It can be chosen empirically by the user, which may be difficult if he there is no clear idea of the growth behavior of the region.

The basic idea of the MRF in computer vision was put forward by Geman and Geman [34] in 1984, when they applied statistical mechanics to image processing. The MRF is a conditional probability model multiplied by a priori probability per se. In most cases, the conditional probability is in Gaussian form, representing the possibility of the observed data given its actual value. The prior probability models the spatial constraint in the neighborhood. Over the past twenty years, extensive efforts have focused on application of an MRF model to various fields [35]. Introduction of the MRF model to medical image segmentation was begun by Wells et al. [8], who used a non-parametric Pazen window to model brain images. One of the most significant contributions of their work is the correction of RF inhomogeneity. Since then, this trend has been most significant [12, 36, 37]. As the MRF is a pixel classification method, the optimization and parameter estimation algorithms are often computationally expensive. Another drawback of the MRF method is its inability to retain topological information. For example, in cortical segmentation the MRF does not preserve its known spherical topology.

An additional cavity or handle-filling step is always required after normal segmentation in order to get the right topology.

Region-based approaches are well known for their robustness, but they can be computationally expensive (e.g., optimization and parameter estimation of the MRF). These techniques can be further classified into many categories (see [26] for the details). It is worth noting that the authors of [26] considered prior knowledge-based techniques to belong to the region-based segmentation class, as the one that we propose below to segment the cardiac valve in echocardiographic sequences.

1.2.2. Boundary-based methods

In traditional boundary-based methods, local discontinuities are detected first (called *edge detection*) and then connected to form complete boundaries (called *edge linking*). There has been a great number of studies on edge detection over the last four decades. Several well-known numerical techniques for intensity edge detection contain Sobel's, Robert's, Kirsh's, and Prewitt and Canny's operators. Several surveys on early edge detection work can be found in [38,39]. The use of edge detection techniques often results in broken edges due to noise. It is generally recognized that boundary detection is therefore finished by edge-linking algorithms. Readers interested in further information about this are referred to [40,41].

The biggest problem of edge detection may be that most traditional gradient operators are sensitive to noise and produce spurious edge elements that make it difficult to construct a reasonable region boundary. In addition, since the two stages of edge detection and edge linking are independent, some missing edge segments in the former stage could never be brought back.

Over the last two decades, probably the most visible approaches brought to maturation in terms of both methodology development and application were boundary-finding strategies based on deformable models [1]. Such a model can obtain an accurate boundary of objects by deforming the initial curve, which is defined in advance. The deformation process is guided by minimizing with respect to the initial curve a functional, whose local minimum is given by the boundary of objects.

Deformable models, though stemming from the computer vision field, are frequently used in medical image processing, and have been widely applied to problems, including segmentation, tracking, and registration. For example, Gupta et al. [2] used deformable model-based techniques to segment the ventricular boundaries in cardiac MR images. Rifai et al. [42] employed a 3D deformable model with variable topology to segment the skull in MRI volumes, where they also tok into account the partial-volume effect to formulate the speed function for the model. Davatzikos and Bryan used an active contour to obtain a mathematical representation of the cortex. These are but a few examples. A more detailed analysis of the use of deformable models in medical image processing can be found in [13].

In contrast to the traditional low-level and model-free image segmentation techniques, such as region growing and edge detection, they offer several advantages for the segmentation of anatomical organs, including the following [13]:

1. Deformable models can be used to obtain closed and smooth contours, even if the images are noisy.

2. Certain deformable models are topology preserving, while others allow changes in the topology without introducing difficulties related to parameterization.

3. Some deformable models (e.g., using Fourier descriptors) allow obtaining an analytic mathematical description of the segmented contour rather than a set of points.

4. Deformable models can be used for 3D reconstruction of anatomical organs.

Since the introduction of the snake model by Kass et al. [43], many researchers have done much work on improving its performance. One of the most interesting issues is extending its capture range and reducing its sensitivity to initial placement. In this aspect, various methods (e.g., the balloon [44], distance transformation [45]) have been proposed. One approach worth mentioning here is Gradient Vector Flow (GVF) [46], which combines almost all the merits of the previous snakes. More importantly, it achieves a large capture range by using a regularization term. It moves snakes into boundary cavities that were unattainable by conventional snakes. In this chapter GVF is applied to refine the contour in tongue segmentation. Snakes are referred to as parametric deformable models in some of the literature [1, 47].

Corresponding to parametric deformable models are geometric deformable models, which were first proposed by Osher and Sethian [48]. The relationship between parametric a deformable model and a geometric deformable model was explored in [47, 49]. Geometric deformable models are in the form of curve evolution within the level set framework, where contour deformation is treated as a propagating wavefront that can be seen as the zero level set of an evolving function. Geometric deformable models have been brought into the medical arena by a variety of researchers [50–52].

1.2.3. Hybrid methods

There has been a significant trend in recent years to fuse region information with a boundary detector [53–55]. One typical example is the level set method with regularizers [56]. Regularizers take in various forms, including shape and clustering. One thing in common for all regularizers is the application of region information.

One intriguing issue in a hybrid level set is minimization of the energy function. The energy function is a natural way to model a preferred segment, and many methods have been put forward to optimize it. Among these methods, one effective way is to convert init to a Partial Differential Equation (PDE), so that handling the segmentation problem corresponds to solution of the associated PDE. Unfortunately, since we often use region integrals to model region information and the integral regions are often variants corresponding to segments, it has to go through an unnatural step of converting region integrals into boundary integrals [54, 57]. Recently, Chan and Vese [58] proposed a similar but more natural method to model region information by introducing the Heaviside function. This excellent strategy is adopted in this chapter to model cortical structures.

Hybrid models driven by both region and boundary information have achieved great success in medical image processing [47, 59]. The main reason behind this success is that it simultaneously takes advantage of local information, which is accurate, and global information, which is robust.

In addition, neural networks have been widely used in medical segmentation problems [30, 60–62]. Chiou and Hwang [60] constructed a two-layer perceptron to train on MR image data to better identify pixels on the boundary of the brain. Alirezaie et al. [61] used Learning-Vector Quantization (LVQ), a typical self-organization map network, for segmenting 2D MR images of the brain, where they treat the segmentation problem as classifying pixels based upon features that are extracted from multispectral images and incorporate spatial information. Shareef et al. [30] utilized a new biologically inspired oscillator network to perform segmentation on 2D and 3D CT and MRI medical-image datasets, and the results were promising. A comparison between the neural network and fuzzy clustering techniques in segmenting brain MR images was presented by Hall et al. [25].

2. DEFORMABLE MODELS

As mentioned earlier, deformable models can be classified as either parametric deformable models or geometric deformable models according to their representation and implementation. In particular, parametric deformable models, also referred to as snakes or active contour models, are represented explicitly as parameterized curves in a Lagrangian formulation. Geometric deformable models are represented implicitly as level sets of two-dimensional distance functions that evolve according to an Eulerian formulation [47].

2.1. Parametric Deformable Models

A snake is a curve driven by using partial differential equations based on the theory of elasticity [13]. The famous external forces for parametric deformable models include Gradient, Balloon [44], the Distance Map [63], and Gradient Vector Flow (GVF) [46]. The goal of modeling an external force is to find one kind of force that has the capability of pushing the curve to significant concavities or convexes, retaining a large capture range, stopping the evolving curve at the edge gaps, and processing high-noise images. For our purposes, we will now give a brief overview of the classic snake model and the GVF snake model.

2.1.1. Classic snake model

Geometrically, a classic snake model is described by $\mathbf{x}(s) = (x(s), y(s))$, where s is the arc length, and $x(s)$ and $y(s)$ are x and y coordinates along the contour, and the energy of the model is given by

$$E_{\text{snake}} = \int_{\text{snake}} E\left(\mathbf{x}(s)\right) ds = \int_{\text{snake}} E_{int}\left(\mathbf{x}(s)\right) + E_{\text{ext}}\left(\mathbf{x}(s)\right) ds, \quad (1)$$

where E_{ext} is the external energy, and E_{int} is the internal energy, given by

$$E_{int} = \frac{1}{2}\left(\alpha(t)\left|\frac{\partial \mathbf{x}(s)}{\partial s}\right|^2 + \beta(t)\left|\frac{\partial^2 \mathbf{x}(s)}{\partial s^2}\right|^2\right), \quad (2)$$

where α and β are the coefficients that control the snake's tension and rigidity, respectively. The goal is to find a snake, $\mathbf{x}^*(s)$, that minimizes E_{snake}. The external energy is in accord with the image features, and for a given image $f(x, y)$,

$$E_{\text{ext}} = -\gamma\left|\nabla\left\{G_{\sigma(x,y)} * f(x, y)\right\}\right|, \quad (3)$$

where $G_{\sigma(x,y)}$ is the two-dimensional Gaussian kernel with σ as the standard deviation.

Solved by the variational method, the minimum of E_{snake} has to satisfy the following Euler-Lagrange equation:

$$-\alpha \mathbf{x}''(s) + \beta \mathbf{x}''''(s) + \nabla E_{\text{ext}} = 0. \quad (4)$$

Discretization of Eq. (4) by the finite-difference method yields a linear system [43]:

$$\mathbf{AP} = \mathbf{L}, \quad (5)$$

where $\mathbf{A}$ is a pentadiagonal matrix depending on α and β, and $\mathbf{P}$ and $\mathbf{L}$ denote the discrete contour points vector and the forces at these points, respectively. From the initial position of the contour, the following associated evolution equation can be solved:

$$\left(\mathbf{I} + \tau \mathbf{A}\right)\mathbf{P}^t = \left(\mathbf{P}^{t-1} + \tau \mathbf{L}\left(\mathbf{P}^{t-1}\right)\right), \quad (6)$$

where t is time, and τ is the time step. The final solution, $\mathbf{x}^*(s)$, can be achieved by solving Eq. (6) iteratively.

2.1.2. GVF snake model

The classical active contour models have several limitations that weaken their practicability in resolving image segmentation problems [46]. One limitation is associated with initialization, that is, the initial contour must be close to the true boundary or it will likely converge to a wrong result. To address this problem, several novel methods have been proposed, including pressure forces [44] and distance potentials [63]. The basic idea is to increase the capture range of the external force fields and guide the contour toward the desired boundary. Another limitation is the poor convergence of classical snakes to boundary concavities. The GVF snake is an effective model that can be employed to solve this problem.

According to the Helmholtz theorem [64], rewriting Eq. (4) and replacing the $-\nabla E_{\text{ext}}$ with Θ, we can obtain

$$\alpha \mathbf{x}''(s) - \beta \mathbf{x}''''(s) + \Theta = 0, \tag{7}$$

where Θ is the gradient vector flow, defined as $\Theta(x, y) = (u(x, y), v(x, y))$, and it is usually generated by the energy functional

$$\varepsilon = \iint \mu \left(u_x^2 + u_y^2 + v_x^2 + v_y^2 \right) + |\nabla f|^2 \cdot |\Theta - \nabla f|^2 \, dx dy, \tag{8}$$

where $|\nabla f|$ is the gradient of the given image $f(x, y)$, and it can also be substituted with its Gaussian smoothing version as Eq. (3). Equation (8) is dominated by the sum of squares of the partial derivatives of the GVF vector field when $|\nabla f|$ is small, yielding a slowly varying field. On the other hand, when $|\nabla f|$ is large, the second term dominates the integrand and is minimized by setting $\Theta = \nabla f$. This results in the desired effect of keeping Θ nearly equal to the gradient of the edge map when it is large, but forcing the field to be slowly varying in homogeneous regions. The parameter μ is a weighting parameter for governing the tradeoff between the two cases.

The physical nature of Eq. (8) is to create an energy field containing both the degree of divergence and curl for a vector field. Using the calculus of variation and the finite-difference method again, Θ can be calculated according to

$$u_{t+1} = \mu \nabla^2 u_t - (u_t - f_x)(f_x^2 + f_y^2),$$
$$v_{t+1} = \mu \nabla^2 v_t - (v_t - f_y)(f_x^2 + f_y^2). \tag{9}$$

Deliberately developed for overcoming the above-mentioned limitations, the GVF snake can expand the capture range remarkably, so the initial contour need not be as close to the true boundary as before. However, proper initialization is still necessary, or else the snake may converge to a wrong result.

2.2. Geometric Deformable Models

In parametric deformable models an explicit parametric representation of the curve is used, which can lead to fast real-time implementation. However, it is difficult for parametric deformable models to adapt the model topology during deformation. On the other hand, the implicit forms, i.e., geometric deformable models, are designed to handle topological changes naturally.

Geometric deformable models were introduced independently by Malladi et al. [52] and Caselles et al. [65]. These models are based on the theory of curve evolution and the level set method, where the evolving curves or surfaces are implicitly represented as a level set of a higher-dimensional scalar function, i.e., a level set function. Thus, geometric deformable models are also called level set methods in much of the literature.

2.2.1. The level set method

The level set method views a moving curve as the zero level set of a higher-dimensional function $\phi(\mathbf{x}, t)$ [48]. Generally, the level set function satisfies

$$
\begin{cases}
\phi(\mathbf{x}, t) < 0 & in \quad \Omega(t), \\
\phi(\mathbf{x}, t) = 0 & in \quad C(t), \\
\phi(\mathbf{x}, t) > 0 & in \quad R^n \backslash \bar{\Omega}(t),
\end{cases}
\tag{10}
$$

where the artificial time t denotes the evolution process, $C(t)$ is the moving curve, and $\Omega(t)$ represents the region (possibly multi-connected) that $C(t)$ encloses. An evolution equation for the curve C moving with speed F in its normal direction is given by

$$
\phi_t = F(\mathbf{x}) |\nabla \phi|.
\tag{11}
$$

Here, the surface $\phi = 0$ corresponding to the propagating hypersurface may change topology, as well as form sharp corners.

A particular case is motion by mean curvature, when $F = \mathrm{div}(\nabla\phi(\mathbf{x})/|\nabla\phi(\mathbf{x})|)$ is the curvature of the level curve of ϕ passing through $\mathbf{x}$. The above equation becomes

$$
\frac{\partial \phi}{\partial t} = |\nabla\phi| \cdot div \left(\frac{\nabla\phi}{|\nabla\phi|} \right),
\tag{12}
$$

with $\phi(0, \mathbf{x}) = \phi_0(\mathbf{x})$ and $t \in (0, \infty)$.

2.2.2. Geometric deformable model

When utilized for image segmentation, the speed function is usually constructed by merging image features. A geometric deformable model based on mean curvature motion is given by the following evolution equation [65]:

$$\frac{\partial \phi}{\partial t} = g\left(|\nabla f|\right) \cdot |\nabla \phi| \cdot \left[div\left(\frac{\nabla \phi}{|\nabla \phi|} \right) + v \right], \qquad (13)$$

where $v \geq 0$ is a constraint on the area inside the curve, increasing the propagation speed; $g\left(|\nabla f|\right)$ is an edge-sensitive speed function and is defined as

$$F(\mathbf{x}) = \frac{1}{1 + |\nabla\{G_\sigma * f(\mathbf{x})\}|^p}, \qquad (14)$$

where $p \geq 1$. From this argument, it is clear that, if the image gradient $|\nabla\{G_\sigma * f(\mathbf{x})\}|$ approaches the local maximum at the object boundaries, the curve gradually attains zero speed. Under the ideal condition that $|\nabla\{G_\sigma * f(\mathbf{x})\}| \rightarrow \infty$, i.e., $F = 0$ at the boundaries, the evolving curve eventually stops and the final zero level set $\Psi(x, \infty) = 0$ corresponds to the segmentation result. In practice, it is impossible for $F = 0$, and the curve will leak as $t \rightarrow \infty$.

Another well-known deformable model [49], the so-called *geodesic snake model*, is employed in our work for cardiac valve segmentation (see below). It also uses the image gradient to stop the curve. Its level set formulation is as follows:

$$\frac{\partial \phi}{\partial t} = |\nabla \phi| \, div\left(g\left(|\nabla f|\right) \frac{\nabla \phi}{|\nabla \phi|} \right) + vg\left(|\nabla f|\right)|\nabla \phi|. \qquad (15)$$

2.2.3. Chan-Vese model

On the other hand, because these classical snake models rely on the edge function $g\left(|\nabla f|\right)$, or say, depend on the image gradient $|\nabla f|$, to stop the curve evolution, these models can detect only objects with edges defined by a gradient. In practice, discrete gradients are bounded, and so the stopping function is never zero on the edges, and the curve may pass through the boundary, even for the geodesic snake model mentioned above. If the image f is very noisy, the isotropic smoothing Gaussian has to be strong, which will smooth the edges as well. To address these problems, Chan and Vese [58] recently proposed a different deformable model, i.e., a model not based on the gradient of the image f for the stopping process. Instead, the evolvement of the curve is based on the general Mumford-Shah formulation of image segmentation [66], by minimizing the functional

$$F^{MS}(f, C) = \mu Length(C) + \lambda \int_\Omega |f - f_0|^2 \, dxdy + \int_{\Omega \backslash C} |\nabla f|^2 \, dxdy, \qquad (16)$$

where $f_0 : \bar{\Omega} \rightarrow R$ is a given image, and μ and λ are positive parameters. The solution image f is formed by smooth regions R_i and sharp boundaries, denoted here by C. A reduced form of this problem is simply the restriction of F^{MS} to piecewise constant functions and finding a partition of Ω such that f in Ω_i equals a constant, and $\Omega = \bigcup_i^n \Omega_i \bigcup C$. Based on Eq. (16), Chan and Vese proposed the following minimization problem for a two-phase segmentation:

$$\min_{C,c_o,c_b} \left\{ \mu \int_\Omega \delta(\phi)|\nabla\phi|\,dxdy + v \int_\Omega H(\phi)\,dxdy \right.$$
$$+\lambda_o \int_{inside(C)} |f - c_o|^2 H(\phi)\,dxdy \qquad (17)$$
$$\left. +\lambda_b \int_{outside(C)} |f - c_b|^2 (1 - H(\phi))\,dxdy \right\}.$$

Here ϕ is the level set function, and $H(\phi)$ is the Heaviside function:

$$H(\phi) = \left\{ \begin{array}{ll} 1, & \phi \geq 0, \\ 0, & \phi < 0. \end{array} \right. \qquad (18)$$

Finding a minimum of (17) is done by introducing an artificial time variable, and moving ϕ in the steepest descent direction to steady state:

$$\phi_t = \delta_\varepsilon(\phi) \left(-(f - c_o)^2 + (f - c_b)^2 - v + \mu \cdot div \left(\frac{\nabla\phi}{|\nabla\phi|} \right) \right), \qquad (19)$$

subject to $\phi(\mathbf{x}, 0) = \phi_0(\mathbf{x})$. Here δ_ε is a globally positive approximation to the δ function (see [58]). The recovered image is a piecewise constant approximation to f_0. We use Chan-Vese model in the application for cortex segmentation below.

Generally, the above deformable models implemented by means of the level set method suffer from a slower speed of convergence than parametric deformable models due to their computational complexity. However, they can automatically handle topology changes and allow for multiple simultaneous boundary estimations, which is the case with most medical imaging.

In the following sections we present our work on medical image segmentation in three different applications, including tongue segmentation within color images used in computerized tongue diagnosis, cerebral cortex segmentation in MR images, and cardiac valve segmentation in echocardiographic sequences. We apply different deformable models for each.

3. TONGUE BODY EXTRACTION BASED ON A COLOR GVF SNAKE

3.1. Introduction

Tongue diagnosis is one of the most important approaches to retrieving significant physiological information on the human body employed in the famous four diagnostic processes of Traditional Chinese Medicine (TCM): inspection, listening and smelling, inquiry, and palpation. TCM doctors have long used information about the color, luster, shape, and movement of a patient's tongue to determine his disease and body condition [67]. However, the clinical competence of traditional

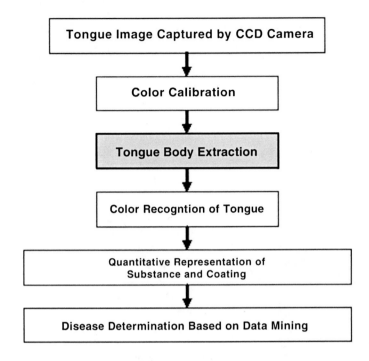

Figure 2. Flowchart of a typical automatic tongue diagnosis system.   See attached CD for color version.

tongue diagnosis is dependent on the subjective experience and knowledge of the doctor, which has inevitably impeded the development of TCM.

To circumvent this problem, some research groups [68–75], especially in China, have designed computerized tongue diagnosis systems based on image analysis techniques that attempt to alleviate the diagnostic discrepancy among doctors and provided systematic and quantitative diagnosis. Figure 2 presents a flowchart of a typical automatic tongue diagnosis system based on image analysis. First, the tongue of a patient or a subject to be examined is captured using a color CCD (Charge Coupled Device) camera under standard imaging geometry conditions. Second, some image analysis techniques are applied to the tongue image: including color calibration, tongue body segmentation and extraction, and color recognition. Third, quantitative representation of the tongue follows to characterize the pathological features defined in TCM, such as the colors of the tongue substance and coating, the thickness and wetness of coating, and the shape of tongue. Finally, the quantitative features obtained are mapped to diseases via data-mining techniques or learning theories, like the Bayesian network adopted in [72]. Here our study is focused on tongue body extraction and segmentation.

The goal of tongue segmentation is to extract the tongue body from the original tongue image, generally including the face, lips, teeth, etc. Only after accurate results of tongue segmentation are achieved can the next steps be effectively continued. Some low-level image processing techniques have been applied in tongue segmentation. Zhao et al. [74] presented a segmentation method based on mathematical morphology and the HIS (Hue, Intensity, and Saturation) color model. Liu et al. [76] proposed an automatic approach for tongue segmentation based on luminance information and the morphology features of the image. Sun et al. [77] presented a method for tongue region segmentation based on a split-and-merge algorithm.

Deformable models have already been adopted in tongue segmentation as well. For example, Pang et al. [71] combined a bi-elliptical deformable template with a snake model to segment a tongue image, where they introduced a novel term, the *template force*, to take the place of internal force. In practice, unfortunately, the methods mentioned above often fail to segment the tongue from out of its surroundings. One of the reasons for this is that most of them do not take the color property into account, which is an essential feature in such a task. In addition, due to the pathological details on the surface of the tongue and the fragmental weakness of the tongue's edge, tongue image segmentation based on deformable models may converge to spurious boundaries.

In this section we propose an automatic segmentation scheme based on a color GVF snake model that is applied directly on the original color tongue image. Note that we do not carry out the segmentation using geometric deformable models because the topology of the tongue is not very complicated and it is the unique object of interest in the original image. Also note that we do not attempt to establish a shape template to guide the convergence of the snake curves, like the case in [16]. The shapes of tongue bodies captured in various diseases or persons are quite different, so it is impossible to properly describe them all with a predefined deformable template. Finally, to refine or correct the segmentation result, an additional interactive segmentation technique is introduced. Now we will discuss the color GVF snake model.

3.2. Color GVF Snake Model

Although having extensive applications in the localization of object boundaries in bi-level and graylevel images, parametric deformable models have been rarely used to find the boundaries of objects in a color image directly using color information. Most researchers have employed the luminance characteristics of the color images to drive the deformation processes, or applied deformable models separately to some/each of the image planes (e.g., RGB [78] or other transformed color spaces [79]), followed by certain combining strategies [80]. A review of boundary localization methods based on parametric deformable models that make use of the color data can be found in [81].

When an edge map is extracted from the original image and then presented to a snake model, the boundary-finding process in color images is quite similar to that in graylevel images. Dumitras and Venetsanopoulos [82] computed an angular map to identify major color changes (edges) in an image, and hence provided a method for object shape description in color images. Similarly, in [83] an affinity map that in nature was a bi-level image was computed and employed in estimation of object boundaries, which were then presented to a parametric deformable model. In our study we directly apply one of the color edge detection techniques, i.e., the Di Zenzo operator, to achieve an edge map of a color image, as in the work of Sapiro [84], where a color geodesic deformable model was established.

3.2.1. Di Zenzo color gradient

In graylevel images the gradient is defined as the first derivative of the image luminance values. It has a high value in those regions that exhibit a high luminance contrast. However, this strategy is not suitable for color images. Both changes in luminance and color between neighboring pixels should be exploited by more efficient color gradient definition. Many robust and complex color gradient operators have been proposed [85–88]. Without loss of generality, we adopt Di Zenzo's definition of gradients for a color image [87] in our study.

Let $\Phi(x, y) : R^2 \to R^3$ be a color image with components $\Phi_i(x, y) : R^2 \to R$, $i = 1, 2, 3$. We look for the local variation $d\Phi^2$, which can be given in matrix form as follows:

$$d\Phi^2 = \begin{bmatrix} dx \\ dy \end{bmatrix}^T \begin{bmatrix} g_{11} & g_{12} \\ g_{21} & g_{22} \end{bmatrix} \begin{bmatrix} dx \\ dy \end{bmatrix}, \tag{20}$$

where $g_{11} = \frac{\partial \Phi}{\partial x} \cdot \frac{\partial \Phi}{\partial x}, g_{12} = g_{21} = \frac{\partial \Phi}{\partial x} \cdot \frac{\partial \Phi}{\partial y}, g_{22} = \frac{\partial \Phi}{\partial y} \cdot \frac{\partial \Phi}{\partial y}$.

Note that the matrix $\mathbf{G} = (g_{i,j})$, also called the *structure tensor* in [89], is symmetric as well as positive definite. The interesting point about $\mathbf{G}$ is that its positive eigenvalues $\lambda_{+/-}$ are the maximum and minimum of $d\Phi^2$, while the orthogonal eigenvectors $\theta_{+/-}$ are the corresponding variation orientations, and are formally given by

$$\lambda_{+/-} = \frac{g_{11} + g_{22} \pm \sqrt{(g_{11} - g_{22})^2 + 4g_{12}^2}}{2}, \tag{21}$$

and the eigenvectors are $(\cos \theta_\pm, \sin \theta_\pm)$, where the angles $\theta_+ = 1/2 \cdot \arctan (2g_{12}/(g_{11} - g_{22})), \theta_- = \theta_+ + \pi/2$. Note that for graylevel images, i.e., $\Phi(x, y) : R^2 \to R$, $\lambda_+ \equiv |\nabla\Phi|^2$, $\lambda_- \equiv 0$ and $(\cos \theta_+, \sin \theta_-) = \nabla\Phi/|\nabla\Phi|$.

In practice, there are three different choices of vector gradient norms [84,89]: $\sqrt{\lambda_+}, \sqrt{\lambda_+ - \lambda_-}$ and $\sqrt{\lambda_+ + \lambda_-}$. Here we select the additive form to define the color gradient in an RGB color space, as shown in Eq. (22). The reason for this is that it is easy to compute and gives preferences to certain corners (see [89]):

$$\nabla \Phi = \sqrt{\lambda_+^{\text{RGB}} + \lambda_-^{\text{RGB}}}, \qquad (22)$$

where

$$g_{11} = \left|\frac{\partial R}{\partial x}\right|^2 + \left|\frac{\partial G}{\partial x}\right|^2 + \left|\frac{\partial B}{\partial x}\right|^2, \quad g_{22} = \left|\frac{\partial R}{\partial y}\right|^2 + \left|\frac{\partial G}{\partial y}\right|^2 + \left|\frac{\partial B}{\partial y}\right|^2$$

and

$$g_{12} = g_{21} = \frac{\partial R}{\partial x} \cdot \frac{\partial R}{\partial y} + \frac{\partial G}{\partial x} \cdot \frac{\partial G}{\partial y} + \frac{\partial B}{\partial x} \cdot \frac{\partial B}{\partial y}.$$

3.2.2. Color GVF snake

Once we achieve the edge map of the color image using Eq. (22), the extension of the graylevel GVF snake to its color counterpart is straightforward. Substituting Θ_{color} for the original GVF vector field Θ in Eq. (7), we have

$$\alpha \mathbf{x}''(s) - \beta \mathbf{x}''\,''(s) + \Theta_{\text{color}} = 0, \qquad (23)$$

where Θ_{color} is the color gradient vector flow, defined as $\Theta_{\text{color}} = (u_{\text{color}}(x, y), v_{color}(x, y))$ that minimizes the following energy function:

$$\varepsilon = \iint \mu \left(u_x^2 + u_y^2 + v_x^2 + v_y^2\right) + |\nabla \Phi|^2 \cdot |\Theta_{color} - \nabla \Phi|^2 \, dx dy, \qquad (24)$$

where $\nabla \Phi$ is given in (22).

The rest of the numerical implementation of color the GVF snake is similar to that for the graylevel GVF snake. The solution of u_{color} and v_{color} can be derived from the iterative algorithm for (9), and the snake curve will move forward to the vicinity of the object boundary.

It is worth mentioning that in (3) larger σ values will cause the boundaries to become blurry if a Gaussian smoothing operation is adopted. Such large σ values are often necessary, however, in order to increase the capture range of the snake. To address this problem, we replaced it with the anisotropic diffusion technique proposed by Sapiro and Ringach [90]. A comparison of these two techniques can be seen in Figure 3, which gives an example of finding the contour of a seed using the proposed color GVF snake.

In Figure 3 we also show the convergence results with different initial curves: one inside the seed (Figure 3e) and the other outside the seed (Figure 3f). Both can arrive at the correct boundary of the seed, which represents the property of initialization insensitivity derived from the graylevel GVF snake. Finally, we compare the closeups of two external force fields in the color GVF snake and a classical snake. It is obvious that, while the external forces of the classical snake are rather disordered, those of the color GVF snake correctly point toward the seed boundary.

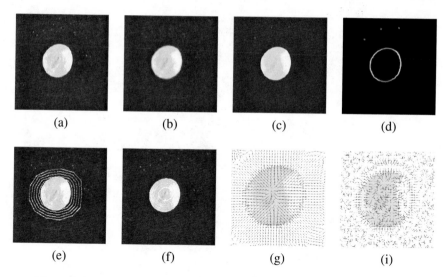

Figure 3. An example of segmenting a seed image using a color GVF snake: (a) original color seed image; (b,c) filtering results from Gaussian kernel and anisotropic diffusion, respectively; (d) edge map using a Di Zenzo color gradient operator; (e,f) convergence of two color GVF snakes with different initial curves; (g,h) closeups of external force fields in a color GVF snake and a classical snake, respectively. See attached CD for color version.

4. TONGUE SEGMENTATION BASED ON A COLOR GVF SNAKE

It seems unreasonable to directly apply the proposed color GVF snake model to tongue image segmentation. There are a lot of pathological details on the surface of the tongue (e.g., tongue fur) with ambiguous colors, cracks, petechia, and highlight areas, which have a strong influence on the convergence of the snake. Although we have adopted the anisotropic diffusion technique to filter a tongue image, sometimes the snake curve still falls into the local minimum. To overcome these problems, a great deal of prior knowledge has been considered to provide an automatic curve initialization method for the color GVF snake.

Generally, in the captured tongue images (see Figures 4a–c), the following classes of colors are contained in the challenging areas: yellow (face skins), white (teeth), black (shadow produced by lips), etc. On the other hand, the color of lips is often red, and the substrate color of the tongue is red as well. According to this observation, we can alleviate the effects of most of the challenging areas first. The following transform of the original tongue image is used for this purpose:

$$I\left(x,y\right) = \left|R\left(x,y\right) + B\left(x,y\right) - 2G\left(x,y\right)\right|, \tag{25}$$

where $R\left(x,y\right)$, $G\left(x,y\right)$, and $B\left(x,y\right)$ are the three components of the color image. This transform may effectively enhance the contrast between the tongue body and

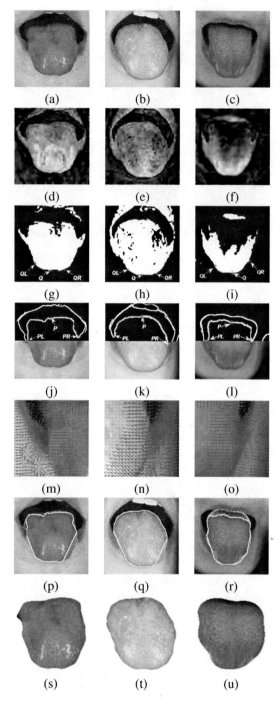

Figure 4. Extraction of tongue bodies using the color GVF Snake on three tongue images. Each column shows an example of tongue segmentation. See attached CD for color version.

the surroundings, as depicted in Fig. 4d–f. Here we pay more emphasis on this transform. First, due to the similar red colors as the tongue body, the lip areas cannot be removed by Eq. (25), which also determines that it is better to initialize the curve of the color GVF snake inside the tongue body area to avoid convergence to the lip edges. Second, many tongue images captured from diseases contain white and yellow colors of fur that are easily weakened. However, we argue that it has no great effect, and our concern is the tongue's contour. Third, someone may note that Eq. (15) is much similar to one of the $I_1 I_2 I_3$ components proposed by Ohta et al. [91], except that the latter is used to construct a color space.

It is not difficult to binarize the transformed images that are actually intensity images. In binary images (Fig. 4g–i), we search for a set of tongue tip points according to the following steps: (a) find the lowest position of the tongue body by scanning line by line from bottom to top and define it as tip feature point Q; (b) beginning with point Q, step left and right over N (here $N = 50$) pixels, respectively, and get left feature point QL and right feature point QR. These feature points are indicated in Figure 4g–i.

Due to the illuminant geometry, some shadows are formed between the upper tip and tongue body in the tongue image. According to this prior knowledge, a set of tongue root feature points can be obtained in the graylevel counterpart of the color tongue image. At first, vertical projections of the graylevel images are performed, and we can find the valley in the formed histogram. Then Sobel operators are used to detect the edge of the tongue root. Searching near the valley pixels, we can obtain tongue root feature point P. Finally, the intersecting points of the tongue root and upper lip, i.e., left feature point PL and right feature point PR at the root of the tongue, can be obtained by boundary tracing techniques.

We now have several feature points at the tip and root boundary of the tongue. A close curve can be formed by linking PL and QL, PR and QR, together with the curves $\overset{\frown}{P\,PL}$, $\overset{\frown}{P\,PR}$, $\overset{\frown}{Q\,QR}$, and $\overset{\frown}{Q\,QR}$. These close curves (the white lines in Figures 4p–r), are used as the initial curves of the color GVF snakes in our work.

The use of prior knowledge makes separation of the tongue body from lower lip the main task. Before deforming the initial curves, Di Zenzo color gradients are computed in the original images and GVF vectors are solved on the basis of them. Figure 4m–o depicts the closeups of the local GVF force fields in the three tongue images. Because the initial curves are relatively close to the true boundaries of the tongue bodies, they are driven by the GVF external forces to converge quickly. Figure 4s–u shows the final segmentation results of the tongue images.

4.1. Snake Pit-Based Interactive Refinement of Segmentation Results

Although these results are promising, the snake curve will sometime fall into unexpected areas. For instance, Figure 5 gives two examples of failure of tongue image segmentation by the color GVF snake. To provide correct segmentation

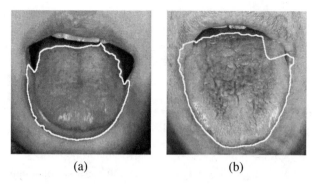

(a)   (b)

Figure 5. Two failure examples of tongue image segmentation by snakes. Notice the white curves are the boundary-finding results. See attached CD for color version.

results for the subsequent analysis, we introduce an interactive refinement technique based on the mechanism of the snake pit.

In essence, a snake is an interactive segmentation model due to manual initialization of curves, although some researchers have attempted to improve its intelligence through setting initial curves automatically in some special applications, such as the case in our work. In the classical snake model proposed by Kass et al. [43], interaction can also be represented by the mechanism of the snake pit.

The snake pit was initially developed by Kass et al. in their experimental user interface, which has proven very useful for semiautomatic image segmentation. The interface allows a user to select starting points and exert forces on snakes interactively as they minimize their energy. In order to specify a particular image feature, the user has only to pull a snake near the feature. Once close enough, the energy minimization will push the snake the rest of the way in. These two cases are characterized with *spring* and *volcano* icons, respectively, in their interface. The pit mechanism can allow the user to accurately control the behavior of the snake with little effort in specifying the feature points of interest. Figure 6 gives a geometric interpretation of the snake pit.

In our implementation, only springs are adopted to pull a snake to the specified true boundary. According to [43], creating a spring between two points x_1 and x_2 simply adds $-k(x_1 - x_2)^2$ to the external energy. A pair of points for the snake pit is shown in Figure 7.

After setting such point pairs on the snakes and the desired boundaries, we choose the existing segmentation results as initial curves, and then deform the snakes with extra spring forces once again. Finally, we can get refined segmentation results, some examples of which are shown in Figure 8.

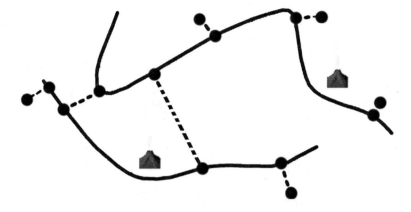

Figure 6. Geometric interpretation of Snake Pit. The two dark curves are different snakes, and the tow springs (dashed line) are connected between them to create a coupling effect. The other springs attach points on the snakes to fixed positions in the image. In addition, two volcanos are set to bend a nearby snake. See attached CD for color version.

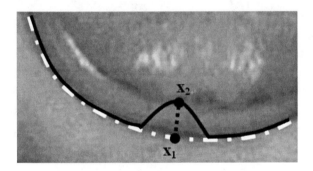

Figure 7. A pair of points for the snake pit. See attached CD for color version.

5. CEREBRAL CORTEX MR IMAGE SEGMENTATION

5.1. Introduction

The cerebral cortex is a thin but convoluted layer of neurons known as Gray Matter (GM) that lies between the White Matter (WM) and the Cerebral Spinal Fluid (CSF) (Figure 9). This layer is only 1–3 millimeters thick and has a total area of about one quarter of a square meter. It is by far the largest portion of the nervous system in the human body. Studies show that many neurological disorders like Alzheimer's disease and schizophrenia are directly related to the pathological state of the cerebral cortex. Therefore, extraction of cerebral cortex from the brain for analysis and measurement is necessary and important.

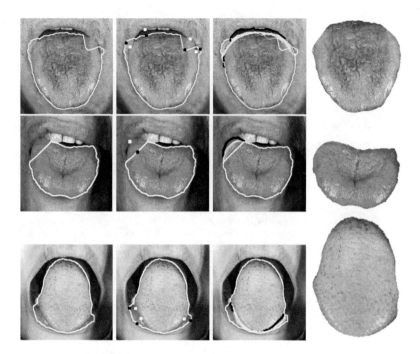

Figure 8. Examples of interactive segmentation on three tongue images. The four columns from left to right are: original segmentation results from the color GVF snakes, point pairs chosen for the snake pit, convergence of the snakes, and final extracted tongue bodies. See attached CD for color version.

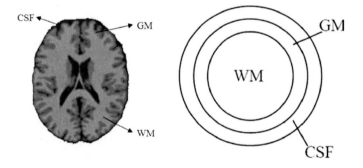

Figure 9. Left: transversal slice of MR brain volume constituting WM, GM, and CSF, as labeled. Right: simplified model with ribbon-like structure. While real cerebral cortex has varying thickness, it is approximated with constant thickness in the simplified model. The motivation for this simplification will be discussed in more depth below.

While manual segmentation of the complicated cortex is time and labor intensive and dependent upon the individual user, semi- or fully automatic segmentation is indispensable. There is a growing number of efforts in this arena. Wells et al. [8] used a non-parametric Pazen window to model brain images, and corrected RF inhomogeneities using an EM algorithm. Kapur [92] extended Wells' work by incorporating spatial information embedded in the raw data in conjunction with an EM-MF estimator to intensively compute inhomogeneities in the RF coil and aid in classification of pixels. Hall et al. [25] employed the FCM in classification of brain images. Xu et al. [93] proposed an Adaptive FCM (ACFM), based on the FCM, for the purpose of correcting the bias field. Bomans et al. [94] applied morphological filters, along with a Marr-Hildreth operator, for 3D cortical segmentation and reconstruction.

In the meantime, deformable models, and level set methods in particular, have become widely recognized for their great potency in segmenting, tracking, and matching anatomic structures by information derived from image data, as well as prior knowledge about the location, size, and shape of structures. Leventhon [95,96] incorporated a priori shape information into the level set framework as the shape force evolving the curve to match the expected shape perfectly. Han et al. [97] proposed topologically preserving the level set, which retains initial topology during evolvution of the curve. Zeng et al. [59] proposed a novel coupled level set and applied it to modeling of the cortical structure. It should be mentioned here that our work is somewhat close to Zeng's work, but the major distinctions between them will be discussed in later sections.

In this section we present a novel approach to cerebral cortex segmentation. We formulate the segmentation problem within the level set framework, the zero level set surface of which is driven by image-derived information, and the a priori knowledge of cortex structures as well. Its efficacy is demonstrated with experiments where this formulation addresses the cortex segmentation problem robustly and accurately.

The outline of this section is as follows. In Section 4.2 we provide a preview of our framework, followed by a detailed description of its components and their integration into the final variational formula, which propagates the surface within the WM and localizes it at WM/GM boundary. The WM/GM surface further evolves into the GM and halts at the GM/CSF boundary. In Section 4.3 we demonstrate our approach with simulated as well as real MR brain data, and provide visual and quantitative results. Finally, we draw our conclusions in Section 4.4.

5.2. Our Approach

In this subsection we develop a two-stage semiautomatic cortex segmentation system, as depicted in Figure 10. Since skulls are part of the brain, we first remove them with the aid of MRIcro software, which is a freeware used for visualization and processing of medical images. We next refine the results through manual intervention. The skull-stripped brain is then fed into the first stage for WM/GM segmentation, followed by GM/CSF segmentation in the next stage.

In the first stage, WM/GM segmentation, we propose a unified variational formula that integrates region and boundary information. Specifically, We modify the Chan-Vese model [58] to describe regional homogeneity of brain tissues, and present a new maximum a posteriori (MAP) framework with which to statistically detect coupled boundaries. The zero level set, which represents the WM/GM surface, is initiated in the WM and evolves until it reaches the WM/GM boundary.

In the second stage the WM/GM surface obtained in the first stage moves out from the WM/GM boundary to fit the GM/CSF boundary. The prior information of approximately constant thickness is also utilized as a constraint.

5.2.1. Define region information

For the sake of clarity of explanation, we first review the original Chan-Vese model [58], which was proposed for segmenting bimodal objects.

Let $\Omega \subset R^2$ be a bounded and open region, C its surface represented by the level set function Φ such that

$$\Phi\left(\mathbf{x}\right) \begin{cases} > 0, \text{ if } \mathbf{x} \text{ is inside } C, \\ = 0, \text{ if } \mathbf{x} \text{ is on surface } C, \\ < 0, \text{ if } \mathbf{x} \text{ is outside } C. \end{cases}$$

Thus, the Mumford-Shah model can be formulated as the minimization of the following functional:

$$\begin{aligned} E &= \lambda_1 \int_\Omega \left|I_0\left(\mathbf{x}\right) - c_1\right|^2 H\left(\Phi\left(\mathbf{x}\right)\right) d\mathbf{x} \\ &+ \lambda_2 \\ &\int_\Omega \left|I_0\left(\mathbf{x}\right) - c_2\right|^2 \left(1 - H\left(\Phi\left(\mathbf{x}\right)\right)\right) d\mathbf{x} \\ &+ \text{some regularizing terms,} \end{aligned} \tag{26}$$

where H is the Heaviside function, c_1 and c_2 are the average intensities inside and outside C, respectively, and λ_1 and λ_2 are two weighting parameters. The first and second terms encode the intensity variations inside and outside C, respectively. This energy functional is thus minimized at the point where both regions inside and outside the surface are most uniform, namely, the boundary of these two regions.

By taking the Euler-Lagrange equation of (26) and minimizing it using the gradient descent method, we obtain the following governing partial differential equation evolving the surface to the minimum of energy functional:

$$\frac{\partial \Phi}{\partial t} = \left\{ \underbrace{-\lambda_1 \left(I_0\left(\mathbf{x}\right) - c_1\right)^2}_{\text{inside force}} \underbrace{\lambda_2 \left(I_0\left(\mathbf{x}\right) - c_2\right)^2}_{\text{outside force}} \right\} \delta\left(\Phi\right)$$

$$+ \text{some regularizing terms.} \tag{27}$$

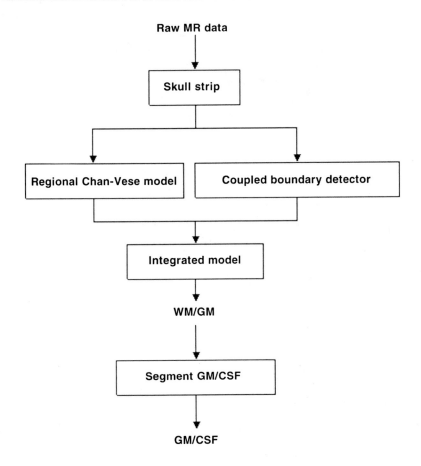

Figure 10. Block diagram of the entire system.

Thus, if we ignore those regularizing terms, the surface is propelled by the coun-
terforces from the outer and inner regions until they completely counteract each
other, which implies a steady-state Eq. (27).

The basic idea of the Chan-Vese model is illustrated for the 2D case in Figure 11. Comparing Figure 11 with the right side of Figure 9, we can recognize
that they are very alike, except for the distinction that this simplified model for the
cortex is trimodal while the Chan-Vese model is designed for bimodal cases.

In order to address this problem, we modify the original formulation by defining two new Heaviside functions to represent the third region in the cortical structure. The thickness of the cerebral cortex in [59] was within the range of 1 to 3
mm, with an average value of $d = 2$mm. Thus, our new Heaviside functions can

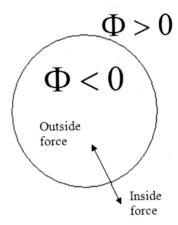

Figure 11. The entire plane is decomposed by the evolving curve into two regions, with $\Phi > 0$ for the outer and $\Phi < 0$ for the inner region. The evolving curve is characterized by $\Phi = 0$. During evolution of the curve, the inside and outside forces compete to determine the speed and direction of curve propagation until a balance between these two forces is established.

be defined as follows:

$$H_1(\Phi) = \begin{cases} 0, \text{ if } \Phi < 0, \\ 1, \text{ if } 0 \leq \Phi \leq d, \end{cases} \quad \text{and} \quad H_2(\Phi) = \begin{cases} 0, \text{ if } \Phi < d, \\ 1, \text{ if } \Phi \geq d. \end{cases}$$

Thus, we modify the original energy functional as follows:

$$\begin{aligned} E &= \lambda_1 \int_\Omega |I_0(\mathbf{x}) - c_1|^2 (1 - H_1(\Phi(\mathbf{x}))) d\mathbf{x} \\ &+ \lambda_2 \int_\Omega |I_0(\mathbf{x}) - c_2|^2 H_1(\Phi(\mathbf{x})) (1 - H_2(\Phi(\mathbf{x}))) d\mathbf{x} \\ &+ \lambda_3 \int_\Omega |I_0(\mathbf{x}) - c_3|^2 H_2(\Phi(\mathbf{x})) d\mathbf{x}, \end{aligned} \quad (28)$$

This notation is consistent with Eq. (27), except for c_3, a new parameter representing the average intensity in the third region, and the new weighting parameter λ_3, which can be tuned during experiments.

Figure 12 depicts our modified Chan-Vese model. The above cortex model is built under the assumption of a constant thickness. Unfortunately, the real cortex is highly folded and convoluted, forming numerous gyri and sulci, thus having different thicknesses throughout the entire brain. Hence, our simplified model, uniformly thick over the entire brain, seems to violate actual situations. One possible solution to this apparent contradiction is to adopt a *multiphase* level

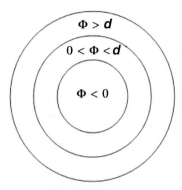

Figure 12. The brain can be simplified and modeled as three concentric spheres (or circles in 2D). The areas of $\Phi < 0$, $0 < \Phi < d$, and $\Phi > d$ represent the WM, GM, and CSF respectively.

set model [98] and construct two level set functions to represent the WM/GM and GM/CSF surfaces. However, this would double computational expenses. However, this issue can be addressed by considering the "average" property of integration calculations. Mathematically, integration can be approximated as a summing-up calculation, which averages out local differences on a global scale. Therefore, in spite of its local inaccuracy, our model is correct globally and does not affect our formulation in Eq. (28). Moreover, compared to a multiphase level set model, our model utilizes only one level set to represent two surfaces, which greatly reduces the 3D computational expense.

5.2.2. Define boundary information

Conventionally, an edge map is determined by voxels and their immediate neighborhoods. Two principal characteristics of an edge map are magnitude and direction. Normally, they are quantified by operators (e.g., the Roberts, Sobel, Prewitt, Kirsch, or Laplacian operators). However, they cannot yield satisfactory results when applied to MR images (see Figure 13). An alternative approach was proposed in [59], and it produced an attractive result. A similar idea was presented in [99], in which a histogram was used to coarsely estimate the parameters and an EM algorithm was adopted to estimate them iteratively. One disadvantage of this method was its high computational complexity, however.

In this section we present a novel approach to edge detection in a Bayesian scheme. It takes into account the ribbon-like nature of the cortex, thus avoiding

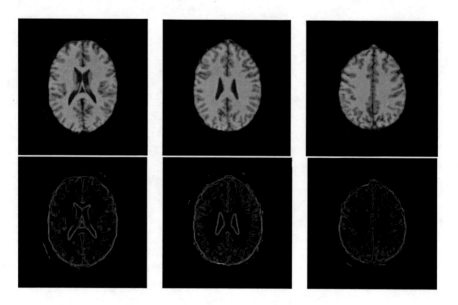

Figure 13. Results from image gradient operators. Top: slices from the original MR data. Bottom: results from a gradient operator.

being trapped in local minima in badly corrupted images. It is therefore the first choice for cortical edge detection.

Let s be a point on the inner boundary, t the other point on the outer boundary (see Figure 14), and N_s the set of points in the normal direction of s. Also, let ∇I_s be the gradient of s in the normal direction, and let ∇I_t be defined similarly. Then the probability that a coupled edge exists in the neighborhood of s that lies in the inner boundary can be represented by

$$P\left(s \in B, \exists t \in B | \nabla I_s, \nabla I_t, t \in N_s\right) = \max_{t \in N_s} P\left(s \in B, t \in B | \nabla I_s, \nabla I_t, t \in N_s\right),$$
(29)

where $s \in B$ means that s lies in the boundary and $t \in B$ means that t lies in the boundary.

Assuming that ∇I_s and ∇I_t are independent variables, we have

$$P\left(\nabla I_s, \nabla I_t | s \in B, t \notin B\right) = P\left(\nabla I_s | s \in B\right) P\left(\nabla I_t | t \in B\right),$$
(30)

where $P\left(\nabla I_s | s \in B\right)$ is the probability of ∇I_s, given the condition that s lies within the boundary.

Using MAP estimation, Eq. (30) can be rewritten as

$$P(s \in B, \exists t \in B | \nabla I_s, \nabla I_t, t \in N_s)$$
$$= \max_{t \in N_s} \frac{P(\nabla I_s | s \in B) P(\nabla I_t | t \in B)}{P(\nabla I_s, \nabla I_t, t \in N_s)} P(s \in B, t \in B)$$
$$\infty \max_{t \in N_s} P(\nabla I_s | s \in B) P(\nabla I_t | t \in B) P(s \in B, t \in B),$$
(31)

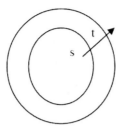

Figure 14. The coupled boundary is defined by a set of coupled points s and t.

where

$$
\begin{aligned}
P\left(\nabla I_s, \nabla I_t, t \in N_s\right) = {} & P\left(\nabla I_s, \nabla I_t, t \in N_s | s \in B, t \in B\right) \cdot P\left(s \in B, t \in B\right) \\
& + P\left(\nabla I_s, \nabla I_t, t \in N_s | s \in B, t \notin B\right) \cdot P\left(s \in B, t \notin B\right) \\
& + P\left(\nabla I_s, \nabla I_t, t \in N_s | s \notin B, t \in B\right) \cdot P\left(s \notin B, t \in B\right) \\
& + P\left(\nabla I_s, \nabla I_t, t \in N_s | s \notin B, t \notin B\right) \cdot P\left(s \notin B, t \notin B\right).
\end{aligned}
$$

The first term of (31) is the conditional boundary probability under the hypothesis that s is on the boundary, the second term under the hypothesis that t is on the boundary, and the last term is the a priori that constrains the distance between s and its associated t within a certain range.

The conditional boundary probability can be modeled as $P\left(\nabla I_s | s \in B\right) = g\left(|\nabla I_s|\right)$ and $P\left(\nabla I_t | t \in B\right) = g\left(|\nabla I_t|\right)$, where $|\nabla I_s|$ and $|\nabla I_t|$ are the magnitude of the gradient at s and t; $g\left(\cdot\right)$ is a monotonically increasing function, which will be defined in the experimental section.

The last term restricts the coupled boundary within a reasonable range. It is an important term that encodes a priori information. We model it as $P\left(s \in B, t \in B\right) = h\left(\mathrm{dist}\left(s, t\right)\right)$, where $h\left(\cdot\right)$ is defined as follows (Figure 15):

$$
h\left(d\right) =
\begin{cases}
\left(\frac{|d|-d_{\min}}{d_1-d_{\min}}\right)^2 \left(0.75 - 0.5\frac{|d|-d_{\min}}{d_1-d_{\min}}\right), & d_{\min} \le |d| \le d_1, \\[2mm]
0.25, & d_1 < |d| < d_2, \\[2mm]
0.25 - 0.75\left(\frac{|d|-d_2}{d_{\max}-d_2}\right)^2 + 0.5\left(\frac{|d|-d_2}{d_{\max}-d_2}\right)^3, & d_2 \le |d| \le d_{\max}.
\end{cases}
$$

Hence, coupled boundary definition greatly enhances the robustness and accuracy of edge detection in three aspects:

1. It models the ribbon structure of the cortex, which moves the surface to cross over noisy points or single lines.

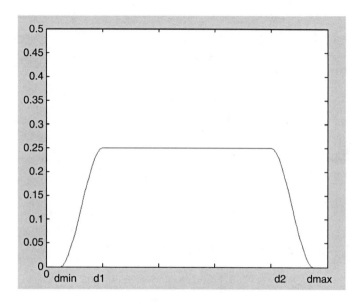

Figure 15. Function h used as a prior constraint: $d_{\min}$ = minimum distance allowed; $d_{\max}$ = maximum distance allowed. See attached CD for color version.

2. It rewards a directional edge, which is another strategy to overcome noise.

3. It has the constraint condition, an effective method for approximately modeling the constant thickness of the cortical layer.

5.2.3. Integrate region and boundary information

In the previous two subsections we independently developed region and boundary forces that propagate the surface to the WM/GM boundary. In theory, both are supposed to converge in the correct position. In practice, however, neither performs well enough because the image data are usually corrupted by noise and RF inhomogeneties. While the region-propagated surface evolves correctly in a global sense, it tends to leak out of weak boundaries. Contrarily, the boundary-propagated surface can localize accurately, but evolves slowly due to its limited capture range. This observation implies that the region and boundary forces can be complementary, thus motivating us to unify them in order to arrive at a robust as well as accurate result.

There have been many attempts at unifying region and boundary information [53, 55, 100]. In this section we employ region information as global criteria and boundary information as a local stopping term. We obtain the following unified evolving equation:

$$\frac{\partial \Phi}{\partial t} = \underbrace{s\left(\mathbf{x}\right)}_{\text{stopping force}}$$

$$\left\{ \underbrace{\lambda_1 \left|I_0 - c_1\right|^2 \delta_1\left(\Phi\right) - \lambda_2 \left|I_0 - c_2\right|^2 \left(\delta_1\left(\Phi\right)\left(1 - H_2\left(\Phi\right)\right) - H_1\left(\Phi\right)\delta_2\left(\Phi\right)\right) - \lambda_3 \left|I_0 - c_3\right|^2 \delta_2\left(\Phi\right)}_{\text{region force}} \right\},$$

$$(32)$$

where $s\left(\mathbf{x}\right)$ is defined as

$$s\left(\mathbf{x}\right) = \frac{1}{1 + \left|H\left(P\left(\mathbf{x}\right)\right)\right|^2}.$$

The terms within the curly braces describe the propagating force from the competition of three regions. The $s\left(\mathbf{x}\right)$ term beyond the curly braces is the stopping term that decreases to zero at coupled boundaries; $H\left(\cdot\right)$ is defined heuristically according to the experimental data. Fortunately, a specific form of $H\left(\cdot\right)$ that is appropriate for most MR brain data is found and given in the experimental section. Thus, this formulation borrows the strength of robustness from the region forces, and simultaneously incorporates the accurate localization ability of the coupled boundary detector.

5.2.4. GM/CSF segmentation

After obtaining the WM/GM surface as described in the previous subsection, we move on to GM/CSF segmentation, where the WM/GM surface is fed as input. GM/CSF segmentation is close to WM/GM segmentation except in one aspect. In GM/CSF segmentation, we replace the coupled edge detector with a conventional single edge detector because only the GM/CSF surface, and not two surfaces, is outside the evolving surface. Thus, we formulate our PDE for GM/CSF segmentation as follows:

$$\frac{\partial \Phi}{\partial t} = H_1\left(\Phi\right) \cdot s\left(\mathbf{x}\right) \cdot \left\{-\lambda_2\left(I - c_2\right)^2 + \lambda_3\left(I - c_3\right)^2\right\} \delta\left(\Phi\right), \qquad (33)$$

where $s\left(\mathbf{x}\right) = \frac{1}{1 + \left|\nabla I(\mathbf{x})\right|^2}$, and all other notations are the same as in the previous subsection.

The right-hand side of Eq. (33) is a propagation term propelled by regional force, but also confined by the boundary detector. The surface is initiated at the WM/GM surface and evolves into the GM until it reaches the GM/CSF surface.

5.3. Experiments

In this section we validate our approach on both simulated and real MR data. We only use T1-weighted scans, which have the best WM/GM contrast, and ignore T2- and PD-weighted scans. Since the skull part of the brain is not included in our model, it is removed by using MRIcro software.

We set $g(x) = 1 - e^{-\frac{x^2}{100}}$ and $H(x) = 1 + 240\left[\log(1-x)\right]^2$, respectively. These two settings proved to have good performance, and are insensitive to different MR brain datasets.

We require a measurement with which to quantify our results in order to evaluate the performance of our method. The Internet Brain Segmentation Repository (ISBR) proposed an Average Overlap Metric (AOM) for comparing segmentations. For any tissue, assuming that V_m denotes the set of voxels assigned for it by manual segmentation and V_α the set of voxels assigned for it by the algorithm, the AOM is defined as the sum of voxels where both segmentations have an assignment relative to the number of voxels that either segmentation has, or is formulated as $\text{AOM} = 2\frac{|V_m \cap V_\alpha|}{|V_m| + |V_\alpha|}$.

5.3.1. Validation on simulated MR brain data

The simulated data used in our experiment were provided by the McConnell Brain Imaging Center at the Montreal Neurological Institute (Brainweb). The images were generated by an MR simulator [101] that allows adjusting some parameters (e.g., noise and intensity inhomogeneities) independently. The most significant advantage of the database is that it allows us to test our algorithm on images of different quality, thus providing a quantitative system to evaluate performance in different situations. The ground truth of the model is provided in the form of membership functions, which indicate the possibility of each voxel belonging to different tissues.

Our work primarily focuses on the WM, GM and CSF of the brain, thus ignoring other brain tissues. To test the accuracy as well as the robustness of the algorithm, we performed experiments on four sets of data with different parameters indicating different the level of corruption by thermal noise and RF inhomogeneities. We began with the most ideal case, with weak noise and no intensity inhomogeneities, and moved on to tougher cases with different levels of noise and intensity inhomogeneities added. We evaluated our results by comparing them with the ground truth of the model, and quantifying them using AOM measurement. The visual performance of our algorithm is illustrated in Figure 16, and the associated quantitative results are listed in Table 1.

We can observe that in the WM the average AOM is 0.89, and in the GM 0.75, with slight fluctuations according to levels of noise and RF inhomogeneities. According to Zijdenbos's statement that results with $\text{AOM} > 0.7$ indicate excellent agreement, our method demonstrates desirable performance in cortical segmenta-

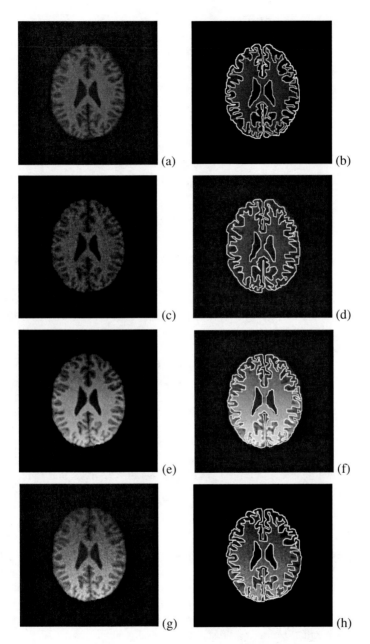

Figure 16. Results on simulated data with our method for four cases. Left: axial slices of original data. Right: automatically detected contours on axial slices. (a,b) noise = 3%, intensity inhomogeities = 0%; (c,d) noise = 9%, intensity inhomogeities = 0%; (e,f) noise = 3%, intensity inhomogeities = 40%; (g,h) noise = 9%, intensity inhomogeities = 40%.

Table 1. Comparison of our Method with
the Phantom Ground Truth

	WM	GM	Overall
pn=3% rf=0%	0.90	0.76	0.83
pn=9%, rf=0%	0.88	0.74	0.81
pn=3%, rf=40%	0.90	0.73	0.82
pn=9%, rf=40%	0.88	0.74	0.81

tion. Moreover, our algorithm performs robustly in the presence of severe thermal noise and RF inhomogeneities.

5.3.2. Validation on real MR brain, data

To further demonstrate the performance of our algorithm under various conditions, we used real MR data as test samples and performed a comparison with manually outlined surfaces. We utilized the MR data provided by the ISBR of center from morphometric analysis done at the Massachusetts General Hospital (20 normal MR brain datasets), along with manual segmentation performed on positionally normalized scans by trained investigators from the ISBR.

The data we obtained and utilized here are 20 normal T1-weighted brains in 8-bit format. The coronal three dimensional T1-weighted spoiled gradient echo MRI scans were performed on two different imaging systems. Ten FLASH scans on four males and six females were performed on 1.5-tesla Siemens magnetic MR systems with the following parameters: TR = 40 ms, TE = 8 ms, flip angle = 50 degrees, field of view = 30 cm, slice thickness = contiguous 3.0 mm, matrix = 256, and averages = 1. Ten 3D-CAPRY scans on six males and four females were performed on a 1.5-tesla General Electric Signa MR System (Milwaukee, WI), with the following parameters: TR = 50 ms, TE = 9 ms, flip angle = 50 degress, field of view = 24 cm, slice thickness = contiguous 3.0 mm, matrix = 256, and averages = 1. The 8-bit version of the 20 normal T1-weighted brains were reduced from 16-bit data by thresholding intensities above or below 99.9% of the total number of different intensities, and scaling the remaining range to $0 \ldots 255$ if and only the range did not already fit within $0 \ldots 255$. All the datasets were positionally normalized by imposing a Talairah coordinate on each 3D MR scan. The repositioned scans were then resliced into normalized 3.0-mm coronal, 1.0-mm axial, and 1.0-mm sagittal scans for subsequent analysis.

The experimental results with our algorithm are depicted in Figure 17 and quantitatively evaluated in Table 2. Fortunately, we can note that the exactly same dataset was extensively used in other published papers, and the results were gathered by Rajapakse and Kruggel [102]. Therefore, it is easy to compare our

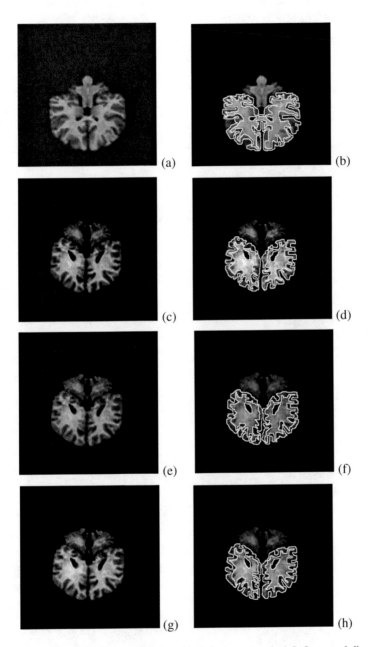

Figure 17. Result on 20 normal T1-weighted brains using our method. Left: coronal slices from original data. Right: automatically detected contours on coronal slices. (a,b) 100_23; (c,d) 111_2; (e,f) 13_3; (g,h) 7_8.

Table 2. AOM for 20 T1-weighted Normal Brains

	WM	GM
1-24	0.75	0.71
100-23	0.79	0.75
11-3	0.76	0.71
110-3	0.73	0.73
111-2	0.83	0.78
112-2	0.79	0.80
12-3	0.84	0.75
13-3	0.84	0.77
15-3	0.70	0.60
16-3	0.70	0.51
17-3	0.80	0.72
191-3	0.84	0.70
2-4	0.79	0.78
202-3	0.80	0.69
205-3	0.80	0.71
4-8	0.76	0.71
5-8	0.68	0.55
6-10	0.76	0.71
7-8	0.79	0.78
8-4	0.77	0.73

results with the ones obtained by other investigators. The results of the comparison are shown in Figures 18 and 19.

We can observe from Figures 18 and 19 that:

1. The overall AOM for WM segmentation is 0.78, which is well above those with six other algorithms, ranging from 0.47 to 0.56. The overall AOM for GM segmentation is 0.71, which is also higher than the six listed algorithms within the range of 0.55–0.58.

2. Our algorithm is persistently robust compared with the other methods. Take WM segmentation, for example. The AOM of our method ranges from 0.68 to 0.84, with a fluctuation of 0.16. Comparatively, the corresponding fluctuation with the six other methods is about 0.6. This shows that our approach has equally excellent performance, even in case of noisy images.

3. The performance for WM segmentation is relatively better than that for GM segmentation. One reason for this is that the GM is much more convoluted than the WM, and the surfaces have difficulty moving into extremely narrow sulci (7 1-2 pixels wide). Another reason is that the GM

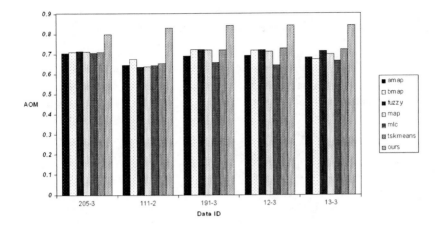

Figure 18. AOM on 20 normal T1-weighted brains for WM segmentation using various methods. See attached CD for color version.

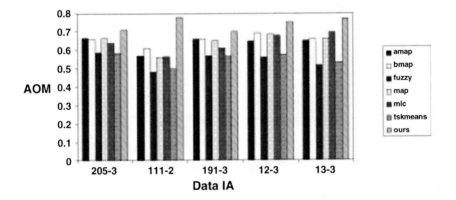

Figure 19. AOM on 20 normal T1-weighted brains for GM segmentation from various methods. See attached CD for color version.

has a much smaller area than the WM, and misclassification of only one pixel thus has a much greater impact on GM segmentation than on WM segmentation.

4. Our algorithm has a relatively lower AOM in some samples, e.g., as 16_3, 5_8, and 15_3. This is due to the fact that these scans have lower WM/GM contrast than other scans. Hence, the edge detector does not perform as

effectively as in other scans, although curves driven by regional information are still robust in segmenting the overall profile.

5. From Figures 18 and 19, we can see that all six methods listed in [102] have approximately the same tendencies. However, our method demonstrates a slightly different performance in some scans. This is mainly because the six other methods are pixel classification-based per se, and our method employs an integration approach, and so it is expected to perform differently from the other six algorithms.

5.4. Conclusions

In this section we have proposed a new approach to segmenting the cerebral cortex. We formulated the segmentation problem using a modified Chan-Vese model, and combined it with statistical coupled edge detection. The knowledge of the thickness of the cortex is considered to improve the accuracy of the results. Convincing results are demonstrated with both simulated and real MR brain data.

It should be mentioned that our approach shares some features with Zeng's approach [59]. Both methods use a level set method ribbon brain model. However, we consider region information and modify the Chan-Vese model to accommodate the ribbon structure of the brain, which improves the robustness the algorithm. Furthermore, we only use one level set function, instead of two, which dramatically decreases the computational expense in 3D cases.

Future work will include explicit modeling of the MR bias field to further improve robustness in case of RF inhomogeneities. Also, it is well known that level set methods are topologically independent, which may be disadvantageous in brain segmentation. Implementation of topology-preserving level set methods [97] may also further improve segmentation results.

6.   PRIOR-BASED CARDIAC VALVE SEGMENTATION USING A GEODESIC SNAKE

6.1. Introduction

The algorithm presented in this section was originally developed for a project for reconstructing the mitral valve leaflet from 3D ultrasound image sequences, which would lead to a better understanding of cardiac valve mechanics and the mechanisms of valve failure. Segmenting the valve efficiently could also aid surgeons in diagnosis and analysis of cardiac valve disease.

Among medical imaging techniques, ultrasound is particularly attractive because of its good temporal resolution, noninvasiveness, and relatively low cost. In clinical practice, segmentation of ultrasound images still relies on manual or semiautomatic outlines produced by expert physicians, especially when it comes to an object as complex as a cardiac valve. The large quantities of data in 3D volume sequences render a manual procedure impossible. Efficient processing of the information contained in ultrasound image calls for automatic object segmentation techniques.

When it comes to echocardiographic sequences, the inherent noise, the similarity of the intensity distribution between object and background, and the complex movements make it difficult to segment the cardiac valve accurately. We could make full use of the valve prior, and segment it under the guidance of prior knowledge to reduce the manual intervention. We can segment the valve automatically guided by the following prior:

1. The valve moves in a relatively fixed region between neighboring images.

2. The valve has a relatively stationary shape at a certain position.

We have developed an algorithm based on a level set framework, and represented the prior as a speed field. The speed field drives the zero level converging on the ideal contour and then the valve of the heart is segmented. Section 5.2 gives an overview of some of the existing prior-based object segmentation methods. The proposed algorithm is described and formulated in Section 5.3. The application results are presented in Section 5.4, and conclusions follow in Section 5.5.

6.2. Related Work

There have been some applications of prior-based image segmentation under the snake framework [43] over the past several years. One can freely incorporate a prior into the function as an energy item. Cremers et al. [103] established a prior Point Distribution Model (PDM) of a certain object, then calculated the contour's posteriori Bayesian probability, and made it an energy item to control the evolving process. Ivana et al. [104] modified the internal energy to preserve the thickness of the cardiac valve leaflet. However, in the snake framework, the object is described as a serial point, which makes it hard to deal with the changing topology. The goal of valve segmentation is to study the mechanism of movement, which makes the cardiac wall that joggles with the valve as important as the valve. The valve leaflet can be divided into several isolated parts in certain slices. All of this means that the topology of the contour changes when the valve moves. So it is too hard for a snake model to be applied to this task. And, what is more, the snake model needs an initial outline close to the contour, which makes an automatic segmentation process impossible.

Level set-based segmentation embeds an initial curve as the zero level set of a higher-dimensional surface, and evolves the surface so that the zero level set converges on the boundary of the object to be segmented. Since it evolves in a higher dimension, it can deal with the topology changing naturally. However, it is difficult to incorporate prior knowledge into the evolution process to make the segment result more robust and efficient. Leventon et al. [105] calculated the difference between the zero level and the statistical prior contours, and embedded it in the evolution process. Chen et al. [106] made it applicable to a linear transform. They all got a more robust result than with the traditional method. However, calculating the difference between the zero level and prior statistical contour at each evolution step is time consuming, and a scalar of the similar contour metric cannot guide the evolution directly. In the following, we present a new algorithm that represents the region and shape prior knowledge in a form of a speed field. The speed vector can drive the zero level set directly to the ideal cardiac valve contour.

6.3. Geodesic Snake Guided by Prior Knowledge

Given a region or shape priors, the information can be folded into the segmentation process. We here represent the region and shape prior as speed fields and embed them to the level set evolution equation to pull the surface to the ideal contour, which could reduce the manual parts procedure to a great extent.

Our approach is based on a geodesic snake [49]:

$$\frac{\partial \phi}{\partial t} = u(x)(k + v_0)|\nabla \phi| + \nabla u \cdot \nabla \phi, \tag{34}$$

where $u(x) = -|\nabla G_\sigma * I|$, and v_0 is an image-dependent balloon force added to force the contour to flow outward. In this level set framework, the surface ϕ evolves at every point perpendicular to the level sets as a function of the curvature at that point and the image gradient.

We add new speed items to the evolution equation of the geodesic snake. The new prior knowledge item forms a total force with an internal and external force of the original image and drives the zero level set to converge to the ideal contour. There are two levels of the additional prior force: one is the lower level of the region prior constraint, which makes the zero level evolve in a certain region, and the other is the higher level of the shape prior constraint, which makes the final contour converge to the prior shape of object. We then obtain a new equation:

$$\frac{\partial \phi}{\partial t} = u(x)(k + v_0)|\nabla \phi| + \nabla u \cdot \nabla \phi + \sum F_i \cdot \nabla \phi, \tag{35}$$

where F_i is the region, shape, or other prior knowledge forces. The speed force is more direct and efficient than the similarity metric of the contour. However, it is difficult to transform the prior knowledge into a speed field. The algorithm for this is presented in detail as follows.

6.3.1. Region prior-based geodesic snake

The movement of a cardiac valve is very complex. It moves with the beating of the heart, turns around the valve root, and creates a great deal of distortion by itself. But the whole valve moves within a relatively stationary region, which is just in the ventricle. When it comes to a 3D echocardiographic sequence, the valve can share the same region in different slices at the same time. So it can be in the same sample position at different times. We can then segment several images under the guidance of the same region. When the zero level set is limited to evolve in the fixed region, the segmenting process will be more robust and efficient. We can segment the whole 3D echocardiographic sequence based on several prior regions.

Consider a prior region Ω within which the valve moves. There is a region function $J(x, y)$:

$$J(x,y) = \begin{cases} 1 & (x, y) \in \Omega, \\ 0 & (x, y) \notin \Omega, \end{cases} \tag{36}$$

A speed field is created outside the prior region. The force of the field is zero inside the prior region and direct to the prior region outside it. The power of the force bears a close relation to the distance from the point to the prior region. So the speed field has a potential to drive the zero level set to the prior region. In addition, the prior force will obtain a balance with the inflating force nearby the boundary of the region. When segmenting the valve, an appropriate contour can be obtained at the root of the valve, lest the zero level set evolve to the whole cardiac wall. The distance from point X to prior region Ω is defined as

$$\gamma(X) = \begin{cases} d(X) & X \notin \Omega, \\ 0 & X \in \Omega, \end{cases} \tag{37}$$

$$d(X) = \min(|X - X_I|) \qquad X_I \in \Omega. \tag{38}$$

Then the speed field of the prior region is

$$F_{region}(X) = [f_r(d) + c_1] \frac{\nabla\gamma}{|\nabla\gamma|}, \tag{39}$$

where c_1 is equal to or a little less than v_0; $f_r(\cdot)$ makes the prior force almost c_1 nearby Ω and to rise to $c_1 + c_2$ far from Ω. We take

$$f_r(d) = c_2\left(1 - \exp\left(-\frac{d^2}{\sigma^2}\right)\right). \tag{40}$$

A speed field is then obtained that can drive the zero level set to Ω.

The final region prior-based geodesic snake equation is

$$\frac{\partial\phi}{\partial t} = u(x)(k + v_0)|\nabla\phi| + \nabla u \cdot \nabla\phi + [f_r(d) + c_1]\frac{\nabla\gamma}{|\nabla\gamma|} \cdot \nabla\phi. \tag{41}$$

We can obtain a final result that includes the cardiac valve, the root of the valve, and the raised cardiac wall that joggles with the valve with some postprocessing.

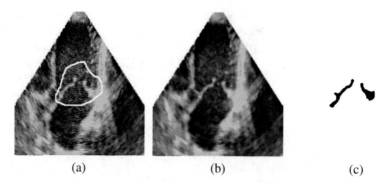

(a)   (b)   (c)

Figure 20. Cardiac valve segmented by region prior-based geodesic snake: (a) image from an echocardiographic sequence and the prior valve region; (b) result of preprocessing; (c) final segmenting result with region prior-based geodesic snake.

We erode the prior region Ω and obtain Ω', and then fill the segmentation result with foreground color outside Ω'. Finally, we perform an intensity reversion and obtain the final result.

Preprocessing is very important because noise is inevitable in an ultrasound image. We adopted a Modified Curvature Diffusion Equation (MCDE) [107,108] to filter the original image, which could preserve the edge and smooth the noise. The equation is given as

$$u_t = |\nabla u| \, \nabla \cdot c\,(|\nabla u|)\, \frac{\nabla u}{|\nabla u|}. \tag{42}$$

We offer an example of a cardiac valve segmented using a region prior-based geodesic snake in Figure 20.

6.3.2. Shape prior-based geodesic snake

Because of the intrinsic noise in an echocardiographic image and the blur caused by movement of the cardiac valve, it is unavoidable that there will be some segmentation errors in the final result. To get a more accurate contour, we need to make full use of the prior shape of the heart valve in the segmenting process.

To that end, we set a speed field nearby the prior shape that directs to the nearest point of the shape. The force F_{shape} pulls all the points near to the prior shape. Consider a prior contour C. We define the distance from point X to contour C as ε:

$$\varepsilon\,(X) = d\,(X) = \min\,(|X - X_I|) \qquad X_I \in C. \tag{43}$$

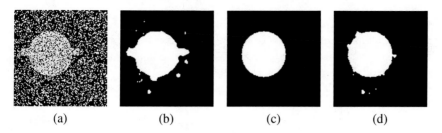

(a)   (b)   (c)   (d)

Figure 21. Circle segmented by the shape prior-based geodesic snake: (a) circle stained by a bar and salt-and-pepper noise; (b) circle segmented by the geodesic snake; (c) prior circle shape; (d) circle segmented by shape prior-based geodesic snake.

Then the speed field produced by the prior contour is

$$F_{\text{shape}}(X) = f_s(d) \frac{\nabla \varepsilon}{|\nabla \varepsilon|}, \tag{44}$$

where F_{shape} directs to the nearest shape point, and the magnitude of F_{shape} is controlled by f_s.

The attributes of the prior shape force are very important. There are two kinds of force: one like the elastic force that would be more powerful far away from prior shape, and the other just like the force in an electric field, so that the closer to the shape, the more powerful it will be. It is hoped that F_{shape} can only take effect in the field nearby the prior contour and leave it alone far from the prior contour, and the closer, the more powerful. So the second choice is taken. It is supposed that the farthest neighborhood distance is δ:

$$f_s(d) = \begin{cases} k(\delta - d) & d \leq \delta, \\ 0 & d > \delta. \end{cases} \tag{45}$$

We then obtain the final shape prior-based geodesic snake equation:

$$\frac{\partial \phi}{\partial t} = u(x)(k + v_0)|\nabla \phi| + \nabla u \cdot \nabla \phi + f_s(d) \frac{\nabla \varepsilon}{|\nabla \varepsilon|} \cdot \nabla \phi. \tag{46}$$

The algorithm was demonstrated on a synthetic image. We found that we could get a better result guided by a prior shape field (Figure 21). We set $\delta = 15$ when segmenting the circle.

6.4. Application and Results

We put the algorithm into practice and efficiently segmented heart valve leaflets from 10 3D echocardiographic sequences, each covering a complete cardiac cycle. The 3D sequences were recorded using a Philips Sonos 750 TTO probe, which scans an object rotationally. There were 13–17 frames per cardiac cycle, and the angular slice spacing was 3 degrees, resulting in 60 images slices in each frame. Therefore, there were about a thousand images in each 3D sequence. The resolution of images was 240×256.

Obviously, it is too tedious to segment all the images manually using the traditional method. Our method deals with all the images without too much manual intervention. Neither it is sensitive to the initial zero level set nor the prior region, as long as it is just between the valve and the cardiac wall. Given several prior regions, our method may segment the whole image sequence automatically without too much parameter choosing or adjusting. The images from the same scanning time can share the same prior region, as do images from neighboring times. Without too many manual processes, segmentation can be as efficient as possible and the segmenting result precise. Some results obtained with the region prior-based geodesic snake are shown below in Figure 22. The images in there are at the same scanning position as a different scanning time from a 3D valve sequence. To facilitate the display, we cut out the valve region.

Most of the above segmentation results may satisfy the needs of 3D reconstruction and diagnosis. Because of contamination of noise and movement blur, there will be inevitable errors in some contours, such as the 8th, 12th, and 13th contours in Figure 23. We can segment this kind of noise-disturbed image guided by a prior shape. The prior shape can either come from an output of a neighboring slice or from a manual outline provided by an expert physician. In the manual outlining process, it is unnecessary to draw out the whole shape: a part of the stained edge is just enough. We depict some results using the shape prior-based geodesic snake in Figure 23. We can alleviate almost all segmentation errors under the guidance of a shape prior.

6.5. Conclusions

The inherent noise, blur, and large quantity of data in echocardiographic sequences make it difficult to segment valve structures, which hinders clinical application. We present a new algorithm to incorporate prior knowledge into the geodesic snake. The priors are expressed as a speed field that directly draws the zero level set to the ideal contour. The region prior limits the zero level set evolving within a certain region and the shape prior draws the curve to the ideal contour. An actual application on 3D echocardiographic sequences demonstrates that the algorithm segments the valve structure accurately and reduces the need for a manual procedure, resulting in a greatly accelerated process.

Prior-based image segmentation is the subject of active interest at present. We can express more prior knowledge as a speed field and embed them in image the segmentation process in future work. Guided by prior information, we can make image segmentation more accurate and efficient.

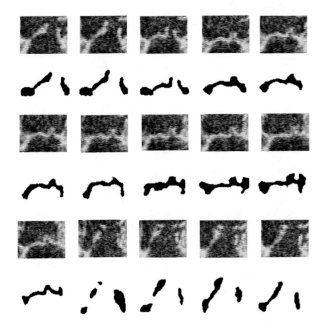

Figure 22. Valves segmented using the region prior-based geodesic snake.

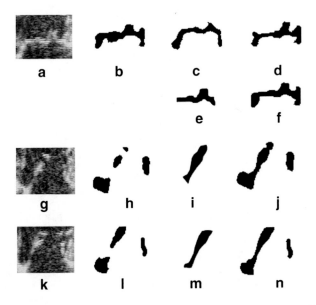

Figure 23. Cardiac valve segmented by the shape prior-based geodesic snake: (a,g,k) initial echocardiographic image; (b,h,l) result guided by region prior; (c) segmentation result of neighbor slice; (d) result guided by shape prior of (c); (e,i,m) manual outline; (f,j,n) result guided by shape prior.

7. REFERENCES

1. Duncan JS, Ayache N. 2000. Medical image analysis: progress over two decades and the challenges ahead. *IEEE Trans Pattern Anal Machine Intell* **22**:85–106.

2. Gupta A, Kurowski Lv, Singh A, Geiger D, Liang CC, Chiu MY, Adler LP, Haacke M, Wilson DL. 1993. Cardiac MR image segmentation using deformable models. In *Proceedings of the 1993 IEEE conference on computers in cardiology*, pp. 747–750. Washington, DC: IEEE Computer Society.

3. Bezdek JC, Hall LO, Clarke LP. 1993. Review of MR image segmentation techniques using pattern recognition. *Med Phys* **20**:1033–1048.

4. Udupa JK, Samarasekera S. 1996. Fuzzy connectedness and object definition: theory, algorithms and applications in image segmentation. *Graphical Models Image Process* **58**:246–261.

5. Pham DL, Prince JL. 1999. Adaptive fuzzy segmentation of magnetic resonance images. *IEEE Trans Med Imaging* **18**:737–752.

6. Simmons A, Tofts PS, Barker GJ, Arridge SR. 1994. Sources of intensity nonuniformity in spin echo images at 1.5 T. *Magn Reson Imaging* **32**:121–128.

7. Pham DL, Xu C, Prince JL. 2000. Current methods in medical image segmentation. *Annu Rev Biomed Engineer* **2**:315–337 .

8. Wells WM, Grimson WEL, Kikins R, Jolesz FA. 1996. Adaptive segmentation of MRI data. *IEEE Trans Med Imaging* **15**:429–442.

9. Guillemaud R, Brady M. 1997. Estimating the bias field of MR images. *IEEE Trans Med Imaging* **16**:238–251.

10. Styner M, Brechbuhler C, Szekely G, Gerig G. 2000. Parametric estimate of intensity inhomogeneities applied to MRI. *IEEE Trans Med Imaging* **19**:153–165.

11. Ahmed MN, Yamany SM, Mohamed N, Farag AA, Moriarty T. 2002. A modified fuzzy c-means algorithm for bias field estimated and segmentation of MRI data. *IEEE Trans Med Imaging* **21**:193–199.

12. Zhang Y, Brady M, Smith S. 2001. Segmentation of brain MR images through a hidden Markov random field model and the expectation-maximization algorithm. *IEEE Trans Med Imaging* **20**:45–57.

13. McInerney T, Terzopoulos D. 1996. Deformable models in medical image analysis: a survey. *Med Image Anal* **1**:91–108.

14. Fischler M, Elschlager R. 1973. The representation and matching of pictoral structures. *IEEE Trans Comput* **22**:67–92.

15. Lipson P, Yuille A, Keefe DO, Cavanaugh J, Taaffe J, Rosenthal D. 1990. Deformable templates for feature extraction from medical images. In *Proceedings of the first European conference on computer vision (ECCV'90)*, pp. 477–484. New York: Springer.

16. Staib LH, Duncan JS. 1992. Boundary finding with parametrically deformable models. *IEEE Trans Pattern Anal Machine Intell* **14**:1061–1075.

17. Staib LH, Duncan JS. 1996. Model-based deformable surface finding for medical images. *IEEE Trans Med Imaging* **78**:720–731.

18. Mortensen EN, Barrett WA. 1998. Interactive segmentation with intelligent scissors. *Graphical Models Image Process* **60**:349–384.

19. Falcþo AX, Udupa JK, Samarasekera S, Sharma S, Hirsch BE, Lotufo RdA. 1998. User-steered image segmentation paradigms: live wire and live lane. *Graphical Models Image Process* **60**(4):233–260.

20. Boykov Y, Jolly M-P. 2000. Interactive organ segmentation using graph cuts. In *Proceedings of the third international conference on medical image computing and computer-assisted intervention (MICCAI'2000). Lecture notes in computer science*, Vol. 1935, pp. 276–286. New York: Springer.

21. Rother C, Kolmogorov V, Blake A. 2004. GrabCut: interactive foreground extraction using iterated graph cuts. *ACM Trans Graphics* **23**:309–314.

22. Haralick RM, Shapiro LG. 1985. Image segmentation techniques. *Comput Vision Graphics Image Process* **29**:100–132.

23. Pal NR, Pal SK. 1993. A review on image segmentation techniques. *Pattern Recognit* **26**(9):1277–1294.

24. Clarke LP, Velthuizen RP, Camacho MA, Heine JJ, Vaidyanathan M, Hall LO, Thatcher RW, Silbiger ML. 1995. MRI segmentation: methods and applications. *Magn Reson Imaging* **13**:343–368.

25. Hall LO, Bensaid AM, Clarke LP, Velthuizen RP, Silbiger MS, Bezdek JC. 1992. A comparison of neural network and fuzzy clustering techniques in segmenting magnetic resonance images of the brain. *IEEE Trans Neural Networks* **3**:672–682.

26. Suri JS, Singh S, Reden L. 2002. Computer vision and pattern recognition techniques for 2d and 3d mr cerebral cortical segmentation (part i): a state-of-the-art review. *Pattern Anal Appl* **5**:46–76.

27. Suetens P, Bellon E, Vandermeulen D, Smet M, Marchal G, Nuyts J, Mortelmans L. 1993. Image segmentation: methods and applications in diagnostic radiology and nuclear medicine. *Eur J Radiol* **17**:14–21.

28. Sahoo PK, Soltani S, Wong AKC. 1988. A survey of thresholding techniques. *Comput Vision Graphics Image Process* **41**:233–260.

29. Lim KO, Pfefferbaum A. 1989. Segmentation of MR brain images into cerebrospinal fulid spaces, white and gray matter. *J Comput Assist Tomogr* **13**:588–593.

30. Shareef N, Wang DL, Yagel R. 1999. Segmentation of medical images using LEGION. *IEEE Trans Med Imaging* **18**:74–91.

31. Adams R, Bischof L. 1994. Seeded region growing. *IEEE Trans Pattern Anal Machine Intell* **16**:641–647.

32. Zucker SW. 1976. Region growing: childhood and adolescence. *Comput Vision Graphics Image Process* **5**:382–399.

33. Cline HE, Dumoulin CL, Hart HR, Lorensen WE, Ludke S. 1987. 3D reconstruction of the brain from magnetic resonance images using a connectivity algorithm. *Magn Reson Imaging* **5**:345–352.

34. Geman S, Geman D. 1984. Stochastic relaxation, Gibbs distributions, and the Bayesian restoration of images. *IEEE Trans Pattern Anal Machine Intell* **6**:721–741.

35. Li SZ. 1995. *Markov random field modeling in computer vision*. London: Springer-Verlag.

36. Held K, Kops ER, Krause BJ, Wells WM, Kikinis R. 1997. Markov random field segmentation of brain MR images. *IEEE Trans Med Imaging* **16**:878–886.

37. Rajapakse JC, Giedd JN, Rapoport JL. 1997. Statistical approach to segmentation of single-channel cerebral MR images. *IEEE Trans Med Imaging* **16**:176–186.

38. Davis LS. 1975. A survey of edge detection techniques. *Comput Vision Graphics Image Process* **4**:248–270.

39. Argyle E. 1971. Techniques for edge detection. *Proc IEEE* **59**:285–287.

40. Farag AA, Delp EJ. 1995. Edge linking by sequential search. *Pattern Recognit* **28**:611–633.

41. Montanari U. 1971. On the optimal detection of curves in noisy pictures. *Commun ACM* **14**:335–345.

42. Rifai H, Bloch I, Hutchinson S, Wiart J, Garnero L. 2000. Segmentation of the skull in MRI volumes using deformable model and taking the partial-volume effect into account. *Med Image Anal* **4**:219–233.

43. Kass M, Witkin A, Terzopoulos D. 1988. Snakes: active contour models. *Int J Comput Vision* **1**:321–331.

44. Cohen LD. 1991. On active contour models and balloons. *Comput Vision Graphics Image Process: Image Understand* **53**:211–218.

45. Leymarie F, Levine MD. 1993. Tracking deformable objects in the plane using an active contour model. *IEEE Trans Pattern Anal Machine Intell* **15**:617–634.

46. Xu C, Prince JL. 1998. Snakes, shapes, and gradient vector flow. *IEEE Trans Image Process* **7**:359–369.

47. Xu C, Anthony Y, Prince JL. 2000. On the relationship between parametric and geometric active contours. In *Proceedings of the 34th Asilomar conference on signals, systems, and computers*, pp. 483–489. Washington, DC: IEEE Computer Society.

48. Osher S, Sethian J. 1988. Fronts propagating with curvature dependent speed: algorithms based on the Hamilton-Jacobi formulation. *J Comput Phys* **79**:12–49.

49. Caselles V, Kimmel R, Sapiro G. 1997. Geodesic active contours. *Int J Comput Vision* **22**:61–79.

50. Yezzi A, Kichenassamy S, Kumar A, Olver P, Tannenbaum A. 1997. A geometric snake model for segmentation of medical imagery. *IEEE Trans Med Imaging* **16**:199–209.

51. Teo PC, Sapiro G, Wandell BA. 1997. Creating connected representations of cortical gray matter for functional MRI visualization. *IEEE Trans Med Imaging* **16**:852–863.

52. Malladi R, Sethian JA, Vemuri BC. 1995. Shape modeling with front propagation: A level set approach. *IEEE Trans Pattern Anal Machine Intell* **17**:158–175.

53. Chakraborty A, Staib L, Duncan J. 1996. Deformable boundary finding in medical images by integrating gradient and region information. *IEEE Trans Med Imaging* **15**:859–870.

54. Zhu S, Yuille A. 1996. Region competition: Unifying snakes, region growing, and Bayes/MDL for multiband image segmentation. *IEEE Trans Pattern Anal Machine Intell* **18**:884–900.

55. Hedden J, Boyce J. 1990. Image segmentation by unifying region and boundary information. *IEEE Trans Pattern Anal Machine Intell* **12**:929–948.

56. Yezzi A, Tsai A, Willsky A. 1999. A statistical approach to snakes for bimodal and trimodal imagery. In *Proceedings of the seventh IEEE international conference on computer vision*, pp. 898–903. Washington, DC: IEEE Computer Society.

57. Paragios NK. 2000. Geodesic active regions and level set methods: contributions and applications in artifical vision, PhD dissertation, University of Nice/Sophie Antipolis, France.

58. Chan T, Vese L. 2001. Active contours without edges. *IEEE Trans Image Process* **10**:266–277.

59. Zeng X, Staib LH, Schultz RT, Duncan JS. 1999. Segmentation and measurement of the cortex from 3D MR images using coupled surfaces propagation. *IEEE Trans Med Imaging* **18**:927–937.

60. Chiou GI, Hwang JN. 1995. A neural network-based stochastic active-contour model (NNS-SNAKE) for contour finding of distinct features. *IEEE Trans Med Imaging* **4**:1407–1416.

61. Alirezaie J, Jernigan ME, Nahmias C. 1997. Neural network-based segmentation of magnetic resonance images of the brain. *IEEE Trans Nucl Sci* **44**:194–198.

62. Suri JS. 1999. Active contours vs. learning: computer vision techniques in CT, MR and x-ray cardiac imaging. In *Proceedings of the fifth conference on pattern recognition and information processing*, pp. 273–277. Washington, DC: IEEE Computer Society.

63. Cohen LD, Cohen I. 1993. Finite element methods for active contour models and ballons for 2d and 3d images. *IEEE Trans Pattern Anal Machine Intell* **15**:1131–1147.

64. Morse PM, Feshbach H. 1953. *Methods of theoretical physics*. New York: McGraw-Hill.

65. Caselles V, Catte F, Coll T, Dibos F. 1993. A geometric model for active contours in image processing. *Num Math* **66**:1–31.

66. Mumford D, Shah J. 1989. Optimal approximation by piecewise smooth functions and associated variational problems. *Commun Pure Appl Math* **42**:577–685.

67. Chien T, Chien M. 1982. *A study on tongue diagnosis*. Shanghai: Shanghai Science Book.

68. Cai Y. 2002. A novel imaging system for tongue inspection. In *Proceedings of the IEEE instrumentation and measurement technology conference*, pp. 159–163. Washington, DC: IEEE Computer Society.

69. Chiu CC. 2000. A novel approach based on computerized image analysis for traditional Chinese medical diagnosis of the tongue. *Comput Methods Prog Biomed* **61**:77–89.

70. Li CH, Yuen PC. 2002. Tongue image matching using color content. *Pattern Recognit* **35**:407–419.

71. Pang B, Wang K, Zhang D, Zhang F. 2002. On automated tongue image segmentation in Chinese medicine. In *Proceedings of the 16th international conference on pattern recognition*, pp. 616–619. Washington, DC: IEEE Computer Society.

72. Pang B, Zhang D, Li NM, Wang K. 2004. Computerized tongue diagnosis based on Bayesian networks. *IEEE Trans Biomed Eng* **51**:1803–1810.

73. Pang JH, Kim JE, Park KM, Chang SO, Kim By. 2002. Development of the digital tongue inspection system with image analysis. In *Proceedings of the second joint EMBS/BMES conference*, pp. 1033–1034. Washington, DC: IEEE Computer Society.

74. Zhao ZX, Wang AM, Shen LS. 1999. An automatic tongue analyzer of Chinese medicine based on color image processing. In *Proceedings of the fourth international conference on electronic measurement and instrumentation*, pp. 830–834. Washington, DC: IEEE Computer Society.

75. Wang Y, Zhou Y, Yang J, Xu Q. 2004. A tongue analysis system for tongue diagnosis in traditional Chinese medicine. In *Proceedings of the international symposium on computational and information sciences (CIS'04). Lecture notes in computer science*, Vol. 3314, pp. 1181–1186. New York: Springer.

76. Guan-Song L, Xu J-G, Gao D-Y. 2003. An automatic approach for tongue image segmentation. *Comput Engineer* **29**:63-64 [in Chinese].

77. Sun Y, Luo Y, Zhou C, Xu J, Zhang Z. 2003. A method based on split-combining algorithm for the segmentation of the image of tongue. *Chinese J Image Graphics* **8**:1395–1399 [in Chinese].

78. Dumitras A, Venetsanopoulos AN. 2000. Multi-colored snakes in the RGB color snake. In *Proceedings of the IEEE Pacific-Rim conference on multimedia (PCM'2000)*, pp. 240–244. Washington, DC: IEEE Computer Society.

79. Hamarneh G, Chodorowski A, Gustavsson T. 2000. Active contour models: application to oral lesion detection in color images. In *Proceedings of the IEEE international conference on systems, man, and cybernetics* pp. 2458–2463. Washington, DC: IEEE Computer Society.

80. DeCarlo D, Metaxas D. 1996. Blended deformable models. *IEEE Trans Pattern Anal Machine Intell* **18**:443–448.

81. Dumitras A, Venetsanopoulos AN. 2001. On the application of parametric snake models to the localization of object boundaries in color images. In *Proceedings of the fourth IEEE workshop on multimedia signal processing* pp. 167–172. Washington, DC: IEEE Computer Society.

82. Dumitras A, Venetsanopoulos A. 2001. Angular map-driven snakes with application to object shape description in color images. *IEEE Trans Image Process* **10**:1851–1859.

83. Jones TN, Metaxas DN. 1998. Image segmentation based on the integration of pixel affinity and deformable models. In *Proceedings of the international conference on computer vision and pattern recongnition (ICCVPR'1998)*, pp. 330–337. Washington, DC: IEEE Computer Society.

84. Sapiro G. 1997. Color snakes. *Comput Vision Image Understand* **68**:247–253.

85. Nevatia R. 1977. A color-edge detector and its use in scene segmentation. *IEEE Trans Syst Mach Cybern* **7**:820–826.

86. Scharcanski J, Venetsanopoulos AN. 1997. Edge detection of color images using directional operators. *IEEE Trans Circ Syst Video Technol* **7**:397–401.

87. Zenzo SD. 1986. A note on the gradient of a multi-image. *Comput Vision Graphics Image Process* **36**:116–125.

88. Ruzon MA, Tomasi C. 2001. Edge, junction, and corner detection using color distribution. *IEEE Trans Pattern Anal Machine Intell* **23**:1281–1295.

89. Tschumperlé D. 2002. *PDEs based regularization of multivalued images and applications*. University of Nice/Sophie Antipolis, France.

90. Sapiro G, Ringach DL. 1996. Anisotropic diffusion of mulitvalued images with applications to color filtering. *IEEE Trans Pattern Anal Machine Intell* **5**:1582–1586.

91. Ohta Y, Kanade T, Sakai T. 1980. Color information for region segmentation. *Comput Graphics Image Process* **13**:222–241.

92. Kapur T. 1999. *Model-based three-dimensional medical image segmentation.* PhD dissertation. Artificial Intelligence Laboratory, Massachusettes Institute of Technology.

93. Xu C, Pham DL, Rettmann ME, Yu DN, Prince JL. 1999. Reconstruction of the human cerebral cortex from magnetic resonance images. *IEEE Trans Med Imaging* **18**:467–480.

94. Bomans M, Höhne K-H, Tiede U, Riemer M. 1990. 3D segmentation of MR images of the head for 3D display. *IEEE Trans Med Imaging* **9**:177–183.

95. Leventon ME. 2000. *Statistical models in medical image analysis.* PhD dissertation, Massachussates Institute of Technology.

96. Leventon ME, Grimson WEL, Faugeras OD. 2000. Statistical shape influence in geodesic active contours. In *Proceedings of the international conference on computer vision and pattern recognition*, pp. 1316–1323. Washington, DC: IEEE Computer Society.

97. Han X, Xu C, Prince JL. 2003. A topology preserving level set method for geometric deformable models. *IEEE Trans Pattern Anal Machine Intell* **25**:755–768.

98. Chan TF, Vese LA. 2000. *Image segmentation using level sets and the piecewise-constant Mumford-Shah model.* CAM Report 00-14, University of California at Los Angeles.

99. Paragios N, Deriche R. 2000. Coupled geodesic active regions for image segmentation: a level set approach. In *Proceedings of the European conference on computer vision (ECCV)*, pp. 224–240. New York: Springer.

100. Bozma HI, Duncan JS. 1994. A game-theoretic approach to integration of modules. *IEEE Trans Pattern Anal Machine Intell* **16**:1074–1086.

101. Kwan RK-S, Evans AC, Pike GB. 1996. An extensible MRI simulator for post-processing evaluation. In *Proceedings of the international conference on visualization in biomedical computing (VBC'96). Lecture notes in computer science*, Vol. 1131, pp. 135–140. New York: Springer.

102. Rajapakse JC, Kruggel F. 1998. Segmentation of MR images with intensity inhomogeneities. *Image Vision Comput* **16**(3):165–180.

103. Daniel C, Florian T, Joachim W, Christoph S. 2002. Diffusion snakes: introducing statistical shape knowledge into the Mumford-Shah function. *Int J Comput Vision* **50**:295–313.

104. Ivana M, Slawomir K, James DT. 1998. Segmentation and tracking in echocardiographic sequences: active contour guided by optical flow estimates. *IEEE Trans Med Imaging* **17**:274–284.

105. Leventon ME, Grimson WEL, Faugeras OD. 2000. Statistical shape influence in geodesic active contours. In *Proceedings of the international conference on computer vision and pattern recognition*, pp. 1316–1323. Washington, DC: IEEE Computer Society.

106. Chen Y, Thiruvenkadam H, Tagare H, Huang F, Wilson D. 2002. Using prior shapes in geometric active contours in a variational framework. *Int J Comput Vision* **50**:315–328.

107. Perona P, Malik J. 1990. Scale space and edge detection using anisotropic diffusion. *IEEE Trans Pattern Anal Machine Intell* **12**:629–639.

108. Whitaker RT, Xue X. 2001. Variable-conductance, level-set curvature for image denoising. In *Proceedings of the international conference on image processing*, pp. 142–145. Washington, DC: IEEE Computer Society.

8

BREAST STRAIN IMAGING:
A CAD FRAMEWORK

Ruey-Feng Chang

Department of Computer Science and Information Engineering
Graduate Institute of Biomedical Electronics and Bioinformatics
Graduate Institute of Networking and Multimedia
National Taiwan University, Taipei, Taiwan

Chii-Jen Chen, Chia-Ling Tsai,
and Wei-Liang Chen

Department of Computer Science and Information Engineering
National Chung Cheng University, Chiayi, Taiwan

Jasjit S. Suri

Biomedical Research Institute, Idaho State University,
Pocatello, Idaho, USA

In 2D ultrasound Computer-Aided Diagnosis (CAD), the main emphasis is extraction of tumor boundaries and its classification into benign and malignant types. This provides a direct tool for breast radiologists and can even prevent breast biopsies, thereby reducing the number of false positives. The prerequisite for accurate breast boundary estimation in 2D breast ultrasound images is accurate segmentation of breast tumors and shape modeling. But this is a challenging task, because there is no set pattern of progression of tumors in the spatiotemporal domain. This chapter adapts a methodology based on geometric deformable models such as the level set, which has the ability to extract the topology of shapes of breast tumors. Using this framework, we extract several features of breast tumors and feed this set of information into a vector machine-based classifier for classification of breast disease. Our system demonstrates accuracy, sensitivity, specificity, PPV, and NPV values of 87, 85, 88, 82, and 89%, respectively.

Address all correspondence to: Ruey-Feng Chang, Department of Computer Science and Information Engineering, National Taiwan University, Taipei 10617, Taiwan. Phone: 886-2-33664888‾331; Fax: 886-2-23628167. rfchang@csie.ntu.edu.tw. http://www.csie.ntu.edu.tw/˜rfchang/.

1. INTRODUCTION

Breast cancer is one of the leading causes of death in women during recent years (see *Cancer Facts and Figures 2004*, published by the American Cancer Society [1]). The role of ultrasound in breast cancer detection has become more prevalent as it offers several advantages for cancer detection, including its low cost and non-ionizing nature (see Ganott et al. [2] and Crystal et al. [3]). For this reason, considerable progress has been made in early cancer detection and diagnosis (see Bassett et al. [4], Jackson [5], and Stavros et al. [6]). Recently, it has begun to yield low false negative rates. Thus, due to all of the above reasons, ultrasound has become and an indispensable modality [7–14].

Today's breast CAD systems require segmentation of breast tumors to analyze the shapes of tumors, and then to classify these types of breast cancer diseases into benign and malignant types. Thus, this introduces the prerequisite of accurate breast boundary estimation in 2D breast ultrasound images and 3D breast ultrasound slices. However, boundary estimation of breast tumors is a challenging task because there is no set pattern of the progression of tumors in the spatiotemporal domain. The shape and structure challenge due to the anatomic nature of breast diseases is just one part of the equation; the other component is the physics involved in imaging these complex structures, as it produces several kinds of artifacts and speckle noise. The anatomic nature of tumors causes blurry boundaries in 2D ultrasound images, and there is considerable signal dropout. This puts an extra burden on CAD (see Rohling et al. [15]).

This chapter adapts a methodology based on geometric deformable models such as level sets that has the ability to extract the topology of the shape of breast tumors. It has been recently shown that medical shape extraction in medical imaging has been dominated by the level set framework (see Suri et al. [16–18]). Recently, many implementations on computer vision and medical imaging have been grounded on this basic concept [16, 19–26].

In the level set paradigm, tracking of the evolution of contours and surfaces is solved using numerical methods. The efficacy of this scheme has been demonstrated with numerical experiments on some synthesized images and some low-contrast medical images (see Malladi [20]). A level set can be used for image segmentation by using such image-based features as mean intensity, gradient, and edges in the governing differential equation. In a typical approach, a contour is initialized by a user and then evolved until it fits the topology of an anatomical structure in the image (see Sethian [19]).

In this chapter we present several studies on using the level set method in breast ultrasound. In order to increase the efficiency of level set-based segmentation within the level set framework, some image preprocessing techniques are adopted prior to application of the geometric level set. For performance evaluation of the proposed studies, we not only show the segmentation results with the level set method but also apply these results to follow-up analysis of breast tumors, so-called progression analysis. All experimental statistics indicate very encouraging results.

The organization of this chapter is as follows. The related work with the level set method is reviewed in Section 2. In Section 3 the overall system and data acquisition are briefly introduced. Section 4 discusses the theory of front evolution for boundary estimation of lesions. Section 5 presents a novel CAD system based on the level set framework, which is proposed to classify breast masses in 2D continuous strain ultrasound. We then offer our conclusions.

2. GENERAL ULTRASOUND IMAGE ANALYSIS ARCHITECTURE

Image analysis in today's world carries a lot of significance, since it is the key to supplying information to clinical practitioners. The value of an image analysis system is enhanced when used for characterization of tissues in breast cancer.

The breast radiologist is increasingly more keen to find if breast lesions are benign or malignant. This provides them with important feedback and helps in deciding whether or not to perform a biopsy. However, classification of a breast lesion is not an easy task, as clinicians do not see the lesion's anatomy during the decision-making process. They are making an interpretation based on image data acquired using ultrasound data, as shown in Figure 1. Thus, they urgently need a reliable tool that can help automatically classify lesions and provide a course of treatment that will bring comfort to the women. This chapter is all about developing such a reliable tool. One such tool is a general-purpose image analysis ultrasound architecture.

As depicted in Figure 1, the key to this scheme is the ultrasound image analysis system. Such a system must have a preprocessor, whose major role is to remove system noise during the physics-based reconstruction process. Along with this is the segmentor, a subsystem in itself that uses a deformable model-based framework for capturing the topology of breast lesions. Note that segmentation of breast lesions is only useful if we have classified the segmented lesions. Thus, we need to extract the features of these lesions and feed them to the classifier, which understands them using their training ability and classifies them into benign and malignant lesions. This is all about a software-based ultrasound image analysis system. Finally, the most important and critical component is the validation system, which helps to design systems for clinical acceptance. This can all be seen in Figure 1.

3. ULTRASOUND DATA ACQUISITION SYSTEM

We now offer an overview of a computer-aided diagnosis system for breast ultrasound. We then describe data acquisition in 2D and 3D.

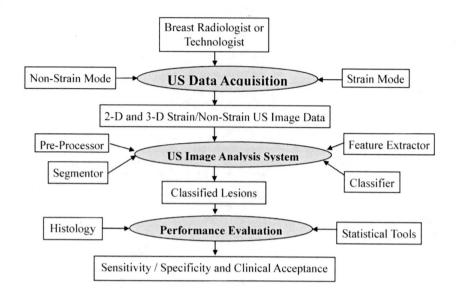

Figure 1. General ultrasound image analysis architecture.

3.1. Typical Setup

Ultrasound has evolved gradually from a limited modality to a sophisticated tool for diagnosis of breast lesions. Its criteria for lesion differentiation include margin irregularity, shadowing, microlobulation, echogenicity, and shape (see Stavros et al. [27]). Palpation is widely used in a screening procedure before a breast imaging study because pathological changes in tissue are generally correlated with changes in elasticity (see Ophir et al. [28, 29]). The tissue elasticity of a lesion could also be a useful diagnosis criterion in the United States. After compression of the probe, a soft lesion will be flattened more than a hard one. Many cancers appear as extremely hard lesions, which is the result of increased stromal density. Fibroadenoma typically has a heterogeneous stiffness; cancers are uniformly stiffer than surrounding tissue.

In the past, an attending physician was the most important personage for patients. When ultrasound images were obtained, the physician would diagnose and analyze the ultrasound data himself, which was very time-consuming work. For this reason, computer-aided diagnosis (CAD) systems were developed to aid physicians in diagnosing ultrasonic abnormalities and possible breast cancers. With the assistance of CAD, physicians can efficiently detect such lesions as spiculations and discriminate more accurately between benign and malignant tumors (see Horsch et al. [30] and Chen et al. [31]). The purpose of this chapter is to

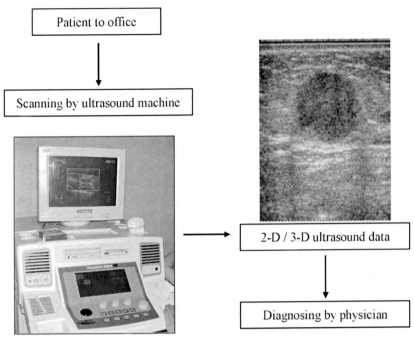

* Photograph source: Voluson 530 (Kretz Technik, Austria) scanner.

Figure 2. Typical automatic image acquisition system. Photographic source: Voluson 530 (Kretz Technik, Austria) scanner.

develop a CAD system based within the level set framework that can classify breast lesions more efficiently. Figure 2 depicts a typical automatic image acquisition system.

3.2. 2D Ultrasound Strain Data Acquisition

In this Section we first introduce the acquisition of 2D ultrasound image data. A Voluson 530 (Kretz Technik, Austria) scanner is used in our proposed CAD system, which allows recording 15 continuous 2D images at per second. Compression is completed within 4 seconds, and 60 images are obtained, which we denote I_s, where $s = 0$–59. Figure 3 illustrates the process of physician compression of a tumor. Because the time for data acquisition is very short, the neighboring images are very similar and variation in elasticity very small. Hence, only one of eight neighboring images is used in our proposed CAD system, and 8 images in total of the original 60 are analyzed, that is, $I_{s \times 8 + 1}$, $0 \leq s \leq 7$.

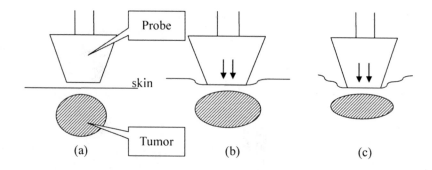

Figure 3. (a) Pre-compression; (b) post-compression (intermediate stage), and (c) post-compression (final stage).

4. THEORY OF FRONT EVOLUTION FOR BOUNDARY ESTIMATION OF LESION

The level set has dominated the field of imaging world for more than a decade. It has features and characteristics that no other mathematical formulations offer. In particular, the role of level sets in imaging and computer vision has been very aggressively advancing, since this field deals with shape changes or morphing. The ability of the level set to capture changes in morphology very well ties in with the adaptation of shape variabilites. The application of the level set has been gaining prominence since the early work by Sethian and colleagues [32,33]. There have since been few books written on the application of level sets (e.g., Suri et al. [34]). We will touch on the basics of the level set framework, which forms the foundation for our proposed method.

4.1. Front Propagation

As a starting point and as motivation for the level set approach, consider a closed curve moving in a plane. Let $\gamma(0)$ be a smooth and closed initial curve in Euclidean plane $\Re^2$, and let $\gamma(t)$ be the family of curves that is generated by the movement of initial curve $\gamma(0)$ along the direction of its normal vector. Moreover, we assume that the speed of this movement is a scalar function F of curvature κ, called $F(\kappa)$.

The central idea of the level set approach [16,20,22,32] is to represent the front $\gamma(t)$ as the level set $\psi = 0$ of a function ψ. Thus, given a moving closed hypersurface $\gamma(t)$, that is, $\gamma(t = 0) : [0, \infty) \to \Re^N$, we hope to produce a formulation for the motion of the hypersurface propagating along its normal direction with speed F, where F can be a function of various arguments, including the curvature,

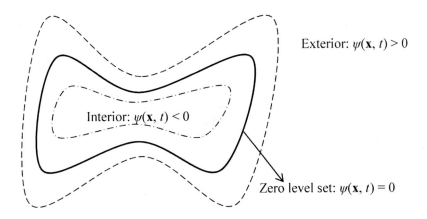

Figure 4. The sign of $\psi(x, t)$ is decided by whether the point is in the interior (minus) or exterior (plus) of the zero level set.

normal direction, etc. The main idea is to embed this propagating interface as the zero level set of a higher-dimensional function ψ. Let $\psi(\mathbf{x}, t = 0)$, where $\mathbf{x}$ is a point in $\Re^N$ be defined by

$$\psi(\mathbf{x}, t = 0) = \pm d, \tag{1}$$

where d is the signed distance from $\mathbf{x}$ to $\gamma(t = 0)$, and the plus (minus) sign is chosen if the point $\mathbf{x}$ is outside (inside) the initial front $\gamma(t = 0)$, as shown in Figure 4. The best discrete approximation of the surface is therefore the set of grid positions closest to the zero-crossings in the image, as shown in Figure 5. Thus, an initial function is $\psi(\rho, t = 0) : \Re^N \to \Re$ with the property that

$$\gamma(t = 0) = (\mathbf{x}|\psi(\mathbf{x}, t = 0) = 0). \tag{2}$$

The goal is to produce an equation for the evolving function $\psi(\mathbf{x}, t)$, which contains the embedded motion of $\gamma(t)$ as the level set $\psi = 0$. Let $\mathbf{x}(t), t \in [0, \infty)$, be the path of a point on the propagating front, i.e., $\mathbf{x}(t = 0)$ is a point on the initial front $\gamma(t = 0)$, and $\mathbf{x}_t = F(\mathbf{x}(t))$ with vector $\mathbf{x}_t$ normal to the front at $\mathbf{x}(t)$ (see Mulder et al. [35]). Since the evolving function ψ is always zero on the propagating front, then

$$\psi(\mathbf{x}(t), t) = 0. \tag{3}$$

According to the chain rule,

$$\psi_t + \sum_{i=1}^{N} \psi_{x_i} x_{i_t} = 0, \tag{4}$$

				2.5	1.9	2.7			
		1.8	1.5	1.3	0.2	0.8	1.9		
	2.1	0.8	0.4	-0.3	-1.1	0.1	0.9	2.2	
2.6	1.1	0.1	-0.8	-1.3	-2.3	-1.6	0	1.1	3.0
1.8	0.1	-1.2	-2.2	-3.1	-4.8	-3.6	-0.9	-0.1	1.8
2.1	0.3	-0.2	-0.7	-1.6	-2.6	-2.9	-0.8	0.4	2.2
2.9	1.6	0.1	0.2	0	-1.5	-1.0	0	1.4	3.2
	2.3	0.9	1.0	0	-0.9	-0.5	0.3	1.2	
		1.8	0.7	-0.3	0.2	0.8	2.8		
			1.9	1.4	1.1	2.5			

Figure 5. Implicit level set surface ψ is the dotted line superimposed over the image grid. The location of the surface is interpolated by the image pixel values. The grid pixels closest to the implicit surface are shown in gray.

where x_i is ith component of $\mathbf{x}$. Since

$$\sum_{i=1}^{N} = (\psi_{x_1}, \psi_{x_2}, \psi_{x_3}, \ldots, \psi_{x_N}) \cdot (x_{1_t}, x_{2_t}, x_{3_t}, \ldots, x_{N_t}) = F(\mathbf{x}(t) \, |\nabla \psi| ,$$

(5)

we have the evolution equation for ψ, namely,

$$\psi_t + F \, |\nabla \psi| = 0,$$

(6)

with a given value of $\psi(\mathbf{x}, t = 0)$. Combining Eqs. (4) and (5), the final curve evolution equation is given as

$$\frac{\partial \psi}{\partial t} = F(\kappa) \, |\nabla \psi| ,$$

(7)

where ψ is the level set function, and $F(\kappa)$ is the speed with which the front (or zero level curve) propagates. This fundamental equation describes the time evolution of the level set function ψ in such a way that the zero level curve of this evolving function is always identified with the propagating interface (see Suri et al. [16]). The

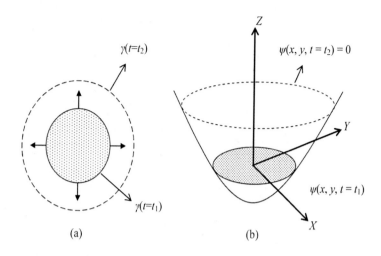

Figure 6. Level set formulation of equations of motion: (a) arrows show the propagating direction of the front $\gamma(t = t_1)$; (b) the corresponding surface $\psi(x, y)$ at time t_2.

above equation is also called an Eulerian Hamilton-Jacobi equation (see [16,32]). Equation (7) for the 2D and 3D cases can be generalized as

$$\frac{\partial \psi}{\partial t} = F_\kappa\,(x, y)\,|\nabla \psi|, \frac{\partial \psi}{\partial t} = F_\kappa\,(x, y, z)\,|\nabla \psi|, \tag{8}$$

where $F_\kappa(x, y)$ and $F_\kappa(x, y, z)$ are curvature-dependent speed functions in 2D and 3D, respectively.

The topological change of the level set segmentation method is illustrated in Figure 6. The arrows in Figure 6a show the propagating direction of the front $\gamma(t = t_1)$. During a period of time t_2, the front $\gamma(t = t_2)$ and the zero level set $\psi(x, y, t = t_2)$ is shown in Figure 6b. In this way, the actual object contour can be obtained using the level set method.

4.2. Analogies of Front Propagation

There are three analogies of the front propagation equation (see Suri et al. [16]). The first is that these equations can be compared with the Euclidean geometric heat equation (see Grayson [36]), given as

$$\frac{\partial C}{\partial t} = \kappa N, \tag{9}$$

where κ is the curvature, N is the inward unit normal, and C are the curve coordinates. The second analogy is that Eq. (7) is also called the curvature motion

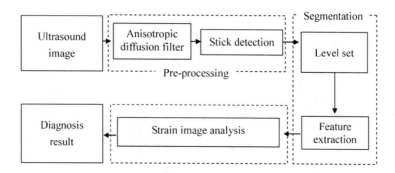

Figure 7. 2D breast leision characterization system.

equation, since the rate of change of the length of the curve is a function of $\partial C/\partial t$. Finally, the above equations can be written in terms of differential geometry using divergence as

$$\frac{\partial\psi}{\partial t} = \nabla \cdot \left(\frac{\nabla\psi}{|\nabla\psi|}\right)|\nabla\psi|,\tag{10}$$

where geometrical properties such as normal curvature N and mean curvature H are given as

$$N = \frac{\nabla\psi}{|\nabla\psi|}\qquad\text{and}\qquad H = \nabla \cdot \left(\frac{\nabla\psi}{|\nabla\psi|}\right).\tag{11}$$

In conclusion, the advantage of the level set approach is that there are no significant differences in following fronts in three space dimensions. By simply extending the array structures and gradients operators, propagating surfaces are easily handled (see Sethian et al. [20]).

5. 2D CONTINUOUS STRAIN MODE SYSTEM

In this Section we describe an elasticity analysis technique based on the level set method (see Moon et al. [22]). In this CAD system, level set segmentation plays the major role in influencing the results of elasticity analysis. Using the proposed preprocessing procedures (including anisotropic diffusion filtering), we employ the stick method to help remove noise from ultrasound images and improve segmentation performance, Acquisition of ultrasonic data is described in Section 3.2. The system flowchart is shown in Figure 7.

5.1. Preprocessors for Ultrasound Images

For medical images, there are some fundamental requirements regarding noise filtering methods that should be noted. First, it is crucial to not lose such important

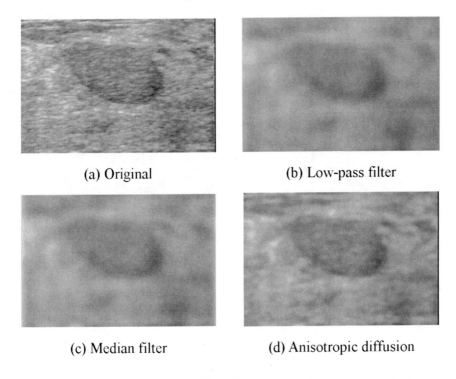

(a) Original   (b) Low-pass filter

(c) Median filter   (d) Anisotropic diffusion

Figure 8. A blurring example with different filters: (a) original benign tumorw; (b) using a low-pass filter; (c) median filter; (d) anisotropic diffusion filter.

information as object boundaries and detailed structures. Second, the noise should be reduced in the homogeneous regions efficiently. In addition, morphological definition by sharpening discontinuities (see Gerig et al. [37]) should be enhanced.

Speckle noise in an ultrasound image must be reduced to improve image quality. Although conventional low-pass filtering and linear diffusion on an ultrasound image can be used to reduce speckle, the edge information may be blurred, which imposes difficulty on segmentation of a tumor. Anisotropic diffusion filtering (see Perona and Malik [38]) can avoid the major drawbacks of the above filters and preserve important information on the object boundary, as depicted shown in Figure 8. It also satisfies the above-mentioned fundamental requirements. Consider the following anisotropic diffusion equation:

$$I_t = \operatorname{div}\left(c(x, y, t)\nabla I\right),\tag{12}$$

where div is the divergence operator, $c(x, y, t)$ is the diffusion coefficient, and t is the time parameter. The anisotropic diffusion equation uses a diffusion coefficient

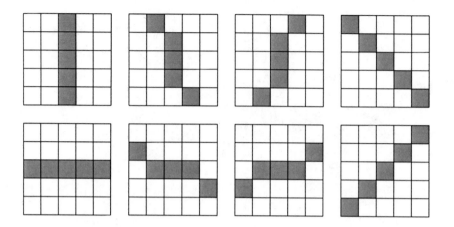

Figure 9. Eight possible orientations of a stick with a length of five (5×5 masks).

that is chosen locally as a function of the magnitude gradient of the intensity function in the image for estimating the image structure. The function

$$c(x, y, t) = f(|\|\nabla I(x, y, t)\||) \tag{13}$$

is chosen to satisfy $f(z) \to 0$ when $z \to \infty$, so that diffusion processing is stopped near the edges. Therefore, the speckle noise within the homogeneous region can be blurred and the region boundary can be preserved.

After anisotropic diffusion, the speckle noise has been reduced effectively. The next step is to enhance the tumor boundary, and we employed edge detection with the stick operation to do so. The edge detection problem can be modeled as a line process, because boundaries between tissue layers will appear as all sorts of lines in an ultrasound image (see Czerwinski et al. [39–41]). The stick is a set of short line segments of variable orientation that can be used to approximate the boundaries and enhance edge information. For a square area with size $N \times N$ in an image, there are $2N - 2$ short lines with a length of N pixels passing through the center. The sums of the pixel values along the lines are calculated for each line with different orientation. Then the largest of these sums is selected, and the value at the center of the square is assigned as this maximum number. After each pixel in an image is replaced by the maximum sum of the lines passing through the pixel, the contrast at the edges is enhanced and speckle is also reduced in the resulting image. Taking the length of five as an example, eight possible line segments are illustrated in Figure 9. Continuing from Figure 8, the result with the stick function is depicted in Figure 10.

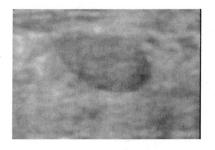   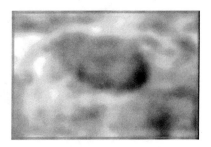

(a) Anisotropic diffusion   (b) Stick detection

Figure 10. (a) The same example as in Figure 8d; (b) after applying stick detection using 5 × 5 masks.

5.2. Segmentation Subsystem for Ultrasound Image Analysis

The level set method (see Sethian and colleagues [19,32]) is a numerical technique for computing and analyzing front propagation. It offers a highly robust and accurate method for tracking interfaces moving under a regime of complex motion. The main idea was introduced in Section 2. During the preprocessing procedure for the eight continuous images extracted from the dataset, we applied 2D anisotropic filtering and a 2D stick-based enhancement method to each image. Because the 2D method is inadequate for calculating the volume of sideslip during compression, the 3D level-set method was used for continuous ultrasound images. Furthermore, changes in the neighboring 2D images were very small and the neighboring images very similar, so that the time axis t can be considered as the z axis in 3D coordinates. With the information of the previous and next frames, the 3D level set method can yield a more accurate segmentation than the 2D method. In Figures 11 and 12, two segmentation results for different tumor cases, both benign and malignant, are illustrated, respectively. It should be noted that malignant cases can be segmented as well as the benign ones.

In order to emphasize the importance of image processing, we compare using the level set method on a non-enhanced image and an enhanced image, as shown in Figure 13. According to the results depicted in Figures 11 and 12, our expectations in terms of accuracy of segmentation were satisfied for both the benign and malignant cases. However, the significance of these preprocessing techniques were still not explicit. Therefore, using the same examples as in Figures 11 and 12, the original ultrasound images were directly processed using the level set approach. Because speckle and noise affect the quality of the ultrasound images, the segmentation results in the middle column of Figure 13 do not seem superior. This shows the importance of the effect of anisotropic diffusion filtering and stick detection.

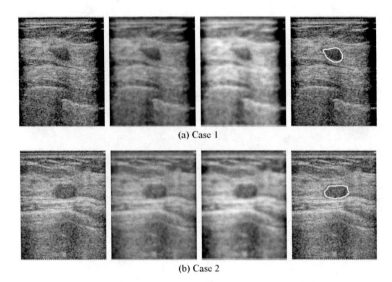

(a) Case 1

(b) Case 2

Figure 11. Two segmentation results for benign tumor cases using the level set method. For each case, the first image is the original one, the second was processed using an anisotropic diffusion filter, the third was enhanced using stick detection and the final one was processed using the level set method.

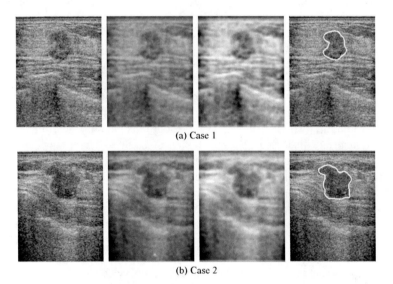

(a) Case 1

(b) Case 2

Figure 12. Two segmentation results for malignant tumor cases using the level set method. For each case, the first image is the original one, the second was processed using an anisotropic diffusion filter, the third was enhanced using stick detection and the final one was processed using the level set method.

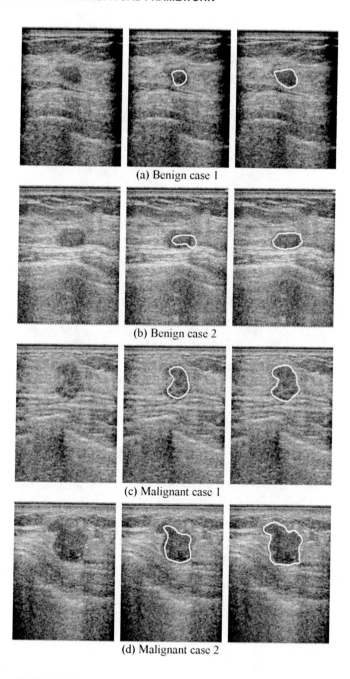

(a) Benign case 1

(b) Benign case 2

(c) Malignant case 1

(d) Malignant case 2

Figure 13. Result of using the level set method on non-enhanced and enhanced images. For each case, the first is the original image, the middle one was processed using the level set method, and the final image was based on image preprocessing, as in Figures 11 and 12.

5.3. Strain Quantification Subsystem

After segmentation of the tumor contours from the continuous ultrasound images, four features are defined for tumor labeling (benign or malignant): contour difference (C_d), shift distance (M_d), area difference (A_d), and solidity (S_o). The first three are related to the strain and the fourth to shape. It is important to review data acquisition (see Section 3.2), because the neighboring images are very similar and the variation in elasticity is very small, as only one of eight neighboring images is used in this work. Therefore, only 8 of 60 total images are analyzed, that is $I_{s \times 8+1}$, where $s = 0$–7. We now discuss the concepts involved of the above four features.

5.3.1. Contour difference (C_d)

The contour difference value is used to evaluate changes in lesion shape between two images. Because of compression, the contours between two neighboring images $\{I_k, I_j\}$ will undergo some slight movement (see Leymarie [42]), where $\{I_k, I_j\}$ is the set $\{s \times 8 + 1, s \times 8 + 9\}$, such that $s = 0$–6. Hence, these contours between I_k and I_j should first be registered, so that the center point of the tumor is used as the reference point. After registering the two images, the pixels in only one contour of I_k or I_j are identified as the different pixels P_d.

The contour difference $C_d(I_k, I_j)$ between two neighboring images $\{I_k, I_j\}$ is defined as the number of different pixels divided by the number of pixels in the image I_k:

$$C_d(I_k, I_j) = \frac{N_{P_d}(I_k, I_j)}{N_{I_k}} \times 100\%, \tag{14}$$

where N_{P_d} is the pixel difference between the two registered contours, and N_{I_k} is the number of tumor pixels in the image I_k. Finally, for each breast case, the average contour difference value is defined as

$$C_d = \frac{1}{N_s - 1} \sum_{(k,j)} C_d(I_k, I_j), \tag{15}$$

where N_s is the number of image slices ($N_s = 8$). For example, in Figure 14 the tumor area in (a) is 12 pixels and the center pixel (black) is at position (4,4), while in (b) the center is at position (5,5) after compression. After registering the two tumor centers, the number of different pixels between (a) and (b) is 5 (slash pixels in Figure 14c). Thus, $C_d = 5/12$.

5.3.2. Shift distance (M_d)

We employ a motion estimation technique (see Richardson [43]) to find the motion of two image contours. For example, in Figure 15, if there is a block

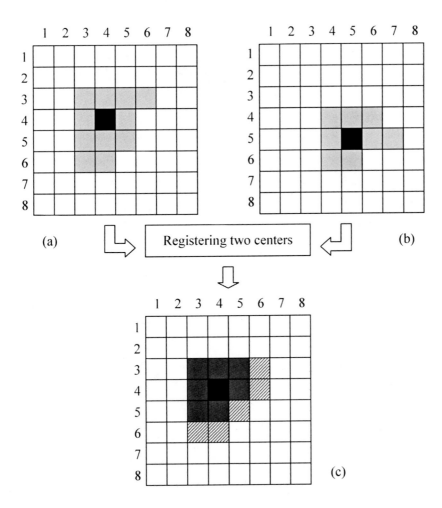

Figure 14. An example of computing C_d: (a) reference image; (b) moving image; (c) after registering (b) to (a) the contour difference is obtained.

(x, y) in the current image, and the most similar block in the previous image is at $(x + m, y + n)$, then the motion vector for block (x, y) is (m, n). Hence, the shift distance $M_d(I_k, I_j)$ between two neighboring images $\{I_k, I_j\}$ can be obtained. (For more details, the reader is referred to Richardson [43].) For each breast case, the total shift distance is defined as the maximum value of each $M_d(I_{s \times 8+1}, I_{s \times 8+9})$:

$$M_d = \max_{\{k,j\}} (M_d(I_k, I_j)). \tag{16}$$

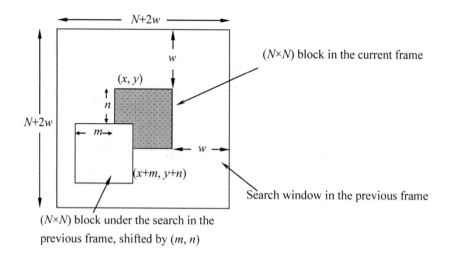

Figure 15. An example of computing shift distance.

5.3.3. Area difference (A_d)

The area difference is used to compare tumor areas between two images, so that for each breast case the area difference is defined as

$$A_d = \frac{1}{N_s - 1} \left(\sum_{(k,j)} \left| \text{Area}_{I_k} - \text{Area}_{I_j} \right| \right) \times 100\%, \qquad (17)$$

where Area_{I_k} is the size of the tumor in image I_k.

5.3.4. Solidity (S_o)

Shape values can be used to distinguish between benign and malignant tumors. Benign tumors usually have smooth shapes, whereas malignant tumors tend to be irregular. The normalized solidity value (see Russ [44]) was used in this study, and is defined as

$$\text{sol} = \frac{\text{Area}_C - \text{Area}_T}{\frac{1}{N_s} \sum_{\{k\}} \left(\text{Area}_C \left(I_k \right) - \text{Area}_T \left(I_k \right) \right)}, \qquad (18)$$

where Area_C is the area of the convex hull of a tumor, and Area_T is the area of the tumor, as shown in Figure 16.

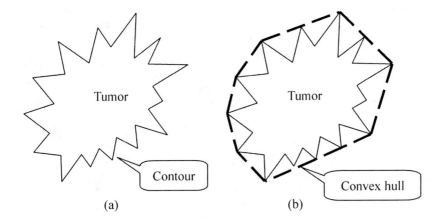

Figure 16. Drawings depict (a) the contour of a tumor, and (b) the convex hull of a tumor. The outer polygon (arrow) is the convex hull of the tumor, while the convex hull is the smallest convex set containing the tumor.

5.4. Experimental Protocol and Results for 2D Strain Data

In the experiments we used 100 pathology-proven cases, including 60 benign breast tumors and 40 malignant ones, to evaluate the classification accuracy of the proposed method. The segmentation results in different compressed images using the level set framework are shown in Figures 17 through 20. The mean values of three strain features—C_d, M_d, A_d—and one shape feature (S_o) in cases of malignant tumors were 3.52 ± 2.12, 2.62 ± 1.31, 1.08 ± 0.85, and 1.70 ± 1.85, whereas those in the cases of benign tumors were 9.72 ± 4.54, 5.04 ± 2.79, 3.17 ± 2.86, and 0.53 ± 0.63, respectively. These values are significantly different, as shown in Table 1 (with p values all smaller than 0.001). The noncontinuous stain values are also given in Table 1. In the noncontinuous strain imaging method, strain values are computed by the first (I_1) and final (I_{57}) frames. All the noncontinuous stain values are also statistically significant. Moreover, the strain values with the noncontinuous method are larger due to the fact that these values are computed from the first and last frames.

In the scatter graph in Figure 21, the three values of the strain features for malignant tumors concentrated around the origin and were smaller than those for the strain features for benign tumors. The receiver operating characteristic (ROC) curves of the four feature values with the support vector machine (SVM) classifier (see Vapnik [45], Pontil et al. [46], and Chapelle et al. [47]) are shown in Figure 22. The A_z values of three strain features were significantly higher than that of the single shape feature ($p < 0.01$). The SVM using all four feature values produced the best performance, with an A_z value of 0.91.

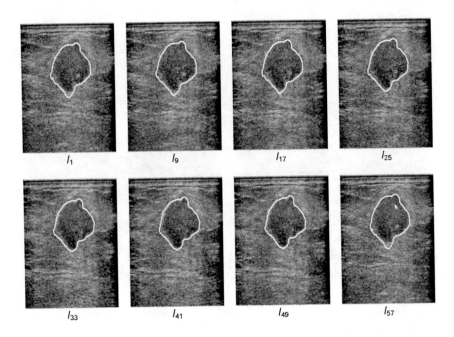

Figure 17. The first segmentation results for the malignant case in different image slices with $C_d = 1.18\%$, $M_d = 1.196$, $A_d = 0.33\%$, and $S_o = 0.8734$.

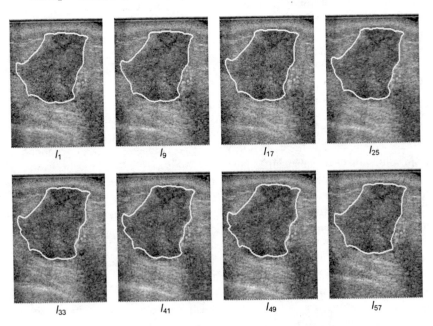

Figure 18. The second segmentation results for the malignant case in different image slices with $C_d = 1.20\%$, $M_d = 1.241$, $A_d = 0.85\%$, and $S_o = 3.6919$.

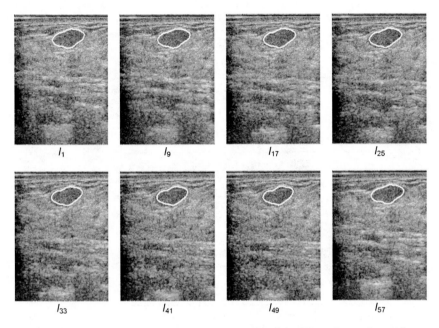

Figure 19. The first segmentation results for the benign case in different image slices with $C_d = 16.90\%$, $M_d = 7.161$, $A_d = 1.71\%$, and $S_o = 0.1876$.

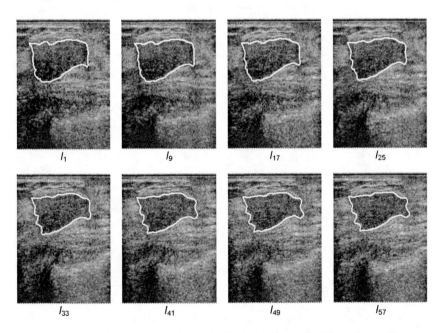

Figure 20. The second segmentation results for the benign case in different image slices with $C_d = 4.73\%$, $M_d = 1.90$, $A_d = 1.78\%$, and $S_o = 1.86$.

Table 1. Mean Value and Standard Deviation of Contour Difference (C_d),
Shift Distance (M_d), Area Difference (A_d), and Solidity (sol)
for Benign and Malignant Nodules for Noncontinuous
and Continuous Strain Imaging Methods

Value	Type	Mean Non-cont.	Mean Cont.	p-value (using t-test) Non-cont.	p-value (using t-test) Cont.
C_d	Benign	56.23% ± 27.53%	9.72% ± 4.54%	< 0.001	< 0.001
	Malignant	22.13% ± 12.44%	3.52% ± 2.12%		
M_d	Benign	5.404 ± 3.047	5.037 ± 2.787	< 0.001	< 0.001
	Malignant	2.855 ± 2.103	2.629 ± 1.309		
A_d	Benign	17.95% ± 16.79%	3.17% ± 2.86%	< 0.001	< 0.001
	Malignant	6.18% ± 6.09%	1.08% ± 0.85%		
S_o	Benign	——	0.532 ± 0.630	——	< 0.001
	Malignant	——	1.702 ± 1.847		

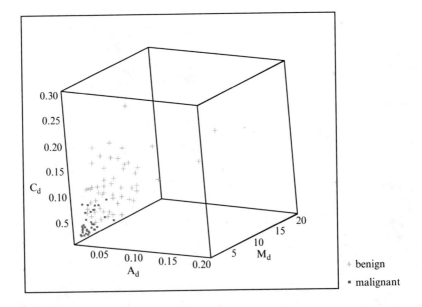

Figure 21. Scatter graph showing contour difference (C_d), area difference (A_d), and shift
distance (M_d) of all the benign and malignant breast tumors. See attached CD for color
version.

Finally, the classification results of breast tumors for the noncontinuous and continuous strain imaging methods are given in Table 2. In order to estimate the performance of the proposed method, five items are compared: accuracy, sensitivity, specificity, positive predictive value (PPV), and negative predictive value (NPV) (see Table 3). According to Tables 2 and 3, continuous strain analysis yields more stable and better results than conventional (noncontinuous) strain analysis, in which only two images were used.

5.5. Discussion on 2D Strain Data Analysis

In this study the level set segmentation approach was used to extract tumor contours from continuous strain images. Because the 2D method was inadequate for calculating the volume of the sideslip during compression, the 3D level set method was used. The results of the automated segmentation were found to be acceptable in all cases with a radiologist's review. According to these satisfying results, we can confirm the feasibility of this proposed framework. However, the accuracy of the CAD system is strongly dependent on an exact segmentation result. In addition to adopting some image preprocessing techniques before using the level set approach, we need to find more robust methods to improve the segmentation result.

The values of all proposed features showed that malignant tumors tend to be more rigid and have more desmoplastic reactions within the surrounding tissue, which means that those features of strain change to a lesser extent on continuous ultrasound images. From the experimental results given in Table 3, the accuracy of continuous strain imaging was 87.00% (87/100), sensitivity 85.00% (34/40), specificity 88.33% (53/60), PPV 82.93% (36/41), and NPV 89.83% (53/59). We can conclude that the proposed method with these strain features is better than conventional noncontinuous strain analysis.

There were limitations in this study. In clinical applications of ultrasound imaging of the strain on tissue from probe compression, the operator must apply constant pressure on the scanning probe to prevent an inclined scanning plane. Otherwise, the tumor may slip out of the scanning plane, which will create inaccuracies. Gradual compression with the ultrasound probe, however, can be performed easily after some practice or by using a compression plate. Compared to the accuracy of elastography with radiofrequency data, the accuracy of our method heavily depends on the results of lesion segmentation. We adjusted some parameters to control the segmented contours and to obtain better results with an expert radiologist's input. Currently, the computerized segmentation in our method is only semi-automated. For tumors with poorly demarcated borders, a good preprocessing technique would be helpful to enhance tumor boundaries. For tumors without a definable boundary or for isoechoic masses, other methods should be developed. For example, some representative reference points could be used to evaluate tissue

Table 2. Classification of Breast Tumors by SVM with the Proposed Features (C_d, M_d, A_d, and S_o) for the Noncontinuous and Continuous Strain Imaging Methods

Classification	Benign*		Malignant*	
	Non-cont.	Cont.	Non-cont.	Cont.
Benign	TN 50	TN 53	FN 10	FN 6
Malignant	FP 10	FP 7	TP 30	TP 34
Total	60		40	

Note: Noncont. = noncontinuous strain imaging;
Cont. = continuous strain imaging;
TP = true positive; TN: true negative;
FP = false positive;
FN = false negative.
An asterisk denotes a histological finding.

Table 3. Result of Performance Items for Noncontinuous and Continuous Strain Imaging Methods Based on the Proposed Features

Items	Performance	
	Noncont.	Cont.
Accuracy	80.00%	87.00%
Sensitivity	75.00%	85.00%
Specificity	83.33%	88.33%
PPV	75.00%	82.93%
NPV	83.33%	89.83%

Note: Noncont. = noncontinuous strain imaging
Cont. = continuous strain imaging
Accuracy = (TP + TN)/(TP + TN + FP + FN)
sensitivity = TP/(TP + FN)
specificity = TN/(TN + FP)
PPV = TP/(TP + FP)
NPV = TN/(TN + FN)

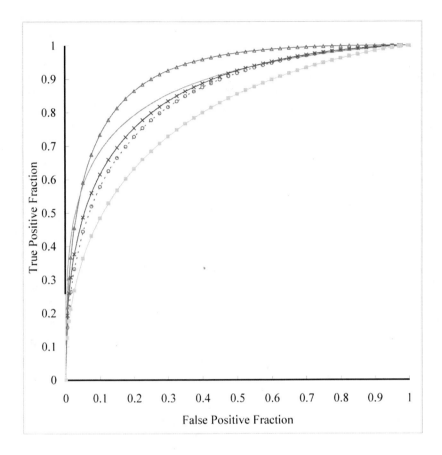

Figure 22. ROC analysis of all 2D strain features. Note that C_d is contour difference, A_d is area difference, M_d is shift distance, S_o is the solidity value, and A_z is the area under the curve. The SVM using all four features produced the best performance, with an A_z value of 0.91. See attached CD for color version.

motion. Moreover, a harmonic imaging technique may improve tumor boundary delineation.

In the future, strain imaging can be extended into 3D ultrasound, because 2D ultrasound can only obtain one cross-section of a tumor and the tumor may slip when the compression force is slanted. However, 3D ultrasound can scan the entire tumor, and its probe is wider. The above drawbacks of 2D ultrasound could thereby be avoided. Hence, the strain imaging technique must be improved for application in 3D ultrasound.

6. CONCLUSION

In this chapter, the level set segmentation framework plays an important role in extracting a tumor contour. All follow-up lesion analyses were based on credible segmentation results. If the adopted segmentation method is not robust, the corresponding tumor analyses will become suspect. In order to increase the accuracy of level set segmentation, some image preprocessing techniques were adopted to reduce the effects from noise and speckle on ultrasound images. In the experiments, the sufficient results proved that the performance of the proposed CAD system was significant.

However, there are some disadvantages of the level set method, the major one being that if some objects are embedded in another object, the level set will not capture all objects of interest. This is especially true if embedded objects are asymmetrically situated. Fortunately, most of the cases from our breast ultrasound sources involved only one tumor. Nevertheless, the above-mentioned problem must be solved in the future if we are to study the level set technique in depth.

7. REFERENCES

1. American Cancer Society. 2004. *Cancer facts and figures 2004*. Arlington, VA: American Cancer Society.
2. Ganott MA, Harris KM, Klaman HM, Keeling TL. 1999. Analysis of false-negative cancer cases identified with a mammography audit. *Breast J.* 5(3):166–175.
3. Crystal P, SD Strano, Shcharynski S, Koretz MJ. 2003. Using sonography to screen women with mammographically dense breasts. *AJR* 181(1):177–182.
4. Bassett LW, Ysrael M, Gold RH, Ysrael C. 1991. Usefulness of mammography and sonography in women less than 35 years of age. *Radiology* 180(3):831–835.
5. Jackson VP. 1990. The role of the US in breast imaging. *Radiology* 177(2):305–311.
6. Stavros AT, Thickman D, Rapp CL, Dennis MA, Parker SH, Sisney GA. 1995. Solid breast nodules: use of sonography to distinguish between benign and malignant lesions. *Radiology* 196(no. 1):123–134.
7. Drukker K, Giger ML, Horsch K, Kupinski MA, Vyborny CJ, Mendelson EB. 2002. Computerized lesion detection on breast ultrasound. *Med Phys* 29(7):1438–1446.
8. Horsch K, Giger ML, Venta LA, Vyborny CJ. 2002. Computerized diagnosis of breast lesions on ultrasound. *Med Phys* 29(2):157–164.
9. Chang RF, Kuo WJ, Chen DR, Huang YL, Lee JH, Chou YH. 2000. Computer-aided diagnosis for surgical office-based breast ultrasound. *Arch Surg* 135(6):696–699.
10. Kuo WJ, Chang RF, Moon WK, Lee CC, Chen DR. 2002. Computer-aided diagnosis of breast tumors with different US systems. *Acad Radiol* 9(7):793–799.
11. Chen DR, Chang RF, Chen WM, Moon WK. 2003. Computer-aided diagnosis for 3-dimensional breast ultrasonography. *Arch Surg* 138(3):296–302.
12. Chen DR, Kuo WJ, Chang RF, Moon WK, Lee CC. 2002. Use of the bootstrap technique with small training sets for computer-aided diagnosis in breast ultrasound. *Ultrasound Med Biol* 28(7):897–902.
13. Chang RF, Wu WJ, Moon WK, Chen DR. 2003. Improvement in breast tumor discrimination by support vector machines and speckle-emphasis texture analysis. *Ultrasound Med Biol* 29(5):679–686.

14. Sawaki A, Shimamoto K, Satake H, Ishigaki T, Koyama S, Obata Y, Ikeda M. 1999. Breast ultrasonography: diagnostic efficacy of a computer-aided diagnostic system using fuzzy inference. *Radiat Med* **17**(1):41–45.

15. Rohling RN, Gee AH, Berman L. 1998. Automatic registration of 3D ultrasound images. *Ultrasound Med Biol* **24**(6):841–854.

16. Suri JS, Liu K, Singh S, Laxminarayan SN, Zeng X, Reden L. 2002. Shape recovery algorithms using level sets in 2D/3D medical imagery: a state-of-the-art review. *IEEE Trans Inf Technol Biomed* **6**(1):8–28.

17. Suri JS, Singh S, Reden L. 2002. Fusion of region and boundary/surface-based computer vision and pattern recognition techniques for 2D and 3D MR cerebral cortical segmentation (Part II): a state-of-the-art review. *Pattern Anal Appl* **5**(1):77–98.

18. Suri JS, Wu D, Reden L, Gao J, Singh S, Laxminarayan S. 2001. Modeling segmentation via geometric deformable regularizers, PDE and level sets in still/motion imagery: a revisit. *Int J Image Graphics* **1**(4):681–734.

19. Sethian JA. 1999. *Level set methods and fast marching methods: evolving interfaces in computational geometry, fluid mechanics, computer vision, and materials science*, 2nd ed. Cambridge: Cambridge UP.

20. Sethian JA, Vemuri BC, Malladi BC. 1995. Shape modeling with front propagation: a level set approach. *IEEE Trans Pattern Anal Machine Intell* **17**(2):158–175.

21. Sussman M, Fatemi E. 1999. An efficient, interface-preserving level set redistancing algorithm and its application to interfacial incompressible fluid flow. *SIAM J Sci Comput* **20**(4):1165–1191.

22. Moon WK, Chang RF, Chen CJ, Chen DR, Chen WL. 2005. Solid breast masses: classification with computer-aided analysis of continuous US images obtained with probe compression. *Radiology* **236**(2):458–464.

23. Chang RF, Wu WJ, Moon WK, Chen DR. 2005. Automatic ultrasound segmentation and morphology based diagnosis of solid breast tumors. *Breast Cancer Res Treat* **89**(2):179–185.

24. Suri JS. 2001. Fast MR brain segmentation using regional level sets. *Int J Eng Med Biol* **20**(4):84–95.

25. Suri JS, Singh S, Reden L. 2002. Computer vision and pattern recognition techniques for 2D and 3D MR cerebral cortical segmentation (part I): a state-of-the-art review. *IEEE Trans Pattern Anal Machine Intell* **5**(1):46–76.

26. Chang RF, Chen DR, Huang YL. 2006. Computer-aided diagnosis for 2d/3d breast ultrasound. In *Recent advances in breast imaging, mammography, and computer-aided diagnosis of breast cancer*, pp. 112–196. Ed JS Suri, RM Rangayyan. Bellingham, WA: SPIE.

27. Stavros AT, Thickman D, Rapp CL, Dennis MA, Parker SH, Sisney GA. 1995. Solid breast nodules: use of sonography to distinguish between benign and malignant lesions. *Radiology* **196**(1):123–134.

28. Cespedes I, Ophir J, Ponnekanti H, Maklad N. 1993. Elastography: elasticity imaging using ultrasound with application to muscle and breast in vivo. *Ultrason Imaging* **15**(2):73–88.

29. Ophir J, Cespedes I, Ponnekanti H, Yazdi Y, Li X. 1991. Elastography: a quantitative method for imaging the elasticity of biological tissues. *Ultrason Imaging* **13**(2):111–134.

30. Horsch K, Giger ML, Vyborny CJ, Venta LA. 2004. Performance of computer-aided diagnosis in the interpretation of lesions on breast sonography. *Acad Radiol* **11**(3):272–280.

31. Chen CM, Chou YH, Han KC, Hung GS, Tiu CM, Chiou HJ, Chiou SY. 2003. Breast lesions on sonograms: computer-aided diagnosis with nearly setting-independent features and artificial neural networks. *Radiology* **226**(2):504–514.

32. Osher S, Sethian J. 1988. Fronts propagating with curvature-dependent speed: Algorithms based on the Hamilton-Jacobi formulation. *J Comput Phys* **79**(1):12–49.

33. Sethian JA. 1990. Numerical algorithms for propagating interfaces: Hamilton-Jacobi equations and conservation laws. *J Differ Geom* **31**:131–161.

34. Suri JS, Laxminarayan SN. 2001. *PDE and level sets: algorithmic approaches to static and motion imagery*. New York: Springer.

35. Mulder W, Osher S, Sethian J. 1992. Computing interface motion in compressible gas dynamics. *J Comput Phys* **100**(2):209–228.

36. Grayson M. 1987. The heat equation shrinks embedded plane curves to round points. *J Differ Geom* **26**:285–314.

37. Gerig G, Kubler O, Kikinis R, Jolesz FA. 1992. Nonlinear anisotropic filtering of MRI data. *IEEE Trans Med Imaging* **11**(2):221–232.

38. Perona P, Malik J. 1990. Scale-space and edge detection using anisotropic diffusion. *IEEE Trans Pattern Anal Machine Intell* **12**(7):629–639.

39. Czerwinski RN, Jones DL, O'Brien Jr WD. 1994. Edge detection in ultrasound speckle noise. In *Proceedings of the IEEE International Conference on Image Processing*, pp. 304–308. Washington, DC: IEEE Computer Society.

40. Czerwinski RN, Jones DL, O'Brien Jr WD. 1998. Line and boundary detection in speckle images. *IEEE Trans Image Process* **7**(12):1700–1714.

41. Czerwinski RN, Jones DL, O'Brien Jr WD. 1999. Detection of lines and boundaries in speckle images: application to medical ultrasound. *IEEE Trans Med Imaging* **18**(2):126–136.

42. Leymarie FL. 1993. Tracking deformable objects in the plane using an active contour model. *IEEE Trans Pattern Anal Machine Intell* **15**(6):617–634.

43. Richardson IEG. 2003. *H.264 and MPEG-4 video compression: video coding for next-generation multimedia*. Chichester, UK: John Wiley & Sons.

44. Russ JC. 2002. *The image processing handbook*, 4th ed. Boca Raton, FL: CRC Press.

45. Vapnik VN. 1999. *The nature of statistical learning theory*, 2nd ed. New York: Springer.

46. Pontil M, Verri A. 1998. Support vector machines for 3D object recognition. *IEEE Trans Pattern Anal Machine Intell* **20**(6):637–646.

47. Chapelle O, Haffner P, Vapnik VN. 1999. Support vector machines for histogram-based image classification. *IEEE Trans Neural Networks* **10**(5):1055–1064.

9

ALTERNATE SPACES FOR MODEL DEFORMATION: APPLICATION OF STOP AND GO ACTIVE MODELS TO MEDICAL IMAGES

Oriol Pujol

Departamento Matemática Aplicada i Análisi
Universidad de Barcelona, Barcelona, Spain

Petia Radeva

Centre de Visió per Computador, Universidad
Autónoma de Barcelona
Barcelona, Spain

1. INTRODUCTION

The role of deformable models [1, 2, 3], in medical image analysis [4] has been increasing over the past two decades. The location of a pathology, the study of anatomical structures, computer-assisted surgery, or quantification of tissue volumes are a few of the applications in which deformable models have proved to be very effective. Due to their importance, the study and improvement of these models is still a challenge [5, 6, 7, 8]. These techniques are used to give a high-level interpretation of low-level information such as contours or isolated regions. These techniques depend on the balance between internal and external constraints. The external constraints are designed to guide the deformable model to the regions

---

Address all correspondence to: Petia Radeva, Centre de Visió per Computador, Edifici O, Universidad Autónoma de Barcelona, 08193 Bellaterra, Barcelona, Spain. Phone: +34-3-581 21 69; Fax: +34-3-581 16 70. petia@cvc.uab.es.

of interest. On the other hand, the internal constraints control the smoothness and continuity of the model.

It is well known that there are two main branches of deformable models according to parametrization of the model. The first, the parametric one, is based on the classical Newtonian mechanics equations that govern the elasticity and stretching of the deformable model. In this branch, the curve defining the deformable model is explicitly parameterized. This fact means that the resulting model is usually restricted to a single object. In this sense, some parametric models [9] try to solve this drawback by re-parameterizing the model at each step of the evolution. The other branch relies on the theory of geodesic curves and level sets [2, 10]. In this formulation the snake is defined using an implicit parametrization. The deformation process is defined by a changing Riemannian surface that minimizes the length of the level set curve under the constraints of the image features. The main advantage of this formulation is that it can naturally deal with topological changes during snake evolution.

In this latter branch, the equation that governs the evolution of the deformable model is divided into two terms. The first is the normal component of the gradient of a potential defined by the image features. The role of this term is to rule the convergence to contours. The second depends on the snake curvature, and endows the snake with a means to deform at null gradient regions while ensuring regularity. However, the role of the curvature has a major impact in the numeric scheme: on one hand, it restricts the maximum speed of the evolution and, on the other, interferes with convergence in concave areas. The usual way to overcome this latter issue is to add a constant motion term, the balloon force [3], that pushes the snake into concave regions.

In general, deformable models were originally designed to be used in a contour space — an image defining the contours of the regions of interest. However, contours are not always available, especially in textured or complex images. Due to this problem, region-based schemes were introduced. They aim at finding a partition of the image such that the descriptors of each of the regions conform to a given "homogeneity" criterion. In this sense, the force guiding the snake is derived from the competition of the descriptors. Several authors address this issue: Ronfard [11] set the velocity function proportional to the difference of simple statistical features. Zhu [12] and Paragios and Deriche [5] defined the region evolution as a quotient of probabilities corresponding to different regions. In Yezzi et al. [13] the difference of mean gray levels inside and outside the evolving front at each iteration defines the motion of the deformable model. Along the same lines, Besson et al. [7] propose a difference of simple statistics, variance, and covariance matrix, inside and outside the evolving curve. Chakraborty et al. [14] consider an evolution using a Fourier parametrization over the original image and previously classified image regions. Probably the most notable technique for complex images is the one proposed by Paragios and Deriche [5] and Samson et al. [15] based on supervised learning of the features of the regions of interest.

However, these approaches require a previous classification or contain implicit classification schemes. In this sense, little control over the false positive and false negative regions is obtained.

Considering the general problem of region-based segmentation, we proposed in [8] a new geodesic snake formulation where the terms ruling convergence and regularity are decoupled. As a result, the curvature term is restricted to the shape regularity at the last stages of the snake deformation. Furthermore, any vector field properly defining the path-to-target contours or regions of interest is suitable to guide the model. In our formulation, we also split the two main motion terms guiding the deformable model to its goal. On one hand, we have the external attractor vector field (GO term), which guides any external curve to the regions of interest. And, on the other hand, a repulsive vector field (STOP term) is used to cancel the forward motion of the GO term at the borders of interest. Due to these two terms, we call this technique the *STOP and GO* active models. In order to use the decoupling strategy, a characteristic function is needed. The characteristic function is defined with the value 1 where the regions of interest are located and 0 in the remainder. To sum up, a mask defining the object of interest would be the ideal tool to bound the scope of the curvature term and perform any decoupling. However, in real applications we do not have this mask. To address this issue, a substitute estimation must be provided. This point is one of the key issues of this formulation. In this chapter we explain a powerful technique that allows any approximation to a mask to be used. In this sense, this technique increases the number of possible definitions of the regions of interest. Therefore, not only the classical region-based definitions or contour images are suitable for deformation of the snakes, but any map ranging from filter responses to likelihood or confidence rate maps can be used. This chapter explains in detail how these alternative deformation spaces are designed and embedded into the deformable model equation. We show results applied to two different medical images: intravascular ultrasound images (IVUS) and intestinal capsule endoscopy. Intravascular ultrasound is an image modality based on the ultrasound technology that provides a unique cross-section display of the morphology and histological properties of the arteries. Figure 1a shows a good example of an IVUS image. In this kind of image we apply deformable models to distinguish between fibrous tissues and the rest. The other kind of images are color intestinal images recorded by a capsule endoscopy. Using this kind of image, we are trying to segment the turbid liquid. Figure 1b shows an example of this modality. We can observe in the image that on the right side we find the turbid liquid — a liquid usually mixed with bubbles.

The layout of the chapter is as follows: First, a mandatory analysis of the current geometric formulations and the basics of the *STOP and GO* formulation are provided. Second, the segmentation pipeline for deformable models is introduced and three different alternative spaces are described. In this section we also provide two tools for enhancing mask estimations. Third, the design of the

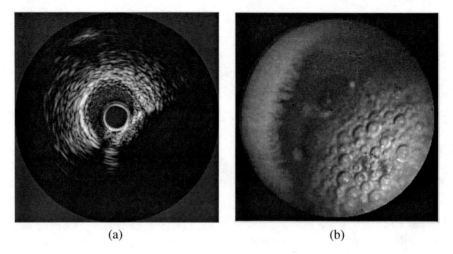

(a)   (b)

Figure 1. The different image modalities used in this chapter: (a) intravascular ultrasound image; (b) intestinal capsule endoscopic image.

STOP and GO model using these new spaces is introduced. Finally, several experiments explaining the behavior of this formulation in the medical environment are provided.

2. ANALYSIS OF CURRENT GEOMETRIC SNAKES

Most of the current snakes define curve evolution within an energy minimization framework. In this context, the energy functional should achieve a compromise between adjusting to image features and achieving curve regularity. There are two main tendencies for the definition of the minimizing energy.

- **Geodesic formulations in a contour space**

    The general geodesic snake formulation defines the evolution of a snake within an energy minimization framework. In particular, the solution to the problem is the curve Γ of minimal length in a Riemannian surface with a metric g depending on the image contrast changes. It follows that the snake, Γ, evolves according to

$$\frac{\partial \Gamma}{\partial t} = (g \cdot \kappa - < \nabla g, \vec{n} >) \cdot \vec{n} \quad \text{with} \quad g = \frac{1}{1 + |\nabla u|^2}, \quad (1)$$

where κ is the curvature of Γ, $\vec{n}$ its inward unit normal, and $<,>$ stands for the scalar product of two vectors.

We can give the following interpretation to each of the terms involved in the above formula. The term $< \nabla g, \vec{n} > \vec{n}$ is a vector field defined on the curve pointing to the region of interest that attracts the snake to the object boundary. Since its computation essentially relies on image edges, from a vector flow point of view, it can be considered as a *Static Vector Field* locally defining the target object. The curvature term, $g \cdot \kappa\vec{n}$, influences different aspects of the snake evolution. On one hand, it defines its motion when it is located far away from the object boundaries. Since it depends on the evolving snake, it acts as a *Dynamic Vector Field* in the convergence process. On the other hand, it serves as a curve-regularizing term, ensuring continuity of the final segmenting snake in a similar fashion [16] as the membrane term of parametric snakes does. Finally, it gives to the process a smooth behavior and ensures continuity during the deformation, in the sense that it prevents shock formation [17]. However, incorporating the curvature term into the convergence scheme has some disadvantages. First, it is difficult to facilitate snake convergence to concave areas. Second, guidance through the curvature is extremely slow, so in spite of giving regularity to the evolution equation, it hinders the numerical scheme since the time increment is bounded by the second-order term [18].

The main problem of (1) is that convergence to the object of interest relies on the properties of the external field. Even considering a regularization [19] of the external force, concave regions such that the unit tangent turns around more than π degrees between consecutive inflexion points of the object contour, cannot be reached [20]. In order to increase convergence to concavities and to speed up the evolution, a constant balloon force velocity term, V_0, corresponding to area minimization is added:

$$\frac{\partial \Gamma}{\partial t} = (g \cdot \kappa + V_0 - < \nabla g, \vec{n} >) \cdot \vec{n}. \qquad (2)$$

Notice that, in order to ensure that the scheme will stop at the boundary of interest, an equilibrium between the constant shrinking velocity, V_0, and the static vector field, ∇g, must be achieved. One easily realizes that, should this condition be satisfied, incorporating the curvature term into the convergence scheme constitutes a significant drawback. V_0 must overpass the magnitude of κ to enter into concave regions but, at the same time, it should be kept under $min|\langle \nabla g, \vec{n}\rangle|$ (minimum taken on the curve to detect!) to guarantee nontrivial steady states. This dichotomy motivates bounding the scope of V_0 to a given image region [7]:

- **Snake formulation in a region-based scheme**

  The "region terms" [7] are added to the minimization scheme as follows:

$$E(\Omega_{in}, \Omega_{out}, \Gamma) = \int\int_{\Omega_{in}} g^{(\Omega_{in})} dx dy + \int\int_{\Omega_{out}} g^{(\Omega_{out})} dx dy + \int_{\Gamma} g^{(\Gamma)} ds,$$

  where Ω_{in} and Ω_{out} refer to the inside and outside of the region of interest. There are two different approaches to determine the region: a "pseudo-static" approach and a dynamic one. In the first case, the attraction term that guides the evolution of each point in the curve is previously computed and kept fixed during the evolution [5, 12]. In the second, measurements of the region descriptors depend on the evolving curve [13, 14], so that all parameters must be updated at each iteration.

  Region-based approaches usually rely on a pseudo-mask behavior [12], which can be implemented by considering:

$$M(x, y) = \begin{cases} \alpha & \text{if} P_{\text{Background}} > P_{\text{Target}} \\ -\alpha & \text{otherwise} \end{cases},$$

  and evolving the snake using

$$\frac{\partial \Gamma}{\partial t} = \text{sign}(I) \cdot \vec{n}. \tag{3}$$

We propose to reformulate (2) decoupling the regularity and convergence terms and embedding the scheme in a region-based framework.

3. STOP AND GO FORMULATION

The evolution of deformable models is basically guided by a compromise achieved by balancing an external force and the inner constraints of the model. The full process of evolution can be decoupled in two stages: a straightforward advancing front defined outside the regions of interest, and an inside region term opposed to it. Evolution stops if these two forces cancel along the curve of interest. A mask defining the object of interest is needed to bound the range of the curvature term and to perform this decoupling. On the other hand, any standard snake vector evolution definition serves to build an outer force ensuring convergence.

3.1. Basics of the STOP and GO Formulation

The formulation of the STOP and GO deformable model needs the definition of two different vector flows: an attractor vector field (GO) moving the curve toward the target and a repulsive one (STOP) making that evolution stop. In order to define this decoupling, a characteristic function defining the region of interest is used. Given the region of interest R, the characteristic function is defined as follows:

$$I(x, y) = \left\{ \begin{array}{ll} 1 & \text{if } (x, y) \in R, \\ 0 & \text{otherwise.} \end{array} \right.$$

Let us assume that the evolving curve is outside the region of interest. In that case, the GO term corresponds to an evolution process that shrinks the model outside of R:

$$V_{GO} = (1 - I) \cdot V_0 \cdot \vec{n}. \tag{4}$$

The above equation creates a constant "inward" motion toward the region of interest. On the other hand, in order to define the "outward" motion we just have to create a STOP field around the region of interest. In this sense, the easiest way to create the STOP term is to use the "outward" gradient of any function, namely g, locally defining the contours of the object of interest:

$$V_{STOP} = I \cdot \langle \nabla g, \vec{n} \rangle \vec{n}. \tag{5}$$

Therefore, combining both terms, the STOP and GO motions, we can define the whole evolution of a deformable model initialized outside the region of interest. Hence, the formulation is as follows:

$$\frac{\partial \Gamma}{\partial t} = \underbrace{< I \cdot \nabla g, \vec{n} > \vec{n}}_{\text{Stop}} + \underbrace{V_0 \cdot (1 - I) \cdot \vec{n}}_{\text{Go}}. \tag{6}$$

Note that the equilibrium solution is obtained if we ensure that the condition $V_0^+ < \nabla g, \vec{n} > \leq 0$ holds along the boundary of R. This formulation is mainly governed by V_0. The change of this parameter allows different behaviors of the curve: on one hand, we can ignore small activations of the potential g; on the other, we can overpass areas with low value.

Figure 2 shows the basic decomposition of the force field in two sets. Figure 2a shows the mask I defining the region of interest. The GO term is represented in Figure 2b and the STOP term in Figure 2c. Joining both terms results in the complete deformation process.

3.2. Improving the Performance of the STOP and GO Basic Formulation

The formulation we have just described leads the curve to the desired boundary defined by the characteristic function. As a result of this process, we will have the borders of the region of interest accurately located. However, one of the attractive features of the deformable models is the possibility of controlling the smoothness and continuity of the resulting model. Since this regularity behavior is only needed in the final stages of the snake deformation, we can bound its scope to

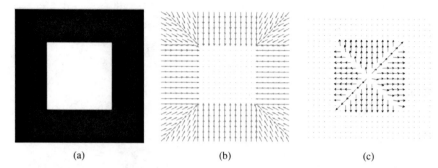

Figure 2. Basic decomposition of the potential field in two terms: (a) characteristic function; (b) static representation of the GO term; (c) STOP term.

a neighborhood of the target object. Such restriction can be performed by means of a smoothed version of the mask $\breve{I} = G_\sigma * I$; for G_σ a gaussian filter with standard deviation σ. Adding this regularity term to (6), the final evolution equation of STOP and GO snakes yields:

$$\Gamma_t = \underbrace{(I < \nabla g, \vec{n} > + V_0(1 - I)) \cdot \vec{n}}_{\text{Stop and Go}} + \underbrace{\alpha \kappa \breve{I} \vec{n}}_{\text{Reg. term}} \, . \tag{7}$$

As one can observe, the formulation given by Eq. (7) resembles that of parametric snakes in the sense that regularity and convergence are distinguished. From a geometric point of view, it can be interpreted as selecting those curves that comply both criteria, to be near the real borders of the region of interest and to obtain a given degree of regularity.

Note the fact that reducing the range of the regularizing term gives to the curvature term a different role than the one it had in classic geodesic snakes. While in geodesic snakes the curvature has a double role, on one hand it allows the snake to shrink providing the inward motion for convergence and, on the other, acts as a regularizing term. This role is drastically different than the one our curvature term has. First, it is strictly a regularizing term — similar to the internal energy of the parametric snakes. Second, since the curvature term is bounded to the environs of the regions of interest, it does not hinder the convergence step of the Euler numeric scheme. When integrating a curvature term into the formulation of the STOP and GO model, we must note that the curvature term competes against a smooth outward vector field created at the borders of the region of interest. This fact endows this formulation with two interesting properties: first, it does not allow the model to leak through small holes. Second, it provides higher smoothness to

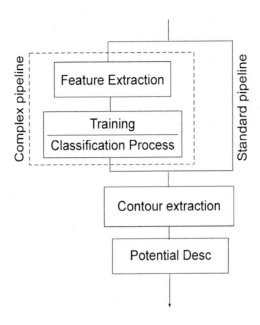

Figure 3. Standard and complex pipelines for deformable models.

the final model. Hence, we can reformulate (7) as:

$$\frac{\partial \Gamma}{\partial t} = \underbrace{(V_0 + I\langle \nabla g, \overrightarrow{n}\rangle)\overrightarrow{n}}_{\text{Convergence}} + \underbrace{I \cdot (\alpha\kappa - V_0)\overrightarrow{n}}_{\text{Regularizing term}}.$$

As we have pointed out, we can observe in the former equation that V_0 ensures convergence, but it also competes with the curvature for regularity near the region of interest.

4. DEFORMABLE MODELS IN THE CLASSIFICATION PIPELINE

Deformable models constitute an important tool for medical image analysis. They are usually involved in segmentation and/or tracking processes. In this section we analyze their application in the segmentation/classification pipeline and provide alternatives to the standard methodology, which can be exploited by our new formulation of the *STOP and GO* model.

Generally, any segmentation process involving deformable models is composed of three stages. First, the graylevel image is described in terms of features in the feature extraction process. Second, a machine learning technique is trained and used to obtain a meaningful set of regions according to our segmentation goal.

Finally, the contours of those regions are used to create the potential for the deformable models evolution. At the end of this chain the deformable model is laid to deform under this potential. Figure 9 shows the usual pipeline for segmentation before using the deformable model.

In simple applications where the structures are clearly defined, the first and second stage of the process can be omitted. However, when the problem is more complex the information obtained from graylevel images cannot suffice to define the regions or contours of interest. It is in these difficult tasks where the full chain must be used. The goal of the first stage, the feature extraction process, is to provide alternate descriptions of the image according to different criteria, e.g., it can be as simple as the variance of the neighboring pixels or as complex as the co-occurrence matrix measures to characterize textures. As a result of applying these different description criteria we obtain a set of N features, $\mathbf{x} = \{x_1, \ldots, x_N\}$, for each pixel in the image.

The features define multiple views of the information contained in the image. These features do not usually define explicitly the region or contours we are looking for as they are. Hence, in order to exploit the new information obtained by the feature extraction process, a machine learning procedure defining which of the areas of interest are needed. This process aims at learning of the rules that allow the discrimination of what we have defined to be useful. In this chapter we will look at this classification stage as a black box in which feature vectors are provided as an input and the box returns a value indicating the belonging to one class or to another. In fact, this value can be just a discrete boolean value that points out if a pixel belongs to the region of interest or a likelihood value that measures the degree of belonging to the area of interest. This difference is important because many deformable model algorithms are defined for clear binary contours. This fact implies that if the classifier returns a likelihood or confidence value a further thresholding process is needed.

At this point a binary image is obtained and the contour detection is straightforward. The last stage of the pipeline consists of the building of the potential field. Most deformable model techniques are applied afterward.

As we have explained, the deformable model process is the last stage in a complex chain. The goal of this process is usually to give continuity and smoothness to the scattered contours obtained in the former stages. In this sense the result of the deformable model can be easily predicted as it is unrelated to the rest. On the other hand, the complexity of the feature extraction and classification process and the parameters involved in such process is usually high. This compartmentalization of tasks is the most commonly used procedure in segmentation tasks involving deformable models.

However, since each stage is unrelated to the others, and in particular, the classification and the deformable model evolution stages, the control of the whole process is difficult to adjust and usually does not generalize well — it is not easily transferred to other environments or can easily degrade its performance if the test

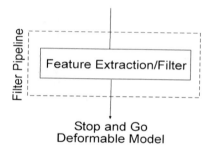

Figure 4. Filter pipeline for STOP and GO active models.

data change a little. Therefore, it looks reasonable that the mixture of classification and evolution could help to improve the control of the processes involved.

In this trend, the most well-known techniques are the region based scheme. However, the main drawback of these techniques is that, although it includes the classification task in its evolutive model, the resulting segmentation does not differ from a batch approximation. Note that the boundaries used in the region competition are those defined by the Bayessian rule: $P(\mathbf{x}|c = A)P(c = A) = P(\mathbf{x}|c = B)P(c = B)$.

From the point of view of the segmentation pipeline, what we propose is a different embedding of the classification task in the evolutive model. In our approach, both tasks are performed at the same time. This means that regions are not *a priori* labeled. On the other hand, we just need a confidence rate of the region belonging to the area of interest. In this sense we observe three main scenarios in which this confidence rate can be obtained: a filter approach, a likelihood map approach and a classification confidence rate approach. The following sections are devoted to the description of these scenarios and possible tools for enhancing the responses if they are not well defined.

4.1. Filter Potentials

Filters are well known tools for enhancing or extracting information from images. Usually, the result of the filtering process of an image shows high values in the areas where the filter has been designed to work, i.e., if we are using a contour detector filter, the values of the filtering process will be higher where the contours are more likely to be found. However, not all filter designs are meant to work in this way, i.e., isotropic filtering just modifies the gray values according to a diffusion criterion. In this section, when we talk about filter potential we just consider those filters in which the premise of having high values at the structures of interest holds. These filters are the ones usually used in feature extraction processes.

Figure 4 shows the pipeline before the deformable model. As one can observe, the response of the filter is used directly as an input to the deformable model. The only minor question is that the filter response has to be normalized between 0 and 1.

In many medical image applications, texture plays a major role in the task of segmentation of regions of interest. Associated with texture features are numerous techniques. Basically, the different methods of feature extraction emphasize different fundamental properties of the texture, such as scale, statistics, or structure. In a very rough way, we can subdivide the texture feature extractors into: complex statistics, with techniques as co-occurrence methods [21] or higher-order statistics represented by moments [22]; multi-resolution strategies, such as derivatives of a gaussian model [23], Gabor filters [24], or Wavelet techniques [25]; and structure related measures, such as Fractal Dimension [26] and Local Binary Patterns [27]. Probably, one of the most well-known techniques is the co-occurrence matrices measures. Due to the popularity of this technique, we have selected it to illustrate the filter approach. The following paragraphs are devoted to give a brief introduction and examples of the co-occurrence matrices measures technique.

The graylevel co-occurrence matrix [28] is a well-known statistical tool for extracting second-order texture information from images [21]. The creation of the matrix involves the computation of the relative frequencies of graylevel pairs of pixels at certain relative displacement. We can look at the co-occurrence matrix as an estimate of the joint probability density function of graylevel pairs in an image for a given angle and distance. For N different gray levels in the image, the co-occurrence matrix $\mathbf{M}$ is of size $N \times N$. Usually, the image is quantified so that the total number of gray levels is smaller than the original image. This is done in order to increase the appearance of pixel pairs contributing to each position of the co-occurrence matrix. Take into account that, if the number of pixel pairs contributing to each element of the matrix $M_{i,j}$ is low, the statistical significance will be poor. On the other hand, if N is small, much of the texture information may be lost in the image quantization.

Given a pixel $p_{(l,m)}$ at position $\{l, m\}$ of the image I, and two parameters $\{D, \theta\}$, a distance and an angle respectively, each element of the co-occurrence matrix is defined as follows:

$$M(i,j) \quad = \quad |\{p_{(l,m)}|I(l,m) = i \text{ and } I(l + D\cos(\theta), m + D\sin(\theta)) = j\}| \\ \forall p_{(l,m)} \in I \qquad (8)$$

The parameter θ is commonly set at $\theta = \{0^0, 45^0, 90^0, 135^0\}$. And the distance D is a scale parameter of the texture we are looking for. This set of four matrices for each distance D is considered to be the minimal set in order to describe texture second-order statistic measures [29].

The co-occurrence matrix is a tool for representing the appearance of the pixel pairs; however, the matrix, as it is, is difficult to use as a descriptor of the texture. Therefore, several measures describing the matrix can be used instead. The most common measures are: Energy, Entropy, Inverse Difference Moment (IDM), Shade, Inertia, and Prominence [29].

Let us introduce some notation for the definition of the features:

$M(i, j)$ is the $(i, j)th$ element of a normalized co-occurrence matrix:

$$
\begin{aligned}
M_x(i) &= \sum_j M(i, j), \\
M_y(j) &= \sum_i M(i, j), \\
\mu_x &= \sum_i i \sum_j M(i, j) = \sum_i i M_x(i) = E\{i\}, \\
\mu_y &= \sum_j j \sum_i M(i, j) = \sum_j j M_y(j) = E\{j\}.
\end{aligned}
$$

With the above notation, the features can be written as follows:

$$
\begin{aligned}
\text{Energy} &= \sum_{i,j} M(i, j)^2, \\
\text{Entropy} &= -\sum_{i,j} M(i, j) log M(i, j), \\
\text{IDM} &= \sum_{i,j} \frac{1}{1 + (i - j)^2} M(i, j), \\
\text{Shade} &= \sum_{i,j} (i + j - \mu_x - \mu_y)^3 M(i, j), \\
\text{Inertia} &= \sum_{i,j} (i - j)^2 M(i, j), \\
\text{Prominence} &= \sum_{i,j} (i + j - \mu_x - \mu_y)^4 M(i, j).
\end{aligned}
$$

In this way, for each measure $m_k : \Re^2 \rightarrow \Re^2$ we obtain an image according to each particular feature of the co-occurrence matrix. Therefore, if we are computing the four orientations, given a single distance D we obtain 24 different filtered images. Those images are the possible inputs to the STOP and GO active model formulation.

Figure 5 shows different filter outputs using the co-occurrence measures in a polar representation of the IVUS images. As we can observe, not all the figures are suitable for use as inputs of the deformable model. Note that Figure 5b,c do not follow the guidelines for the filter to be used, since the regions of interest (the textured tissue) is not defined by high values. Note also that the rest of the images comply with this requisite in different ways.

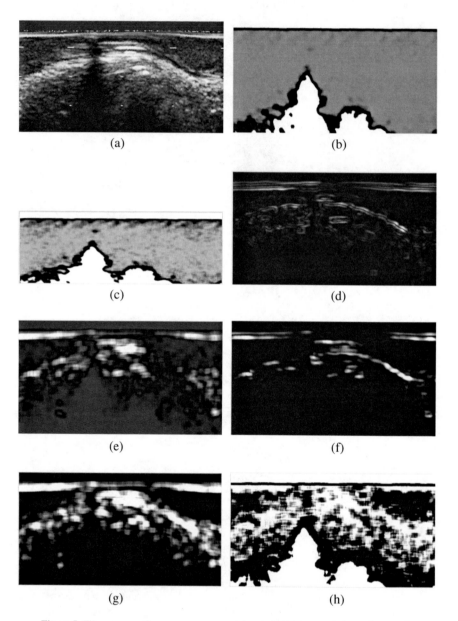

Figure 5. Filter spaces using co-occurrence matrices in IVUS images (using polar coordinates): (a) original image; (b) energy measure map; (c) entropy measure map; (d) inverse Differential Moment measure map; (e) inertia measure map; (f) prominence measure map; (g) inertia measure map at 90 degrees; (h) shade measure map at 135 degrees.

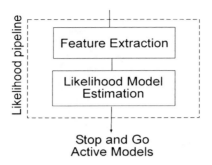

Figure 6. Likelihood map pipeline for STOP and GO active models.

4.2. Likelihood Potentials

A likelihood function, in statistics, is a function proportional to the conditional probability function of its second argument while keeping the first fixed. Extrapolating from this definition and using the Bayes theorem, we consider the likelihood function to be any conditional probability density function with one parameter fixed. In segmentation/classification environments the likelihood function depends on two random variables, $\mathbf{x}$ and c that represent the feature vector data and the class label, respectively. Therefore, the likelihood function that we consider corresponds to the conditional probability function holding the random variable c constant to a certain label of interest (LOI).

$$L(\mathbf{x}) = \alpha p(\mathbf{x}|c = \text{'LOI'})$$

Using the former definition, we define the *likelihood map* as the set of corresponding likelihood values for each of the elements of a given space. In our case, the likelihood map is composed by the likelihood values for each of the pixel feature vectors of an image. Likelihood maps contain information related to the probability of how much an area of the image represents the class of interest.

Figure 6 shows the place where the deformable model is used in this approach. The use of likelihood maps to guide a deformable model evolution is important when an area of interest is under the influence of noise or subject of great variations. In those scenarios the use of the certainty of a given area belonging to the region of interest can be exploited. This approach opposes the most traditional trend of classification techniques that rely on the *a posteriori* probability equality given by $p(\mathbf{x}|c = \text{'LOI'}) = p(\mathbf{x}|c = \text{'NOT LOI'})$. Note that in this last technique the boundaries are strictly fixed by the equality disregarding the value of the probability. In this sense the one-class approach via likelihood maps has the desirable effect of avoiding false positive segmented/classified regions. Our approach exploits this fact to guide the deformation of the deformable model to the most probable regions.

4.2.1. Likelihood map estimation

Likelihood maps require estimation of the conditional probability density function. In this section we provide a brief introduction to one of the multiple approaches available for density estimation, and we will use it, for illustration, in our experiments with gaussian mixture models.

A gaussian mixture model is a semi-parametric technique that allows estimation of an approximation to a density function by combining gaussian functions. One of the main advantages of this technique is that is able to smooth over gaps given a sparse data set:

$$G(\mathbf{x}, \mu, \Sigma) = \frac{1}{2\pi|\Sigma|^{1/2}} \exp^{-\frac{1}{2}(\mathbf{X}-\mu)\Sigma^{-1}(\mathbf{X}-\mu)}.$$

The model is formulated as a linear model in the following way:

$$MG(\mathbf{x}, \Theta) = \sum_{r=1}^{K} \alpha_r G(\mathbf{x}, \mu_r, \Sigma_r),$$

where $G(\mathbf{x}, \mu_r, \Sigma_r)$ is a multidimensional gaussian function, k is the number of gaussians involved, $\Theta = (\mu_1, \ldots, \mu_K, \Sigma_1, \ldots, \Sigma_K)$ are the gaussian's mean values and standard deviation matrices.

In order to adjust the parameters of the model Θ, we will use the *expectation maximization* process. This process assumes that we know the number K of gaussian functions that will approximate the probability density function. Given the number of gaussian functions desired, a pre-initialization is performed using a k-means algorithm. This algorithm looks for a certain number of cluster representatives in an unsupervised manner. Once the initial parameters are set θ^0, the expectation maximization algorithm optimizes the model parameters given a set of features points. The basic idea is to iteratively estimate the likelihood of the data. This is done in two steps: the first, *expectation*, is concerned with the probability model building assuming that the current parameters are the optimal ones; the second, *maximization*, looks for the optimal parameters assuming that the model is the one obtained in the expectation step.

As a result of this process an accurate estimate of an approximation to the likelihood is computed. This model is used to find the likelihood values of the whole working image, resulting in the likelihood map. The likelihood map for a pixel located at (x, y) is computed using the following expression:

$$L(x, y, \Theta) = MG(\mathbf{x}(x, y), \Theta)$$

However, the likelihood maps suffer form several drawbacks: First, there is a lack of accuracy at the real boundaries of the regions. It is easy to see that due to the

Table 1. Expectation Maximization Algorithm

Initialization: $\theta^0, \epsilon, i = 0$

do $i \leftarrow i + 1$ E step: compute $M(\theta^i)$
$\quad\quad$ M step: $\theta^{i+1} = \underset{\theta}{argmax}M(\theta)$

until $M(\theta^{i+1}) - M(\theta^i) \leq \epsilon$

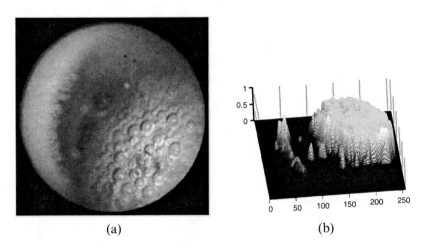

(a) $\quad\quad\quad\quad\quad\quad\quad\quad\quad\quad$ (b)

Figure 7. Likelihood map extraction using color information: (a) original image; (b) likelihood map for the bubbles region.

smoothing effect of the gaussian functions, neighboring pixels are likely to have similar likelihood values, leading to smooth transitions. On the other hand, the higher likelihood values in a region of interest occur in the inner part of the region and decrease in the borders. This effect is what we call the "safety region effect" — due to the fact that it has a high value on "safety" areas, and low likelihood values elsewhere. The safety areas are usually sub-regions of the regions desired. Due to both drawbacks, the boundary information must be improved for better results. There are several ways to improve the technique. In the following subsection we describe one that is intimately related to the process we have described.

Figure 7 shows the original image and the three-dimensional representation of the likelihood map for the bubbles region. Observe that the likelihood map has higher values at the regions where the estimation is more confident about the presence of bubbles.

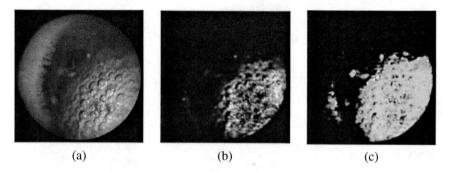

(a)   (b)   (c)

Figure 8. Likelihood map enhancement using the two-class approach: (a) original image; (b) original likelihood map; (c) enhanced likelihood taking into account the bubbles region and the background region.

4.2.2. Two-class enhancement of the likelihood map

In several applications the knowledge of the domain allows for definition of two classes: the first one, related to the region of interest, and the second, related to everything else. This can be done if the non-desired areas are well known and a model of them can be built. Therefore, if a two-class problem arises, the likelihood map can be improved provided that an *a priori* knowledge about the desired properties of the different regions is available. In this case, we can enhance the likelihood map using the following expression:

$$\tilde{L}(x,y,\Theta,\overline{\Theta}) = \left(\frac{\lambda}{\lambda + |L(x,y,\Theta) - L(x,y,\overline{\Theta})|}\right) \cdot L(x,y,\Theta), \qquad (9)$$

where $L(x,y,\Theta)$ is the likelihood map for image $I(x,y)$ using a likelihood model with parameters Θ. The parameter Θ corresponds to the parameters of the likelihood model for the region of interest, and the parameter $\overline{\Theta}$ are the model parameters of the complement of the target region. λ is a weighting parameter. Note that when both likelihood values are similar ($L(x,y,\Theta) \sim L(x,y,\overline{\Theta})$), the likelihood map ($L(x,y,\Theta)$) is emphasized. It remains smooth elsewhere. This enhancement highlights the likelihood map in a range near the border given by $L(x,y,\Theta) = L(x,y,\overline{\Theta})$. In this way, we enhance edges near the classification border weighted by their likelihood value in the map. The proposed enhanced likelihood map ($\tilde{L}(x,y,\Theta,\overline{\Theta})$) partially overcomes one of the drawbacks of the likelihood map, giving better accuracy and removing non-prominent edges.

Figure 8 shows the procedure when taking into account the background information. Figure 8a shows the original image, (b) displays the likelihood map for the region of interest (the bubbles), and (c) shows the enhanced likelihood map. We can see that the definition of the region of interest is much more accurate.

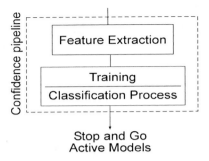

Figure 9. Filter pipeline for the confidence rate approach of the STOP and GO active models.

4.3. Confidence Rate Approach

The confidence rate approach is based on the output of a classifier. Several classification techniques are able to provide the confidence of the output label. The confidence rate is a measure of the certainty that the algorithm has in its label choice. According to this confidence rate we can build a *confidence map* in the same way we created the likelihood map. Given a classification technique $h(\mathbf{x})$, we consider that the output of this function is $y = \{C, \mathbf{c_r}\}$, where C is the label assigned to each feature vector $\mathbf{x}$ and $\mathbf{c_r}$ is a vector of the confidence rates associated with each of the class labels. Of course, the label selected is the label associated with the maximum value of confidence rate. The confidence map is the result of classifying each feature vector associated with each pixel $I(x, y)$ of a given image I,

$$C(x, y) = h(\mathbf{x}(I(x, y)))$$

Many classification schemes are able to produce these confidence rates — e.g., adaptive boosting (adaboost), support vector machines, etc. In this section we introduce the one we have selected to demonstrate the performance of the STOP and GO models with confidence rate spaces.

We will focus the following paragraphs on the adaboost process. The adaboost algorithm is an ensemble method for supervised classification. The basic idea of the method is to combine a set of *weak* classifiers until some desired low training error has been achieved. The combination of the *weaks* is done using a weight independent of error associated with that weak.

Adaboost defines a systematic way to create these *weaks*: each feature point in the training set has a weight associated with it. This weight depends on how accurate the data point is being classified up to that point by the combination of weaks — the combination of weaks will be called **strong** from now on. If a data point is accurately classified, then its probability of being used by subsequent

Table 2. Adaboost Algorithm

[Initialization] $w_{1,i} = \frac{1}{2m}, \frac{1}{2l}$ for $c_i = \{-1, 1\}$ respectively.

Step 1. Normalize weights

$$w_{t,i} \leftarrow \frac{w_{t,i}}{\sum_{j=1}^{n} w_{t,i}}$$

Step 2. For each dimension j, train a classifier, h_j which is restricted to using that single random variable.

The error is evaluated with respect to w_t, $\epsilon_j = \sum_i w_i |h_j(x_i) - c_i|$.

Step 3. Choose the classifier, h_t with the lowest error ϵ_t.

Step 4. Update the weights:

$$w_{t+1,i} = w_{t,i} \beta_t^{e_i}$$

where $e_i = 1$ for each well-classified feature and $e_i = 0$ otherwise. $\beta_t = \frac{\epsilon_t}{1-\epsilon_t}$.

Step 5. Calculate the parameter $\alpha_t = -log(\beta_t)$.

Step 6. $t = t + 1$.
    If $t \geq T$ go to Step 1

The final *strong* classifier is:

$$h(x) = \begin{cases} 1 & c_r = \sum_{t=1}^{T} \alpha_t h_t(x) \geq 0 \\ 0 & \text{otherwise} \end{cases}$$

where c_r is the confidence rate associated with the label.

---

learners is reduced, or increased otherwise. As a result, each classifier is centered in the most difficult data up to that point.

Let the training set be composed by N pairs $\{x_i, c_i\}$, where $c_i = \{-1, 1\}$ is the class of each multidimensional data point x_i. Let $w_{t,i}$ be the weighting factor at time t for data point x_i. Also, let l and m be the number of data points for each class. The adaboost algorithm is described in the Table 2.

Parameter α_t is the weighting factor of each of the classifiers of the ensemble. The loop ends whether the classification error of a the *weak* classifier is over 0.5;

the estimated error for the whole *strong* classifier is lower than a given error rate, or if we achieve the desired number of *weaks*. The final decision is the result of the weighted classification results of the *weaks*.

The most commonly used weak learner is the *decision stumps*. This simple learner looks for the most discriminant feature of the training set and classifies using a threshold. Formally, the weak classifier, $h_j(x)$, consists of a feature f_j, a threshold θ_j, and a parity value p_j. The classifier is trained using ROC curve evaluation. Note that, although the threshold separates the two classes, it is not enough to identify which class is on either side of the threshold. Therefore, a parameter p_j (parity) is needed to indicate the direction of the inequality sign when classifying:

$$h_j(x) = \begin{cases} 1 & \text{if } p_j f_j(x) < p_j \theta_j, \\ 0 & \text{otherwise.} \end{cases}$$

Observe that the label resulting from the evaluation of the strong classifier is based on the comparison of the weighted combination of weak results with a threshold. If we omit this last comparison, we can consider that the number resulting from this process is related to the confidence rate of that output. In fact, the greater the number of weak classifiers that agree, the more extreme the value is. The output of this process can be used to feed a STOP and GO active model.

4.4. Geometry-Based General Enhancement of Continuous Potentials

Up to this point we have seen several scenarios with different spaces in which STOP and GO active models can be used. However, several of them do not provide maps accurate enough for feeding the STOP and GO models. In this sense, general tools for further enhancing the results are useful. In this subsection we provide an independent method for image and local contour enhancement based on the geometry. The method is based on a new representation of an image proposed in the work of Salembier and Garrido [30].

In their approach, Salembier and Garrido represent an image as a tree (**Max-Tree**) composed by flat regions and linking information among regions. Each flat region is a node C_h^k in the tree. The process for creating the tree is divided into two steps:

- *Binarization step:* For each temporary node TC_h^k, the set of pixel belonging to the local background is defined and assigned to the max-tree node C_h^k.

- *Connected components definition step:* The set of pixels belonging to the complement of the local background ($TC_h^k \backslash C_h^k$, where $\backslash$ is the set difference defined on connected components) are analyzed and its connected components create the temporary child nodes TC_{h+1}^k.

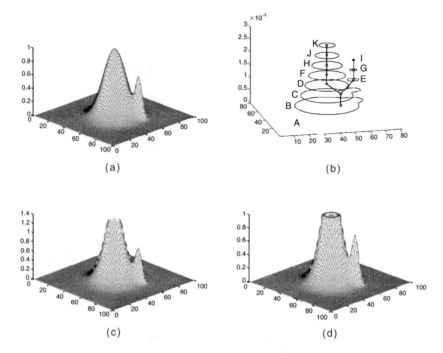

Figure 10. Creation of the topological enhanced likelihood map: (a) original likelihood map; (b) Max-Tree representation; (c) enhanced likelihood map without constraining maximum values; (d) final enhanced likelihood map.

    The idea underlying the above formalization is to create a tree recursively by analysis of the relationships among connected components of the thresholded versions of the image. Figure 10 illustrates the process for *max-tree* creation. The following explanation of the creation of the max-tree uses the notation for the flat zones depicted in Figure 10b. In the first step, a threshold is fixed to the gray value 0, and all the pixels at level $h = 0$ are assigned to the root node $C_0^1 = \{A\}$. The pixels with values strictly superior to $h = 0$ form the temporal nodes (in our case, $TC_1^1 = \{B, C, D, E, F, G, H, I, J, K\}$). Each temporal node is processed as if it was the original image, and the new node will be the connected components associated with the next level of thresholding $h = 1$, $C_1^1 = \{B\}$. Let's illustrate a split. Suppose the process goes on until processing node $C_2^1 = \{C\}$. The temporal nodes at that point are the connected components strictly superior to $h = 2$, $TC_3^1 = \{E, G, I\}$ and $TC_3^2 = \{D, F, H, J, K\}$, and the associated nodes at $h = 3$ are $C_3^1 = \{E\}$ and $C_3^2 = \{D\}$.

    Taking advantage of that concept, we now use the *Max-Tree representation* to describe the function maps (characteristic function estimations). This representation allows further processing to be done keeping topological issues unchanged.

The function map topological enhancement can be described as follows. Given the *max-tree representation* of the function map T and a parameter θ that represents a value that we consider to be high enough to determine a set of seed connected components, a safety set is defined $S_T = \{C_h^k \mid h > \theta\}$. For instance, we can assume that regions with values over 90% are reliable enough to represent safety areas that are used to initialize the method. The method enhances topologically all the connected components that contain any of the safety areas by weighting the value of the connected component by a function $f(h)$, where h is the threshold parameter for the connected component. The function f is monotonically increasing and is desired to be S-shaped. Let's define the set of connected components that have a node in S_T:

$$S_N = \{C_h^k \mid C_h^k \supset C_i^j, \quad \forall \quad C_i^j \in S_T\}.$$

Then, the topologically enhanced function map is defined as:

$$\check{L}(h) = (f(h) \cdot S_N(h)) \cup \overline{S_N}(h),$$

where $(f(h) \cdot S_N(h))$ is the product of the value of each of the connected components of S_N at level h with the value of a function at the threshold level. The result of the product is an "enhanced" set of components in which the value of each of the components has been increased. $\overline{S_N}$ is the complementary set of S_N. The resulting enhanced map $\check{L}$ is the union of the enhanced set and the complementary set. The effect of this enhancing process is to increase topologically the value of the neighboring connected components of the high likelihood value areas while preserving the rest of the map intact. A final step is performed so that the resulting values after enhancing never surpass the value of the connected component at level θ. Therefore, each connected component the value of which is over θ is constrained to the value at level θ. Remember that Figure 10c shows the non-constrained enhanced map, and Figure 10d depicts the final result. As can be observed in Figure 10d, the topologically enhanced area has steeper slopes and therefore defines better the contours of the region. On the other hand, the low-value region is kept at the same level. The shape of the function $f(h)$ determines the degree of enhancement. Usually this function parameters are related to the inflexion point and the slope. In our experiments we have used an exponential function.

Figure 11 shows the result of the enhancing process when applied to the original likelihood map. Figure 11a shows the original image, Figure 11b depicts the likelihood map, and Figure 11c shows the enhanced map. Note that the process enhances the regions near the areas of maximum likelihood while preserving the rest of the regions untouched.

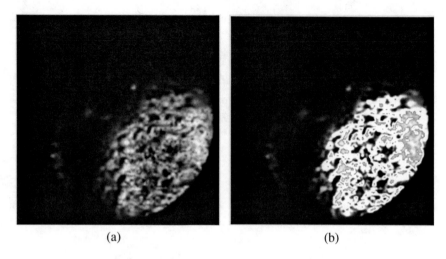

(a)   (b)

Figure 11. Likelihood map extraction using color information: (a) original image; (b) likelihood map for the bubbles region.

5.   STOP AND GO SNAKES DESIGN

5.1. Term Decoupling

The hypothesis we consider in the creation of our formulation is that we can obtain a characteristic function of the region of interest. However, this does not happen in practical applications. At this point, alternate schemes must be used as approximations of the characteristic function to perform the decoupling needed for the STOP and GO models. The only requirement for this approximation is that the region of interest be defined as a local extremum while having small values outside this area. At this point the use of the filter spaces, likelihood maps, and confidence rate maps come into play. Recall that all these techniques comply with the above requirement and therefore can be used as estimations of the characteristic function.

Let $\check{L}$ be the estimate of the characteristic function normalized between 0 and 1. Therefore, replacing I by $\check{L}$ in the *Stop and Go* equation, we obtain the following:

$$\frac{\partial \Gamma}{\partial t} = \alpha \kappa \check{L} \cdot \vec{n} + \check{L} < \nabla g, \vec{n} > \cdot \vec{n} + V_0 (1 - \check{L}) \cdot \vec{n}.$$

At this point, it only remains to define the STOP term, $\check{L} \cdot \nabla g$, which defines the object of interest.

5.2. Using Characteristic Function Estimates to Define the STOP and GO Field

The choice of the function g depends on the particular segmenting problem we handle. Classic applications of deformable models deal with contour-based spaces. Note that contour spaces are a degenerate version of the characteristic function. In this sense they can be used in a STOP and GO formulation without altering the scheme. However, in more complex problems the use of alternate spaces like the filter space, likelihood map, or confidence rate spaces allow the use of deformable models at any step of the classic classification pipeline. Take, for instance, a color or texture feature space. In these spaces it is nearly unthinkable to use a contour-based approach; however, it is simple to create either of the alternatives introduced in this chapter. Therefore, we define the STOP term based on the characteristic function estimate as $\nabla(1 - \check{L})$. Moreover, since the former gradient is negligible outside a band around the contours, we can merge the two STOP factors as follows:

$$\frac{\partial \Gamma}{\partial t} = \alpha \kappa \check{L} \cdot \vec{n} + \beta < \nabla(1 - \check{L}), \vec{n} > \cdot \vec{n} + V_0(1 - \check{L}) \cdot \vec{n}. \qquad (10)$$

5.3. STOP and GO Numeric Formulation

Evolution of an initial snake Γ_0 under (10) is implemented using the Level Sets [10] formulation. That is, given any initial surface (ϕ_0) properly defining the interior of Γ_0, the snake evolution at time t coincides with the 0 level contour of the solution to:

$$\frac{\partial \phi}{\partial t} = (\alpha \check{L} \text{div}(\frac{\nabla \phi}{|\nabla \phi|}) + V_0(1 - \check{L}))|\nabla \phi| + < \nabla(1 - \check{L}), \nabla \phi > .$$

The explicit Euler scheme we use in the numeric implementation of the former equation is given by

$$\phi_{t+1} = \phi_t + (\alpha \check{L} \frac{u_{xx}u_y^2 - 2u_{xy}u_x u_y + u_{yy}u_x^2}{|\nabla u|^2} + $$
$$+ V_0(1 - \check{L})|\nabla \phi_t| + < \nabla(1 - \check{L}), \nabla \phi_t >)\Delta t, \qquad (11)$$

where ϕ_t stands for the solution at time t and derivatives are computed using centered finite differences. Notice that the speed of convergence hinges upon the magnitude of the time step Δt; the higher it is, the less iterations the algorithm requires. Accuracy is determined by V_0.

6. EXPERIMENTAL RESULTS

In this section we provide different experiments results. In the first subsection the general behavior of the STOP and GO active models is shown. The next

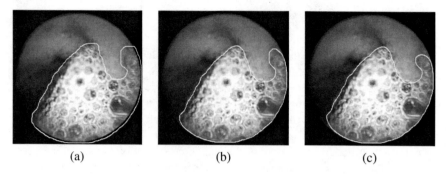

(a)   (b)   (c)

Figure 12. Different results when changing the parameters controlling the smoothness of the model: (a) rough model; (b) average smooth model; (c) smooth model. See attached CD for color version.

subsection shows experiments designed to compare other deformable models with the STOP and GO snake. Finally, the third subsection shows the application of this deformable model to different domains and spaces in medical image processing.

6.1. Behavior of the STOP and GO Models

In this section we provide several experiments showing the behavior of the STOP and GO active models. The first experiment shows how we can change the degree of smoothness of the final model.

Figure 12 shows the results of changing the parameters governing the smoothness of the model. In order to do so we just have to decrease the value of parameter V_0 and the time increment Δt. Note that for convergence issues around using this numerical scheme, the condition $\alpha \cdot \Delta t \leq 0.4$ must hold. As we can see, we can obtain very smooth results; in particular, in [8] we show that the smoothness obtained using these models is greater than that using classical deformable models. This is due to the fact that we have two terms competing: on one hand, the curvature term that tries to shrink the model; on the other, an area term repulsing the model. Typical values for very smooth results are $\alpha = 0.75$, $\Delta t = 0.5$, $V_0 = 0.5$.

Figure 13 displays the number of iterations needed to obtain different degrees of smoothness. As we can observe, there is a trade-off between the number of iterations and the degree of smoothness. We need more iterations to create a smoother model.

The final experiment of the STOP and GO behavior reflects control of the model for leaking through small gaps. Figure 14a shows the original image. Figure 14b displays a co-occurrence feature space map where the deformable model will evolve. Figures 14c,d show the final segmentation controlling leakage through small holes. Figure 14c is obtained if we increase the value of V_0 to force the model to get inside the concave region. Figure 14d uses small values for V_0.

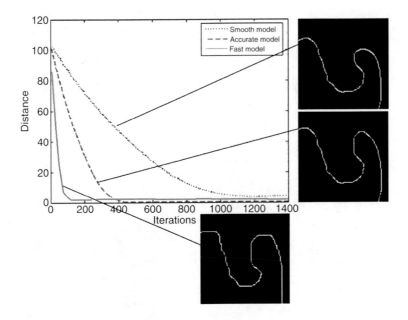

Figure 13. Convergence speed versus degree or smoothness.

In this case, the model stops at the entrance of the concave area and can be used to close gaps in the shape of unconnected regions or contours.

6.2. Comparing STOP and GO with Other Deformable Models

In this section we compare the performance and advantages of the STOP and GO active model with the classic geodesic formulation and the region-based approach of Paragios and Deriche [5] or Zhu [12].

The first experimental results are depicted in Figure 15. This graphic shows convergence speed with the parameters for the geodesic and STOP and GO models set at their fastest. As we can observe, the results using STOP and GO have a faster convergence than with the classic snakes. This is due to the fact that we are removing the constraint imposed by the curvature term along the deformation. In our case, the curvature term only has effects in the last steps of the deformation, thereby speeding up the process.

One of the most important and well-known problems of the geodesic snakes is a lack of convergence in the concave regions. Figure 16 shows a real problem where this occurs. Figure 16a shows the original image segmented by experts, and Figures 16b,c show the geodesic model segmentation and the STOP and GO segmentation, respectively. Observe that the geodesic model is unable to get into

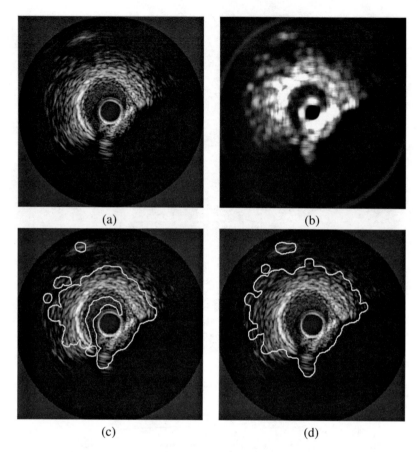

Figure 14. Segmentation of an IVUS image. Example of leaking control: (a) original image; (b) filter space for deformation using co-occurrence matrix measures; (c) example of STOP and GO model with a fast configuration: (d) example of STOP and GO model with anti-leak configuration.

the concave region, while the STOP and GO model actually converges to the desired borders.

In the next experiment we are comparing the advantages of using a likelihood map instead of other implicit classification schemes, such as that used in [5] or [12]. These approaches rely on a pseudo-mask behavior [12], which can be implemented by considering:

$$M(x,y) = \begin{cases} \alpha & \text{if } P_{\text{Background}} > P_{\text{Target}}, \\ -\alpha & \text{otherwise}, \end{cases}$$

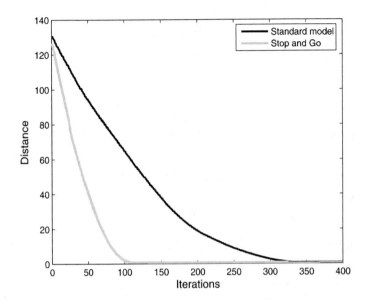

Figure 15. Convergence speed (in number of iterations) for classical geodesic snakes and STOP and GO models.

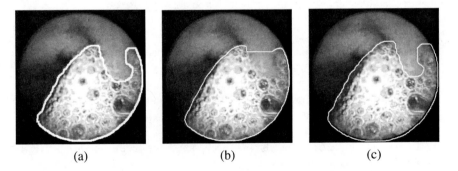

(a)   (b)   (c)

Figure 16. Creation of the topological enhanced likelihood map: (a) original likelihood map; (b) Max-Tree representation; (c) enhanced likelihood map without constraining maximum values; (d) final enhanced likelihood map. See attached CD for color version.

Table 3. Mean and Maximum Errors in Pixels per Model Point

	Standard models	STOP and GO
Mean error	40	14
Max error	130	55

where $P_{Background}$ is the probability density function for the non-desired region and P_{Target} is the pdf for the region of interest. Using the former equation we can evolve the snake as follows:

$$\frac{\partial \Gamma}{\partial t} = \text{sign}(I) \cdot \vec{n}. \tag{12}$$

The last equation is a simplification of the real one, which takes into account the curvature term. However, the effect of guiding the snake to the border where $P_{Background} = P_{Target}$ is the same as the complete equation, except for the regularity of the final model. Figure 17 shows an example where the condition of equiprobability fails to define the regions of interest. Figure 17a,b shows the probability estimation of the region of interest and the background, respectively. Figure 17c shows the mask obtained by the inequality $P_{Background} \leq P_{Target}$. The edges of this mask are the attraction contours. As we can see, since the value of the probabilities is not being taken into account, the regions in which both probabilities have small values are also being classified as desired regions. Figure 17d shows the resulting segmentation using a region scheme. Figure 17e displays the geometrically enhanced likelihood map, and, finally, Figure 17f shows the resulting segmentation using the STOP and GO models. As we can observe, the resulting region is much closer to the real one than the one obtained using classic schemes.

The next experiment was performed using 100 intestinal endoscopy images. We compare the error achieved using *STOP and GO* and Geodesic Region Based models with the segmentation made by experts. Table 3 shows the resulting errors in pixels per model point. As we can observe, the mean error for the standard region-based technique is 40 pixels per model point. This huge difference between automatic segmentation and expert segmentation is mainly due to the fact that all errors in the embedded "classification" have a lot of impact on the deformation result. As an example of this effect, the reader can check Figure 17. On the other hand, *STOP and GO* models seem to overpass most of the errors and converge more accurately to the real borders achieving a mean error of 14 pixels per model point.

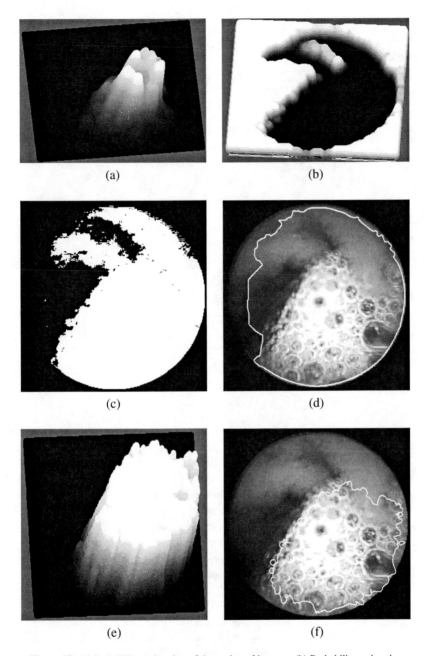

Figure 17. (a) Probability estimation of the region of interest. (b) Probability estimation of the background. (c) Mask created using the inequality $P_{\text{Background}} \leq P_{\text{Target}}$. (d) Resulting segmentation using region schemes. (e) Geometrically enhanced likelihood map. (f) Resulting segmentation using STOP and GO models. See attached CD for color version.

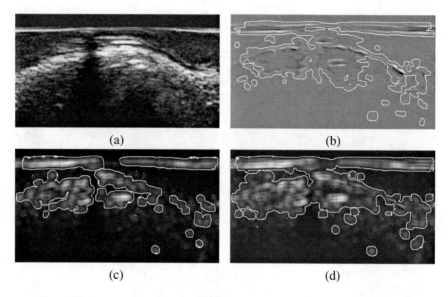

Figure 18. Segmentation of a polar IVUS image. Example using different filter spaces and a combination of filters: (a) original image; (b) filter space for deformation using co-occurrence matrix measures (IDM); (c) filter space for deformation using co-occurrence matrix measures (Inertia); (d) filter space composed by the linear combination of IDM and Inertia.

6.3. Applying STOP and GO to Medical Images

The following section includes several examples of STOP and GO active models applied to different medical images and with different space maps.

Figure 18 shows an example of tissue detection on polar transformation of intravascular ultrasound images using different filter spaces. Figure 18a shows the original image, while Figure 18b shows the segmentation using the inverse differential moment of the co-occurrence matrix at zero degrees, Figure 18c shows the final snake using the inertia of the co-occurrence matrix, and Figure 18d depicts the result using a linear combination of the inertia and inverse different moment.

Figure 19 shows the segmentation of turbid liquid in endoscopic images acquired by a wireless capsule using a confidence rate space. We have trained a 40-round adaboost with decision stumps using general bubble data. Figure 19a shows the original image, while Figure 19b displays the confidence rate of the classifier. As we can observe, the confidence rate at the regions of interest is higher than in rest of the areas. Figure 19c shows a geometric enhancement of the confidence rate map, and Figure 19d displays the resulting segmentation.

Figure 20 shows another example of the segmentation of bubbles using a confidence rate spaces. Using the same model and classifier, we built a 40-round

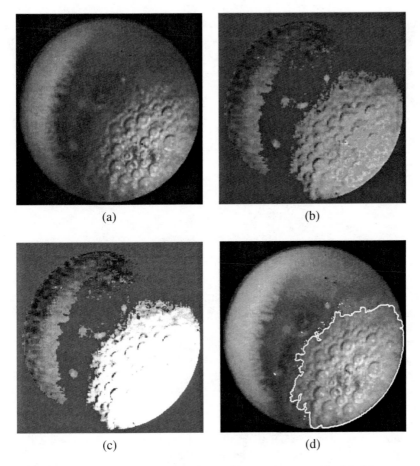

Figure 19. Segmentation of bubbles using confidence rate spaces: (a) original image; (b) confidence rate of an adaboost classifier trained with a bubble model; (c) geometric enhancement of the confidence rate map; (d) resulting segmentation. See attached CD for color version.

adaboost. Figure 20a shows the original image, while Figure 20b displays the confidence rate of the classifier. In this case, we fed the deformable model with this map without further improvement. Figure 20c displays the resulting segmentation.

7. CONCLUSIONS

In this chapter we consider a novel geodesic snake formulation, termed *STOP and GO*, for more efficient convergence to shapes. The formulation is based on restricting the regularizing term to the last stages of the snake deformation

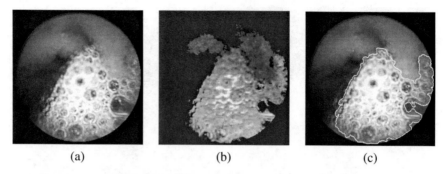

Figure 20. Another segmentation of bubbles using confidence rate spaces: (a) original image; (b) confidence rate of an adaboost classifier trained with a bubble model; (c) resulting segmentation. See attached CD for color version.

by decoupling the convergence from the regularity. This decoupling has several advantages over existing geodesic formulations. On one hand, the numeric scheme is more efficient since it admits arbitrary large time increments, except for the last regularizing steps. On the other hand, we built a robust vector field ensuring convergence but, at the same time, snake stabilization. Convergence is achieved by defining separately a dynamic attractive term and an image feature-based repulsive one. We also introduce likelihood maps to decouple as well as to define the STOP term of the external potential vector field. By using likelihood maps as an external force, the particular version of *STOP and GO* presented in here is suited to feature space-based image segmentation (texture, motion, color schemes).

We have also introduced three different alternate spaces that can be used in conjunction with our formulation: the filter space maps, the likelihood maps, and the classification confidence rate map. We have applied these techniques in two different image modalities — intravascular ultrasound images and intestinal images — with great success.

8. ACKNOWLEDGMENTS

This work was partly supported by GivenImaging, Israel.

9. REFERENCES

1. Kass M, Witkin A, Terzopoulos D. 1988. Snakes: active contour models. *Int J Comput Vision* **1**:321–331.
2. Caselles V, Catte F, Coll T, Dibos F. 1993. A geometric model for actives contours. *Num Math* **66**:1–31.
3. Cohen LD. On active contour models and ballons. *Comput Vision Graphics Image Process: Image Understand* 53(2):211–218, 1991.

4. McInerney T, Terzopoulos D. 1996. Deformable models in medical images analysis: a survey. *Med Image Anal* **1**(2):91–108.

5. Paragios N, Deriche R. 1999. Geodesic active contours for supervised texture segmentation. In *Proceedings of the IEEE conference on computer vision and pattern recognition*, Vol. 2, pp. 422–427. Washington, DC: IEEE Computer Society.

6. Pujol O, Radeva P. 2004. Texture segmentation by statistic deformable models. *Int J Image Graphics* **4**(3):433–452.

7. Jehan-Besson S, Barlaud M, Aubert G. 2003. DREAMS: deformable regions driven by an Eulerian accurate minimization method for image and video segmentation. Submitted to *Int J Comput Vision*.

8. Pujol O, Gil D, Radeva P. 2005. Fundamentals of stop and go active models. *J Image Vision Computing* **23**(8):681–691.

9. McInerney T, Terzopoulos D. 2000. T-Snakes: topology adaptative snakes. *Med Image Anal* **4**:73–91.

10. Osher S, Sethian JA. 1988. Fronts propagating with curvature-dependent speed: algorithms based on Hamilton-Jacobi formulations, *J Comput Phys* **79**:12–49.

11. Ronfard R. 1994. Region-based strategies for active contour models. *Int J Comput Vision* **13**(2):229–251.

12. Zhu SC. 1994. *Region competition: unifying snakes, region growing, and Bayes/MDL for multi-band image segmentation*. Technical Report 94-10, Harvard Robotics Laboratory.

13. Yezzi A, Tsai A, Willsky A. 1999. A statistical approach to snakes for bimodal and trimodal imagery. In *Proceedings of the seventh IEEE international conference on computer vision*, pp. 898–903. Washington, DC: IEEE Computer Society.

14. Chakraborty A, Staib L, Duncan J. 1996. Deformable boundary finding in medical images by integrating gradient and region information. *IEEE Trans Med Imaging* **15**:859–870.

15. Samson C, Blanc-Féraud L, Aubert G, Zerubia J. 1999. A level set model for image classification. In *Proceedings of the second international conference on scale-space theories in computer vision. Lecture notes in computer science*, Vol. 1682, pp. 306–317.

16. Xu C, Yezzi A, Prince J. 2000. On the relationship between parametric and geometric active contours. In *Proceedings of the 34th Asilomar conference on signals, systems, and computers*, pp. 483–489. Washington, DC: IEEE Computer Society.

17. Evans LC. 1993. *Partial differential equations*. Berkeley Mathematics Lecture Notes, vol. 3B. Berkeley: UCB Press.

18. Tveito A, Winther R. 1998. *Introduction to partial differential equations*. Texts in Applied Mathematics, no 29. New York: Springer.

19. Xu C, Prince JL. 1998. Generalized gradient vector flow: external forces for active contours. *Signal Process Int J* **71**(2):132–139.

20. Gil D, Radeva P. 2005. Curvature vector flow to assure convergent deformable models. *Comput Vision Graphics Image Process* **99**(1):118–125. EMMCVP'03.

21. Haralick R, Shanmugam K, Dinstein I. 1973. Textural features for image classification. *IEEE Trans Syst Mach Cybern* **3**:610–621.

22. Tuceryan M. 1994. Moment based texture segmentation. *Pattern Recognit Lett* **15**:659–668.

23. Lindeberg T. 1994. *Scale-space theory in computer vision*. New York: Kluwer Academic.

24. Jain A, Farrokhnia F. 1990. Unsupervised texture segmentation using gabor filters. *Proceedings of the international conference on systems, man and cybernetics*, pp. 14–19. Washington, DC: IEEE Computer Society.

25. Mallat S. 1989. A theory for multiresolution signal decomposition: the wavelet representation. *IEEE Trans Pattern Anal Machine Intell* **11**(7):674–694.

26. Mandelbrot B. 1983. *The fractal geometry of nature*. New York: W.H. Freeman.

27. Ojala T, Pietikainen M, Maenpaa T. 2002. Multiresolution grayscale and rotation invariant texture classification with local binary patterns. *IEEE Trans Pattern Anal Machine Intell* **24**(7):971–987.

28. Julesz B. 1962. Visual pattern discrimination. *IRE Trans Inf Theory*, **8**:84–92.
29. P. Ohanian, Dubes R. 1992. Performance evaluation for four classes of textural features. *Pattern Recognit* **25**(8):819–833.
30. Salembier P, Garrido L. 2000. Binary partition tree as an efficient representation for image processing, segmentation, and information retrieval. *IEEE Trans Image Process* **9**(4):561–576.
31. Duda R, Hart P. 2001. *Pattern classification*, 2d ed. New York: Wiley-Interscience.
32. Paragios N, Deriche R. 1999. Unifying boundary and region-based information for geodesic active tracking. In *Proceedings of the IEEE conference on computer vision and pattern recognition*, Vol. 2, pp. 300–305. Washington, DC: IEEE Computer Society.
33. Pujo O. *A semi-supervised statistical framework and generative snakes for IVUS analysis*. PhD dissertation, Universidad Autónoma de Barcelona.
34. Hofmann T, Puzicha J, Buhmann JM. 1998. Unsupervised texture segmentation in a deterministic annealing framework. *IEEE Trans Pattern Anal Machine Intell* **20**(8):803–818.
35. Sapiro G. 1997. Color snakes. *Comput Vision Image Understand* **68**(2):247–253.

10

DEFORMABLE MODEL-BASED SEGMENTATION
OF THE PROSTATE FROM ULTRASOUND
IMAGES

Aaron Fenster

Robarts Research Institute, London, Ontario, Canada

Hanif Ladak

Department of Medical Biophysics
The University of Western Ontario, London, Ontario, Canada

Mingyue Ding

Institute for Pattern Recognition and Artificial Intelligence
Huazhong University of Science and Technology, Wuhan, China

1. INTRODUCTION

Prostate cancer is the most commonly diagnosed malignancy in men, and is the second leading cause of death due to cancer in men [1, 2]. It has been found at autopsy that 30% of men at age 50, 40% at age 60, and almost 90% at age 90 have prostate cancer [3, 4]. Over the past decade, the prostate-specific antigen (PSA) blood test has become well established for early detection of prostate cancer, particularly for monitoring of prostate cancer after treatment [5–10]. The wide availability of the PSA test [7,10], the public's increased awareness about prostate cancer, and the growing number of men over 50 have all combined to increase the proportion of prostate cancer diagnosed at an early stage [11]. Currently, 77%

Address all correspondence to: Aaron Fenster, Robarts Research Institute, 100 Perth Drive, London, Ontario, N6G 4N9, Canada. Phone: 519-663-3834; Fax: 519-663-3900. afenster@imaging.robarts.ca.

of men are diagnosed to have early stage prostate cancer, compared to only 57% between 1975 and 1979 [12,13].

When diagnosed at an early stage, the disease is curable; however, once the tumour has extended beyond the prostate, the risk of metastases increases [5,14,15]. Nevertheless, treatment options vary depending on the extent of the cancer, and the prognosis worsens when diagnosed at an advanced stage. Thus, the challenges facing physicians managing patients with possible prostate cancer are to: (a) diagnose clinically relevant cancers at a stage when they are curable, (b) stage and grade the disease accurately, (c) apply appropriate therapy accurately to optimize destruction of cancer cells while preserving normal tissues [16,17], and (d) follow patients to assess side effects and the effectiveness of the therapy.

While radical prostatectomy is a highly effective surgical method to treat prostate cancer, over the past 10 years improvements in imaging technology, computer-aided dosimetry, and new treatment options have stimulated investigators to search for minimally invasive therapies for localized prostate cancer, e.g., brachytherapy [17,18], cryosurgery [19–23], hyperthermia, interstitial laser photocoagulation (ILP), and photodynamic therapy (PDT).

Effective delivery of therapy in all these techniques requires accurate dose planning based on images of the prostate anatomy and its surrounding structures. The most common method for acquisition of images for dose planning and guiding the minimally invasive procedure is the use of 2D or 3D transrectal ultrasound (TRUS). Typically, a biplane TRUS transducer is used, which contains a side-firing linear transducer array and a curved array positioned near the tip, producing an axial view perpendicular to the linear array. The probe is covered with a water-filled condom to allow good contact with the rectal wall, inserted into the rectum, and attached to the mechanical assembly used to guide and deliver the therapy.

Two imaging acquisition approaches are currently being used for dose and therapy planning: 2D TRUS and 3D TRUS. For 2D TRUS, the US transducer is typically withdrawn in 5-mm steps, while a 2D image is acquired at each step, resulting in about 7 to 10 2D transverse images. For 3D TRUS, a motorized assembly is attached to the transducer to rotate it around its long axis. While the transducer rotates, 2D images are acquired at about $0.7r$ intervals at 30 Hz and immediately reconstructed into a 3D image. While accurate and high-quality 2D and 3D images of the prostate can be acquired rapidly, accurate and reproducible segmentation of the prostate boundary is an important step in effective guidance and delivery of treatment. Manual delineation of the margins of the prostate has been shown to be time consuming and tedious, leading to increased variability and an inability to use it effectively in intraoperative procedures [24]. Hence, many investigators have been developing automatic and semiautomatic prostate boundary segmentation techniques using 2D and 3D TRUS images [25–30]. Although various image processing methods have been used for 2D and 3D prostate segmentation, the Deformable Model approach has been most successful and is the subject of this chapter.

2. PROSTATE BOUNDARY SEGMENTATION FROM 2D TRUS IMAGES

2.1. Discrete Dynamic Contour (DDC)

2.1.1. Overview of the DDC

Our 2D segmentation algorithm [31] is described in Section 2.2, and is based on the Discrete Dynamic Contour (DDC) developed by Lobregt and Viergever [32]. We utilized the DDC because of its proven performance on noisy medical images and because of its simplicity of implementation. The DDC is represented by a sequence of vertices connected by straight-line segments that automatically deform to fit features in an image. When using the DDC to segment the boundary of an object from an image, the user must first initialize the DDC by drawing an *approximate* outline of the object. This initial outline defines the DDC, and is automatically and iteratively deformed to fit nearby features (e.g., edges) that presumably lie on the object's boundary. In principle, less user effort is required to outline an object using the DDC than to outline the object manually because the initial definition need only be approximate and can be drawn quickly with only a few vertices. Furthermore, because the deformation of the contour drives it toward edges automatically, there is a potential for less intra- and interoperator variability compared to manual outlining. Intuitive editing mechanisms can also be incorporated to allow the user to modify the DDC in problematic areas, where it is not able to find the object's boundary. Mathematical details of the operation of our DDC approach used to segment the prostate boundary from ultrasound images are given below.

2.1.2. Structure of the DDC

The structure of the DDC at a particular iteration t (analogous to time) during the deformation process is depicted in Figure 1a. The DDC consists of vertices (V_i) with coordinates (x_i, y_i) that are connected by straight-line segments. A unit edge vector $\hat{d}_i$ is defined such that it points from vertex i to vertex $i + 1$. A local tangential unit vector at vertex i, denoted $\hat{t}_i$, is defined from the two edge vectors associated with the vertex by the vector addition of $\hat{d}_i$ and $\hat{d}_{i-1}$, and then normalizing the sum. A local outer radial unit vector at vertex i, denoted $\hat{r}_i$, is defined from $\hat{t}_i$ by rotating $\hat{t}_i$ by $\pi/2$ radians.

The position of each vertex at $t = 0$ (i.e., at the beginning of the iterative deformation process) is specified by the user-drawn contour.

2.1.3. Dynamics

Once initialized, the DDC is iteratively and automatically deformed. The deformation process is based on Newtonian mechanics. At a particular iteration t, a net force, $\vec{f}_i$, is computed for each vertex i; the force serves to drive each vertex

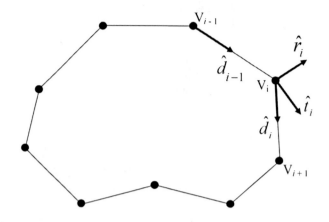

Figure 1. Configuration of the DDC. See the text for symbols. Reprinted with permission from the AAPM.

to the closest features while keeping the DDC smooth, and is fully described in Section 2.1.4. This net force causes the vertex to accelerate according to a well-known formula:

$$\vec{a}_i(t) = \frac{1}{m_i}\vec{f}_i(t), \qquad (1a)$$

where m_i is the mass of the vertex. For simplicity, the mass of each vertex is taken to be unity.

Next, the velocity, $\vec{v}_i$, and position, $\vec{p}_i = (x_i, y_i)^T$, of each vertex i are computed and updated for the next iteration at time $t + \Delta t$ using explicit Euler integration:

$$\vec{v}_i(t + \Delta t) = \vec{v}_i(t) + \vec{a}_i(t)\,\Delta t, \qquad (1b)$$

and

$$\vec{p}_i(t + \Delta t) = \vec{p}_i(t) + \vec{v}_i(t)\,\Delta t, \qquad (1c)$$

where Δt is the time step. The initial velocity of each vertex, i.e., the velocity at $t = 0$, is taken to be zero. The deformation process continues until all vertices come to rest, which occurs when the velocity and acceleration of each vertex become approximately zero. A time step of unity is used for the iterations.

During deformation, the distance between neighboring vertices can become larger, and the DDC may no longer accurately represent the local geometry of the boundary. Therefore, after each iteration, the DDC is "re-sampled" so that the distance between vertices is maintained at a uniform value. Linear interpolation of the vertices as a function of curve length was found to work well. A sampling distance of 20 pixels was found to provide a good representation of the prostate boundary.

2.1.4. Forces

The net force $\vec{f}_i$ is critical to operation of the DDC. It consists of a weighted vector sum of an image force ($\vec{f}_i^{\,img}$), an internal force ($\vec{f}_i^{\,int}$), and a damping force ($\vec{f}_i^{\,d}$):

$$\vec{f}_i = w_i^{int} \vec{f}_i^{\,int} + w_i^{img} \vec{f}_i^{\,img} + \vec{f}_i^{\,d}, \qquad (2)$$

where w_i^{img} and w_i^{int} are relative weights for the image and internal forces, respectively. Image forces drive vertices toward the closest features. Their design is application dependent and depends on the particular feature that defines the object's boundary. For TRUS images of the prostate, image forces act to drive vertices toward edges. Image forces are defined in terms of an "energy" field, E, associated with each pixel in an image [33]:

$$E(x,y) = \left\| \vec{\nabla} (G_\sigma * I(x,y)) \right\|, \qquad (3a)$$

where (x,y) are coordinates of a pixel in the image I and G_σ is a Gaussian smoothing kernel with a characteristic width of σ. The operator denoted by an asterisk represents convolution, $\vec{\nabla}$ is the gradient operator, and $\| \ \|$ denotes the magnitude of a vector. An image force field can then be computed from E at each pixel in the image using [33]:

$$\vec{f}_i^{\,img}(x,y) = \frac{2\vec{\nabla}E(x,y)}{\max \left\| \vec{\nabla}E(x,y) \right\|}. \qquad (3b)$$

The energy field as defined by Eq. (3a) consists of local maxima at the edges, and the force field computed at a pixel near an edge will point toward the edge.

The energy and force fields defined by Eqs. (3a) and (3b) are defined at pixel locations within the image. The image force acting on vertex i of the DDC with coordinates (x_i, y_i) can be obtained from the force field represented by Eq. (3b) using bilinear interpolation. As noted by Lobregt and Viergever [32], the tangential component of the image force can cause vertices on the DDC to cluster together, thus resulting in a poor representation of the prostate boundary. In order to prevent this, only the radial component of the field, i.e., the component in the direction of $\hat{r}_i$ in Figure 1a, is applied to the vertex.

The internal force minimizes local curvature at each vertex, and attempts to keep the DDC smooth in the presence of image noise. The internal force at vertex i is defined by the following equations:

$$\vec{f}_i^{\,int} = \left(\vec{c}_i \cdot \hat{r}_i - \frac{1}{2} (\vec{c}_{i-1} \cdot \hat{r}_{i-1} + \vec{c}_{i+1} \cdot \hat{r}_{i+1}) \right) \hat{r}_i, \qquad (4a)$$

$$\vec{v}_i(t + \Delta t) = \vec{v}_i(t) + \vec{a}_i(t) \Delta t, \qquad (4b)$$

where $\vec{c}_i$ is the local curvature vector at vertex i. The definition of $\vec{f}_i^{\text{int}}$ as in Eq. (4a) prevents the DDC from collapsing to a point in the absence of image forces. Such a collapse would occur if $\vec{f}_i^{\text{int}}$ were simply taken to be proportional to $\vec{c}_i$.

The damping force $\vec{f}_i^d$ is used to prevent oscillation of the DDC and to ensure convergence to the desired equilibrium state. $\vec{f}_i^d$ is taken to be proportional to the velocity $(\vec{v}_i)$ at vertex i:

$$\vec{f}_i^d = w_i^d \vec{v}_i, \tag{5}$$

where w_i^d is a negative weighting factor.

2.2. Prostate Segmentation Algorithm

2.2.1. Modifications to the DDC

Our experience shows that it is difficult to apply the DDC directly to 2D TRUS images of the prostate because the images suffer from speckle, shadowing, and refraction. Moreover, the contrast between the prostate and surrounding tissues is low and dependent on the system's transducer and ultrasound frequency. In order to overcome these effects, the user must draw the initial outline accurately if the DDC is to converge to the correct boundary features, and not to nearby non-prostate edges. However, accurate initialization requires substantial user effort since many points may need to be entered. Therefore, we have focused our efforts on developing an initialization routine that uses prostate-specific shape information to obtain a good estimate of the prostate boundary with very little user input. To aid the deformation algorithm in converging on the prostate boundary rather than edges corresponding to surrounding tissues, we have incorporated edge direction information into the image force field. Finally, we have developed editing tools to allow the user to guide the DDC in problematic regions. Each of the modifications is described below and in detail in the literature [31].

2.2.2. Initialization

Our initialization routine requires the user to select only four seed points, labeled from (1) to (4) in Figure 2a. Points (1) and (3) form the approximate axis of symmetry, and points (2) and (4) lie at the extremities in a direction perpendicular to the axis of symmetry. An $x - y$ coordinate system is defined with the y-axis directed from point (1) to point (3). The x-axis is perpendicular to the y-axis, and is oriented toward point (2). The origin of the coordinate system is at the average of points (1) and (3).

The four seed points subdivide the prostate boundary into four unique segments: segment 1–2 starting from point 1 and ending on point 2, as well as segments 2–3, 3–4, and 4–1. The initial shape is estimated by cubic interpolation of the endpoints to automatically generate points within each segment. The initial

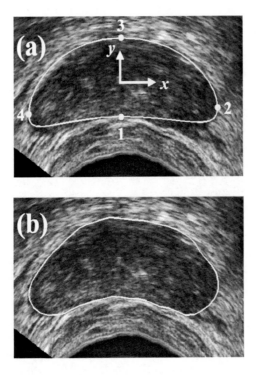

Figure 2. Initialization and deformation stages of the prostate segmentation algorithm. (a) Initial outline showing the four user-selected points, labeled (1)–(4) along with the local $x - y$ coordinate system defined from these points. (b) Final outline obtained after deforming the DDC. Reprinted with permission from the AAPM. See attached CD for color version.

shape within each segment is estimated using the following parametric equations:

$$\vec{p}(s) = \begin{cases} x\,(s) = a_3 s^3 + a_2 s^2 + a_1 s + a_0, \\[2mm] y\,(s) = b_3 s^3 + b_2 s^2 + b_1 s + b_0, \end{cases} \tag{6}$$

where $\vec{p} = (x, y)^T$ is the position of a point on the DDC having coordinates (x, y), s is a parameter that varies from 0 at the starting point of the segment to 1 at the ending point, and a_i and b_i ($i = 0, 1, 2, 3$) are unknown coefficients. The coefficients can be calculated using Eqs. (14a) and (14b) and Table 1 in Ladak et al. [31]. After calculating the coefficients, points are uniformly generated within each segment at every $\Delta s = 0.1$ units. Figure 2a shows an example initialization.

Table 1. Average Distance- and Area-Based
Metrics for all 117 Images

Metrics	Average	Standard Deviation
Distance-based		
MD (pixels)	-0.5	2.3
MAD (pixels)	4.4	1.8
MAXD (pixels)	19.5	7.8
Area-based		
Sensitivity (%)	94.5	2.7
Accuracy (%)	90.1	3.2

Reprinted with permission from the AAPM.

2.2.3. Use of edge direction information during deformation

In TRUS images of the prostate, the interior of the prostate appears darker than the exterior. We have chosen to only apply the radial component of the image force at any vertex if the gray levels in the vicinity of a vertex vary from dark to light in the direction of the outer radial vector, $\hat{r}_i$; otherwise, no force is applied. Figure 2b shows the final deformed DDC for the image in Figure 2a.

2.2.4. Editing

Intuitive editing mechanisms are easy to incorporate into the segmentation algorithm, and permit the user to guide the algorithm if the segmentation is deemed inadequate. Figure 3b shows a segmentation result in which the DDC converged to incorrect features because of poor initialization in the localized regions, indicated by the arrows in Figure 3a. The editing tools allow the user to move a few vertices onto the prostate boundary, clamp the vertices into place and re-deform the boundary. Only a few vertices (as indicated in Figure 3c) need to be moved because re-deformation will initially cause neighboring vertices to move under the influence of internal forces so that the DDC becomes smoother. As these neighbors move to minimize local curvature, they may come under the influence of image forces around the desired prostate edge and become attracted to it, as shown in Figure 3d.

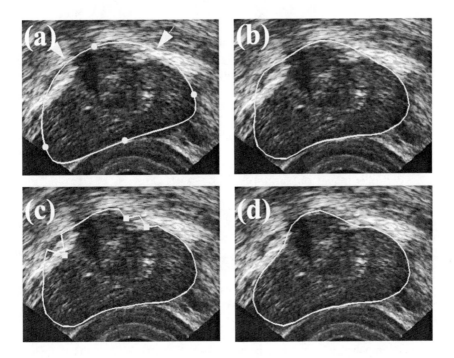

Figure 3. Illustration of interactive editing. (a) Initial DDC showing the four user-selected points. The portions of the DDC that do not follow the prostate boundary very well are indicated by arrows. (b) After first deformation. (c) Three vertices (squares) are dragged to new positions and clamped, and the DDC is deformed again. (d) After re-deformation. Reprinted with permission from the AAPM. See attached CD for color version.

2.2.5. Parameter selection

The main parameters affecting segmentation quality are the parameters w_i^{img} and w_i^{int} in Eq. (2), and σ in Eq. (3a). For simplicity, w_i^{img} and w_i^{int} were assumed to have the same value for each vertex. The weights were taken to be $w_i^{img} = 1.0$ and $w_i^{int} = 0.3$ for the images used in our work [31]. These values were empirically selected; however, the larger value for w_i^{img} relative to w_i^{int} favors deformation of the contour toward edges rather than smoothing due to internal forces. For noisier images, a larger value for w_i^{int} relative to w_i^{img} would be preferable. The exact value for the damping parameter w_i^d appears to be less critical, and $w_i^d = -0.5$ was found to provide good stability.

The image forces in Eq. (3b) are based on Eq. (3a). These forces act over a limited spatial range around an edge. A vertex on the DDC can only be driven to the closest edge in the image if the vertex is within this range. The parameter σ in

Eq. (3a) controls this range, with the spatial extent becoming larger as σ becomes larger. A large range may be desirable if the initial outline of the DDC formed by the user is poor (e.g., some vertices lying outside the range); however, a large σ can result in poor localization of the desired edge. Increasing σ also has the advantage of increasing noise suppression. For our TRUS images of the prostate, we empirically selected a value of $\sigma = 5$ pixels (which is 0.63 mm in our images) as a compromise.

2.3. Algorithm Evaluation

2.3.1. Prostate images and outlining

The performance of the algorithm was tested with 117 transverse 2D TRUS images. The 2D images were extracted from 3D TRUS images at 5-mm intervals from the base of the prostate to the apex using a multi-planar reformatting approach [34,35]. The 3D images were acquired using our 3D TRUS system [22,24,36,37] from 19 patients who were candidates for brachytherapy.

An expert radiologist manually outlined all images in one session. The same images were presented in random order at another session, and the radiologist outlined them using the algorithm. When using the algorithm, the radiologist visually evaluated the outcome, and edited the DDC as required. Each image was classified into the following three categories depending on how much editing was required:

1. "easy" if no editing was required;

2. "moderate" if the DDC had to be edited and re-deformed only once;

3. "difficult" if more than one editing/re-deformation operation was required.

2.3.2. Metrics

2.3.2.1. Distance-based metrics   Distance- and area-based metrics were used to compare the manual and algorithm outlines. Both local and global comparisons of the outlines can be made using distance-based metrics. For each image j, the signed distance, $d_j(\theta_i)$, between corresponding points on the manual and algorithm outlines was computed as a function of angle for discrete angles $0° \leq \theta_i < 360°$ ($i = 1, 2, \ldots, N$, where N is the total number of angles), as illustrated in Figure 4b for the image in part (a) of the figure. The signed distance $d_j(\theta_i)$ is negative when the algorithm outline is inside the manual outline, and it is positive when the algorithm outline is outside the manual outline. Finally, $d_j(\theta_i)$ is zero wherever the two outlines coincide. A plot of $d_j(\theta_i)$ as a function of θ_i for the prostate image in Figure 4a is shown in part (c) of the figure. The metric $d_j(\theta_i)$ provides a local measurement of the performance of the algorithm relative to the

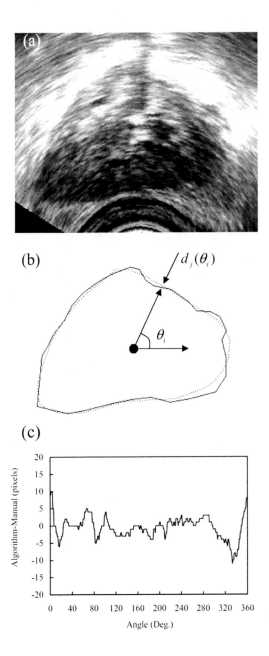

Figure 4. Local signed distance, $d_j(\theta_i)$, between two boundaries. (a) Sample prostate image. (b) Manual- (solid) and algorithm- (dotted) outlined boundaries. (c) $d_j(\theta_i)$ calculated for boundaries in (b). Reprinted with permission from the AAPM.

expert's performance. We also used three global distance-based metrics to provide an overall indicator of the performance of the algorithm. The mean difference (MD) is a measure of the segmentation bias. The mean absolute difference (MAD) quantifies the error in segmentation. The maximum difference (MAXD) indicates the maximum error in segmentation. These global distance-based metrics are computed for each image j using the following equations:

$$MD_j = \sum_{i=1}^{N} d_j(\theta_i)/N, \tag{7a}$$

$$MAD_j = \sum_{i=1}^{N} |d_j(\theta_i)|/N, \tag{7b}$$

$$MAXD_j = \max_i\{|d_j^{\theta_i}|\}. \tag{7c}$$

2.3.2.2. Area-based metrics Prostate volume is often used in prescribing the appropriate radiation dose and in interpreting the Prostate-Specific Antigen (PSA) test for diagnostic purposes and for treatment evaluation. This involves outlining the prostate in 2D images that span the length of the prostate, then adding up the areas enclosed by the individual outlines and multiplying by the distance between slices. Since area calculations affect volume estimates, we used three area-based metrics — (1) fractional area difference, P_d, (2) sensitivity, C_s, and (3) accuracy, C_a — to compare the algorithm outlines to manual outlines, which were taken to be the "true" outlines of the prostate. The three metric are defined as

$$P_d = A_d/A_m, \tag{8a}$$

$$C_s = TP/A_m, \tag{8b}$$

$$C_a = 1 - (FP + FN)/A_m, \tag{8c}$$

where TP is the true positive area that is the common region between the manual outline and the algorithm outline, FP is the false positive area that is defined as the region enclosed by the algorithm outline but outside of the manual outline, FN is the false negative area that is the region enclosed by the manual outline that is missed by the algorithm, $A_m = TP + FN$ is the area enclosed by the manual outline, and $A_d = (TP+FP)-(TP+FN) = FP-FN$ is the area difference.

2.4. Results and Discussion

2.4.1. Classification and examples

Approximately 36% of the images were classified as being "easy" to segment, 51% "moderate," and the remaining 13% difficult. The left-hand column in Figure 5 gives examples of manually outlined boundaries in the (a) easy, (b) moderate,

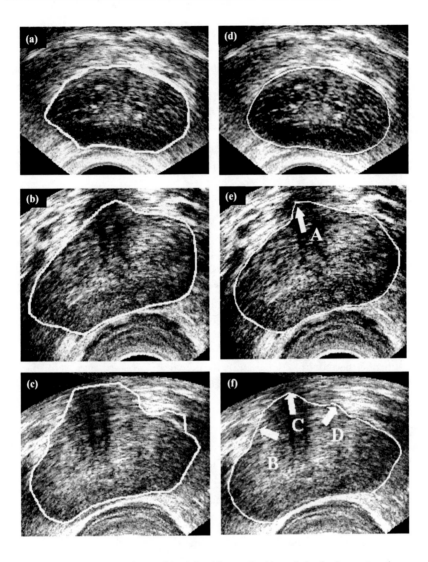

Figure 5. Comparison of manual- and algorithm-outlined boundaries for three categories: (a,d) easy; (b,e) moderate; (c,f) difficult. Reprinted with permission from the AAPM.

and (c) difficult categories, whereas the right-hand column gives corresponding algorithm-outlined boundaries in the (d) easy, (e) moderate, and (f) difficult categories for the same images. For these particular images, editing operations were required at the locations indicated by the arrows and are in or near areas of shadow. Furthermore, the time to segment an image increased as the difficulty increased, but in all cases less time was required to segment the image using the algorithm than the manual approach [31].

Good initialization is required for the DDC to converge to the desired boundary; however, to reduce the burden on the user in comparison to manual outlining, the amount of input required for initialization should be kept as small as possible. The four-point method works well for prostate shapes that are approximately elliptical. These are generally in the "easy" and "moderate" categories, representing 87% of our images. For the "difficult" cases, initialization is poorer but could be improved by requiring the user to initialize the DDC with a *few* additional points.

2.4.2. Metrics

Table 1 lists the mean values and standard deviations for each of the metrics described above: MD, MAD, MAXD, C_s, and, C_a. The means and standard deviations were computed from the corresponding metric for each of the 117 images. The mean value of MD is close to zero, that of MAD less than 5 pixels (0.63 mm), and that of MAXD less than 20 pixels (2.5 mm), indicating good overall agreement between the manual "gold standard" and semiautomatic segmentation methods. However, the values of these metrics generally increase as the segmentation complexity increases from "easy" to "moderate" to "difficult." The mean sensitivity and accuracy are greater than 90%.

Whereas the above metrics quantify the global performance of the algorithm as compared to manual outlining by an expert, the local metric $d_j\left(\theta_i\right)$ provides insight as to locations, specified by the angle θ_i, where the manual "gold standard" and algorithm outlines deviate or agree well with each other. The segmented prostate boundaries are generally similar in areas where the contrast is high, such as the lower boundary of the prostate defined approximately by $240° \leq \theta_i < 320°$. The segmented prostate boundaries deviate from each other at $\theta_i = 190°$ and $\theta_i = 350°$, where the ultrasound reflection is weak because the prostate boundary is locally parallel to the ultrasound beam. Deviation also occurs in areas of shadow caused by calcifications in the prostate.

Figure 6 is a plot of the area enclosed by the algorithm-generated outline versus that enclosed by the corresponding manual outline for all 117 images. A line passing through the coordinate origin was fitted to the data in a least-squares sense, and has a slope of 0.987 ($R = 0.993$), suggesting that areas enclosed by the manual and algorithm outlines agree over a large range of prostate cross-sectional areas from 1.5 to 15.6 cm^2.

3. TESTING AND OPTIMIZATION USING VIRTUAL OPERATORS

3.1. Introduction

Two parameters are critical to the performance of our algorithm for segmenting 2D TRUS images: σ in Eq. (3a) and w^{int} in Eq. (2). The value of w^{img} is also

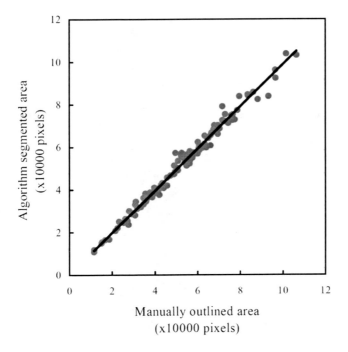

Figure 6. Area enclosed by algorithm-segmented outline versus corresponding area enclosed by manually outlined area. Reprinted with permission from the AAPM.

important, but can be constrained to be $1 - w^{\text{int}}$, as it should be balanced with w^{int}. As described in Section 2.2.5, the values used for these parameters were selected empirically, and their effects on segmentation quality were not investigated or optimized. Here, we describe a method for testing the effects of these parameters using "virtual operators" [38]. The method described here can also be applied to testing and optimization of other segmentation algorithms.

Chalana and Kim [39] have proposed a method for evaluating the single output produced by automatic segmentation algorithms. The single algorithm-generated boundary is compared to a "gold standard" formed by averaging together multiple boundaries that are manually segmented by several observers, rather than comparing to a single boundary outlined by a single observer, as done in Section 2.3. Forming a "gold standard" from multiple outlines reduces the effects of observer bias and accounts for intra- and inter-observer variability. In our semiautomatic algorithm, the output is dependent on the selection of the four control points and is also subject to observer bias and intra- and inter-observer variability. Therefore, multiple algorithm-generated boundaries, rather than a single boundary, should be compared to multiple manually generated boundaries. However, applying our algorithm (or other segmentation algorithms) many times (e.g., 100 times in this work) to generate multiple outputs requires a dedicated user and a significant effort. In order to avoid the need for a dedicated user, we developed "virtual operators" that automatically initialize the algorithm being tested for a particular image. The construction of virtual operators requires an initial investment of time from several users. However, once the virtual operators are constructed, they can be used as often as required to automatically initialize the segmentation algorithm without further user interaction.

Mathematically, a virtual operator for our TRUS-generated prostate image i is denoted VO_i and consists of four probability distributions, $p_{c,i}^{VO}(x,y)$, one for each control point $c = 1, 2, 3, 4$. Each $p_{c,i}^{VO}(x,y)$ describes the spatial distribution of selections made by the average user for control point c in image i. A separate virtual operator should be constructed for each type of image because the choice of control points depends on the image.

3.2. Constructing and Using Virtual Operators

The construction of a virtual operator requires four steps, as outlined by Ladak et al. [38] and as summarized here. First, each user u ($u1, 2, \ldots, U$, where U is the total number of users) selects each control point c in image i. This is repeated a total of R times by each user, yielding a population of $R \times U$ selections per control point when all user selections are pooled together.

Second, the parameters of a "population" distribution, $p_{c,i}^{pop}(x,y)$, are computed to describe the spatial distribution of the $R \times U$ selections for control point c in image i. $p_{c,i}^{pop}(x,y)$ is analytically represented by a bivariate Gaussian distribution. The parameters of $p_{c,i}^{pop}(x,y)$ are $\bar{x}_{c,i}^{pop}$, the mean x coordinate of control point c; $\bar{y}_{c,i}^{pop}$, the mean y coordinate; and the variances $\left(\sigma_{Xc,i}^{pop}\right)^2$ and $\left(\sigma_{Yc,i}^{pop}\right)^2$ along the major and minor principal axes of the distribution ($X_{c,i}^{pop}$ and $Y_{c,i}^{pop}$, respectively). The variances and principal axes are calculated using principal component analysis [40].

Third, the parameters the of "individual" distributions, $p_{u,c,i}^{ind}(x,y)$, which describe the spatial distribution of user u selections of control point c in image i, are computed from the R selections made by that user. $p_{u,c,i}^{ind}(x,y)$ is also described by a bivariate Gaussian distribution. Each of the U distributions $p_{u,c,i}^{ind}(x,y)$ for control point c in image i can have different mean x and y coordinates, $\bar{x}_{u,c,i}^{ind}$ and $\bar{y}_{u,c,i}^{ind}$, variances $\left(\sigma_{Xu,c,i}^{ind}\right)^2$ and $\left(\sigma_{Yu,c,i}^{ind}\right)^2$, and principal axes $X_{u,c,i}^{ind}$ and $Y_{u,c,i}^{ind}$; the differences arise due to inter-observer variability.

Fourth, the parameters of the bivariate Gaussian distributions $p_{c,i}^{VO}(x,y)$ are computed from the individual distributions $p_{u,c,i}^{ind}(x,y)$ and the population distribution $p_{c,i}^{pop}(x,y)$. $\left(\sigma_{Xc,i}^{VO}\right)^2$ denotes the variance of $p_{c,i}^{VO}(x,y)$, and is computed as the average of the variances $\left(\sigma_{Xu,c,i}^{ind}\right)^2$ for all U users. Similarly, $\left(\sigma_{Yc,i}^{VO}\right)^2$ is the average of all U variances $\left(\sigma_{Yu,c,i}^{\text{ind}}\right)^2$. $\bar{x}_{c,i}^{\text{VO}}$ denotes the mean x coordinate of $p_{c,i}^{\text{VO}}(x,y)$, and is taken to be $\bar{x}_{c,i}^{\text{pop}}$, and $\bar{y}_{c,i}^{\text{VO}}$ is taken to be $\bar{y}_{c,i}^{\text{pop}}$. The principal axes of $p_{c,i}^{\text{VO}}(x,y)$ are $X_{c,i}^{\text{VO}}$ and $Y_{c,i}^{\text{VO}}$, and are set to $X_{c,i}^{\text{pop}}$ and $Y_{c,i}^{\text{pop}}$, respectively. The distributions $p_{c,i}^{\text{VO}}(x,y)$ were meant to represent the spatial distribution of selections made by an average individual user. Therefore, the variability of $p_{c,i}^{\text{VO}}(x,y)$ was set to the average variability of the individual distributions $p_{u,c,i}^{\text{ind}}(x,y)$ rather than that of the population distribution $p_{c,i}^{\text{pop}}(x,y)$, which would contain more variability than found in any one user because $p_{c,i}^{\text{pop}}(x,y)$ is constructed from the pooled selections of all observers.

When using virtual operator VO$_i$ to initialize our 2D segmentation algorithm for a particular TRUS prostate image i, the coordinates of control point c, i.e., $(x_{c,i}, y_{c,i})$, are generated from the corresponding distributions $p_{c,i}^{\text{VO}}(x,y)$. Because x and y are prineipal axes, $p_{c,i}^{\text{VO}}(x,y)$ is separable, and can be written as $p_{c,i}^{\text{VO}}(x,y) = p_{c,i}^{\text{VO}}(x)\,p_{c,i}^{\text{VO}}(y)$, where $p_{c,i}^{\text{VO}}(x)$ is a univariate Gaussian distribution with a mean of $\bar{x}_{c,i}^{\text{VO}}$ and a variance of $\left(\sigma_{Xc,i}^{\text{VO}}\right)^2$, and $p_{c,i}^{\text{VO}}(y)$ has a mean of $\bar{y}_{c,i}^{\text{VO}}$ and a variance of $\left(\sigma_{Yc,i}^{\text{VO}}\right)^2$. $x_{c,i}$ is generated from $p_{c,i}^{\text{VO}}(x)$ using any standard algorithm for random number generation. Similarly, $y_{c,i}$ is generated from $p_{c,i}^{\text{VO}}(y)$. This method of using VO$_i$ as well as the method for constructing VO$_i$ assumes that there are no correlations in the selection of control points.

3.3. Example of Virtual Operator Construction

We have constructed 15 virtual operators, one for each of 15 mid-gland 2D TRUS images extracted from the 3D images described in Section 2.3.1. To form the virtual operators, five trained operators (i.e., $U = 5$) each selected all four control points in each of the 15 images in one session. Each session was repeated 10 times (i.e., $R = 10$) to yield a total population of 50 selections for each control point c in image i. The sessions were separated by 3 days each, and the images were presented in random order at each session in order to minimize the effects of memory. The outputs of the four steps involved in constructing a virtual operator are illustrated in Figures 7 through 9. Figure 7a illustrates the output of the first step. The Figure shows a typical image of the prostate with the population of 50 selections per control point superimposed on the image. The output of the second step is four population distributions, $p_{c,i}^{\text{pop}}(x,y)$, describing the selections for each control point c ($c = 1, 2, 3, 4$). The spatial extent of each $p_{c,i}^{\text{pop}}(x,y)$ is depicted by an ellipse in Figure 7b; the original selections are omitted for clarity. Figures 7c–f show closeups of all four distributions $p_{c,i}^{\text{pop}}(x,y)$, and include the original selections. The ellipse for control point c is centered at $(\bar{x}_{c,i}^{\text{pop}}, \bar{y}_{c,i}^{\text{pop}})$. The direction of the semi-major axis of the ellipse is specified by $X_{c,i}^{\text{pop}}$, and the length of the semi-major axis is two times $\sigma_{Xc,i}^{\text{pop}}$. The length of the semi-minor axis ($Y_{c,i}^{\text{pop}}$) is two times $\sigma_{Yc,i}^{\text{pop}}$. Hence, the ellipse includes 95% of the samples along each axis.

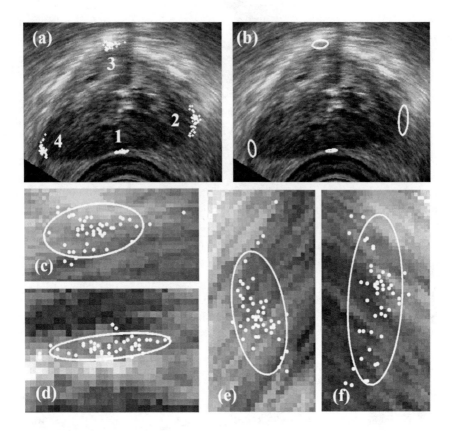

Figure 7. Construction of population distributions $p_{c,i}^{\text{pop}}(x, y)$. Shown are (a) all 50 selections per control point made by five users on 10 different occasions; (b) ellipses enclosing 95% of selections along the principal axes of distributions $p_{c,i}^{\text{pop}}(x, y)$ that are fitted to samples in (b); closeup views of selections for control points (c) 3, (d) 1, (e) 4, and (f) 2 along with ellipses enclosing the corresponding $p_{c,i}^{\text{pop}}(x, y)$ are also shown. Reprinted with permission from the AAPM.

Figure 8 shows sample outputs of the third step, the formation of the individual distributions $p_{u,c,i}^{\text{ind}}(x, y)$ describing how user u selects control point c in TRUS prostate image i. The four panels show closeup views of the spatial extent of the individual distributions as well as the 10 selections made for control point 1 by: (a) user 1 and (b) user 2 for the image in Figure 7a, and for control point 2 for: (c) user 1 and (d) user 2. In total, there are five individual distributions for each control point in an image because $U = 5$ users constructed the distributions. Each distribution has slightly different centers, variances, and principal axes.

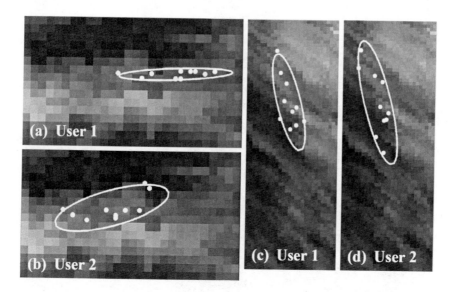

Figure 8. Sample individual selections and distributions $p_{u,c,i}^{\text{ind}}(x,y)$ for 2 control points in Figure 1a. (a) Control point 1, user 1; (b) control point 1, user 2; (3) control point 2, user 1; (4) control point 2, user 2. Each user made 10 selections of the control point for the same image as in Figure 1a. The ellipses enclose 95% of samples along the principal axes of $p_{u,c,i}^{\text{ind}}(x,y)$. Reprinted with permission from the AAPM.

The output of the fourth and last step is the four distributions $p_{c,i}^{\text{VO}}(x,y)$ that comprise the virtual operator VO_i for image i, as shown in Figure 9a for the image of Figure 7a, with closeups for control points 1 and 2 shown in parts (b) and (c). For each control point, the smaller ellipse indicates the spatial extent of $p_{c,i}^{\text{VO}}(x,y)$, whereas the larger ellipse encompassing it depicts $p_{c,i}^{\text{pop}}(x,y)$. By design, both ellipses have the same centers and axes. However, the extent of $p_{c,i}^{\text{VO}}(x,y)$ is smaller than the extent of $p_{c,i}^{\text{pop}}(x,y)$ because $p_{c,i}^{\text{VO}}(x,y)$ describes how a single average user selects control point c, whereas $p_{c,i}^{\text{pop}}(x,y)$ describes how all users select the same control point. This shows that the population of users would have more variability in their selections than would a single average user.

The ellipses representing all of the various distributions generally exhibit lower variance in the direction perpendicular to the edge, and higher variance in the direction tangential to the edge. This is reflected by the narrower width of the ellipses in the direction perpendicular to the edge. In this direction, the sharp transition in gray levels at the edge provides a clue to the user as to where to select the control point; however, there is no such clue in the tangential direction, resulting in increased variance. The variance in both directions is also higher for control points 2 and 4 than it is for control points 1 and 3. As noted in Section 2.4.2

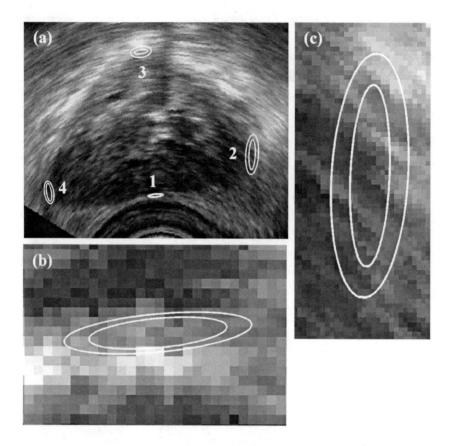

Figure 9. (a) Population, $p_{c,i}^{\text{POP}}(x, y)$, and virtual operator, $p_{c,i}^{\text{VO}}(x, y)$, distributions for the image shown in Figure 1. The larger ellipses represent the spatial extent of $p_{c,i}^{\text{POP}}(x, y)$, whereas the smaller ones represent $p_{c,i}^{\text{VO}}(x, y)$. (b) Closeup of control point 1. (c) Closeup view of control point 2. Reprinted with permission from the AAPM.

above, in these two areas the ultrasound reflection from the prostate boundary is weak, resulting in low boundary contrast and variable selection of the location of the prostate boundary.

3.4. Example Application of Virtual Operators

We have used virtual operators to evaluate the sensitivity of our algorithms to the choice of parameters and also to optimize the choice of their values [38]. In this section, we present an example of evaluating the sensitivity of our segmentation algorithm to the parameter σ in Eq. (3a).

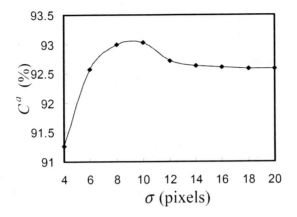

Figure 10. C_i^a computed for values of σ from 4 pixels to 20 pixels for the image in Figure 7a: $w^{\text{int}} = 0.25$ and $w^{\text{img}} = 0.75$. Reprinted with permission from the AAPM.

To evaluate the algorithm, we created a "gold standard" outline with which to compare algorithm-segmented outlines. The five trained operators who assisted in the construction of the virtual operators each manually outlined all 15 TRUS prostate images in one session. Each session was repeated 10 times, so there was a total of 50 manual outlines for each image. Again, the sessions were separated by 3 days each, and the images were presented in random order at each session in order to minimize the effects of memory. All 50 manual outlines were averaged together to form the "gold standard" prostate boundary outline.

We applied our DDC-based segmentation algorithm to all 15 images 100 times each for each value of $\sigma = 4, 6, 8, \ldots, 20$. For each value of σ, virtual operator VO_i was used to initialize our algorithm on image i. The 100 algorithm-segmented outlines for a specific image and a specific value of σ were then averaged, and the average algorithm outline was compared to the "gold standard" outline corresponding to that image. For purposes of illustrating the sensitivity of algorithm-generated outlines to variations in the choice of the parameter values, we computed the area-based accuracy metric, C_a, defined by Eq. (8c) for each image and for each value of σ.

Figure 10 shows C_a plotted against σ for the TRUS prostate image shown in Figure 7a. In this case, C_a is greater than 91% for all values of σ, and has a peak for σ between 8 and 10. For several of the other images, C_a peaked at about the same σ values. Yet, in others, C_a generally decreased with increasing σ, but in these cases, C_a was generally higher than 90%. We have utilized plots of C_a versus σ, and w^{int} versus σ, to optimize the performance of our algorithm and reported the results in [38].

For the optimization example discussed above, each of the 15 images was segmented 100 times for a particular value of σ. This would require anywhere from 3.3 to 10 hours if done manually by a user. The time requirement to segment many images many times is prohibitive if virtual operators are not available. Although the construction of each virtual operator requires some investment of time, the virtual operator can then be applied as many times as needed without the need for the user to be present.

4. 3D SEGMENTATION

In many therapy and surgery applications such as prostate brachytherapy and cryosurgery, the 2D segmentation techniques described in Section 2 are inadequate, as they do not provide the required 3D description of the prostate. To obtain the 3D information, such as the volume or the 3D boundary of the prostate, a 3D prostate segmentation method must be used. 3D prostate segmentation methods can be categorized into two classes: propagation of a 2D slice based-segmentation to 3D, and direct 3D segmentation. In Section 3.1, a 2D slice-based 3D prostate segmentation method is described [41, 42]. In order to overcome the potential segmentation error accumulation problem observed in the 2D slice-based 3D segmentation method, a modified slice-based 3D segmentation method using continuity constraint implemented with an AR model is described in Section 3.2. In Section 3.3, a direct 3D prostate segmentation method using an ellipsoid deformable model is described [43].

4.1. Slice-Based 3D Prostate Segmentation

The basic idea of 2D slice-based 3D prostate segmentation method is to solve the 3D prostate segmentation problem by re-slicing the 3D prostate image into a series of uniformly spaced contiguous 2D images and segment the prostate in these 2D images. Differentiating from the 2D prostate segmentation method that requires manual initiating the initial contour of the prostate in each 2D image, the slice-based 3D segmentation method only requires initialization of one contour in an initial slice, then, iteratively propagating the refined contour to its adjacent slice and deforming it to the boundary of the prostate. The procedure is repeated until all slices are segmented. After the segmentation of all re-sliced 2D images is obtained, a 3D surface mesh of the prostate is reconstructed from the contours in all 2D slices. The details of the slice-based 3D prostate segmentation method is described in the following steps:

Step 1: Re-slicing. First we re-slice the 3D US image of the prostate into a series of slices using one of two possible methods [41]. In the first — called parallel re-slicing — the prostate is cut into a series of parallel slices with a uniform spatial interval, usually in the transverse plane (Figure 11a).

Using the parallel re-slicing, a good segmentation in the slices close to the middle of the prostate is possible. But when the slice is nearly tangential to the boundary of prostate, i.e., at the ends of the prostate, only a small portion of the prostate appears in the image and the segmentation is more difficult (see Figure 12). Considering that the prostate is approximately ellipsoidal shaped, an alternative re-slicing technique — called rotationally re-slicing — is superior. In this method, the 3D US image of the prostate is re-sliced rotationally about an axis approximately through the center of the prostate into N rotational slices separated by π/N (Figure 11b). Hence, the prostate shapes and sizes in the re-sliced 2D images are similar (see Figure 13).

Step 2: Initialization. The contour initialization in the initial slice requires the operator to select four points on the prostate boundary as described in Section 2. The 4-point-based model generates useful prostate initialization models for simple prostate shapes but not for complex abnormally shaped prostates. In order to represent an abnormal prostate more accurately, an alternative model based on cardinal-spline interpolation can be used [42]. Using this model, a number of initial points (usually 3–8 depending on the complexity and contrast of the prostate) are chosen on the prostate boundary to obtain an initial contour.

Step 3: Refinement in 2D image. Refinement of the prostate contour is performed using the DDC method described in Section 2. If the refined contour in the initial slice is far from the "true" boundary of the prostate, it may be edited by adding or moving its vertices. Then, the edited contour is refined again as the initial contour. The procedure is repeated until the final refined contour matches the prostate boundary.

Step 4: Propagation to three dimensions. The refined contour in the initial slice can be propagated to its adjacent slice and used as a good initial approximation of the prostate contour in the distance between the two slices is small. For the rotational re-slicing method, the distance between slices increases with the distance to the rotational axis. In order to decrease the spatial interval located at the boundary of the prostate, a small angular step has to be used in the rotationally re-slicing, which can be typically $2r$ [42]. Thus, for a large prostate with a 40-mm diameter, the largest spatial interval at the prostate boundary in rotational re-slicing is about 0.7 mm, which is the approximate resolution of the US images and is less than the parallel re-slicing spacing of 1.0 mm used in [41].

Step 5: 3D reconstruction. Steps 3 and 4 are repeated until all the prostate boundaries in the 2D slices have been segmented. The 3D prostate boundary surface can then be reconstructed by interpolation of the contours obtained in the 2D segmentations of all the 2D slices.

348   AARON FENSTER et al.

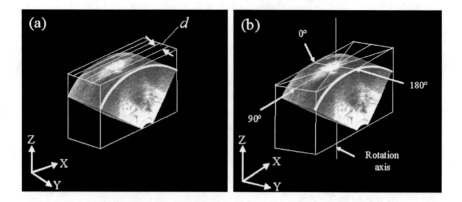

Figure 11. Two different re-slicing methods: (a) parallel re-slicing along the y-axis with spatial spacing (d); (2) rotationally re-slicing along the z-axis with uniform angular spacing. Reprinted with permission from the AAPM.

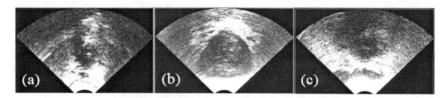

Figure 12. Three different slices in parallel re-slicing: (a) at the front end of the prostate; (b) in the middle of the prostate; (b) at the back end of the prostate. Reprinted with permission from the AAPM.

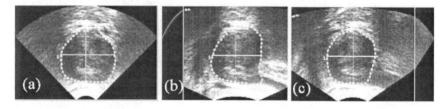

Figure 13. Three different slices in rotationally re-slicing of the same prostate: (a) slice at $0°$; (b) slice at $45°$; (b) slice at $90°$. The dotted contour is the prostate boundary outlined by the operator. Reprinted with permission from the AAPM.

4.1.1. Evaluation of the slice-based 3D segmentation method

In order to demonstrate the feasibility of the slice-based 3D prostate segmentation method, the segmentation experiments have been conducted using the 3D transrectal ultrasound (TRUS) images of six patients scheduled for prostate brachytherapy (see Figure 14). The 3D US images were acquired with a 3D

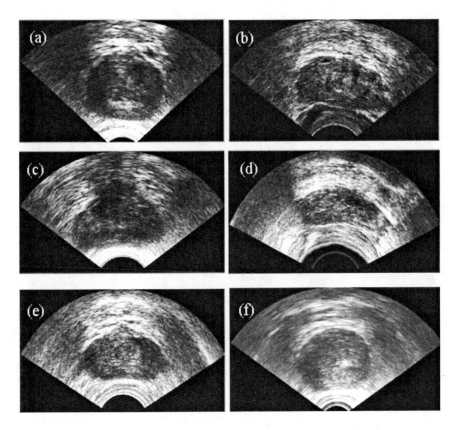

Figure 14. Initial segmentation slices of six different 3D TRUS prostate images obtained from different patients. (a) This 3D TRUS image was used to determine the classification criterion for selection of the vertex on the clockwise or anti-clockwise contours. (b–f) These 3D TRUS images were used to evaluate the segmentation algorithms. Reprinted with permission from the AAPM. See attached CD for color version.

US imaging system developed in our laboratory, using a tilt scanning mechanism [24, 35, 36]. This system is used in both 3D US guided cryosurgery and brachytherapy, as well as in the development of our 3D US guided breast biopsy system [22, 44]. We used an Aloka 2000 ultrasound machine (Aloka, CN) with a biplane side-firing transrectal ultrasound (TRUS) transducer, mounted in a motorized scanning mechanism [22, 24, 35, 36]. The transducer was rotated about its axis tilted through a total scanning angle of about $120°$ while a series of 120 conventional 2D B-mode images were acquired with an 8-bit video frame grabber operating at 15 fps. For each scan, the acquired 2D images were reconstructed into a 3D image with the z-axis oriented parallel to the transducer axis [24, 35].

Each 3D image contained $294 \times 184 \times 176$ voxels of approximate size $0.34 \times 0.34 \times 0.31$ mm.

4.1.2. Evaluation of slice-based segmentation

In evaluation of the accuracy of the slice-based segmentation method, the manual volume estimates generated by the parallel re-slicing method, V_{mp}, and by the rotational re-slicing method, V_{mr}, were used as the "true" volume estimates. Thus, the percentage error E_k in the volume estimate V_k is given by

$$E_k = \left(\frac{V_k}{V_{mk}} - 1 \right) \times 100\%, \qquad k = p, r. \tag{9}$$

While both methods can produce useful prostate volume estimates, it is instructive to examine which is better for prostate segmentation. This can be examined by investigating the accuracy and precision of the parallel segmentation method relative to manual planimetry by calculating the mean and standard deviation of the parallel error E_p, given by Eq. (10). Similarly, the mean and standard deviations for the rotational error E_r can also be calculated. The systematic "error" E_{rp} resulting with the use of the rotational segmentation method rather than the parallel segmentation method is then given by

$$E_{rp} = \left(\frac{V_{mr}}{V_{mp}} - 1 \right) \times 100\%. \tag{10}$$

Table 2. Summary of Prostate Volume Errors and Editing Rate for Parallel and Rotational Segmentation Algorithms (mean $\pm$ standard deviation).

Segmentation Method	Volume error	Volume |error|	Editing rate
Parallel	-5.42±4.43%	6.49±2.07%	19.7±5.4%
Rotational	-1.74±3.51%	3.13±2.06%	14.4±5.4%

Errors in the volume estimates are measured relative to manual planimetry, done in the same geometry as the corresponding segmentation method. Reprinted with permission from the AAPM.

4.1.3. Evaluation results of slice-based segmentation

A comparison of the volume error and editing rate for the parallel and rotationally re-slicing segmentation methods are listed in Table 2. This table shows that the average volume error of the parallel re-slicing method is 5.4% of the volume, and it is 1.7% for the rotationally re-slicing method. The average editing rate of the parallel re-slicing is about 20%, and 14% for the rotationally re-slicing method. The variability in volume error and editing rate of the two methods is almost the same. This demonstrates that the rotational re-slicing method is superior to the parallel re-slicing method, and that accurate and reproducible results can be obtained.

4.1.4. Segmentation time

Both segmentation methods required a four-point initialization lasting about 3 seconds. After initialization, both algorithms were able to segment a complete prostate within about 3 seconds. Contour editing, when required, added about 6 or 7 seconds per edited slice to the procedure. This time included the time required to deform the boundary in the edited slice and to propagate the correction through the subsequent slices in the segmentation series.

4.2. Slice-Based 3D Segmentation Using an AR Model Continuity Constraint

4.2.1. Error accumulation and continuity constraint

The slice-based 3D segmentation described in Section 4.1 is efficient and can produce accurate results, but it can fail when the evolving contour approaches shadows at the prostate boundary or bright regions inside the prostate produced by intra-prostatic calcifications or implanted brachytherapy seeds. As discussed in Section 4.1, manual editing is helpful for solving the problem; however, the following problems limit the utility of the slice-based segmentation methods.

1) Because the 3D boundary evolves from sequential 2D boundaries, it is difficult to choose from which slice to start editing. In addition, manual editing increases the variability of the final segmented prostate boundary.

2) Manual editing is performed by the user, who must decide when to start editing. This adds time to the segmentation procedure and takes much longer than a method that would not require manual editing.

Figure 15 shows an example of error accumulation in the segmentation of a prostate using the rotational slice-based segmentation. In the 45th slice, the refined prostate contour matches the manually segmented boundary, as shown in Figure 15a. Then, the segmentation error increases and accumulates (Figure 13–15b), and finally reaches its maximum deviation from the manually segmented prostate boundary in the 56th slice (Figure 15c). This error accumulation can be observed at the intersection between the 2D segmented contours and the coronal plane passing through the approximate center of the prostate (with the rotational

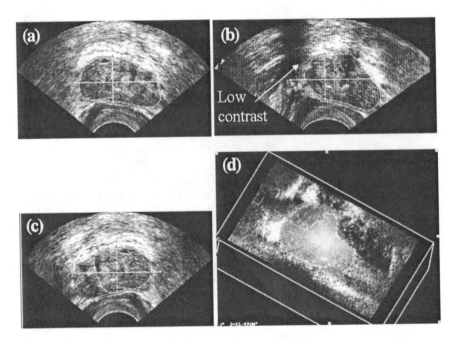

Figure 15. Illustration of error accumulation in the slice-based 3D prostate segmentation method. The 3D prostate was rotationally re-sliced into 90 slices, and their 45th, 48th, and 56th slices are shown in (a)–(c). In each slice the manual (GRAY) and automatically (WHITE) segmented contours are presented. In the center of these slices, the vertical line is the rotational axis while the horizontal line represents the coronal cross-sectional plane. (d) Coronal cross-sectional view of the manually and algorithm-segmented prostate contours. See attached CD for color version.

axis in the longitudinal direction, as shown in Figure 15a–c). In Figure 15d, each line corresponds to an intersection of the segmented prostate in a 2D slice with the coronal cross-sectional plane. The white line was generated by the slice-based rotational 3D segmentation method, and the gray line was generated using manual segmentation. The intersections of the 2D prostate boundary in 2D slice with the coronal cross-sectional plane are called the start and endpoints, respectively. Figure 15d shows that the start point in the initial slice is geometrically adjacent to the endpoint in slice $J - 1$, where J is the number of slices used in re-slicing. Thus, their distances to the origin, the intersection of the rotational axis with the coronal cross-sectional plane, should be constrained to be the same using a continuity consideration. This *continuity constraint* is satisfied in the manually segmented contour (gray contour) but not in the slice-based rotational 3D segmentation algorithm contour (white contour).

4.2.2. Slice-based segmentation using AR model-based continuity constraint

To ensure that the surface of the segmented prostate is smooth, a continuity constraint must be imposed in the contour propagation phase of the slice-based 3D segmentation procedure. In [44], we described how to apply a so-called zero-order autoregressive (AR) model to impose a continuity constraint on the start and endpoints associated with the first and last propagated 2D contours. The following is a description of the continuity constrained method used in conjunction with the slice-based 3D prostate segmentation.

Suppose that the start and endpoints are represented by $X_s(j)$ and $X_e(j)$ for slice j, $j = 0, 1, \ldots, J - 1$. $R_s(j), R_e(j)$ are the radial lengths between $X_s(j), X_e(j)$ and O, the origin of a chosen coronal cross-sectional plane. Because $R_s(j), R_e(j)$ can be calculated, a linear equation model in Eqs. (3) and (4) can be used to represent the smoothed radial length so that the computational cost for the estimation of the model parameters is minimized:

$$R'_s(j) = \beta_s(j) \cdot R_s(j) = \|X'_s(j), O\|, \tag{11}$$

$$R'_e(j) = \beta_e(j) \cdot R_e(j) = \|X'_e(j), O\|. \tag{12}$$

In Eqs. (11) and (12), $\|A, B\|$ is the Euclidean distance between A and B; $\beta_s(j)$ and $\beta_e(j)$ are the coefficients used in the estimation of $R'_s(j), R'_e(j)$. $R'_s(j), R'_e(j)$ are the radial lengths that satisfy the continuity constraint. In the following, we discuss how the coefficients $\beta_s(i)$ and $\beta_e(i)$ are used to impose bounds on the rate of change of $R'_s(j)$ and $R'_e(j)$ during the propagation phase of the segmentation.

The following two continuity constraints are imposed in the estimation of the two rates of change, $R'_s(j), R'_e(j)$:

$$R'_s(J) = R_e(0), \tag{13}$$

$$R'_e(J) = R_s(0). \tag{14}$$

Empirical experiments demonstrated that most segmentation errors occurred near the end of the propagation phase of the slice-based segmentation due to error accumulation, as shown in Figure 15(d). Thus, a continuity constraint is imposed by restricting the rate of change of both $R'_s(j)$ and $R'_e(j)$ with respect to $R'_s(J)$ and $R'_e(J)$, i.e., $R_e(0)$ and $R_s(0)$, to a maximum $\tan(\theta_{max})$ based on Eqs. (15) and (16):

$$\frac{R'_s(J) - R'_s(j)}{J - j} = \frac{R_e(0) - R'_s(j)}{J - j} \leq \tan(\theta_{max}), \quad j = 1, \ldots, J - 1, \tag{15}$$

$$\frac{R'_e(J) - R'_e(j)}{J - j} = \frac{R_s(0) - R'_e(j)}{J - j} \leq \tan(\theta_{max}), \quad j = 1, \ldots, J - 1, \tag{16}$$

where $\theta_{\max}$ is the angle of the largest slope allowed, which is used to satisfy the continuity constraint. The value of $\theta_{\max}$ is dependent on the value of J and the desired smoothness of the segmented prostate. For a smooth segmented prostate or using a large J, a small $\theta_{\max}$ should be selected, which can be determined empirically. In our experiments with $J = 90$, we used $\theta_{\max} = 15°$.

We define $E_s(j)$, $E_e(j)$ to be the square differences between estimated distances $R'_s(j)$ and $R'_e(j)$ and original distances $R_s(j)$ and $R_e(j)$:

$$E_s(j) = [\beta_s(j) - 1]^2 R_s^2(j),\qquad(17)$$

$$E_e(j) = [\beta_e(j) - 1]^2 R_e^2(j).\qquad(18)$$

It can be shown that $\beta_s(i)$ and $\beta_e(i)$ can be determined using Eqs. (19) and (20) so that Eqs. (7) and (8) are satisfied, and $E_s(i)$ and $E_e(i)$ are kept to a minimum. According to Eqs. (17) and (18), $E_s(i)$ and $E_e(i)$) attain their minimum when $\beta_s(i)$ and $\beta_e(i)$) are as close to 1 as possible:

$$\beta_s = \begin{cases} 1 & \text{if } \left|\frac{R'_s(J)-R_s(j)}{J-j}\right| \le \tan(\theta_{\max}), \\ \frac{R'_s(J)-(J-j)\cdot\tan(\theta_{\max})}{R_s(j)} & \text{if } \frac{R'_s(J)-R_s(j)}{J-j} > \tan(\theta_{\max}), \\ \frac{R'_s(J)+(J-j)}{R_s(j)} & \text{if } \frac{R'_s(J)-R_s(j)}{J-j} < \tan(\theta_{\max}), \end{cases}\qquad(19)$$

$$\beta_e = \begin{cases} 1 & \text{if } \left|\frac{R'_e(J)-R_e(j)}{J-j}\right| \le \tan(\theta_{\max}), \\ \frac{R'_e(J)-(J-j)\cdot\tan(\theta_{\max})}{R_e(j)} & \text{if } \frac{R'_e(J)-R_e(j)}{J-j} > \tan(\theta_{\max}). \\ \frac{R'_e(J)+(J-j)}{R_e(j)} & \text{if } \frac{R'_e(J)-R_e(j)}{J-j} < \tan(\theta_{\max}), \end{cases}\qquad(20)$$

The start and endpoints on the initial segmentation slice, $X_s(0)$, $X_e(0)$; the origin of the coronal cross-sectional plane, O; and the estimated start point of the segmented prostate contour in the jth slice, $X'_s(j)$, will form two adjacent triangles, $(X_s(0), O, X'_s(j))$ and $(X'_s(j), O, X_e(0))$, in the coronal cross-sectional plane (see Figure 14d). The desired coordinates of $X'_s(j)$ can be determined using the cosine rule. Similarly, the coordinate of $X'_e(j)$ can be determined from triangles $(X_e(0), O, X'_e(j))$ and $(X'_e(j), O, X_s(0))$.

After determining the start and endpoints, $X'_s(j)$, $X'_e(j)$, $j = 0, 1, \cdots, J-1$, on each slice of the re-sliced 3D prostate image, these coordinates can be inserted into the propagated contour as new vertices to obtain a new initial contour. From this contour, a new prostate boundary can be refined by deformation using the DDC model.

4.2.3. Choice of coronal cross-sectional plane

The use of the continuity constraint as described above requires selection of a coronal cross-sectional plane. While multiple planes may be selected, the use of one plane will minimize the computational cost of the procedure, ensuring that the segmentation time is short. Since the prostate is approximately ellipsoidal, the cross-sectional plane passing through the approximate center of the prostate will result in a large and smooth boundary, which is better than the cross-sectional planes near the ends of the prostate.

4.2.4. Propagation in two opposite directions

The modified slice-based 3D prostate segmentation method described above can generate a smooth prostate surface that matches the actual prostate boundary in most cases, i.e., when the segmentation errors occur near the end of the propagation. However, it is possible that segmentation errors will occur near the beginning of the propagation, usually due to the loss of prostate boundary contrast produced by shadowing from calcifications, brachytherapy seeds, or needles. To overcome this problem, the modified slice-based 3D segmentation method is repeated in the opposite propagation direction. Thus, the slices near the beginning of one propagation (e.g., the clockwise direction with respect to the coronal view) will appear near the end of the other propagation in the anti-clockwise direction.

It is important to note that the worst case will occur when segmentation errors occur at both ends of the propagations. To handle this case, the bidirectional contours can be combined, as described by Ding et al. [44], to obtain the final optimal contour.

4.2.5. Evaluation

Our slice-based 3D segmentation method using a continuity constraint implemented with an AR model has been used to segment 3D TRUS images of 15 patients' prostates obtained using the 3D TRUS system described above. Some of the 3D TRUS images are shown in Figure 15, and others can be found in [44]. Each 3D TRUS prostate image was segmented five times manually and using four slice-based segmentation algorithm methods: the original as described by Wang et al. [41] (SB), clockwise (CP), anti-clockwise (AP), and a combination of both CP and AP (OPT).

Figure 16 shows a segmentation example of the 3D TRUS prostate image shown in Figure 14b. Figure 16a shows the segmentation results in the 0th slice (i.e., the initial slice) and the three contours obtained using the CP (green), AP (blue), and OPT (purple) methods. It is evident that these contours are almost the same as the contour produced by manual segmentation red. Figure 16b shows the segmentation results in the 17th slice. In this slice, the OPT contour (purple) on the left side of the prostate is based on a selection rule described in [44] of the CP and AP contours, and the OPT contour on the right side was obtained from the AP contour alone. Figure 16c is the segmentation result in the 59th slice. The OPT contour on the right side of the prostate is based on a selection rule described in

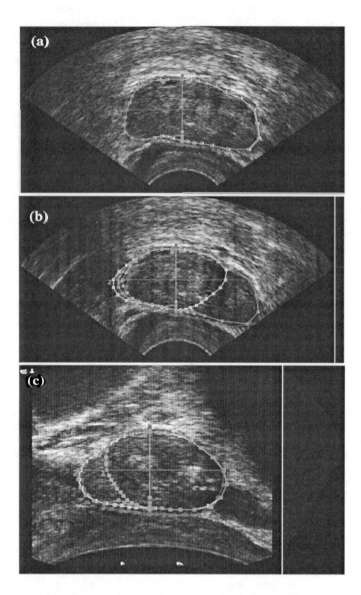

Figure 16. Optimal combination of clockwise and anti-clockwise propagated prostate contours of Figure 5b. The vertical line is the rotational axis of re-slicing and the horizontal line is the cross-sectional plane. Four contours are shown: manual (red), clockwise propagation (green), anti-clockwise propagation (blue), and optimal contour (purple). (a) 0th slice, i.e., the initial slice; (b) 17th slice, the blue contour is optimal; (c) 59th slice, green contour is optimal. See attached CD for color version.

[44] of the CP and AP contours, and the OPT contour on the left was obtained from the CP contour alone. These examples show qualitatively that our algorithm, which combines the CP and AP contours, generates a result that is closer to manual segmentation than any of the other slice-based 3D segmentation approaches.

Table 3. Prostate Volume Measurements (cm^3) Associated with Study 1 for the Manual Segmentation Method (MAN) and the Four Slice-Based Segmentation Methods

	METHOD	$\overline{V_{i1}}$	$\overline{V_{i2}}$	$\overline{V_{i3}}$	$\overline{V_{i4}}$	$\overline{V_{i5}}$	$\overline{V_i}$	$\hat{\sigma}_i^2$	$F = \frac{\hat{\sigma}_i^2}{\hat{\sigma}_1^2}$	p-value	Reject Null Hypothesis $(H_o : \sigma_i^2 = \sigma_1^2)$
	1	20.9	30.9	21.9	24.2	50.7	29.7	1.21	–	–	–
Volume	2	16.0	24.8	16.6	18.4	41.8	23.5	1.92	1.59	0.1550	No
(cm^3)	3	16.7	27.1	17.5	20.1	42.8	24.6	2.52	2.08	0.0545	No
	4	15.4	22.9	13.0	18.6	39.0	21.8	5.19	4.29	0.0010	Yes
	5	19.3	29.0	18.5	21.7	46.6	27.0	1.21	1.00	0.5000	No

SB = slice-based segmentation method described by Wang et al. [41];
CP = clockwise propagating; AP = anti-clockwise propagating;
OPT = optimal AR model-based segmentation, which are labeled respectively from methods 1 to 5.
The prostates depicted in Figure 14a–f are labeled prostates 1 to 5, respectively. For each segmentation method i and prostate j, segmentation was performed five times and the volume computed. $\overline{V_{ij}}$ was computed by taking the mean for the five repeated volume measurements. The average volume associated with each segmentation method i, $\overline{V_i}$, was computed by averaging the mean volume $\overline{V_{ij}}$ associated with prostates 1 to 5. Using the one-way ANOVA model, the variance of the volume measurement for each segmentation method i, $\hat{\sigma}_i^2$, was computed and tabulated. The F-test was used to compare the estimated variance associated with each algorithm and manual segmentation. The p-value, the probability that the two population variances are the same while the ratio of two estimated variances are greater than the computed f-value associated with each comparison set, was also tabulated.

Table 3 lists the mean volume measurements of the prostates, with the MAN, SB, CP, AP, and OPT segmentation methods labeled $i = 1$ to 5 respectively. For each segmentation method i, the average volume $\overline{V_i}$ and its associated variance, $\hat{\sigma}_i^2$, wwere calculated from the multiple segmentations. By computing the ratio between the variances associated with the algorithm segmentation methods, $\hat{\sigma}_i^2$, and the variance associated with the manual segmentation method, $\hat{\sigma}_1^2$, and using the F-test, we found, with a 95% confidence interval, that the variance of the AP method, σ_4^2, is higher than that with the MAN method, whereas the variances associated with the other three algorithm segmentation methods are not statistically different from the manual method. Using a one-way ANOVA, we have also calculated the p-value: the probability that the two population variances are the same while the F-statistics were greater than the computed f-value. From the tabulated p-value, it is apparent that the null hypothesis $H_o : \sigma_3^2 = \sigma_1^2$ is unlikely to be true (p-value $= 0.0545$), although we are not able to reject the hypothesis with 95% confidence.

Prostate segmentation from 3D TRUS images is a critical step in planning prostate intervention procedures such as brachytherapy. The slice-based 3D prostate segmentation method is fast, and therefore suitable for clinical application. However, this method requires manual editing of the boundary when the image contrast is poor or in the presence of intra-prostatic calcification artifact. To solve this problem, we developed a modified slice-based prostate segmentation method based on the continuity constraint implemented as a zero-order AR model. This modified slice-based segmentation method propagates in the clockwise and anticlockwise directions, and the resulting segmented contours are combined. The continuity constrained slice-based 3D prostate segmentation method can be used in other applications when segmentation of ellipsoidal objects are required. Possible applications are solid tumors, the kidney, and heart chambers. Statistical analysis of the results obtained using volume- and distance-based metrics verified that an optimal segmentation can be achieved by combining the clockwise and anti-clockwise contours. This results with this approach are closer to manual segmentation than with any other slice-based segmentation method, and with low local variability compared to the other algorithms we studied in this chapter, and with lower inter-observer variability for manual segmentation than that described by Tong et al. [37].

4.3. Direct 3D Segmentation

4.3.1. Algorithm

An alternative to the slice-based DDC segmentation methods is to find the surface of the prostate directly from a 3D TRUS image using a 3D deformable model [45]. The direct 3D segmentation algorithm we developed is based on a deformable model that is represented by a mesh of triangles connected at their vertices [46,47]. The direct 3D segmentation algorithm is an extension of our 2D algorithm presented in Section 2, and involves three major steps: (1) initialization of the 3D mesh; (2) automatic deformation toward the prostate surface; and (3) interactive editing if required.

The user selects six control points in the 3D TRUS image in order to initialize the mesh: four points in an approximate mid-gland transverse 2D slice, as in our 2D segmentation algorithm, one point at the prostate apex, and one point at the base. A sample 3D TRUS image with user-selected control points is shown in Figure 17a. An ellipsoid is estimated from the control points, and has center (x_0, y_0, z_0) and semi-major axes with lengths a, b, and c in the x, y, and z directions, respectively; this assumes that the length, width, and height of the prostate are approximately

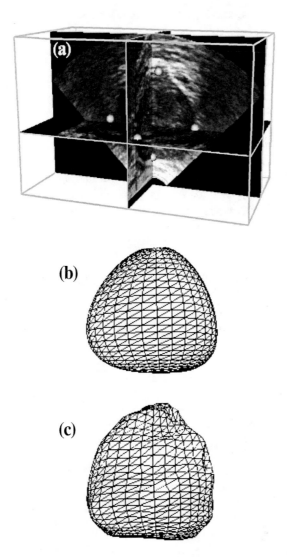

Figure 17. Illustration of steps in the operation of the 3D deformable model based segmentation algorithm: (a) 3D TRUS image with 5 of the 6 user-selected control points shown as white spheres; (b) initial mesh; (c) deformed mesh. Reprinted with permission from the AAPM.

oriented along the x, y, and z axes of the 3D image. The value of x_0 is the average of the x coordinates of the two control points with extreme x values. Similarly, y_0 and z_0 are estimated by averaging the two control points with extreme y and z

values, respectively. The semi-major axes (a, b, and c) are set to halve the distance between the two control points with extreme x, y, and z values, respectively. The resulting ellipsoid generally does not pass through the six control points, nor does it follow the prostate boundary well. To obtain a better initialization, the ellipsoid is warped using a thin-plate spline transformation, so the six ends of the semi-major axes of the ellipsoid map into the corresponding control points. Figure 17b shows the initial mesh for the 3D prostate image shown in Figure 17a.

The deformation of the mesh is described by Eqs. (1) and (2); however, for the 3D case, the position vector of each vertex has three components, as opposed to two in the 2D case, i.e., $\vec{p}_i = (x_i, y_i, z_i)^T$, instead of $\vec{p}_i = (x_i, y_i)^T$. Similarly, velocity, acceleration, and force vectors all have three components as well.

As in the 2D case, image forces in the 3D case drive vertices toward closest edges and are described by Eq. (3). The values of energy E and image forces $\vec{f}_i^{\,\mathrm{img}}$ are calculated at 3D voxel coordinates (x, y, z). The forces are sampled using trilinear interpolation to obtain their values, $\vec{f}_i^{\,\mathrm{img}}$, at vertex i. In order to prevent bunching of vertices during deformation, only the component of $\vec{f}_i^{\,\mathrm{img}}$ that is locally normal to the surface is applied.

The internal force, $\vec{f}_i^{\,\mathrm{int}}$, at each vertex i keeps the model smooth in the presence of noise and is simulated by treating each edge of the model as a spring. It is defined by

$$\vec{f}_i^{\,\mathrm{int}} = -\frac{1}{M} \sum_{j=1}^{M} \frac{\hat{e}_{ij}}{\|\hat{e}_{ij}\|}, \tag{21}$$

where $\hat{e}_{ij} = \hat{p}_i - \hat{p}_j$ is a vector representing the edge connecting vertex i with coordinate $\vec{p}_i$ to an adjacent vertex j with coordinate $\vec{p}_j$, and M is the number of edges connected to vertex i. Again, only the normal component of $\vec{f}_i^{\,\mathrm{int}}$ is applied at each vertex.

The damping force is again defined by Eq. (5). The values for w_i^{img}, w_i^{int}, and w_i^d were set at 1.0, 0.2, and –0.5, respectively, for each vertex. The initial mesh of Figure 17b is again shown in Figure 17c after deformation.

We have also developed 3D interactive editing tools, similar to tools used in the 2D prostate segmentation approach, to allow the user to edit the mesh in 3D. Specifically, the user can drag vertices to desired locations and optionally clamp them and re-deform the mesh. To keep the mesh smooth when a vertex is dragged, vertices within a sphere of a user-defined radius centered at the displaced vertex are automatically deformed using the thin-plate spline transformation. A larger radius has the effect of applying this smoothing to more neighboring vertices.

4.3.2. Algorithm evaluation

The algorithm was tested with six 3D TRUS images acquired from patients who were candidates for prostate brachytherapy. The surface of each prostate was outlined from the 3D images by a trained technician who is a representative of typical users in a radiation oncology department. Each 3D image was re-sliced into a set of 2D transverse slices along the length of the prostate, and each slice was manually outlined. The resulting 2D stack of contours for each prostate was then tessellated into a 3D meshed surface using the NUAGES program [48] generating the "gold standard" prostate boundary mesh. On a separate occasion, the same technician used the direct 3D segmentation algorithm to segment the prostate in each 3D TRUS image.

To compare the manual- ("gold standard") and algorithm-segmented 3D surfaces, the signed distance d_j was computed between corresponding points on the two meshes for each prostate. The distance d_j provides a local measure of the agreement between the two meshes. >From d_j, the global metrics MD_k, MAD_k, and $MAXD_k$ were computed using a modification of Eqs. 7a–c so that the summation for image k occurs over all vertices ($j = 1, 2, \ldots, N$) rather than specific angles, i.e.,

$$MD_k = \frac{1}{N} \sum_{j=1}^{N} d_j, \tag{22a}$$

$$MAD_k = \frac{1}{N} \sum_{j=1}^{N} |d_j|, \tag{22b}$$

$$MAXD_k = \max |d_j|. \tag{22c}$$

We also calculated the percent difference in prostate volume, $\Delta V_k\%$, computed from the manually "gold standard" segmented surface ($V_{m,k}$) and that computed from the algorithm-segmented surface ($V_{a,k}$) for the prostate image k ($k = 1, 2, \ldots, 6$):

$$\Delta V_k\% = \frac{V_{m,k} - V_{a,k}}{V_{m,k}} \times 100. \tag{23}$$

The algorithm requires a user to initialize it, and this gives rise to variability in the segmented boundaries because of potential variability in the choice of control points. To quantify this variability, one 3D image was segmented 10 times by the same technician using both manual and semiautomatic segmentation techniques. The local standard deviation of the position of each vertex in the set of 10 manually segmented meshes was computed at each vertex in the average manually segmented mesh. Similarly, the local standard deviation for the set of 10 algorithm-segmented meshes was computed at each vertex in the average algorithm-segmented mesh.

4.3.3. Results and discussion

The algorithm and manually segmented meshes for a typical 3D TRUS image are plotted in Figure 18. Figure 18a shows the algorithm-segmented mesh embedded in the 3D TRUS image, with (b) transverse, (c) coronal, and (d) sagittal

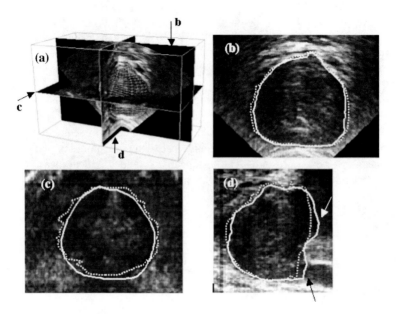

Figure 18. Cross-sections through the image in Figure 17 along with the algorithm segmentation (solid line) and manual segmentation (dotted line). (a) 3D TRUS image of the prostate with transverse, coronal, and sagittal cutting planes indicated by (b–d), respectively, to show 2D cross-sectional images. (b) Transverse cross-section of the image and the boundaries corresponding to the plane shown in (a). (c) Coronal cross-section of the image and the boundaries. (d) Sagital cross-section of the image and boundaries. Reprinted with permission from the AAPM.

cutting planes to show 2D cross-sectional images. Figures 18b–d show the same 2D cross-sections, respectively, with cross-sectional contours through the manually and algorithm-segmented meshes superimposed. The manual and algorithm contours are similar and follow the prostate boundary well in regions where the contrast is high. In regions of low ultrasound image signal and ultrasound image shadowing, the prostate boundary is difficult to discern in the images, and the manual and algorithm-segmented contours differ from each other. This is particularly apparent in regions near the bladder (indicated by the white arrow) and the seminal vesicle (indicated by the black arrow), as shown in Figure 18d.

The complete direct 3D semiautomatic DDC-based segmentation procedure required less than a minute to segment a prostate in a 3D TRUS image on a Pentium III 400 MHz personal computer. Of this total time, approximately 5–6 sec were required to initialize the algorithm, and 20 sec were taken up by the deformation algorithm. Editing was required for only one 3D image, and took approximately 30 sec. In contrast, 1 to 1.5 hours were required to segment a single 3D TRUS image manually.

Table 4. Comparison Between Manual and Algorithm Segmentation for the Six Prostates (Permission granted by the AAPM)

Prostate k	Volume (cm^3)		$\Delta V_k\%$	MD_k (mm)	MAD_k (mm)	$MAXD_k$ (mm)
	Manual $V_{m,k}$	Algorithm $V_{a,k}$				
1	36.93	33.63	8.95	-0.45	1.16	8.45
2	27.36	26.33	3.75	-0.10	1.03	5.69
3	22.87	20.80	9.05	-0.32	1.39	7.04
4	24.22	22.42	7.41	0.13	1.03	6.59
5	23.54	20.85	11.42	-0.48	1.33	7.58
6	21.58	21.06	2.39	-0.12	1.17	7.32
Average	26.08	24.18	7.16	-0.20	1.19	7.01
Standard Deviation	5.65	5.08	3.45	0.28	0.14	1.04

Reprinted with permission from the AAPM.

Table 4 lists the volumes calculated from the manually and algorithm-segmented boundaries for each prostate k as well as $V_k\%$. The volumes calculated from the manually segmented (i.e., "gold standard") boundaries are larger than those calculated from algorithm-segmented boundaries, and this is reflected in positive values for $V_k\%$. This table also shows the global metrics MD, MAD, and MAXD for each prostate as well as their averages and standard deviations. It is not clear whether the differences between the two methods are caused by inaccuracies in semiautomatic segmentation, or by manual segmentation, and it is not possible to resolve this in the absence of a true gold standard.

Figures 19a,b show the local standard deviation in the manually segmented meshes that were repeatedly segmented from the same 3D image by the same technician. For clarity, the local standard deviation is mapped on top of the average manually segmented mesh. Figure 19a is a view that is perpendicular to the transverse plane in the direction from the base of the prostate to the apex, and Figure 19b is a view perpendicular to the sagittal plane in the direction from the patient's right to left. Figures 19c,d show the same views as in Figures 19a,b, respectively, but for the algorithm-segmented meshes. The average standard deviation (averaged over all vertices) for the manual segmentation was 0.98 ± 0.01 mm, whereas the average standard deviation was lower for the algorithm, with a value of 0.63 ± 0.02 mm. The local variability in algorithm-segmented boundaries is lowest in regions where the prostate boundary is clearly visible. In these regions, automatic deformation can guide vertices toward the prostate boundary even when there is variability in

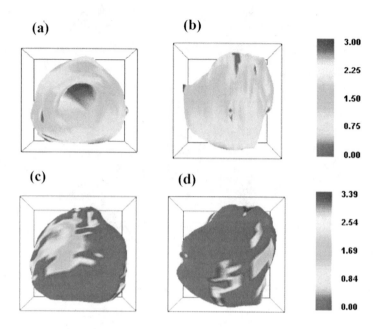

Figure 19. Local standard deviation maps: (c,d) Local standard deviation mapped on the average manually segmented boundary. (e,f) Local standard deviation mapped on the average algorithm-segmented boundary. Red regions indicate zero standard deviation and blue regions represent maximum standard deviation, which was 3.0 for manual and 3.4 mm for algorithm segmentation. The left-hand column is a view of the prostate perpendicular to the transverse plane in the direction from the base to the apex, whereas the right-hand column is a view perpendicular to the sagital plane in the direction from the patient's right to left. Reprinted with permission from the AAPM. See attached CD for color version.

the initialization and in editing. In areas where the prostate boundary is weaker or there is complete signal dropout (shadowing), the variability is increased for both segmentation approaches because the user must decide where to place vertices.

5. SUMMARY AND DISCUSSION

Advances in medical imaging over the past decade allow real-time or fast 3D acquisition, real-time reconstruction, and 3D visualization with real-time image manipulation, as well as the availability of commercial 3D US systems that have been shown to be clinically useful by allowing users to focus on demonstrating clinical utility in a variety of diagnostic and therapeutic applications. Advanced visualization and measurement tools are allowing the examination of complex anatomical structures and accurate measurement of complex volumes. These tools have been particularly important in obstetrics, cardiology, and urology. Although 3D US has been shown to be useful and is used clinically in a variety of applications, progress is still required in various aspects of this imaging modality for it to achieve its full potential. In this chapter we have examined one application of 3D ultrasound that requires fast, accurate, precise, and robust segmentation of the prostate for use in prostate brachytherapy.

As discussed above, a DDC-based prostate segmentation tool may allow the development of an intraoperative prostate therapy technique in which all steps are carried out at one session. Some of the necessary aspects of the complete procedure have already been developed and have been reported elsewhere. A 3D US image of the prostate can be obtained quickly and a dose plan can be calculated with that image. The location of the implantation needles used to implant the radioactive seeds can be accurately localized in 3D and can be verified using fast 3D US imaging tools. However, for the procedure to be effective and accurate, fast segmentation of the prostate is required for all aspects of the procedure, including dose planning prior to radioactive seed implantation, re-planning during the procedure due to changes in the prostate, and post-implantation dose calculation to determine if any regions of the prostate are underdosed. The DDC-based segmentation tool described in this chapter has been demonstrated to be an excellent candidate to achieve these goals. We have shown that the segmentation in 3D can be achieved within seconds, and the results are accurate and precise. Nontheless, some improvements are still necessary to make this approach better.

DDC-based segmentation requires good initialization of the prostate to converge to the desired boundary. We described a method of initialization requiring the user to input four or more initialization points. However, to minimize the workload on the user, interactive initialization should require minimal input or perhaps no input at all. Most prostate shapes are approximately ellipsoidal; however, deviations from a simple shape exist, especially in diseased prostates. To handle these difficult cases, our approach has been to provide the user with boundary editing capabilities for interactive editing of the boundary. However, manual editing may result in inaccuracy and variability and can be time consuming if many editing operations are required. Since the difficult cases occur often enough, it is important to develop alternate initialization approaches that require no user interactions.

Even with automated and accurate initialization, boundary editing facilities are necessary since boundary segmentation errors may occur because the prostate boundary is either missing or very weak. Although the current editing tools are effective, they require the user to employ a mouse and select the erroneous points on the computer screen for editing. This operation has been found to be difficult in a busy and sometimes crowded operating room, where the physician may have difficulty in manipulating a computer mouse to edit points a screen. Thus, improved approaches for editing would be of great benefit.

Since segmentation tools are to be used clinically, validation of the segmentation is critical. While a great deal of effort has been spent on the development of segmentation algorithms, a lesser emphasis has been placed on appropriate evaluation of segmentation algorithms. Investigators continue to develop yet more advanced and computationally complex segmentation algorithms but often fail to evaluate them using uniform or standard performance measurement metrics. As a result, finding the appropriate segmentation algorithm for a particular task as well as choosing the optimal parameters internal to the segmentation algorithm is often a problem. Thus, it is necessary to identify appropriate tools for evaluating and comparing segmentation algorithms.

In this chapter we have reported on the evaluation of our approaches using distance-, area-, and volume-based metrics to compare the performance of the DDC-based semiautomatic prostate segmentation algorithms to manual outlining. Since therapy planning often requires knowledge of the prostate volume or cross-sectional area, area-, and volume-based metrics are important. These types of metrics are easy to compare, as a single value is obtained for each segmentation of each prostate. Accuracy and variability metrics can be used as discussed above and statistical comparisons between segmentation methods can be performed. In addition, area- and volume-based metrics can also be used to optimize the choice of the DDC parameters. Examples of the use of these metrics are given in the sections above.

Distance-based metrics provide both local and global methods for comparison. Global distance-based metrics such as the MAD and MAXD averaged across the ensemble of images indicate overall agreement between the two outlining methods. Since the values of these metrics may vary locally due to ultrasound imaging artifacts, a local plot of the error supplements this global information by indicating regions where the two methods agree or disagree the most. This approach is useful to identify consistent segmentation errors where the prostate boundary may be weak or missing altogether either because of the orientation of the prostate with respect to the ultrasound beam or because of shadowing. Identification of these regions will guide the developer where improvements are necessary.

In summary, we have described a DDC-based segmentation tool to be used to segment the prostate from 3D US images. We have described a 2D method to segment cross-sectional images of the prostate and have described methods to extend this technique to 3D. In addition to the development of the algorithms, we have used evaluation metrics and statistical tests to validate the segmentation results and optimize the algorithm parameters. Based on our results, it is clear that a DDC-based segmentation approach can provide fast, accurate, precise, and robust 3D segmentations of the prostate from 3D US images and can be used for intraoperative prostate brachytherapy procedures.

6. REFERENCES

1. Silverberg E, Boring CC, Squires TS. 1990. Cancer statistics, 1990 [see comments]. *CA Cancer J Clin* **40**:9–26.

2. Abbas F, Scardino PT. 1997. The natural history of clinical prostate carcinoma [editorial; comment]. *Cancer* **80**:827–833.

3. McNeal JE, Bostwick DG, Kindrachuk RA, Redwine EA, Freiha FS, Stamey TA. 1986. Patterns of progression in prostate cancer. *Lancet* **1**:60–63.

4. Garfinkel L, Mushinski M. 1994. Cancer incidence, mortality and survival: trends in four leading sites. *Stat Bull Metrop Insur Co* **75**:19–27.

5. Terris MK, McNeal JE, Stamey TA. 1992. Estimation of prostate cancer volume by transrectal ultrasound imaging. *J Urol* **147**:855–857.

6. Guinan P, Bhatti R, Ray P. 1987. An evaluation of prostate specific antigen in prostatic cancer. *J Urol* **137**:686–689.

7. Drago JR, Badalament RA, Wientjes MG, Smith JJ, Nesbitt JA, York JP, Ashton JJ, Neff JC. 1989. Relative value of prostate-specific antigen and prostatic acid phosphatase in diagnosis and management of adenocarcinoma of prostate: Ohio State University experience. *Urology* **34**:187–192.

8. Benson MC. 1994. Prostate specific antigen [editorial comment]. *J Urol* **152**:2046–2048.

9. Waterhouse RL, Resnick MI. 1989. The use of transrectal prostatic ultrasonography in the evaluation of patients with prostatic carcinoma. *J Urol* **141**:233–239.

10. Kirby RS. 1997. Pre-treatment staging of prostate cancer: recent advances and future prospects. *Prostate Cancer Prostatic Dis* **1**:2–10.

11. Rifkin MD. 1997. *Ultrasound of the prostate: imaging in the diagnosis and therapy of prostatic disease*, 2d ed. Philadelphia: Lippincott-Raven.

12. Mettlin C, Jones GW, Murphy GP. 1993. Trends in prostate cancer care in the United States, 1974-1990: observations from the patient care evaluation studies of the American College of Surgeons Commission on Cancer. *CA Cancer J Clin* **43**:83–91.

13. Middleton RG, Thompson IM, Austenfeld MS, Cooner WH, Correa RJ, Gibbons RP, Miller HC, Oesterling JE, Resnick MI, Smalley SR. 1995. Prostate cancer clinical guidelines panel summary report on the management of clinically localized prostate cancer: The American Urological Association. *J Urol* **154**:2144–2148.

14. Shinohara K, Scardino PT, Carter SS, Wheeler TM. 1989. Pathologic basis of the sonographic appearance of the normal and malignant prostate. *Urol Clin North Am* **16**:675–691.

15. Lee F, Torp-Pedersen ST, McLeary RD. 1989. Diagnosis of prostate cancer by transrectal ultrasound. *Urol Clin North Am* **16**:663–673.

16. Pouliot J, Taschereau R, Cote C. 1999. Dosimetric aspects of permanents radioactive implants for the treatment of prostate cancer. *Phys Can* **55**:61–68.

17. Nath R, Anderson LL, Luxton G, Weaver KA, Williamson JF, Meigooni AS. 1995. Dosimetry of interstitial brachytherapy sources: recommendations of the AAPM Radiation Therapy Committee Task Group No. 43, American Association of Physicists in Medicine [published erratum appears in *Med Phys* 1996 **23**(9):1579]. *Med Phys* **22**:209–234.

18. Edmundson GK, Yan D, Martinez AA. 1995. Intraoperative optimization of needle placement and dwell times for conformal prostate brachytherapy. *Int J Radiat Oncol Biol Phys* **33**:1257–1263.

19. Downey DB, Fenster A. 1995. Three-dimensional power Doppler detection of prostate cancer [letter]. *AJR* **165**:741.

20. Onik GM, Downey DB, Fenster A. 1996. Three-dimensional sonographically monitored cryosurgery in a prostate phantom. *J Ultrasound Med* **15**:267–270.

21. Chin JL, Downey DB, Onik G, Fenster A. 1996. Three-dimensional prostate ultrasound and its application to cryosurgery. *Tech Urol* **2**:187–193.

22. Chin JL, Downey DB, Mulligan M, Fenster A. 1998. Three-dimensional transrectal ultrasound guided cryoablation for localized prostate cancer in nonsurgical candidates: a feasibility study and report of early results. *J Urol* **159**:910–914.

23. Downey DB, Fenster A. 1998. Three-dimensional ultrasound: a maturing technology. *Ultrasound Q* **14**:25–40.

24. Tong S, Downey DB, Cardinal HN, Fenster A. 1996. A three-dimensional ultrasound prostate imaging system. *Ultrasound Med Biol* **22**:735–746.

25. Liu YJ, Ng WS, Teo MY, Lim HC. 1997. Computerised prostate boundary estimation of ultrasound images using radial bas-relief method. *Med Biol Eng Comput* **35**:445–454.

26. Richard WD, Keen CG. 1996. Automated texture-based segmentation of ultrasound images of the prostate. *Comput Med Imaging Graphics* **20**:131–140.

27. Shen D, Zhan Y, Davatzikos C. 2003. Segmentation of prostate boundaries from ultrasound images using statistical shape model. *IEEE Trans Med Imaging* **22**:539–551.

28. Kwoh CK, Teo MY, Ng WS, Tan SN, Jones LM. 1998. Outlining the prostate boundary using the harmonics method. *Med Biol Eng Comput* **36**:768–771.

29. Ghanei A, Soltanian-Zadeh H, Ratkewicz A, Yin FF. 2001. A three-dimensional deformable model for segmentation of human prostate from ultrasound images. *Med Phys* **28**:2147–2153.

30. Chiu B, Freeman GH, Salama MM, Fenster A. 2004. Prostate segmentation algorithm using dyadic wavelet transform and discrete dynamic contour. *Phys Med Biol* **49**:4943–4960.

31. Ladak HM, Mao F, Wang Y, Downey DB, Steinman DA, Fenster A. 2000. Prostate boundary segmentation from 2D ultrasound images. *Med Phys* **27**:1777–1788.

32. Lobregt S, Viergever MA. 1995. A discrete dynamic contour model. *IEEE Trans Med Imaging* **14**:12–24.

33. McInerney T, Terzopoulos D. 1995. A dynamic finite element surface model for segmentation and tracking in multidimensional medical images with application to cardiac 4D image analysis. *Comput Med Imaging Graphics* **19**:69–83.

34. Fenster A, Downey DB. 1996. 3-dimensional ultrasound imaging: a review. *IEEE Eng Med Biol* **15**:41–51.

35. Fenster A, Downey DB, Cardinal HN. 2001. Topical review: three-dimensional ultrasound imaging. *Phys Med Biol* **46**:R67–99.

36. Tong S, Cardinal HN, Downey DB, Fenster A. 1998. Analysis of linear, area and volume distortion in 3D ultrasound imaging. *Ultrasound Med Biol* **24**:355–373.

37. Tong S, Cardinal HN, McLoughlin RF, Downey DB, Fenster A. 1998. Intra- and inter-observer variability and reliability of prostate volume measurement via two-dimensional and three-dimensional ultrasound imaging. *Ultrasound Med Biol* **24**:673–81.

38. Ladak HM, Wang Y, Downey DB, Fenster A. 2003. Testing and optimization of a semiautomatic prostate boundary segmentation algorithm using virtual operators. *Med Phys* **30**:1637–1647.

39. Chalana V, Kim Y. 1997. A methodology for evaluation of boundary detection algorithms on medical images. *IEEE Trans Med Imaging* **16**:642–652.

40. Oliveira LF, Simpson DM, Nadal J. 1996. Calculation of area of stabilometric signals using principal component analysis. *Physiol Meas* **17**:305–312.

41. Wang Y, Cardinal HN, Downey DB, Fenster A. 2003. Semiautomatic three-dimensional segmentation of the prostate using two-dimensional ultrasound images. *Med Phys* **30**:887–897.

42. Ding M, Chen C, Wang Y, Gyacskov I, Fenster A. 2003. Prostate segmentation in 3D US images using the Cardinal-spline based discrete dynamic contour. *Proc SPIE* **5029**:69–76.

43. Hu N, Downey D, Fenster A, Ladak H. 2003. Prostate boundary segmentation from 3D ultrasound images. *Med Phys* **30**:1648–1659.

44. Ding M, Gyacskov I, Yuan X, Drangova M, Fenster A. 2004. Slice-based prostate segmentation in 3D US images based on continuity contraint. *Proc SPIE* **5367**:151–160.

45. Hu N, Downey DB, Fenster A, Ladak HM. 2003. Prostate boundary segmentation from 3D ultrasound images. *Med Phys* **30**:1648–1659.

46. Gill JD, Ladak HM, Steinman DA, Fenster A. 2000. Accuracy and variability assessment of a semiautomatic technique for segmentation of the carotid arteries from three-dimensional ultrasound images. *Med Phys* **27**:1333–1342.

47. Chen Y, Medioni G. 1995. Description of complex objects from multiple range images using an inflating balloon model. *Comput Vision Image Understand* **61**:325–334.

48. Geiger B. 1993. *Three-dimensional modeling of human organs and its application to diagnosis and surgical planning*. Technical report No. 2105. Institut National de Rechereche en informatique et automatique, Sophia-Antipolis, France.

11

SEGMENTATION OF BRAIN MR IMAGES USING J-DIVERGENCE-BASED ACTIVE CONTOUR MODELS

Wanlin Zhu, Tianzi Jiang, and Xiaobo Li

National Laboratory of Pattern Recognition
Institute of Automation, Beijing, China

In this chapter we propose a novel variational formulation for brain MRI segmentation. The originality of our approach is on the use of J-divergence (symmetrized Kullback-Leibler divergence) to measure the dissimilarity between local and global regions. In addition, a three-phase model is proposed to perform the segmentation task. The voxel intensity value of all regions is assumed to follow Gaussian distribution. It is introduced to ensure the robustness of the algorithm when an image is corrupted by noise. J-divergence is then used to measure the "distance" between the local and global region probability density functions. The proposed method yields promising results on synthetic and real brain MR images.

1. INTRODUCTION

Image segmentation plays a major role in medical applications since segmentation results often influence further image analysis, diagnoses, and therapy. Manual delineation of brain tissues performed by an expert is time consuming and does not allow reproducibility of segmentation results. Thus, interactive semi-automatic or automated and reliable methods are desirable. However, medical images acquired from different imaging systems or machines often suffer from different artifacts, such as noise and the partial volume effect (due to imaging

Address all correspondence to: Tianzi Jiang, Department of Medical Imaging and Computing, National Laboratory of Pattern Recognition, Institute of Automation, P.O. Box 2728, Beijing 100080, PR China, Phone: +86 10 8261 4469; Fax: +86 10 6255 1993. jiangtz@nlpr.ia.ac.cn. http://www.nlpr.ia.ac.cn/jiangtz.

resolution, different tissue signals may be present in one voxel). Moreover, some anatomical structures may have different signal intensities, which is an inherent property of brain tissue [1], and increases the difficulty of accurate segmentation. To precisely extract objects from medical images, robust and efficient algorithms that are insensitive to noise and poor image contrast are required.

There are many segmentation algorithms in the literature. Some have been successfully applied in medical image analysis. Classification techniques group voxels into different subsets. The fundamental principle of such algorithms is to partition images in desired features space, under prior knowledge constraints. For brain MR images segmentation, the fuzzy C-means (FCM) algorithm [2, 1] has been successfully applied. The algorithm is fast and effective but difficult to combine with prior knowledge and is prone to be affected by outliers. The edge detection technique similarly distinguishes voxels with features (e.g., gradient) prominently different from others. In the present work, we consider active contour models that are techniques used to move the segmenting hypersurface toward the boundaries of the objects to be segmented in the image. Although they have been developing for many years, these models are still in use and are quite popular. As in [3], active contour models can be classified into two categories: one parametric and the other geometric. Parametric active contour models (e.g., snakes [4]) represent shapes explicitly in their parametric form. Thus, motion of parametric points represent evolution of the hypersurface. The models experience difficulty in handling topology changes and are hard to be implemented for 3D image applications. Another drawback is the numerical instability when two parametric points are very close. Moreover, the energy functional is dependent on the parameterization, which is counterintuitive. On the other hand, geometric active contour models can overcome these shortcomings, as they use an implicit function to represent the hypersurface. The hypersurface is embedded into a higher-dimension function. The geometric active contour models are based on the level set theory [5], which was first developed in fluid dynamics. With the long development of computational fluid dynamics, numerous numerical techniques have been proposed to solve conservation-type partial differential equations (PDEs). The evolution equation of a level set is a conservation form of the Hamilton-Jacobi equation, which can be solved using numerical techniques developed in computational fluid dynamics (CFD). The authors of [6] first applied the level set method to solve segmentation problems. In that work the level set motion equation was obtained directly by analogy with interface motion in physics. At the same time, the authors of [7, 8] independently derived a curve evolution equation represented with a level set function from a variational approach.

Many well-known segmentation methods are formulated for minimization of energy functional. Early geometric deformable models only considered edge information to move the hypersurface toward the object boundary. The segmentation results based on these models are very sensitive to noise and highly dependent on initialization. To overcome these shortcomings, region information is then introduced into variational segmentation frameworks [9, 10, 11, 12, 13]. The authors of [9] propose an energy functional that is a piecewise constant Mumford-Shah functional. This is equivalent to representing a region by its mean intensity value. A voxel is assigned to a region if its intensity is close to the region's mean intensity value. Without a curve length constraint, the method reduces to K-means clustering [14]. Another more general variational segmentation model is obtained from observed data by the Maximum Likelihood principle [11, 12, 13]. According to the assumptions that regions are independent, voxels follow identical an independent distribution in a region, and given that the prior probability is uniform, it becomes the Maximum Likelihood of observed data. In addition, edge information can be incorporated into the model. The models employed in [9, 11, 12, 13] behave very well when the noise level is not too high. However, when the image is corrupted with prominent noise, the results are not satisfactory. In [13], the authors suggest multiscale preprocessing to filter the noise and accelerate evolution of the hypersurface. This is equivalent to using a voxel's neighborhood weighted mean instead of its own intensity. This method improves the results. However, it is ineffective if regions have similar means but different variances. To solve this problem, more information should be considered, such as prior shape knowledge. However, shape prior data are not guaranteed to be easily available in all cases. Incorporation of variance information is another natural way to deal with this issue [15, 16]. The authors of [16] use average probability in the neighborhood of a voxel so that second-order statistics are considered. Besson and Barlaud [15] propose a general region-based variational segmentation framework where any information from the region and boundary can be generalized as descriptors.

In this chapter, we propose an energy functional using voxels' neighborhood information. The variational framework can be derived from the Minimum Description Length (MDL) criterion, as in [16], or as a special case of region-based segmentation using active contours [15]. The major contribution of the present work is the formulation of an energy measuring the distribution discrepancy between local and global regions in the sense of J-divergence. With the Gaussian distribution hypothesis, the proposed energy is formulated with local and global region mean and variance, respectively.

It is worth noticing that in the work of [17], where segmentation is based on region competition and implemented within a level set framework, it is deduced that the average probability distribution function (PDF) is equivalent to Kullback-Leibler (KL) divergence between the PDF of the local and global regions. Recently, [18, 19] proposed a variational segmentation framework incorporating mean and variance in the same manner as we do. However, as their application is to extract objects from natural images, the distribution of regions is assumed to be a Generalized Laplacian. We make the assumption that each region follows a Gaussian distribution. In addition, the dissimilarity between distributions in their work is KL divergence, which is a directional but not symmetric form like ours; therefore, their derived evolution equation is completely different. In this chapter we apply the proposed J-divergence-based active contour model to brain tissue segmentation for MR images. A lot of contributions [20, 21, 22, 23] have been made in this area.

The remainder of the chapter is organized as follows. In Section 2 we briefly introduce the variational segmentation model using J-divergence and derive the corresponding evolution equation. Experimental results are demonstrated in Section 3, and we conclude our work in Section 4.

2. METHODS

In this section, we first introduce the energy functional based on J-divergence, as well as its level set representation. The evolution equation coupled with the level set is then derived and numerical implementation is briefly presented.

2.1. Variational Segmentation Model

The proposed energy functional is composed of region- and edge-based energies, which are complementary during the evolution of the hypersurface, as suggested in [24, 10]. In our work, the regional energy is well suited for voxels far from the object boundary, but degenerated in the vicinity of the boundary because that local region may contain pixels sampled from more than one region. Hence, edge-based energy is needed to reduce segmentation errors.

We first introduce the definition of region homogeneity. We follow the definition from [16]: "A region R is considered to be homogeneous if its intensity values are consistent with having been generated by one of a family of prespecified probability distributions $p(I|\theta)$, where θ are the parameters of the distribution." A global region defined in this chapter is a homogeneous region. An image is made up of global regions and their boundaries. A local region is the neighborhood of a voxel, including itself. We confine our approach to the intensity image. It can be extended easily to a vector image by using a multidimensional probability distribution.

Next, let $I : \Omega \in \mathbb{R}^p \to \mathbb{R}^q$ be an input image, where Ω is an open and bounded image domain ($p = 2$ or $p = 3$) in Euclidean space, q is the dimension of the observed data. For example, $q = 1$ is an intensity image, $q = 3$ is a color image. Image I is composed of non-overlapping regions $\{R_i\}$ and their boundaries $\{\Gamma_i = \partial R_i\}$. They satisfy $R_i \cap R_j = \emptyset$ when $i \neq j$, $\bigcup_{i=1}^{m} R_i = \Omega/\Gamma$, and $\Gamma = \bigcup_{i=1}^{m} \Gamma_i = \bigcup_{i=1}^{m} \partial R_i$.

Based on the aforementioned definitions, we make the following assumptions:

1. The voxel intensity value in every global region R_i and local region that is not nearby the object boundary are homogeneous. In other words, voxel

intensity values in any region are independent and sampled from one distribution. As a consequence we can represent a region with a distribution.

2. For brain MR Images, we assume that each global region follows a Gaussian distribution. This hypothesis has been extensively used in brain tissue segmentation [25, 26]. Another reason for using this assumption is computational efficiency. Indeed, active contour evolution can be achieved solely by computation of the region mean and variance. It is efficient and very easy to implement.

3. The local region statistics are most similar to the global region to which the voxel belongs. The assumption is intuitive; however, it will be degenerated in the vicinity of the object boundary, where voxels are sampled from two different Gaussian distribution. As a result, the region information is not reliable, but the complementary edge-based information will reduce segmentation errors in this situation.

With these hypotheses, each region corresponds to one Gaussian distribution. In other words, for a voxel we use a Gaussian distribution (local region) to replace its intensity value. For a global region, it is also represented with a Gaussian distribution. Next, for the sake of measuring which region a voxel should belong to, we need to measure the difference between two probability distributions. From information theory, information divergence measures have been widely used in image segmentation [18, 19, 10]. In this chapter we choose symmetric Kullback-Leibler divergence, which is also named J-divergence:

$$D\big(p_1(x) \parallel p_2(x)\big) = \frac{1}{2} \int \Big(p_1(x) \log \frac{p_1(x)}{p_2(x)} + p_2(x) \log \frac{p_2(x)}{p_1(x)}\Big) dx, \quad (1)$$

The J-divergence is convex, and $D(p_1 \parallel p_2) \geq 0$ with $D(p_1 \parallel p_2) = 0$ if and only if p_1 and p_2 have the same value everywhere. For Gaussian probability density functions $p_1(x)$ and $p_2(x)$, the J-Divergence can be reduced to a simple form when the base is the irrational number e:

$$
\begin{aligned}
D\big(p_1(x) \parallel p_2(x)\big) &= \frac{1}{2} \int \Big(p_1(x) \ln \frac{p_1(x)}{p_2(x)} + p_2(x) \ln \frac{p_2(x)}{p_1(x)}\Big) dx \\
&= \frac{1}{2} \int p_1(x) \Big[\ln \frac{\sigma_2}{\sigma_1} + \frac{(x - \mu_2)^2}{2\sigma_2^2} - \frac{(x - \mu_1)^2}{2\sigma_1^2} \Big] dx \\
&\quad + \frac{1}{2} \int p_2(x) \Big[\ln \frac{\sigma_1}{\sigma_2} + \frac{(x - \mu_1)^2}{2\sigma_1^2} - \frac{(x - \mu_2)^2}{2\sigma_2^2} \Big] dx \\
&= \frac{\sigma_2^2 + (\mu_2 - \mu_1)^2}{4\sigma_1^2} + \frac{\sigma_1^2 + (\mu_1 - \mu_2)^2}{4\sigma_2^2} - \frac{1}{2}. \quad (2)
\end{aligned}
$$

Based on the aforementioned definition, we propose the region-based energy functional as follows:

$$E(\Gamma, \theta) = \sum_{i=1}^{n} \left[\int_{R_i} D(p(N(x)) \parallel p(R_i \mid \theta_i)) dx \right], \quad (3)$$

where $p(N(x))$ is the PDF of the local region around voxel $I(x)$, $p(R_i \mid \theta_i)$ is the PDF of the ith global region with statistical parameters θ_i. $D(\cdot)$ is the dissimilarity measure between two distributions. Equation (3) can be derived from Zhu's [16] united regions competing segmentation framework. From another viewpoint, it is also a special case of the Mumford-Shah functional, where the image fidelity term is replaced by the dissimilarity between the local and global regions. The region intensity smooth constraint is discarded to allow strong noise to be present. Intuitively, the region-based energy functional is a weighted volume; when the optimal contour is obtained, each voxel has a minimum weight that measures the dissimilarity between it and the region it belongs to. Obviously, this happened only when a voxel is correctly classified with regard to a region. For the sake of simplicity and interpretation, we first consider the bipartitioning segmentation and will later extend the scheme to the multiphase case.

We use the geodesic length constraint [8] as the edge-based energy. The edge energy is equivalent to finding the minimal-length smooth curve in Riemannian space and given by

$$E(\Gamma) = \oint g(I(\Gamma)) ds, \quad (4)$$

where ds is the Euclidean arc length, and $g(\cdot)$ is the function indicating boundaries in the image. When $g(\cdot) = 1$, the geodesic length constraint reduces to a Euclidean curve smooth constraint. A very common choice of $g(\cdot)$ is:

$$g(I(\Gamma)) = \frac{1}{1 + \parallel \nabla I(\Gamma) \parallel^2}, \quad (5)$$

where $\parallel \nabla I(\Gamma) \parallel^2$ is the norm of the image intensity gradient.

2.2. Representation with a Level Set

In this study, the level set technique [5] is used because of its topological flexibility, numerical stability, and parameterization-free nature, in contrast to parametric representation. The key idea is that hypersurface representation with the implicit function provided it is Lipschitz continuous. A common choice of level set function ϕ is the signed distance function. It is defined as follows:

$$\begin{cases} \phi(\mathbf{x}) = -\mathbf{D}(\mathbf{x}, \Gamma) & \text{if } \mathbf{x} \in R^-, \text{ exterior of } \Gamma, \\ \phi(\mathbf{x}) = 0 & \text{if } \mathbf{x} \in \Gamma, \\ \phi(\mathbf{x}) = \mathbf{D}(\mathbf{x}, \Gamma) & \text{if } \mathbf{x} \in R^+, \text{ interior of } \Gamma, \end{cases} \quad (6)$$

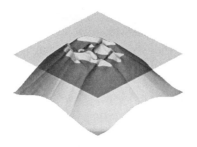
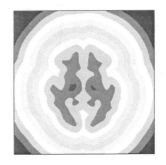

(a) Level set function in 3D   (b) Color representation of distance function

Figure 1. (a) Representation in three dimensions of the intersection of a level set with the zero plane. (b) Color contour of the level set function in (a). Colors represent the Euclidean distance. See attached CD for color version.

where $R^- \cup R^+ \cup \Gamma = \Omega$, hypersurface Γ is the zero level of ϕ, and $D(\mathbf{x}, \Gamma)$ is the Euclidean distance between $\mathbf{x}$ and Γ. The gradient of the signed distance function is $|\nabla \phi| = 1$. It is a good property that can assure numerical stability. The geometrical quantities of the hypersurface can be easily represented in terms of level set function ϕ. In this chapter we define the normal of Γ in the direction of increasing values of ϕ. Thus, the unit normal vector is

$$\mathbf{N} = \frac{\nabla \phi}{|\nabla \phi|}. \tag{7}$$

The mean curvature of the hypersurface is the divergence of the unit normal vector:

$$\kappa = div\left(\frac{\nabla \phi}{|\nabla \phi|}\right). \tag{8}$$

To represent regions and the hypersurface with a level set function, Heaviside and Dirac functions [9] are used:

$$H(z) = \begin{cases} 1 & z \geq 0 \\ 0 & z < 0 \end{cases} \qquad \delta_0(z) = \frac{dH(z)}{dz}. \tag{9}$$

2.2.1. Two-phase segmentation

For a bipartitioning problem, only one level set function is needed to represent the boundaries and regions. We denote R_1 as regions with negative values of the level set function and R_2 those with positive values of the level set function. Their interface is Γ:

$$
\begin{cases}
R_1: & \phi < 0, & 1 - H(\phi), \\
\Gamma: & \phi = 0, & |\nabla H(\phi)|, \\
R_2: & \phi > 0, & H(\phi).
\end{cases}
$$

The energy functional of Eq. (3) incorporating region and edge information is rewritten in terms of level sets as follows:

$$
\begin{aligned}
E(\phi, \theta_1, \theta_2) = & \lambda_1 \cdot \int_\Omega D_1 \cdot (1 - H(\phi)) dx + \lambda_2 \cdot \int_\Omega D_2 \cdot H(\phi) dx + \\
& \nu \cdot \int_\Omega g(|\nabla I|)|\nabla H(\phi)| dx,
\end{aligned} \tag{10}
$$

where $D_1 = D(p(N(x)) \parallel p(R_1 \mid \theta_1))$ is the J-divergence between the probability distributions of region R_1 and the local region. $D_2 = D(p(N(x)) \parallel p(R_2 \mid \theta_2))$. λ_i is the weight of the energy based in region R_i and ν is the coefficient of the geodesic length constraint.

2.2.2. Multiphase segmentation

For multiple region segmentation, we follow the method introduced in [27], where the authors present an elegant way of representing n regions with $\log_2 n$ level set functions. Their multiphase level set model has no vacuum or overlap among the phases, in contrast with other multiphase models, where one region is represented by one level set function. Using the level set representation [11], Eq. (3) can be rewritten as

$$
\begin{aligned}
E(\phi_1, \phi_2, \ldots, \phi_n) = & \sum_{i=1}^{s} \lambda_i \cdot \int_\Omega D_i \cdot G_i(\phi_1, \phi_2, \ldots, \phi_n) dx \\
& + \sum_{j=1}^{n} \nu_j \cdot \int_\Omega g(|\nabla I(\Gamma_j)|)|\nabla H(\phi_j)| dx,
\end{aligned} \tag{11}
$$

where n is the number of level set functions and s is the number of regions. They satisfy $n \leq s \leq 2^n$. G_i is the characteristic function representing the region R_i with n level set functions. They satisfy

$$
\begin{cases}
G_i(\mathbf{x}) = 1, & \text{if } \mathbf{x} \in R_i, \\
G_i(\mathbf{x}) = 0, & otherwise.
\end{cases} \tag{12}
$$

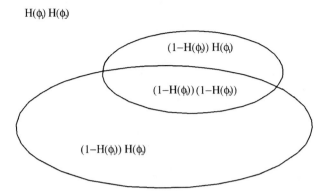

Figure 2. Four-phase level set model illustration. There are four regions in the image, using two level set functions. They can be represented by $H(\phi_1)H(\phi_2)$, $(1 - H(\phi_1))H(\phi_2)$, $H(\phi_1)(1 - H(\phi_2))$ and $(1 - H(\phi_1))(1 - H(\phi_2))$.

A four-phase representation using characteristic functions of the level set is presented in Figure 2. Here, with the Gaussian distribution assumption, the dissimilarity measure D_i can be simplified as follows:

$$D_i = \frac{\sigma_w^2 + (\mu_w - \mu_i)^2}{4\sigma_i^2} + \frac{\sigma_i^2 + (\mu_i - \mu_w)^2}{4\sigma_w^2} - \frac{1}{2}, \tag{13}$$

where σ_i is the variance of the region R_i and σ_w is the variance of a neighborhood region.

For MR image brain tissue segmentation, scalped brain MR images consist of three regions: gray matter (GM), white matter (WM), and cerebrospinal fluid (CSF). They have very complex topology and shape. In [28, 27], the authors applied a four-phase level set model to brain tissue segmentation. During the evolution of the curve, one region will reduce its size and finally disappear. However, as the intensity values of the real MR Images are not strictly composed of three regions due to the partial volume effect and inherent tissue class-related intensity variations [1], the four-region initialization may lead to erroneous results. We propose to use a three-phase level set representation, whose region definitions are as follows:

$$\begin{cases} \text{CSF:} & \phi_1 > 0, \quad \phi_2 < 0, \quad G_1 = H(\phi_1)(1 - H(\phi_2)), \\ \text{WM:} & \phi_1 < 0, \quad \phi_2 < 0, \quad G_2 = (1 - H(\phi_1))(1 - H(\phi_2)), \\ \text{GM:} & \phi_2 > 0 \qquad\qquad G_3 = H(\phi_2) \end{cases} .$$

Then the energy functional of Eq. (11) can be written as

$$
\begin{aligned}
E(\phi_1, \phi_2) \;=\; & \lambda_1 \cdot \int_\Omega D_1 \cdot H(\phi_1)(1 - H(\phi_1))dx + \lambda_2 \\
& \cdot \int_\Omega D_2 \cdot (1 - H(\phi_1))(1 - H(\phi_2))dx \\
& + \lambda_3 \cdot \int_\Omega D_3 \cdot H(\phi_2)dx + \nu_1 \cdot \int_\Omega g(|\nabla I|)|\nabla H(\phi_1)|dx \\
& + \nu_2 \cdot \int_\Omega g(|\nabla I|)|\nabla H(\phi_2)|dx,
\end{aligned}
\tag{14}
$$

where D_i is the J-divergence between a voxel's neighborhood probability distribution and the PDF of the global region $H(\phi_1)(1 - H(\phi_2))$, $(1 - H(\phi_1))(1 - H(\phi_2))$, and $H(\phi_2)$, respectively. ν_1 and ν_2 are coefficients of the smoothing constraint of two level set functions.

2.3. Gradient Flow

To minimize the energy functional, Eq. (10), a two-step algorithm is performed. First, the statistical parameters of the regions are fixed, and one calculates the Euler-Lagrange equation of the proposed energy functional with respect to the level set function. For of differentiation of Eq. (11) and numerical implementation, regularized versions of the Heaviside and Dirac functions are used. We choose the approximations introduced in [9]:

$$
\begin{aligned}
H_\varepsilon(z) \;&=\; \frac{1}{2}\left(1 + \frac{2}{\pi}\arctan(\frac{z}{\varepsilon})\right), \\
\delta_\varepsilon(z) \;&=\; \frac{\varepsilon}{\pi(\varepsilon^2 + z^2)}.
\end{aligned}
$$

Using the gradient descent flow, we obtain the following curve evolution equation:

$$
\begin{aligned}
\frac{\partial \phi}{\partial t} = \delta_\varepsilon(\phi)\Big[& \nu \cdot \left[g(|\nabla I|) \cdot div\left(\frac{\nabla \phi}{|\nabla \phi|}\right) + \nabla g(|\nabla I|) \cdot \left(\frac{\nabla \phi}{|\nabla \phi|}\right)\right] \\
& + \lambda_1 \cdot D_1 - \lambda_2 \cdot D_2 \Big].
\end{aligned}
\tag{15}
$$

The details of the calculations leading to Eq. (15) can be found in Appendix A. Second, we update the regions' statistical parameters with fixed level set functions. This is done to find the optimal parameters that minimize the energy functional with a constant ϕ. As in [29], we can update the parameters of these corresponding regions by simply evaluating their sample means and variances:

$$\mu_1 = \frac{\int_{R_1} I(\mathbf{x})d\mathbf{x}}{V_1} = \frac{\int_{\Omega} I(\mathbf{x})(1 - H_\varepsilon(\phi(\mathbf{x})))d\mathbf{x}}{\int_{\Omega}(1 - H_\varepsilon(\phi(\mathbf{x})))d\mathbf{x}}, \tag{16}$$

$$\mu_2 = \frac{\int_{R_2} I(\mathbf{x})d\mathbf{x}}{V_2} = \frac{\int_{\Omega} I(\mathbf{x})H_\varepsilon(\phi(\mathbf{x}))d\mathbf{x}}{\int_{\Omega} H_\varepsilon(\phi(\mathbf{x}))d\mathbf{x}}, \tag{17}$$

$$\sigma_1^2 = \frac{\int_{R_1}(I(\mathbf{x}) - \mu_1)^2 d\mathbf{x}}{V_1} = \frac{\int_{\Omega} I^2(\mathbf{x})(1 - H_\varepsilon(\phi(\mathbf{x})))d\mathbf{x}}{\int_{\Omega}(1 - H_\varepsilon(\phi(\mathbf{x})))d\mathbf{x}} - \mu_1^2, \tag{18}$$

$$\sigma_2^2 = \frac{\int_{R_2}(I(\mathbf{x}) - \mu_2)^2 d\mathbf{x}}{V_2} = \frac{\int_{\Omega} I^2(\mathbf{x})H_\varepsilon(\phi(\mathbf{x}))d\mathbf{x}}{\int_{\Omega} H_\varepsilon(\phi(\mathbf{x}))d\mathbf{x}} - \mu_2^2. \tag{19}$$

Finally, the curve evolution equation can be rewritten as follows:

$$\frac{\partial \phi}{\partial t} = \delta_\varepsilon(\phi)\left[\nu \cdot \left[g(|\nabla I|) \cdot div\left(\frac{\nabla \phi}{|\nabla \phi|}\right) + \nabla g(|\nabla I|) \cdot \left(\frac{\nabla \phi}{|\nabla \phi|}\right)\right]\right.$$

$$+ \frac{\sigma_1^2 + (\mu_1 - \mu_w)^2}{4\sigma_w^2} + \frac{\sigma_w^2 + (\mu_1 - \mu_w)^2}{4\sigma_1^2}$$

$$\left. - \frac{\sigma_2^2 + (\mu_2 - \mu_w)^2}{4\sigma_w^2} - \frac{\sigma_w^2 + (\mu_2 - \mu_w)^2}{4\sigma_2^2}\right], \tag{20}$$

where (μ_w, σ_w) are the local region statistical parameters. When KL divergence is used, Eq. (20) becomes Paragios's [11, 12, 13] geodesic active regions evolution equation. Moreover, setting $\sigma_1 = \sigma_2$, the geodesic active regions reduce to Tony Chan's [9] level set evolution equation. For the proposed energy functional (14), the two level set evolution equations Eq. (27)–(28) can be found in Appendix A.

2.4. Numerical Implementation

The numerical scheme we used is the finite-difference implicit scheme introduced in [9, 27]. It is unconditionally stable for any time step. Considering numerical accuracy, let the time step $\Delta t = \max(\Delta x_1, \Delta x_2, \ldots, \Delta x_m)$, that is, the time step is equivalent to the largest space step. When image intensity values vary drastically, due to the fact that the speed of active contours is dependent on the voxel intensity value, the velocity discrepancy is large, and thus the convergence rate is slow. We use normalized velocity to obtain a smooth and slowly varying velocity as follows:

$$g(z) = \frac{2}{\pi}\left(\arctan\left(\frac{z}{\theta}\right)\right) \qquad z \in \mathbb{R}, \tag{21}$$

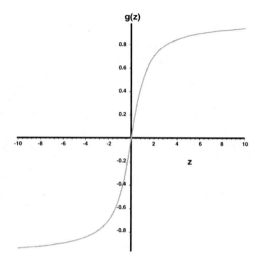

Figure 3. Normalized velocity.

where θ is a parameter to control the smoothing rate of the velocity. Figure 3 shows the profile of the function. For all numerical experiments, we choose $\theta = 1$. The signed distance function cannot be preserved during the level set evolution, and it becomes numerically unstable when the level set function becomes too flat or steep. Hence, the re-initialization step needs to be applied to keep the level set function close to a signed distance function. We implemented the method proposed in [30] to re-distance the level set during the hypersurface evolution:

$$\phi(\mathbf{x}, 0) = \phi_0,$$
$$\frac{\partial \phi}{\partial t} + sign(\phi_0)(|\nabla \phi| - 1) = 0. \tag{22}$$

However, it should be implemented carefully as it slows down the convergence rate of the active contour in a sense. Another drawback is that it may change the location of the zero level set slightly. As a result, the final level set functions should not be reinitialized.

3. EXPERIMENTAL RESULTS

In this section, segmentation experiments are conducted on both synthetic and real data to illustrate the effectiveness of our approach. Comparisons with Paragios's method ([11, 12, 13]) with synthetical data are also presented. Real data are first preprocessed by skull-stripping before applying our segmentation scheme. All experiments were run on a PC (PentiumIV 2.4 GHz, 512Mb RAM).

3.1. Synthetic Data

Three synthetic datasets are used with the same square pattern and different levels of Gaussian and salt pepper noise. We performed experiments using the two-phase model and different region information to extract the square objects from the image. The results given in Figure 4 demonstrate the stability and robustness of our algorithms. As the image regions have different mean intensity and variance, the results obtained using our method (Figure 4b) and the geodesic active regions [11, 12, 13] (Figure 4c) have similar results. When the image is corrupted by high noise and has diffuse boundary, region-based energy plays a more important role in curve evolution. When the regions have the same mean intensity and different variance, geodesic active regions seem to be prone to converge to local minima as the velocity is dependent on voxel intensity and regional statistical parameters. Opposite to this, when the proposed method applied both local mean and variance, one can reduce the risk of converging to the local minima. Figure 4e,f shows the robustness of the proposed method. We give experiments for region intensity corrupted by salt-and-pepper noise and show the results in Figure 4h,i.

3.2. Real Data

In this subsection we use two 3D real data sets to validate our approach. The first is MRI data obtained on a 1.5T GE Signa Twin Speed scanner with a 3D Spoiled Gradient-Recalled (SPGR). The imaging parameters are as follows: $TR = 11.3$ ms, $TE = 4.2$ ms, and $FlipAngle = 15°$. At first, we perform our two-phase model to delineate brain lateral ventricles from the 3D image data. In order to delineate lateral ventricles, a necessary preprocessing that manually crops the third ventricle is performed to satisfy bipartitioning condition. The local neighborhood size is $3 \times 3 \times 3$. WM and GM will be classified to the same region during surface evolution. Both 2D and 3D results are shown in Figure 5. The initialization surface is a sphere centered at the centroid of the two lateral ventricles. The gray matter and CSF nearby the cortex are discarded during preprocessing.

The second test using two-phase model are performed on DT-MRI data acquired on a 1.5T Siemens Sonata with high-speed gradients. The diffusion sensitizing gradients are applied along six non-collinear directions with a b value = 900 s/mm^2. The imaging parameters are: $TR = 8000$ ms, $TE = 106$ ms, number of excitations = 3, and voxel size is $0.9 \times 0.9 \times 4.0$ mm^3.

The Diffusion Tensor matrix is calculated according to the Stejskal and Tanner equation [31]. Our algorithm is performed on the fractional anisotropy (FA) image computed from the diffusion tensor image. In order to extract the corpus callosum using the two-phase model, we cropped the FA image around the region of interest so as to assure a bimodal condition. The initial surface is a sphere centered in the image with a radius equal to 20 voxels. Figure 6 shows the evolution process and the final result. A three-phase segmentation model is applied to brain tissue

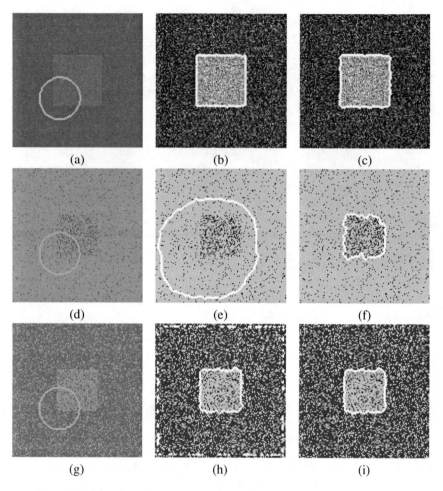

Figure 4. Segmentation of a square pattern from background. The first row shows initial-
izations for both algorithms. The second row shows the results of geodesic active regions
[11, 12, 13]. The third row shows results of the proposed algorithm. (a–c): Gaussian noise,
background mean/variance = 10/100, square mean/variance = 10/225. (d–f): Gaussian
noise, background mean/variance = 0/0.1, square mean/variance = 0/1 (the curve in (e) will
not stop and expands out of the image domain). (g–i): salt and pepper noise, background
and square mean = 1 noise density = 0.5.

segmentation for scalped brain MR images. Figure 7 shows the 3D segmentation
results. The zero level set of two level set functions are both initialized as multiple
spheres. In Figure 7a, 27 small spheres (gray) are initialized for level set function
ϕ_0, four larger (deep gray) spheres are initialized for level set function ϕ_1. Both
level set functions are updated according to Eq. (27)–(28). The final results are

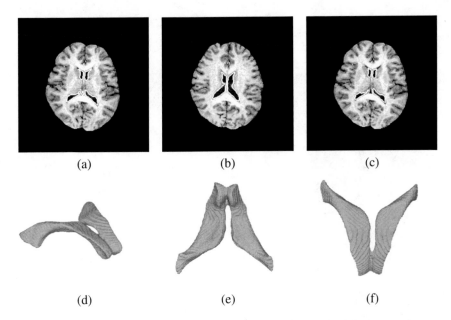

Figure 5. Segmentation of lateral ventricles from MRI brain data: (a–c) final contour in different axial slices; (d–f) segmentation results represented by a 3D surface.

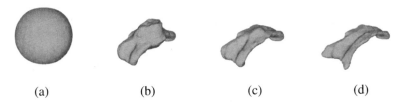

Figure 6. Segmentation of corpus callosum from 3D DTI data: (a) initial surface, a sphere; (b,c) intermediate evolution results; (d) final result.

shown for the gray matter surface (Figure 7b), the white matter surface (Figure 7c), and the cerebrospinal fluid surface (Figure 7d).

From Figures 4–7, we can see that our method can successfully delineate brain tissues and the corpus callosum from 3D real images. The two-phase model requires image preprocessing to obtain satisfying results. On the other hand, the three-phase model can obtain very good results for scalped MR images. They both demonstrate the potential of the proposed approach for medical image segmentation.

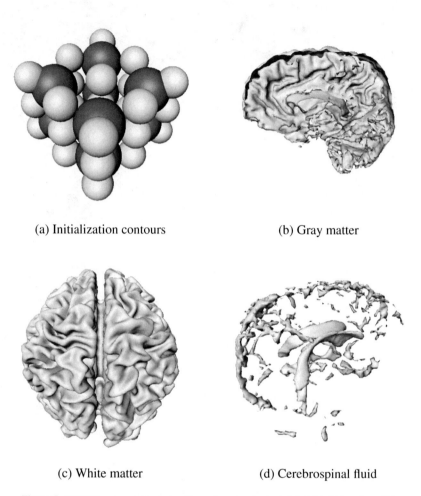

     (a) Initialization contours   (b) Gray matter

       (c) White matter   (d) Cerebrospinal fluid

Figure 7. 3D MRI segmentation using three-phase level set model: (a) initial surface; 27 small spheres are initialized for ϕ_0, 4 larger spheres are initialized for ϕ_1; (b) final GM segmentation result; (c) final WM segmentation result; (d) final CSF segmentation result.

4. CONCLUSIONS AND FUTURE RESEARCH

We proposed a variational segmentation algorithm that measures the dissimilarity between local and global regions. Region boundaries were modeled as a regular hypersurface implicitly represented by level set functions. The image regions were assumed to follow Gaussian distributions. A geodesic curve-based energy was imposed on the energy functional to reduce segmentation errors when the hypersurface is in the vicinity of the object boundary. The hypersurface evolution can be obtained by calculating the gradient flow of the proposed energy functional. In the chapter, both two-phase and multiphase methods have been investigated. In particular, for brain MR images segmentation, we performed segmentation using a three-phase level set model. We obtained a united form of the evolution equation from which we can derive geodesic active regions model when we replace J-divergence with KL-divergence. Setting the region variance to a constant gives the same evolution equation as in [9]. Besides, only mean and variance need to be calculated for the Gaussian distribution assumption. It is straightforward in terms of implementation and computing efficiency. Experimental results have been validated for the proposed algorithm.

Future work will focus on using nonparametric statistical methods instead of the Gaussian distribution hypothesis, although the latter can fulfill most of the MRI segmentation requirements. To reduce computation time, a new energy term $\int_{\Omega}(|\nabla\phi|-1)^2 d\mathbf{x}$ from [32] will be added to our proposed energy, which will force the level set close to a signed distance function and therefore completely eliminate the need for re-initialization during evolution.

5. ACKNOWLEDGMENTS

The authors wish to thank Dr. T. Bailloeul for his many valuable suggestions and comments about the chapter and pleasant discussions about the level set method.

APPENDIX A

1. DERIVATION OF LEVEL SET EVOLUTION EQUATION

We now deduce the gradient flow minimizing the functional of Eq. (11). The energy functional consists of region- and edge-based energy. To obtain the gradient flow, one can directly compute the first variation by the shape derivative introduced in [33]. Another approach is to calculate the first variation with the level set representation [9]. The proposed energy functional is as follows:

$$
\begin{aligned}
E(\phi_1, \phi_2, \ldots, \phi_n) &= \sum_{i=1}^{s} \lambda_i \cdot \int_{\Omega} D_i \cdot G_i(\phi_1, \phi_2, \ldots, \phi_n) d\mathbf{x} \\
&+ \sum_{j=1}^{n} \nu_j \cdot \int_{\Omega} g(|\nabla I(\Gamma_j)|)|\nabla H(\phi_j)| d\mathbf{x},
\end{aligned}
$$

where D_i is the J-divergence between the probability of region R_i and local region probability, n is the number of the level set function, and s is the number of regions.

It satisfies $n \leq s \leq 2^n$. With the Gaussian distribution assumption, D_i can be simplified as follows:

$$D_i = \frac{\sigma_w^2 + (\mu_w - \mu_i)^2}{4\sigma_i^2} + \frac{\sigma_i^2 + (\mu_i - \mu_w)^2}{4\sigma_w^2} - \frac{1}{2},$$

where σ_i is the variance of region R_i, and σ_w is the variance of a neighborhood region. G_i is the characteristic function used to represent region R_i with n level set functions. The evolution equation can be obtained directly from an Euler-Lagrange formulation. Let

$$F(\phi_1, \phi_2, \ldots, \phi_n) = \sum_{i=1}^{s} \lambda_i \cdot D_i \cdot G_i(\phi_1, \phi_2, \ldots, \phi_n) + \sum_{j=1}^{n} \nu_j$$
$$\cdot \cdot g(|\nabla I(\Gamma_j)|) \cdot |\nabla H(\phi_j)|. \tag{23}$$

Equation (11) can be written as

$$E(\phi_1, \phi_2, \ldots, \phi_n) = \int_\Omega F(\phi_1, \phi_2, \ldots, \phi_n) d\mathbf{x}.$$

For any ϕ_j, keeping μ_j and σ_j fixed, the Euler-Lagrange equation of Eq. (11) is

$$\frac{\partial F}{\partial \phi_j} - \sum_{k=1}^{m} \frac{d}{dx_k} \left(\frac{\partial F}{\partial \phi_{jk}} \right)$$

$$= \sum_{i=1}^{s} \lambda_i \cdot D_i \cdot \frac{\partial G_i}{\partial \phi_j} - \nu_j \cdot \delta(\phi_j) \cdot \sum_{k=1}^{m} \frac{d}{dx_k}(g(|\nabla I|) \cdot \frac{\partial |\nabla \phi_j|}{\partial \phi_{jk}})$$

$$= \sum_{i=1}^{s} \lambda_i \cdot D_i \cdot \frac{\partial G_i}{\partial \phi_j} - \nu_j \cdot \delta(\phi_j) \cdot \sum_{k=1}^{m} \frac{d}{dx_k}(g(|\nabla I|) \cdot \frac{\phi_{jk}}{|\nabla \phi_j|})$$

$$= \sum_{i=1}^{s} \lambda_i \cdot D_i \cdot \frac{\partial G_i}{\partial \phi_j} - \nu_j \cdot \delta(\phi_j) \cdot div\left(g(|\nabla I|) \cdot \frac{\nabla \phi_j}{|\nabla \phi_j|}\right)$$

$$= \sum_{i=1}^{s} \lambda_i \cdot D_i \cdot \frac{\partial G_i}{\partial \phi_j} - \nu_j \cdot \delta(\phi_j) \cdot \left[g(|\nabla I|) \cdot div\left(\frac{\nabla \phi_j}{|\nabla \phi_j|}\right)\right.$$

$$\left. + \nabla g(|\nabla I|) \cdot \left(\frac{\nabla \phi_j}{|\nabla \phi_j|}\right)\right], \tag{24}$$

where m is the number of the space dimension, and $\partial\phi_{jk}$ is the partial derivation of ϕ_j in the kth dimension. Keeping $\phi_1, \phi_2, \ldots, \phi_n$ fixed, the statistical parameters μ_i and σ_i can be directly estimated from the samples in the corresponding region:

$$\mu_i = \frac{\int_{R_i} I(\mathbf{x})d\mathbf{x}}{V_i} = \frac{\int_\Omega I(\mathbf{x})G_i(\phi_1, \phi_2, \ldots, \phi_n)d\mathbf{x}}{\int_\Omega G_i(\phi_1, \phi_2, \ldots, \phi_n)d\mathbf{x}}, \tag{25}$$

$$\sigma_i^2 = \frac{\int_{R_i} (I(\mathbf{x}) - \mu_i)^2 d\mathbf{x}}{V_i} = \frac{\int_\Omega I^2(\mathbf{x})G_i(\phi_1, \phi_2, \ldots, \phi_n)d\mathbf{x}}{\int_\Omega G_i(\phi_1, \phi_2, \ldots, \phi_n)d\mathbf{x}} - \mu_i^2. \tag{26}$$

For the two-phase problem, the characteristic functions are

$$\begin{aligned} G_1 &= 1 - H(\phi), \\ G_2 &= H(\phi). \end{aligned}$$

The evolution equation is

$$\frac{\partial\phi}{\partial t} = \delta(\phi)\Bigg[\nu \cdot \Big[g(|\nabla I|) \cdot div\Big(\frac{\nabla\phi}{|\nabla\phi|}\Big) + \nabla g(|\nabla I|) \cdot \Big(\frac{\nabla\phi}{|\nabla\phi|}\Big)\Big]$$

$$+ \lambda_1 \cdot D_1 - \lambda_2 \cdot D_2\Bigg].$$

For the three-phase problem, the characteristic functions are

$$\begin{aligned} G_1 &= H(\phi_1)(1 - H(\phi_2)), \\ G_2 &= (1 - H(\phi_1))(1 - H(\phi_2)), \\ G_3 &= H(\phi_2). \end{aligned}$$

From Eq. (24), the evolution equations for three-phase segmentation are given by

$$\frac{\partial\phi_1}{\partial t} = \delta(\phi_1)\Bigg[\nu_1 \cdot \Big[g(|\nabla I|) \cdot div\Big(\frac{\nabla\phi_1}{|\nabla\phi_1|}\Big) + \nabla g(|\nabla I|) \cdot \Big(\frac{\nabla\phi_1}{|\nabla\phi_1|}\Big)\Big]$$

$$+ (\lambda_2 \cdot D_2 - \lambda_1 \cdot D_1)(1 - H(\phi_2))\Bigg], \tag{27}$$

$$\frac{\partial\phi_2}{\partial t} = \delta(\phi_2)\Bigg[\nu_2 \cdot \Big[g(|\nabla I|) \cdot div\Big(\frac{\nabla\phi_2}{|\nabla\phi_2|}\Big) + \nabla g(|\nabla I|) \cdot \Big(\frac{\nabla\phi_2}{|\nabla\phi_2|}\Big)\Big]$$

$$+ (\lambda_1 \cdot D_1 - \lambda_3 \cdot D_3) \cdot H(\phi_1)$$

$$+ (\lambda_2 \cdot D_2 - \lambda_3 \cdot D_3) \cdot (1 - H(\phi_1))\Bigg]. \tag{28}$$

6. REFERENCES

1. Zhu C, Jiang T. 2003. Multicontext fuzzy clustering for separation of brain tissues in magenetic resonance images. *NeuroImage* **18**685–696.
2. Pham DL, Prince JL. 1999. Adaptive fuzzy segmentation of magnetic resonance images. *IEEE Trans Med Imaging* **18**(9):737–752.
3. Xu C, Pham DL, Prince JL. 2000. Medical image segmentation using deformable models. In *Handbook of medical imaging*, Vol. 2: *Medical image processing and analysis*. pp. 129–174. Bellingham, WA: SPIE Press.
4. Kass M, Witkin A, Terzopoulos D. 1987. Snakes: active contour models. In *Proceedings of the IEEE international conference on computer vision*, pp. 259–268. Washington, DC: IEEE Computer Society.
5. Osher S, Sethian JA. 1988. Fronts propagating with curvature-dependent speed: algorithms based on Hamilton-Jacobi formulations. *J Comput Phys* **79**(1):12–49.
6. Malladi R, Sethian JA, Vemuri BC. 1995. Shape modeling with front propagation: a level set approach. *IEEE Trans Pattern Anal Machine Intell* **17**(2):158–175.
7. Caselles V, Catte F, Coll T, Dibos F. 1993. A geometric model for active contours. *Num Math* **66**:1–31.
8. Caselles V, Kimmel R, Sapiro G. 1997. Geodesic active contours. *Int J Comput Vision* **22**(1)61–72: .
9. Chan TF, Vese LA. 2001. Active contours without edges. *IEEE Trans Image Process* **10**(2)266–277.
10. Hibbard LS. 2004. Region segmentation using information divergence measures. *Med Image Anal* **8**(3):233–244.
11. Paragios N. 2000. Geodesic active regions and level set methods: contributions and applications in artifical vision, PhD dissertation, University of Nice, Sophia Antipolis, France.
12. Paragios N, Deriche R. 2000. Coupled geodesic active regions for image segmentation: a level set approach. In *Proceedings of the European conference on computer vision (ECCV)*, pp. 224–240. New York: Springer.
13. Paragios N, Deriche R. 2002. Geodesic active regions and level set methods for supervised texture segmentation. *Int J Comput Vision* **46**(3):223–247.
14. Gibou F, Fedkiw R. 2003. A Fast hybrid k-means level set algorithm for segmentation. *Int J Comput Vision* **50**(3):271–293.
15. Besson SJ, Barlaud M. 2003. DREAM2S: Deformable regions driven by an eulerian accurate minimization method for image and video segmentation. *Int J Comput Vision* **53**(1):45–70.
16. Zhu S, Yuille A. 1996. Region competition: unifying snakes, region growing, and Bayes/MDL for multiband image segmentation. *IEEE Trans Pattern Anal Machine Intell* **18**(9):884–900.
17. Kadir T, Brady M. 2003. Unsupervised non-parametric region segmentation using level sets. In *Proceedings of the IEEE international conference on computer vision*, pp. 1267–1274. Washington, DC: IEEE Computer Society.
18. Heiler M, Schnorr C. 2003. Natural image statistics for natural image segmentation. In *Proceedings of the IEEE international conference on computer vision*, Vol. 2, pp. 1259–1266. Washington, DC: IEEE Computer Society.
19. Heiler M, Schnorr C. 2005. Natural image statistics for natural image segmentation. *Int J Comput Vision* **63**(1):5–19.
20. Goldenberg R, Kimmel R, Rivlin E, Rudzsky M. 2002. Cortex segmentation: a fast variational geometric approach. *IEEE Trans Med Imaging* **21**:1544–1551.
21. Han X, Xu C, Prince JL. 2003. A topology preserving level set method for geometric deformable models. *IEEE Trans Pattern Anal Machine Intell* **25**(6):755–768.
22. Han X, Pham D, Tosun D, Rettmann ME, Xu C, Prince JL. 2004. CRUISE: cortical reconstruction using implicit surface evolution. *NeuroImage* **23**(3):997–1012.

23. Zeng X, Staib L, Schultz R, Duncan J. 1999. Segmentation and measurement of the cortex from 3D MR images using coupled surfaces propagation. *IEEE Trans Med Imaging* **18**(10):927–937.

24. Chakraborty A, Staib LH, Duncan JS. 1996. Deformable boundary finding in medical images by integrating gradient and region information. *IEEE Trans Med Imaging* **15**(6):859–870.

25. Van Leemput K, Maes F, Vandermeulen D, Suetens P. 2003. A unifying framework for partial volume segmentation of brain MR images. *IEEE Trans Med Imaging* **22**(1):105–119.

26. Rajapakes J, Frugges F. 1998. Segmentation of MR images with intensity inhomogeneities. *Image Vision Comput* **16**(3):165–180.

27. Vese LA, Chan TF. 2002. A multiphase level set framework for image segmentation using the Mumford and Shah model. *Int J Comput Vision* **50**(3):271–293.

28. Kim J, Fisher III JW, Yezzi A, Cetin M, Willsky AS. 2005. A nonparametric statistical method for image segmentation using information theory and curve evolution. *IEEE Trans Image Process* **14**(10):1486–1502.

29. Lenglet C, Rousson M, Deriche R. 2004. Segmentation of 3D probability density fields by surface evolution: application to diffusion mr images. In *Proceedings of the international conference on medical image computing and computer-assisted intervention (MICCAI 2004). Lecture notes in computer science*, Vol. 3216, pp. 18–25. Berlin: Springer.

30. Sussman M, Smereka P, Osher S. 1994. A level set approach for computing solutions to incompressible two-phase flow. *J Comput Phys* **199**:146–159.

31. Stejskal EO, Tanner JE. 1965. Spin diffusion measurements: spin echoes in the presence of a time-dependent field gradient. *J Chem Phys* **42**:288–292.

32. Li C, Xu C, Gui C, Fox MD. 2005. Level set evolution without re-initialization: a new variational formulation. In *IEEE international conference on computer vision and pattern recognition (CVPR)*, pp. 430–436. Washington, DC: IEEE Computer Society.

33. Aubert G, Barlaud M, Faugeras O, Jehan-Besson S. 2003. Image segmentation using active contours: calculus of variations or shape gradients? *SIAM J Appl Math* **63**(6):2128–2154.

34. Sethian JA. 1999. *Level set methods and fast marching methods: evolving interfaces in computational geometry, fluid mechanics, computer vision and materials science*. Cambridge: Cambridge UP.

35. Tai X, Chan T. 2004. A survey on multiple level set methods with applications for identifying piecewise constant functions. *Int J Num Anal Model* **1**(1):25–47.

36. Wang Z, Vemuri BC. 2004. Tensor field segmentation using region based active contour model. In *Proceedings of the European conference on computer vision (ECCV)*, Vol. 4, pp. 304-315. Washington, DC: IEEE Computer Society.

37. Yezzi A, Tsai A, Willsky A. 1999. *A statistical approach to curve evolution for image segmentation*. MIT LIDS Technical Report.

38. Zhu W, Jiang T, Li X. 2005. Local region based medical image segmentation using J-divergence measures. In *Proceedings of the 27th annual international conference on engineering in medicine and biology*, pp. 7174–7177. Washington, DC: IEEE Computer Society.

12

MORPHOMETRIC ANALYSIS OF NORMAL AND PATHOLOGIC BRAIN STRUCTURE VIA HIGH-DIMENSIONAL SHAPE TRANSFORMATIONS

Ashraf Mohamed and Christos Davatzikos

Section of Biomedical Image Analysis, Department of Radiology
University of Pennsylvania, Philadelphia,
Pennsylvania, USA

1. INTRODUCTION

The widespread use of neuroimaging methods in a variety of clinical and basic science fields has created the need for systematic and highly automated image analysis methodologies that extract pertinent information from images, in a way that enables comparisons across different studies, laboratories, and image databases. Quantifying the morphological characteristics of the brain from tomographic images, most often from magnetic resonance images (MRIs), is important for understanding the way in which a disease can affect brain anatomy, for constructing new diagnostic methods utilizing image information, and for longitudinal follow-up studies evaluating potential drugs.

The conventional type of morphological analysis of brain images has relied on manual tracings of regions of interest (ROI) [5–22]. These methods typically require that the reliability and repeatability of manual tracings across different raters, but also within the same rater at different times, be established first. However, methods based on manually defined ROIs are limited in many ways. First,

---

Address all correspondence to: Christos Davatzikos, Section of Biomedical Image Analysis, Department of Radiology, University of Pennsylvania, 3600 Market Street, Suite 380, Philadelphia, PA, 19104; Phone: 215-349-8587. Christos.Davatzikos@uphs.upenn.edu, http://www.rad.upenn.edu/sbia/.

they rely on the need for a priori knowledge of the regions that are affected by a disease, so that respective ROIs can be defined, and therefore they might fail to discover new findings. Although a good hypothesis might be available in the beginning of a morphometric study, one would typically want to discover new knowledge that, by definition, is not part of the hypothesis. As an example selected from the neuroimaging of dementia literature, although the role of hippocampal and entorhinal cortical atrophy in early prediction of Alzheimer's Disease (AD) is widely accepted, relatively little is known about the potential involvement of other brain regions, which could help construct more sensitive methods for detection of and differentiation among different types dementia. The complete investigation of the role of all brain structures in a disease and its diagnosis would be prohibitively labor intensive for an adequately large sample size, if manual methods are employed. Moreover, inter- and intra-rater reliability issues would become crucial limiting factors, particularly in longitudinal studies in which it is extremely difficult to maintain intra- and inter-rater reliability over time. Second, the spatial specificity of ROI-based methods is limited by the size of the ROIs being measured, which is typically rather coarse. A region that might be affected by disease may be only part of a pre-defined ROI, or it might span two or more ROIs, which inevitably washes out the results and reduces the statistical power of the measurement method. Alternative methods, such as stereology, are also limited in a similar way. Although in principle one could define the size of the ROIs measured to be as small as desired, in order to increase spatial specificity, this would decrease rater reliability for measurement methods that are based on human raters. Finally, manual ROI tracing is severely limited in many modern studies, for which it is not unusual to include over a thousand scans per study.

In order to address the limitations of ROI-based approaches, image analysis methods based on shape analysis have been studied in the literature during the past 15 years [23–38]. One very promising approach for morphometric analysis is based on *shape transformations*, and the associated methods are often called unbiased, or hypothesis-free methods. A shape transformation is a spatial map that adapts an individual's brain anatomy to that of another. The resulting transformation measures the differences between the two anatomies with very high spatial specificity, and ultimately the specificity allowed by the image voxel size. More generally, a template of anatomy is first selected, which serves as a measurement unit. The shape transformation that maps other brains to the template is determined via some sort of image analysis algorithm, and it is used as a means of quantifying the individual anatomies. Inter-individual comparisons are then performed by applying standard statistical methods to the respective shape transformations. Voxels that display significant group differences or longitudinal changes are grouped into regions. Therefore, there is no need to define ROIs in advance. Instead, the ROIs are determined retrospectively via the voxel-wise statistical analysis of the shape transformations. The concept of this approach is shown in Figure 1a, which is based on some of the second author's earlier work on the corpus callosum [25].

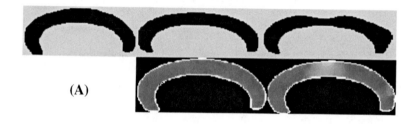

(A)

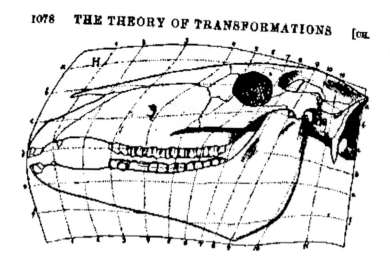

1078 THE THEORY OF TRANSFORMATIONS [CH.

Figure 1. Using a shape transformation for morphometric measurements: (a) Top left: a template of the cross-section of the corpus callosum, a brain structure connecting the two hemispheres. Top middle and right: two individual shapes. Bottom: respective color-coded maps of the determinant of the Jacobian of the shape transformation mapping the template to the two shapes. Contraction is colored green and expansion red. Voxel-wise comparison of these images reveals local shape differences of the respective shapes. (b) Seminal work by D'Arcy Thompson in 1917 using shape transformations to make comparisons among species. See attached CD for color version.

Although this approach has gained widespread attention only within the past decade, it has its roots in the seminal work by D'Arcy Thompson [39], who studied differences among species by measuring deformations of coordinate grids from images of one species to images of another (see Figure 1b). At that time, very limited manual drawing methods were available to D'Arcy Thompson, which imposed limits on the spatial specificity of this approach. The approach was later adopted by Bookstein in the landmark-based morphometrics literature [23] and further extended by Grenander's pattern theory [40] and Miller's work on diffeomorphisms [24], and by P. Thompson's work on tensor mapping [27], among several other investigators. One of the first applied studies was performed by our group by focusing on sex differences in the corpus callosum [25, 41].

In addition to allowing the mophometric analysis of brain structure, the availability of shape transformations from an anatomical brain template to various brain images provides an additional important benefit. Through the inverse of such shape transformations, information defined on the domains of individual brain images can now be mapped onto the domain of the template. Thus the template acts as a stereotactic space where structural, functional, and pathological information from large databases of brain images can be collected and used for construction of statistical atlases of normal and pathological variability. Through the use of multivariate statistical analysis methods, it is also possible to discover correlates between all variables stored in the atlas and to link this information to normal, pathological and aging processes.

Despite the mathematical subtleties involved in the morphometric analysis via shape transformations, the basic principle is simple and follows three standard measurement steps, similar to the steps one would perform in order to measure, for example, the lengths of objects:

1. A measurement unit is first selected to be used as reference; this might be the meter or the yard in standard length measurements; and the measurement unit is a typical brain image in shape measurements and is referred to as the template.

2. The template is stretched over the extent of an individual's brain, so that homologous features are mapped to each other; the shape transformation quantifies exactly this stretching, and is analogous to stretching the meter or the yard over the full length of an object, if one seeks to obtain a length measurement.

3. Inter-individual comparisons are performed by comparing respective shape transformations, exactly as one would compare a 2.3-m object to a 2.8-m object. Of course, obtaining and comparing three- or four-dimensional shape transformations is far more complicated than obtaining and comparing scalar length measurements, but the fundamental principle is the same.

This chapter is dedicated to describing an approach for extracting shape transformations based on medical images and the use of these shape transformations to obtain voxel-based morphometric measurements of the anatomy in the images. The selection of a suitable template that acts as a standard unit of measurement is an important decision that affects subsequent steps. This active research topic is not dealt with here, but the interested reader may wish to refer to recent articles on the topic [42, 43].

Many methods have been proposed in the literature for obtaining shape transformations between a template shape and shape instances in images. This is usually achieved through a method for deformable image registration. In Section 2 we describe recent efforts in deformable image registration by our group. Section 3 is dedicated to explaining approaches for voxel-based morphometry and the use of these approaches in the study of normal and pathological changes in brain structure.

Available methods for brain image morphometry would also be very useful in quantifying and understanding changes in brain structure due to the presence of a brain tumor. In addition to these benefits that voxel-based morphometric methods can provide, deformable registration between brain tumor images and a brain template (Step 2 above) will make the construction of statistical brain tumor atlases possible. These statistical atlases will be able to link structural and functional information to variables such as the tumor size, type, location, and response to therapy or the success of surgery. Such statistical brain tumor atlases will be extremely useful in neurosurgery and radiotherapy planning and in the study of brain tumor development and mechanisms.

The presence of tumors and their associated effects on the brain images significantly complicate the deformable registration and make the results of current image registration methods inaccurate in the vicinity of the tumor. In Section 4 we describe recent efforts by our group for deformable registration of brain tumor images. Two main components have been developed to solve this deformable registration problem. The first is a biomechanical model of brain tumor mass-effect. The second is a statistical model that links deformation caused by tumors to variables such as the tumor size, location, and the amount of peri-tumor edema. These components and their integration into a method for deformable registration of brain tumor images are described in detail in Section 4.

2. SHAPE TRANSFORMATIONS AND DEFORMABLE REGISTRATION OF BRAIN IMAGES

The goal of the deformable registration between two brain images is to find the transformation that maps every point in the first image to its matching point in the second image. Matching points should correspond to the same anatomical feature or structure. The shape transformation found is usually required to be a diffeomorphism — a differentiable and invertible mapping between the domains of the two images. In mathematical terms, let D_1 be the domain of the first image, and let D_2 be the domain of the second image. The sought shape transformation is a differentiable and invertible mapping $\varphi : D_1 \rightarrow D_2$ such that for every point $\mathbf{x} \in D_1$, the point $\varphi(\mathbf{x}) \in D_2$ corresponds to the same anatomical feature or structure as that of point $\mathbf{x}$.

Early approaches for morphometric analysis in the medical imaging literature required a human rater to define a number of reliability identifiable landmark points on a shape template and to manually locate their corresponding points on each of the images subject to the analysis. The beginning of the modern phase of this approach in medical imaging could perhaps be dated back to 1989 with Bookstein's work on landmark-based morphometrics [23]. Shape transformations are obtained by interpolating the mapping on the landmarks everywhere else in the brain, using a thin plate spline model. This approach has been mainly used in 2D neuroimaging studies, often restricted to the corpus callosum, since not many anatomical structures lend themselves to 2D analysis. Moreover, defining landmarks in 3D with high accuracy and reproducibility is often a very difficult and impractical task, especially in large studies.

Finding shape transformations from 3D medical images requires the use of an automated or semi-automated method for finding the deformation map φ. Algorithms based on maximizing the similarity between an image treated as template and other images in the study have been widely used for solving this deformable registration problem [24, 33, 44–50]. These methods assume that if a shape transformation renders two images similar, it implies anatomical correspondence between the underlying anatomies. This is a reasonable assumption, but it can easily be violated in practice, since two images can be made similar via shape transformations that do not respect the underlying anatomical correspondences. For example, one can simply flow gray matter into gray matter, white matter into white matter, and CSF into CSF, thereby creating images that look alike, since these three tissue types have similar intensity distributions throughout the brain, without the underlying shape transformations reflecting true anatomical measures, since, for example, it could morph the precentral gyrus to the postcentral gyrus.

An important issue with intensity-based transformations is that of inverse consistency. In particular, if we attempt to match Image1 to Image2, then Image2 to Image1, we should get shape transformations that are the inverses of each other. This condition is not necessarily met in practice, especially by image similarity measures. Therefore, techniques that specifically impose inverse consistency have also been examined in the literature [44, 51, 52].

Somewhat related to image intensity matching are methods optimizing information theoretic criteria, in order to find appropriate shape transformations. The main advantage of these methods over image similarity methods is that they can potentially be used across different imaging modalities, i.e., when tissue intensities are different in two images to be matched. The most popular criterion of optimality has been mutual information [46, 53, 54], which is maximized when the "predictability" of the warped image based on the template is maximized, and which tends to occur when the different tissue types in two images are well registered.

A different class of algorithms is based on some form of feature matching [26, 48, 55–60]. A number of features, such as edges or curves or surfaces, are typically extracted from the images via an image analysis algorithm, or simply drawn manually, and are then used to drive a 3D deformable registration method, which effectively interpolates feature correspondence in the remainder of the brain. Related are medialness models [30], which use the medial axes of anatomical shapes as features, instead of boundaries themselves. Feature-based methods pay more attention to the biological relevance of the shape matching procedure, since they only use anatomically distinct features to find the transformation, whereas image matching methods seek transformations that produce images that look alike, with little warranty that the implied correspondences have anatomical meaning. However, the latter approaches take advantage of the full dataset, and not only of a relatively sparse subset of features.

A method that has been previously developed by our group attempts to bridge between these two extremes by developing attribute vectors that aim at making each voxel a feature [52,61,62], and it was called the Hierarchical Attribute Matching Mechanism for Elastic Registration (HAMMER). HAMMER is a hierarchical warping mechanism that has two key characteristics. First, it places emphasis on determining anatomical correspondences, which in turn drive the 3D warping procedure. In particular, we have used feature extraction methods whose goal is to determine a number of parameters from the images, which can characterize at least some key anatomical features as distinctively as possible. In [52], we used geometric moment invariants (GMIs) as a means for achieving this goal. GMIs are quantities constructed from images that are first segmented into GM, WM, and CSF, or any other set of tissues of interest. They are determined from the image content around each voxel, and they quantify the anatomy in the vicinity of that voxel. GMIs of different tissues and different orders are collected into an attribute vector, for each voxel in an image. Ideally, we would like for each voxel to have a distinctive attribute vector; of course, this is not possible in reality. Figure 2 shows a color-coded image of the degree of similarity between the GMI-based attribute vector of a point on the anterior horn of the left ventricle and the attribute vectors of every other point in the image. The GMI attribute vector of this point, as well as of many other points in the brain, is reasonably distinctive, as Figure 2 shows. HAMMER was constructed to solve an optimization problem that involves finding a shape transformation that maximizes the similarity of respective attribute vectors, while being smoothed by a standard Laplacian regularization term (a detailed description can be found in [52]). We have recently explored more distinctive attribute vectors, aiming at constructing even more distinctive morphological signatures for every image voxel. Toward this goal we used wavelet-based hierarchical image descriptions of large neighborhoods centered on each image voxel [63,64].

A second key characteristic of HAMMER addresses a fundamental problem encountered in high-dimensional image matching. In particular, the cost function being optimized typically has many local minima, which trap an iterative optimization procedure into solutions that correspond to poor matches between

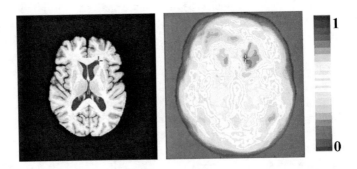

Figure 2. The point marked by a cross has a relatively distinctive GMI-based attribute vector. The color-coded image on the right shows the degree of similarity between the attribute vector of the marked (by crosses) point and the attribute vector of every other point in the brain. 1 is maximum and 0 minimum similarity. See attached CD for color version.

the template and the individual. This is due, in part, to the ambiguity in finding point correspondences. For example, if many candidate points in an individual image have similar attribute vectors to that of a particular template voxel, then this introduces an ambiguity that results in local minima of the corresponding energy function. In contrast, consider the situation in which there are a few anchor points for which correspondence (the value of the shape transformation) can be determined rather unambiguously, perhaps because each anchor point's attribute vector is very different for all but its corresponding anchor point. In that case, the shape transformation on all other (non-anchor) points could be determined via some sort of interpolation from the anchor points. This problem would not have local minima. Of course, the cost function being minimized would be only a lower-dimensional approximation, compared to a cost function involving every single voxel in the image. HAMMER is based on this fact, and forms successive lower-dimensional cost functions, based initially only on key anchor points, and gradually involving more and more points. More points are considered as a better estimate of the shape transformation is obtained, and potential local minima are avoided. Anchor points are defined based on how distinctive their attribute vectors are.

A third feature of HAMMER is that it is inverse consistent, in terms of the driving correspondences. This means that if the individual is deformed to the template, instead of the converse, the mapping between any two driving points during this procedure would be identical. This feature is a computationally fast approximation to the problem of finding fully 3D inverse consistent shape transformations originally proposed by Christensen [65]. Representative results elucidating HAMMER's performance are shown in Figures 3 and 4.

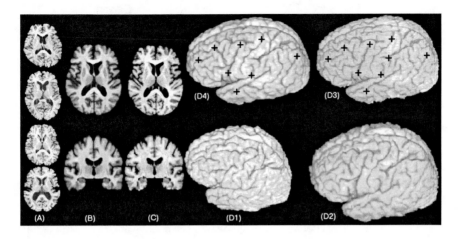

Figure 3. Results using the HAMMER warping algorithm. (a) Four representative sections from MR images of the BLSA database. (b) Representative sections from the image formed by averaging 150 images warped by HAMMER to match the template shown in (c). (d1–d4) 3D renderings of a representative case, its warped configuration using HAMMER, the template, and the average of 150 warped images, respectively. The anatomical detail seen in (b) and (d4) is indicative of the registration accuracy. The red crosses in (d3–d4) are identically placed, in order to allow visualization of point correspondences. See attached CD for color version.

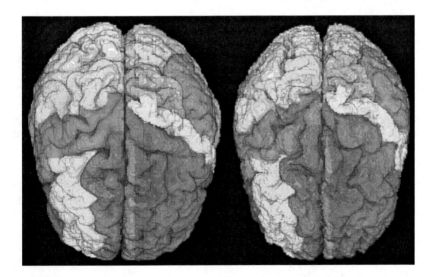

Figure 4. Representative example of automated definition of regions of interest, by warping a pre-labeled atlas (left) to an individual's MR images (the warped atlas is shown on the right as a color-coding of a volume rendering of the target brain). This automated ROI definition makes it possible to apply the method to studies with large sample sizes in a streamlined way. See attached CD for color version.

3. VOXEL-BASED MORPHOMETRIC ANALYSIS

3.1. Deformation-Based Methods

This is the most popular family of methods, and it derives directly from the principles described above, namely that the shape transformation from a template to an individual anatomy is a quantitative measure of the individual anatomy. A variety of methods that rely on the analysis of shape transformations have been presented in the literature. Many of these methods deal directly with the deformation fields generated at each voxel in the template image. Examples of this approach include Bookstein's work on landmark-based morphometrics [23], the work of Grenander [40], Miller [24], and earlier studies by our group focusing on sex differences in the corpus callosum [25,41].

Quantities that are derived from shape transformations have been studied in the literature and proposed for morphometric analysis. A deformation field that maps one image to another may be treated as a discrete vector field. Taking the gradients of this field at each element produces a Jacobian matrix field in which each element is a tensor. The use of this tensor field in shape analysis is sometimes called Tensor-Based Morphometrey (TBM) [27]. The determinant of this Jacobian field has also been suggested for mophometric analysis [66]. This scalar field describes local differences in the volume of structures relative to their corresponding structures in the template image.

3.2. The VBM Method Used by the SPM Software

An alternative to the approach of measuring a deformation field that accurately maps a template to an individual has been adopted by the SPM group [67] and used in several studies (e.g., [68]). The main rationale behind that method is that one does not necessarily need to accurately match all images in a study to the template. A coarse match, which removes some but not all variability across subjects, is used to spatially normalize images into a stereotaxic coordinate system. Then, residual differences in tissue types encountered in the vicinity of an image voxel are assumed to reflect underlying morphological differences across individuals and groups. For example, if a particular brain disease causes a selective loss of tissue in a particular region of the brain, the residual density, after spatial normalization, of brain tissue in a diseased population will be lower than that in a population of healthy controls. This approach is a reasonably effective approach when the tissue atrophy is spread over a large region of the brain, in which case accurate registration should not be critical. However, for diseases that affect brain tissue relatively focally, this approach is limited. Moreover, some of the morphological characteristics of interest are removed by the spatial normalization transformation, and therefore they are never measured by the residual density. This is in contrast to deformation-based methods. Even more importantly, the amount of information

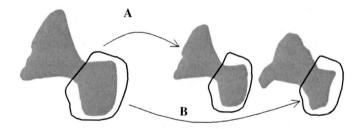

Figure 5. Schematic representation of the mass-preserving framework of the RAVENS analysis. A shape transformation (a) that causes contraction of the structure as it maps it to a stereotaxic space increases the tissue density within the structure, so that the total amount of tissue is preserved. The transformation (b) is different (e.g., it might correspond to a result with greater error in the shape transformation). However, the total amount of tissue is preserved under both transformations, (a) and (b). For example, integrating the tissue density within the outlined regions gives exactly the same result, and is equal to the area of the outlined region in the original shape. This property is lacking in direct measurements of the shape transformation.

that is lost during spatial normalization is not controlled in any way, but might actually vary from one image to another, depending on how similar the template is to the respective individuals and what the limitations of the spatial normalization algorithm are. Despite these limitations, VBM has been freely available via the SPM software and has used quite widely and successfully, especially in studies that do not seek subtle and spatially localized brain abnormalities.

3.3. The Mass-Preserving Principle for Regional Volumetric Analysis

Morphometric analysis based solely on the shape transformation that maps a template to an individual anatomy is affected by errors in determining the shape transformation. If the warping mechanism used by a particular method is not able to perfectly match the anatomy of each individual with the anatomy of the template, then subtle structural characteristics are lost and never recovered in subsequent stages of the analysis. These errors can be significant obstacles in studying subtle differences between two or more individuals or time points. In order to address this problem, we developed a mass-preserving framework for shape transformations that is relatively more robust, for reasons that are explained below. Our approach is shown schematically in Figure 5.

In the mass-preserving framework of RAVENS [2, 69, 70] (Regional Analysis of Volumes Examined in Normalized Space), if the shape transformation applies an expansion to a structure, the density of the structure decreases accordingly to warranty that the total amount of tissue is preserved. Conversely, tissue den-

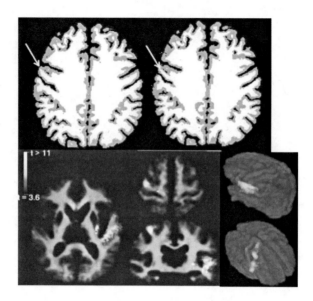

Figure 6. Top: representative slices from the level of the precentral gyrus, with simulated atrophy indicated by the arrows (left = before, right = after uniform 30% atrophy within the gyrus was applied). Bottom: regions detected by the RAVENS analysis, overlaid on the average WM RAVENS maps of the 24 individuals. The two detected regions were exactly where atrophy was simulated. Reprinted with permission from [2]. Copyright ©2001, Academic Press. See attached CD for color version.

sity increases during contraction. Consequently, tissue density in the template's (stereotaxic) space is directly proportional to the volume of the respective structure in its original form. Therefore, regional volumetric measurements and comparisons are performed via measurements and comparisons of the respective RAVENS density maps. One RAVENS map is generated for each tissue of interest, typically GM, WM, and CSF. In [2] we validated RAVENS on 24 MR images having synthetic atrophy. Specifically, we randomly selected standard SPGR images of 12 BLSA subjects, and we outlined the precentral and superior temporal gyri in all of them. We then introduced a uniform 30% volumetric contraction in these two outlined gyri, thereby generating another 12 images with synthesized atrophy in them. Figure 6 (top) shows cross-sections of a typical image before and after contraction of the precentral gyrus (segmented images are shown).

We then used RAVENS to determine the 24 respective brain tissue density maps, and applied a pointwise statistical analysis to them via paired t-tests. Regions of statistically significant differences between the two sets of 12 are shown in Figure 6 (bottom), overlaid on the average WM RAVENS map of the 24 subjects (used for reference). The highlighting of the two regions in which atrophy was introduced shows the spatial specificity of RAVENS. In [2] we also compared the sensitivity of RAVENS with the widely used VBM approach of the SPM package [67], and we found that RAVENS performed significantly better in this validation study.

3.4. Longitudinal Stability

With a growing interest in longitudinal studies, which are important in studying development, normal, aging, early markers of Alzheimer's disease, and response to various treatments, amongst others, securing longitudinal stability of the measurements is of paramount importance. However, in a longitudinal morphometric study, we would typically measure the shape transformation during each time point, and then examine longitudinal changes in the shape transformation. This approach is valid in theory, but limited in practice. This is because small error measurements are dramatically amplified when we calculate temporal differences. Although temporal smoothing can be applied retrospectively to shape measurements, it is far better if temporal smoothing is actually incorporated into the procedure for finding the shape transformation, when the image information is available to the algorithm, rather than retrospectively adjusting a noisy shape transformation. The issue of longitudinal measurement robustness is particularly important in measuring the progression of a normal older adult into mild cognitive impairment, which makes it important to have the ability to detect subtle morphological changes well before severe cognitive decline appears. To further illustrate the difficulties that the current 3D method is facing, in Figure 7 we have shown some representative longitudinal volumetric measurements from single subjects as well as from averages obtained from 90 older individuals over 6 years.

In order to address this issue and be able to obtain longitudinally stable measurements, we have developed an approach to finding the shape transformation in 4D, with the 4th dimension being time [71]. The formulation is readily reduced to a 3D problem, if only cross-sectional data are available. We should note that a step toward this proposed direction was proposed in [37], in which the image at one time-point was used as the template for shape reconstruction in another frame. However, that approach still measures longitudinal differences independently for different time-points, and therefore it does not apply temporal smoothing other than by using the same anatomy of a different time-point as the template.

The 4D warping approach of [71] simultaneously establishes longitudinal correspondences in the individual as well as correspondences between the template and the individual. This is different from the 3D warping methods, which aim at establishing only the inter-subject correspondences between the template and the individual in a single time-point. Specifically, 4D-HAMMER uses a fully automatic four-dimensional atlas matching method that constrains the smoothness in both the spatial and temporal domains during the hierarchical atlas matching procedure, thereby producing smooth and accurate estimations of longitudinal changes. Most importantly, morphological features and matches guiding this deformation

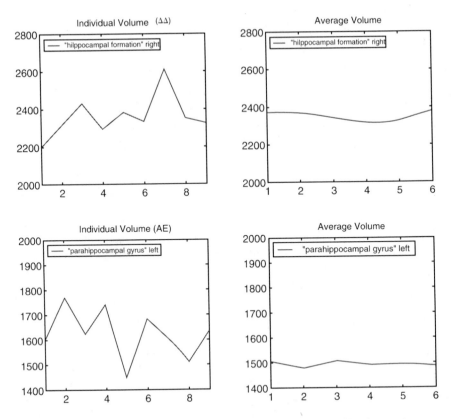

Figure 7. Example illustrating the problems faced when applying a 3D atlas warping method independently to each time-point in a longitudinal study. Left: plots of volumetric measurements from two representative BLSA participants and two structures, using 3D HAMMER (right hippocampal formation and left parahippocampal gyrus). Right: analogous plots showing average volumes of these two structures, obtained by averaging the volumetric measurements of 90 BLSA participants for each of 6 years. Considerable variation is apparent. For example, the standard deviation around the baseline is about 5% for the left hippocampus of subject AD. Although a difference of 5% cannot be appreciated by visual inspection (see Figure 8, below), it can adversely affect the accuracy of longitudinal measurements. As should be expected, variation of the average hippocampal volume is much lower (less than 1%) because of the averaging over 90 individuals. See attached CD for color version.

process are determined via 4D image analysis, which significantly reduces noise and improves robustness in detecting anatomical correspondence. Put simply, image features that are consistently recognized in all time-points guide the warping procedure, whereas spurious features, such as noisy edges, appear inconsistently at different time-points and are eliminated. In [71] this 4D approach was found

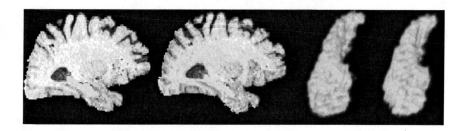

Figure 8. Automated segmentation results using 3D HAMMER for subject AD, years 3 and 4 (see Figure 15, top left). The 5% difference in volumes, in this case, is not readily appreciated visually from these images. (The sections are only approximately corresponding, since the scans were at slightly different orientations. 3D renderings are shown on the right.) Reprinted with permission from [3]. Copyright ©2001, Society for Neuroscience. See attached CD for color version.

to yield both stable and accurate longitudinal measurements, compared to 3D warping.

3.5. Diagnosis: Putting It All together

The voxel-based morphometric analysis methods described above have enjoyed widespread acceptance in the past decade, since they do not rely on any a priori hypotheses regarding the structures to be measured, but rather apply unbiased analyses of the entire set of data on a voxel-by-voxel basis. Accordingly, they highlight regions in which there is a statistically significant difference between two groups, for example. However, the existence of significant differences in certain brain regions does not necessarily imply that volumetric measurements of those regions are sufficient to diagnose disease. For example, say that normal control older subjects differ from patients developing mild cognitive impairment (MCI) in the volumes of the hippocampus and the entorhinal cortex (ERC), but volumes of normal and MCI individuals are highly overlapping. In this case, diagnosis based solely on volumes of the hippocampus and the ERC could be unreliable. In recent years, interest in integrating voxel-wise mophometric measurements into tools that can be used for diagnosis has gained interest [31,72,73]. One of the motivating factors behind these developments is the complex and spatiotemporally distributed nature of the changes that most diseases cause, particularly in the brain. For example, the anatomical structures that carry most discriminative power are likely to depend on the stage of the disease, as the disease progressively spreads throughout various brain [74], but also on age and other demographic and genetic [75], since disease is to be distinguished from complex and progressively changing background normal variations in anatomy and function that may depend on demographic and/or genetic background. Moreover, disease might cause changes of the image characteristics beyond those measured by volumetrics, such as brightening or darkening of an MR image due to demyelination, deposition of minerals, or other macro- or microstructural changes caused by disease. Vascular disease also causes well-known MR signal changes, for example in the white matter of the brain (e.g., brightening of a T_2-weighted signal). It is thus becoming clear that multiple modalities and multiple anatomical regions must be considered jointly in a multivariate classification fashion, in order to achieve the desirable diagnostic power. Moreover, regions that are relatively less affected by disease should also be considered along with regions known to be affected (which for the example of Alzheimer's Disease might include primarily temporal lobe structures, in relatively early disease stages), since differential atrophy or image intensity changes between these regions are likely to further amplify diagnostic accuracy and discrimination from a background of normal variation.

The approach described in [72] is based on the RAVENS mass-preserving morphological representation described earlier in this chapter. It hierarchically decomposes a RAVENS map into images of different scales, each capturing the morphology of the anatomy of interest at a different degree of spatial resolution. The most important morphological parameters are then selected and used in conjunction with a nonlinear pattern classification technique to form a hypersurface, the high-dimensional analog to a surface, which is constructed in a way that it optimally separates two groups of interest, for example, normal controls and patients of a particular disease. Effectively, that approach defines a nonlinear combination of a large number of volumetric measurements from the entire brain, each taken at a different scale that typically depends on the size of the respective anatomical structure and the size of the region that is most affected by the disease. This nonlinear combination of volumetric measurements is the best way to distinguish between the two groups, and therefore to perform diagnosis via classification of a new scan into patients or normal controls.

3.6. Neuroimaging Studies of Aging, Schizophrenia, and Genetic Influences on Brain Development

Voxel-based morphometric analysis has been adopted in a variety of studies. Here, we briefly summarize three studies in which we have applied these techniques, in order to illustrate their use.

3.6.1. Baltimore Longitudinal Study of Aging(BLSA)

The neuroimaging arm of the BLSA was initiated in 1993, and it is now in its 11th year [3,76]. Approximately 150 healthy older adults have been followed annually over this period with structural, functional (PET-^{15}O), and neuropsychological evaluations. Analysis and integration of these data aims at determining early markers of Alzheimer's disease (AD) in a background of structural and functional changes occurring in normal aging. The RAVENS methodology described

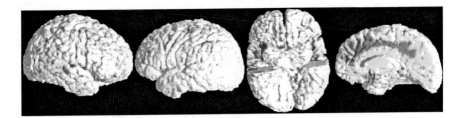

Figure 9. Regions displaying significant longitudinal gray matter atrophy over a 4-year period. Estimates of longitudinal atrophy were determined by segmentation into GM, WM and CSF, then applying the mass-preserving RAVENS methodology described in the text, which deforms each individual's brain into alignment with a template brain, while preserving tissue mass by converting it to density. Voxel-based analysis of the resultant tissue density maps is equivalent to voxel-based volumetric analysis and therefore of atrophy quantification. Reprinted with permission from [3]. Copyright ©2001, Society for Neuroscience. See attached CD for color version.

above has been applied to structural images from this study, in order to measure patterns of significant longitudinal atrophy in normal healthy adults. Figure 9 displays a 3D rendering of the regions displaying significant longitudinal atrophy over a 4-year period.

In addition to atrophy and other shape changes, signal changes are very pronounced even in normal aging. Most importantly, the white matter tends to get darker in standard T1-SPGR images, perhaps due to underlying vascular disease, demyelination, mineral deposition, or other degenerative processes. The methods described in this chapter can also be used in voxel-based analysis of signal changes. In [1] we studied WM darkening in the BLSA sample. Figure 10 displays a statistical parametric map of voxel-wise analysis of longitudinal change. Quantification of signal changes is just as important as measurement of atrophy, for many reasons. First, many degenerative changes can be first manifested as signal changes, prior to tissue atrophy. Second, in early AD stages, vascular disease or demyelination of WM can have an additive effect on cognitive decline to that of AD pathology. Therefore, structural and functional changes caused by vascular disease, and which most often change MR signal characteristics, must be well characterized in order to isolate the imaging signatures that are specific to AD. Moreover, our previous work suggests that, from certain perspectives, signal changes carry orthogonal information to atrophy [1].

3.6.2. Neuroimaging of schizophrenia

We have performed voxel-based analysis of the RAVENS tissue density maps in a study of 158 normal controls and schizophrenia patients. Using voxel-based analysis of the RAVENS maps, we have identified spatially complex patterns of tissue volume differences between healthy controls and patients. Moreover, using

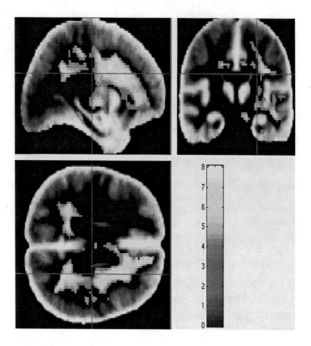

Figure 10. Statistical parametric maps of T1 signal darkening with normal aging, obtained using the RAVENS methodology for elastic registration. T1 darkening might be due to a variety of factors, such as vascular disease, demyelination, mineral deposition, or other degenerative processes. Reprinted with permission from [1]. Oxford UP. See attached CD for color version.

multivariate nonlinear classification methods described in Section 4 above, we have identified morphological signatures that are unique to the disease, and which can potentially be used for early diagnostic purposes.

3.6.3. Neuroimaging of XXY children

In [4] we examined brain morphometry variation associated with XXY males (Klinefelter's syndrome) by using an automated whole-brain volumetric analysis method. The application to 34 XXY males and 62 normal male controls reveals pronounced volume reduction in the brains of XXY males, relative to the brains of normal controls, localized at the insula, temporal gyri, amygdala, hippocampus, cingulate, and occipital gyri. Most of these statistically significant regions are located in the gray matter structures, with the exception of one cluster of atrophy involved in white matter structure, i.e., right parietal lobe white matter. Figure 11. shows some representative results from the statistical analysis of the RAVENS tissue density maps obtained in this study.

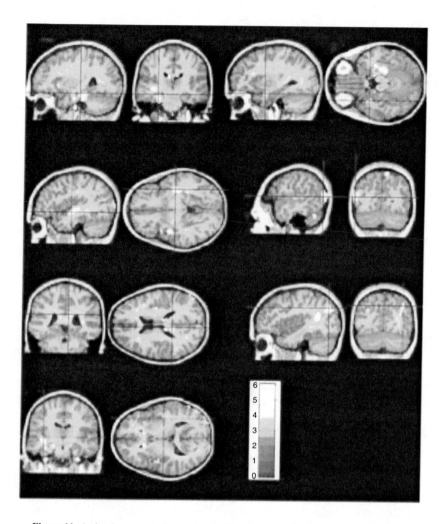

Figure 11. A visual summary of several detected regions with significant group differences between XXY brains and normal control brains. The underlying image is the template that we used to normalize individual brains. Color-coding was based on the values of the t-statistic. Only the voxels with significant group differences, i.e., the corrected p-values exceeding a significance threshold 0.005, are shown. (a) left hippocampal formation; (b) left superior temporal gyrus; (c) cingulate region; (d) left insula; (e) right amygdala; (f) left middle temporal gyri; (g) right parietal lobe WM. Reprinted with permission from [2]. Copyright ©2001, Academic Press. See attached CD for color version.

4. DEFORMABLE REGISTRATION OF BRAIN ATLASES TO BRAIN TUMOR IMAGES

4.1. Introduction and Background

Today, radiologists, neurosurgeons, and neurooncologists use 3D brain images of brain tumor patients for diagnosis, therapy, and surgery planning. In addition to this everyday use of brain tumor images at clinical centers, the deformable registration of these images into a common stereotactic space has the potential of making a significant positive impact on brain cancer research and therapeutic outcome. First, this deformable registration will make it possible to apply the morphometric analysis methods described above in this chapter to brain tumor images. Perhaps more importantly, solving this deformable registration problem will allow the pooling of data from a large number of patients into a common stereotactic space, which will make possible the construction of statistical atlases that are based on collective morphological, functional, and pathological information. These atlases will be useful in planning neurosurgical operations and therapeutic approaches that deal with brain tumors by statistically linking the functional and structural information provided by multimodality radiological images to variables such as tumor size, grade, progression, therapeutic approach, and outcome. The registration of such atlases to a patient's tumor-bearing images will augment the images with the rich information available in the atlases and therefore will act as tools for optimal planning of tumor treatment.

Since current anatomical brain atlases are based on images of normal human subjects, tumors are absent from these atlases. The direct application of currently available deformable registration methods to adapt the images of a neuroanatomy atlas to a patient's tumor-bearing images is therefore inundated by inaccuracies near the tumor due to the substantial dissimilarity between the two images. These dissimilarities arise from topological differences between the atlas and the patient's images, severe deformation in the vicinity of the tumor, tumor infiltration, tissue death and resorption, and the confounding effects of edema.

To account for topological differences between the atlas and the patient's images, Dawant et al. [77] suggested an approach that introduces a tumor "seed" in the brain atlas, which is subsequently grown to match the patient's tumor via the used deformable image registration method. Although this approach is successful in producing qualitatively acceptable results, the seed deformation is strongly dependent on the parameters of the image-matching method, as well as the seed location and size, which are only chosen in an approximate manner. To overcome the problems of this approach, Bach Cuadra et al. [78] suggested the use of a simplified, radially symmetric model of tumor growth coupled with the image-matching forces. In spite of this improvement, the approach in [78] was still not able to achieve acceptable atlas registration accuracy for patients with large tumors and substantial brain tissue deformation. Such inaccuracies can be traced back to the inability of the suggested tumor growth model in reproducing physically realistic brain tissue deformations, which therefore derails the image matching process.

A good model for deformations induced by tumor growth is essential for achieving a registration with accuracy that is acceptable for purposes of surgery and therapy planning. Although Kyriacou et al. [79] used a biomechanical model of the deformation caused by tumors to register images of tumor patients to anatomical atlases, this approach was only implemented in 2D and relied on a computationally expensive regression procedure to solve the inverse problem of estimating the tumor location in the atlas.

Here an approach for establishing the deformable registration of a normal anatomical atlas to a tumor-bearing brain scan is presented. This approach requires the integration of three components. The first is a biomechanical 3D model for the soft-tissue deformation caused by the bulk tumor and peri-tumor edema. This model is implemented using the finite-element (FE) method and is used to generate a number of examples of deformed brain anatomies due to tumors starting from normal brain images. The second component is a statistical model of the desired deformation map that approximates this map via the sum of two components in orthogonal subspaces with different statistical properties. For any particular tumor case that should be registered to the atlas, a partial observation of the desired deformation map is obtained via a deformable image registration method developed for dealing with two normal brain images (HAMMER), which is the third component of the presented approach. Based on the constructed statistical model of the deformation, this partial observation is used to estimate the corresponding mass-effect model parameters that would have produced such a deformation. Finally, the desired deformation is obtained by applying the mass-effect model to the atlas image and the use of deformable image registration to match it to the subject's image.

The rest of this section is organized as follows. In Section 4.2 we provide a detailed overview of the whole approach. In Section 4.3 we provide a description of the biomechanical model for tumor mass-effect and show the results of comparisons between the actual deformations and deformations predicted by this model in four real brain tumor cases. In Section 4.4 we describe the developed statistical approach for estimating the biomechanical model's parameters. Deformable registration results for a real and a simulated brain case are presented in Section 4.5. We conclude with a discussion of the approach and suggestions for future work.

4.2. Overview of the Approach

The proposed deformable registration approach is best explained with the aid of Figure 12. The subject's brain B_{SD} includes regions T_{SD} (bulk tumor), and possibly D_{SD} (peri-tumor edema). The main goal of the deformable registration

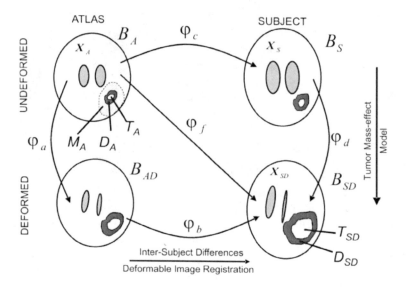

Figure 12. Illustration of the deformation maps involved in the proposed approach. φ_f is the map from the atlas to a subject's tumor-bearing image. Regions T_{SD} and D_{SD} denote the bulk tumor and edema regions in the subject's images, and T_A, D_A are the corresponding regions in the atlas. φ_c is the mapping from the atlas to the subject's image before tumor mass-effect simulation (B_S is not known for non-simulated cases), and φ_d is that obtained through simulation of the tumor mass-effect. Simulating the tumor mass-effect on the atlas results in φ_a and a deformed atlas image that can then be registered to the deformed subject's image through φ_b. Copyright ©2006, Elsevier B. V. See attached CD for color version.

approach is to find the transformation

$$\varphi_f : B_A \backslash T_A \rightarrow B_{SD} \backslash T_{SD} \tag{1}$$

that maps points with coordinates X_A in the atlas image to points with coordinates X_{SD} in the subject image. Here, the $\backslash$ is used to denote the set difference operator. Another goal of the deformable registration approach is to identify T_A, which corresponds to brain tissue that is no longer present in the subject's image (died or invaded by tumor).

As will be illustrated with an example later in Section 4.5, the direct use of deformable image registration to obtain φ_f results in an inaccurate warping in and around tumor due to a substantial dissimilarity between the normal atlas image and the patient's tumor-bearing image. The approach proposed here precedes this deformable registration step with a simulation of the tumor mass-effect on the atlas image.

In Section 4.3 a biomechanical FE model for the deformation induced by brain tumors is described and partially validated via real serial tumor scans. This model can be used to simulate deformation induced by the tumor in the atlas and obtain φ_a, followed by the use of a deformable image registration method to get φ_b, and therefore also the desired deformation map:

$$\begin{aligned} \varphi_f(\mathbf{X}_A) &= \varphi_b \circ \varphi_a(\mathbf{X}_A) \\ &= \varphi_b\left(\varphi_a(\mathbf{X}_A)\right). \end{aligned} \tag{2}$$

The behavior of the biomechanical model is controlled by a number of parameters, such as the location of the tumor, its size, and the extent of peri-tumor edema. We will collectively refer to these variables as Θ. The values of these parameters are not known for real tumor cases, and therefore they must be estimated for each new tumor case. This inverse estimation problem is solved via a statistical model that exploits the relationship between φ_f and the mass-effect model parameters. The overall procedure for deformable image registration between the normal brain image of an atlas and a patient's tumor-bearing image can be summarized as follows:

1. A readily available deformable brain image registration approach (such as HAMMER [52]) is used to obtain an approximation of the desired deformation map φ_f between the atlas image (with no tumor) and the patient's tumor-bearing image. The resulting deformation map will be inaccurate in and around the tumor area (denoted by M_A in the atlas image in Figure 12).

2. Although the approximation of φ_f obtained in Step 1 is incorrect in region M_A, the pattern of this deformation outside M_A can guide the estimation of the mass-effect model parameters Θ. This is achieved here via a statistical model, which is trained on examples of the map $\varphi_f = \varphi_d \circ \varphi_c$ for different values of the tumor parameters. These deformation maps are obtained through the use of HAMMER to register the atlas to brain images of normal subjects, followed by tumor mass-effect simulations on the images of these normal subjects. The details of the statistical model training and estimation stages are provided in Sections 4.4.1 and 4.4.2, respectively.

3. With the estimated biomechanical tumor model parameters, a simulation of tumor mass effect is performed on the atlas images to obtain an estimate of the deformation map φ_a and to generate an atlas image with a simulated tumor.

4. A deformable image registration approach, such as HAMMER, is then used to obtain an estimate of the deformation map φ_b between the atlas image with the simulated tumor and the image of the real tumor patient.

5. The composition of the obtained deformation maps in Steps 3 and 4 provides an estimate of the desired deformation map φ_f. The estimate of the

region T_A in the atlas is provided by the tumor model parameters obtained in Step 2.

4.3. Biomechanical Finite-Element Model of Tumor Mass-Effect

The aim of the proposed model is to simulate only the mass-effect component of the tumor growth process via a mechanical FE model constructed from 3D medical images. Since tumor growth is not purely a mechanical process, but involves a host of interacting biological, biochemical, and mechanical mechanisms at different scales, it is essential to initialize the model simulations with a configuration for the brain from which the target configuration (that deformed by the tumor at the desired stage of tumor growth) is reachable by solving a mechanical boundary value problem (BVP).

The proposed model for tumor-induced deformation may be understood with the aid of Figure 13. Let κ_o be the initial configuration of the brain at a reference time point $t = 0$ before tumor emergence. The stresses in κ_o are assumed negligible. Let κ_t be the configuration of the brain at the target macroscopic stage of tumor development. The bulk tumor, denoted by T_t, is assumed to be composed of proliferative, quiescent, and necrotic tumor cells [80–82]. A region D_t of brain tissue swollen by edema may also be associated with the tumor in κ_t.

If T_t is resected, the edema is diffused, and the stresses in κ_t are allowed to relax to zero, the brain tissues will reach a relaxed configuration κ_r. There is a relaxed configuration associated with every κ_t, and it is, in general, different from both κ_t and κ_o. Given κ_r, the stresses caused by the tumor, and the amount of

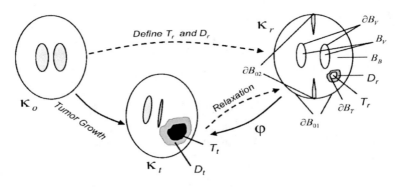

Figure 13. A schematic showing the three configurations involved in the model. κ_o is the brain before tumor development, κ_t is the brain at the desired stage of tumor growth, and κ_r is the corresponding relaxed configuration. T_t and D_t are the bulk tumor and peri-tumor edema regions in κ_t, respectively, while T_r and D_r are the corresponding regions in κ_r. In κ_r, the ventricles are denoted by B_V. ∂B_{01} denotes the outer surface of the brain except for ∂B_{02}, where the falx meets the skull.

swelling due to edema, the deformation map φ can be obtained by solving the mechanical BVP problem.

For real tumor cases, T_r and D_r are not known but are estimated via a statistical approach as explained in Section 4.4. To simulate the mass-effect of tumors starting with normal brain images, approximations of these parameters must be used as explained next.

4.3.1. Defining the relaxed configuration

Defining κ_r involves specifying the geometry of the brain and that of T_r (which corresponds to brain tissue that had died and is no longer present in κ_t or is infiltrated by tumor cells) and D_r (which corresponds to brain tissue that is swollen by edema in κ_t). These regions are highly variable for different tumor cases and types. In order to make the problem tractable, herein, T_r and D_r are approximated with two concentric spheres. The center, c_t and radii r_t and r_e of T_r and D_r, respectively, are treated as model parameters.

It is worth noting that the shape of the final tumor depends on the generated surrounding stresses and need not be spherical [79]. Furthermore, the goal of the biomechanical model described here is, for a given definition of T_r and D_r, to predict brain tissue deformation in a normal brain image. Having built such a forward model for the deformation caused by tumors, the estimation of the unknown model parameters, including T_r and D_r, for a real tumor case will be dealt with in the context of inverse problem solving. This is explained in detail in Section 4.4.

4.3.2. Tumor mass-effect and edema

To account for the mass-effect of the bulk tumor, following the work of Wasserman and Acharya [81], the expansive force of the neoplasm is assumed to be generated by the proliferative tumor cells only. Accordingly, in model simulations, brain tissue in region T_r is removed and a constant outward pressure P is applied normal to the boundary of T_r. P is a model parameter that determines the mass effect exerted by the bulk tumor, and therefore, to a large extent, the final tumor size.

Depending on the type of tumor and its aggressiveness, T_r may be surrounded with a peri-tumor edema region D_r. Since expansion due to edema occurs in white matter (WM) only [83,84], D_r is restricted to WM tissues. Edema expansion in WM is mostly perpendicular to the direction of the fibers. Here, no knowledge of WM fiber orientation is assumed, and, therefore, an isotropic expansive strain e is applied to D_r by using analogy to thermal expansion. A thermal conductivity value of zero for brain tissues prevents this expansion from spreading outside D_r. Studies of brain edema that measured a volume expansion of 200 to 300% in WM [83,84] imply $e \in [0.26, 0.44]$. For simulations starting with normal brain scans a value of $e = 0.35$ is adopted.

4.3.3. Brain tissue constitutive material models

Depending on the area of application, researchers studying the mechanics of brain tissue have used a number of different material constitutive relationships. The brain tissue behavior has been modeled as linear elastic [81, 85–89], hyperelastic [79], hypervisco elastic [90–93], and poroelastic [94]. Given the time scale of the tumor growth process, inertial effects can be ignored and the deformation of brain tissues may be modeled as a quasi-static process. Furthermore, with such a large time scale any viscoelastic effects of the brain tissues would have abated since viscoelastic time constants of living soft tissues, such as the brain, do not exceed a few hours [90,92,93]. Therefore, in this work, the viscous component of the brain tissue's response will be ignored.

Clearly, the brain is heterogeneous, since it is composed of white and gray matter, with a different molecular makeup. A difference in material properties between white and gray matter has been reported in the literature [89,93], although the exact material parameter values vary widely. Directional property differences were also reported for brain white matter [93]. Based on experiments on the porcine brain, Miga et al. [95] observed that the use of a heterogeneous model of the brain tissue did not significantly improve the accuracy of their brain-shift model. Therefore, in simulations reported in this chapter, a homogeneous and isotropic material model for the brain tissue is adopted. The simulations can easily be adapted to deal with the heterogeneous anisotropic case if accurate material property values and white matter orientation information are available and reliable.

Using the dataset described later in this chapter, experiments were performed to compare the behavior of the linear material model and four hyperelastic material models [79,90,92,93] suggested for modeling brain tissue. All FE simulations were performed using the commercial package ABAQUS [96], and nonlinearities arising from large deformations were taken into account. The testing of the poroelastic material model was deferred to future work since ABAQUS requires the use of second-order finite elements with this material model, which is one order higher than the one used in simulations reported here for the tested materials. The stability of the different material models at strain levels encountered during mass-effect simulations, the ability of the simulations to reach convergence, and the error in predicting deformations caused by real tumors were the factors used to select the most suitable material model to use for brain tissues. Based on these experiments, which are described in [97], we adopted the isotropic and homogeneous material model proposed by Miller and Chinzei [92] while relaxing the perfect incompressibility assumption and ignoring viscous effects. Under these conditions, the strain energy density function of the material becomes [96]:

$$W = \frac{2\mu}{\alpha^2} \left(\bar{\lambda}_1^\alpha + \bar{\lambda}_2^\alpha + \bar{\lambda}_3^\alpha - 3 \right) + \frac{1}{D_1} \left(J/J^{th} - 1 \right)^2, \tag{3}$$

where $\bar{\lambda}_i = J^{-1/3} \lambda_i$, $\lambda_i, i = 1, 2, 3$, are the principal material stretches,

$J = \det(\mathbf{F})$ is the volume ratio, $\mathbf{F}$ is the deformation gradient, $J^{th} \left(1 + e^{th}\right)^3$ is the thermal volume ratio, and e^{th} is the thermal strain. The constants μ and D_1 are related to the Young's modulus at zero strain E_o, and Poisson's ratio v by

$$\mu = \frac{E_o}{2(1 + v)} \quad \text{and} \quad D_1 = \frac{6(1 - 2v)}{E_o} \tag{4}$$

The value $\alpha = -4.7$ determined in [92] was adopted here. Since the brain bio-mechanics literature includes varying accounts of brain tissue compressibility and stiffness, in the experiments described below the effects of μ and D_1 (equivalently μ and v) on the proposed model were investigated.

4.3.4. Boundary conditions and interactions

The brain is surrounded by three meninges — the pia, the arachnoid, and the dura mater — which are enclosed within the cranium that constrains the brain deformation. The falx cerebri, which is the extension of the dura mater to in between the two cerebral hemispheres, is more rigid than the brain tissue, and is attached anteriorly and posteriorly to the skull. A large range of values for the stiffness of the falx compared to that of brain tissue is present in the literature. Here, as suggested by the experiments of Miga et al. [94], the brain is assumed to be fixed at the points where the falx meets the skull, and the same material properties assigned for the brain is used for the falx. Assuming negligible friction between the brain meninges and the skull, all other points on the outer surface of the brain are allowed to slide freely in the plane tangent to the surface of the brain, with constrained motion in the normal direction. Initial experiments confirmed that this choice of the boundary conditions for the brain makes the deformation simulations more realistic and produce much lower errors compared to the use of fixed boundary conditions over the whole brain surface [79,81,98].

The brain ventricles are assumed void since normal CSF circulation allows it to leave the ventricles when pressure is imposed by the neighboring tissues. However, for many large brain tumors, the opposite walls of the ventricles may come in contact with each other, leading to propagation of the stresses and displacements to the other side of the ventricle. In such cases, an appropriate model for the contact between the ventricle walls is necessary.

The use of a model of contact in the FE package ABAQUS requires satisfying a number of conditions on the involved self-contacting surface, including that every edge in that surface must be part of exactly two triangular surface patches in the used FE mesh. Satisfaction of this condition was not possible in many cases since the topology of the ventricular FE surface mesh depends on the input segmentation of the ventricles, and on the meshing approach. To avoid this problem, for simulations in which contact of ventricles is anticipated, the ventricles are assumed to be filled with hyperfoam material [96]. This material responds by little resistance for values of nominal strain up to 0.9, after which there is a rapid increase in the stress with the strain. Such a material also allows the use of a zero Poisson's ratio, which prevents coupling of side strain to the axial strain and therefore makes it ideal for approximating the contact in the ventricles. The first-order strain energy density function for this material is given by [96]

$$W_{\text{hyperfoam}} = \frac{2\mu_h}{\alpha_h^2} \left(\lambda_1^{\alpha_h} + \lambda_2^{\alpha_h} + \lambda_3^{\alpha_h} - 3\right) + \frac{1}{\beta_h} \left(J^{\beta_h \alpha_h} - 1\right). \quad (5)$$

Here, the stiffness of this material is chosen to be a fraction of that used for the brain tissue, $\alpha_h = -4.7$ (the same as the value of α used by Miller et al. [92] for the brain tissue with a similar energy function), and $\beta_h = 0$ (for fully compressible behavior, i.e., $v_h = 0$). Initial experiments have shown that using this material model for the ventricles, displacements propagated to the ventricle wall opposite to that which proximal to the simulated tumor were minimal.

4.3.5. boundary value problem statement

If body forces, such as gravity, are ignored, the desired deformation mapping $\varphi : \kappa_r \rightarrow \kappa_t$ can be found by solving the static equilibrium equation:

$$\nabla_o \cdot \mathbf{P} = \mathbf{0}, \quad (6)$$

where $\mathbf{P}$ is the first Piola-Kirchhoff tensor, which is related to strain via the material constitutive law [96]. For brain tissues, simulations are performed with the constitutive law described in Section 4.3.3. The following boundary conditions (BCs) complete the statement of the BVP (refer to Figure 13):

$$\varphi(\mathbf{X}) \cdot \mathbf{N}(\mathbf{X})) = 0, \mathbf{X} \in \partial B_{01}, \quad \text{and} \quad \varphi(\mathbf{X}) = 0, \mathbf{X} \in \partial B_{02}, \quad (7)$$
$$e^{th}(\mathbf{X}) = e, \mathbf{X} \in D_r \quad \text{and} \quad e^{th}(\mathbf{X}) = 0, \mathbf{X} \in \partial B, \quad (8)$$
$$\mathbf{SNX} = PJ\mathbf{F}^{-T}\mathbf{N}(\mathbf{X}), \quad \mathbf{X} \in \partial B_T, \quad (9)$$
$$\mathbf{SN}(\mathbf{X}) = 0, \quad \mathbf{X} \in \partial B_V, \quad (10)$$

where $\mathbf{N}(\mathbf{X})$ is the outward surface normal at $\mathbf{X}$ in the relaxed configuration. Equation (7) implies a sliding BC over the brain surface, except for locations where the falx meets the inner surface of the skull which are pinned. Equation (8) implies that the expansive strain due to edema is restricted to D_r. Equation (9) is the traction BC implied by the tumor pressure, expressed in terms on normals inκ_r. In simulations where no contact in the ventricles is anticipated, Eq. (10) implies that the ventricles are assumed void with zero intraventricular pressure. If hyperfoam material is used for approximating ventricle contact, Eq. (10) should be replaced with the constitutive model for this material (Eq. (4)).

4.3.6. Finite-element mesh generation

Solving the system of equations in Section 4.3.5 requires the use of a numerical method such as the FE method. An important initial step in FE analysis is mesh generation, which involves discretization of the multidimensional domain of the problem into small elements of simple geometry, such as tetrahedra or hexahedra for 3D problems. Although hexahedra are known to have higher accuracy than tetrahedra for the same computational cost, tetrahedra are more popular in mesh generation for complicated geometries, such as the brain, because they are easier to generate and automatically refine.

We developed a tetrahedral mesh generator capable of automatically creating FE meshes from segmented medical images [99]. The input to the mesh generator is an image that is segmented into brain tissue (both white and gray matter), ventricular CSF, tumor, and edema, if present. The output meshes satisfy a number of requirements for accurate FE simulations. For example, tetrahedra in the mesh conform to the boundaries of the underlying segmented image, have sizes that vary across the domain according to a user-defined sizing function, and have an element quality that is sufficient for accurate FE computations. Since ABAQUS was used in solving the FE problem, the tetrahedral quality measure used by ABAQUS was adopted. The quality of a tetrahedron T is therefore given by

$$q_T = \frac{V_T}{V_r}, \tag{11}$$

where V_T is the volume of T, and V_r is the volume of the equilateral tetrahedron that can be inscribed in the circumsphere of T. For an equilateral tetrahedron, q_T is 1.0, and it approaches 0 as the tetrahedron becomes degenerate.

The mesh generation approach starts by casting a regular grid of cubes over the domain of the input image. The size of the cubes is a user-defined input parameter. Cubes totally outside the input image labels are removed, and each of the remaining cubes is tesselated into 5 tetrahedra. Mesh refinement is then performed to make the tetrahedra satisfy the sizing function, which is defined over the domain of the input image. Values of the sizing function reflect the maximum acceptable length of an overlying edge of a tetrahedron. Values of the sizing function may be specified for each label in the image, derived from the surface curvature, or defined by the user arbitrarily. Mesh refinement is carried out via the longest edge propagation path algorithm [100], which guarantees a lower bound on the quality of the generated tetrahedra after subdivision.

After mesh refinement, tetrahedra that straddle a boundary in the segmented image are forced to conform to this boundary by attempting a number of local mesh operations and choosing the one that produces the best quality of the associated tetrahedra. These local mesh operations are relocation of a mesh node to the boundary, splitting of an edge at the point where it crosses the boundary, or its collapse to that point. As the result of these operations, the quality of the elements near the boundaries may be affected; therefore, postprocessing is used as a final step in order to produce meshes with no degenerate or poor quality elements. Postprocessing operations involve optimization of the mesh node locations and the use of edge-split and edge-collapse operations where necessary to improve element quality.

Based on brain tumor simulations conducted initially, severe distortion occurs in the FE mesh due to the large deformation associated with growing large tumors. This affects the convergence of the FE solution and may cause early termination of the simulation before the desired realistic tumor sizes are reached. To deal with this issue, we have included an ability to conduct the tumor growth simulations in a stepped fashion, and correct the distorted mesh (remesh) between steps. Details of the employed FE mesh generation and remeshing methods can be found in [99].

4.3.7. Experiments and results

Here, deformations predicted by the described tumor mass-effect model are compared to deformations observed in four real brain tumor cases. These experiments serve two purposes. First, this dataset of real tumor cases is used to guide the selection of the parameters of the adopted constitutive material model for brain tissues. Second, the accuracy of the model in reproducing deformations in real tumor cases is evaluated.

The rest of this section is organized as follows. A description of the used dataset is provided in Section 4.3.7.1. In Section 4.3.7.2 the steps involved in applying the proposed biomechanical model to this dataset are explained. Experiments performed to select the material constitutive parameter values for brain tissues are described in Sections 4.3.7.3 and 4.3.7.4. Using the material model parameters and mass-effect model parameters providing the best agreement with the observed deformation in the real cases, partial validation experiments were performed. The results of these experiments are reported in Section 4.3.7.5. Finally, a tumor mass-effect simulation starting with an MR brain image of a normal subject is demonstrated in Section 4.3.7.6.

4.3.7.1. Dataset   Four brain tumor cases with serial MRI scans were used in the experiments described here. Some parameters of this dataset can be found in Table 1, and example 2D images are shown in Figure 14, and later in Figure 18.

Assuming that canine brain tissue properties and tumor growth process are reasonably representative of their counterparts in humans, three of the studied tumor cases were dogs with surgically transplanted glioma cells. These dog models were prepared according to the protocol first described by Wodinsky et al. [101]. (The procedure was carried out by Dr. James Anderson and Carolyn Magee at the Johns Hopkins University School of Medicine and was approved by the Animal Care and Use Committee. The animal welfare act and guidelines for the ethical and humane treatment of animal were observed at all times.) A baseline

Table 1. Description of MRI Scans for
the Dataset Used in This Study

Identifier	Image Size	Voxel Size (mm)	Scan Type
DC1	256x256x100	0.391x0.391x0.7	MPRAGE+Gd
DC2	256x256x100	0.391x0.391x0.7	MPRAGE+Gd
DC3	256x256x124	0.46875x0.46875x1.0	T1+Gd
HC	256 × 256 × 124	0.9375 × 0.9375 × 1.5	T1

Identifiers DC1, DC2, and DC3 stand for dog cases 1, 2, and 3. Identifier HC refers to the human case.
All scans for each case have the same parameters.

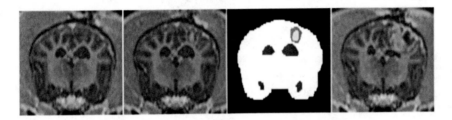

Figure 14. Corresponding 2D images from volumetric gadolinium-enhanced MPRAGE
scans of DC1. Left to right: before tumor implantation, 6 days post-implantation, segmentation of the 6 days post-implantation image, and 10 days post implantation

scan was acquired before implantation of the tumors, followed by scans on the
sixth and tenth days post-implantation. Gadolinium-enhanced high-resolution
T1-weighted images were acquired (MPRAGE sequences were acquired for the
DC1 and DC2). The tumor grows rapidly to a diameter of 1–2 cm by the tenth
day post-implantation, beyond which the animals were sacrificed and prior to
the presentation of significant neurological complications. The fourth dataset
comes from T1-weighted serial MRI scans of a human subject with a low-grade
astrocytoma (LGA) undergoing malignant transformation before the final scan.
Two scans of this patient were used with approximately 2 years in between. An
increase in the tumor mass and significant tissue swelling due to edema were
observed in between the two scans.

4.3.7.2. Experimental Procedure   To compare the model predictions to actual
deformations in the available datasets, values of the parameters (c_t, r_t, r_e, and P)
must be determined for each case. As noted above, for real tumor cases, these
parameters should be estimated through inverse problem solving. To conduct the
experiments needed here, an alternative approach involving the optimization of
the model parameters is used.

To avoid optimizing all model parameters for each tumor case in the used dataset, the first images after tumor growth (6th-day scan for dog cases, and the first scan for the HC) are used to approximate κ_r. This approximation involves the assumption of negligible edema spread, tumor infiltration, and tissue death between this and the final scan, which corresponds to κ_t. Additionally, since tumors in the starting images are small, the stresses and deformation due to the tumor may be assumed negligible. The small deformation assumption was confirmed for the dog cases by measuring the deformation of landmark points around the tumor in the pre-transplantation and the 6th-day scans. These landmark points were selected manually by an expert in the area around the tumor. Under the above-mentioned assumptions, regions D_r and T_r were obtained from segmentations of the tumor and edema in the starting images. The starting images already had some peri-tumor edema. Therefore, e was treated as a parameter with $e \in [0.1, 0.4]$.

In addition to performing simulations with different values of P and e for each tumor case, simulations were also performed with varying material parameter values for the brain tissues. For each simulation, the error in the deformation predicted by the model compared to the actual deformation was computed. This error calculation performed through the use of corresponding landmark points that were found by a human expert in the used two images for each tumor case. The overall procedure is summarized in the following steps.

1. Rigid registration of the target (final) scan to the respective starting scan (used to define κ_r) was performed. Registration was carried out using a stepped multiresolution minimization of normalized mutual information via the CISG registration package [102].

2. Pairs of corresponding landmarks were manually identified by a human expert (rater) in the starting and target images. The number of landmarks for each case varied between 20 and 25 (see Table 2) and were selected in the region around the tumor, where large deformation is observed.

3. A combination of manual and automatic segmentation of the starting image into brain, ventricles, falx, tumor, and edema was performed. The falx cerebri was also manually segmented in order to use it for the boundary condition as explained above.

4. The automatic mesh generation approach explained in Section 4.3.6 was used to generate tetrahedral FE meshes for each of the datasets. For visual illustration, views of the mesh generated for DC1 are shown in Figure 15.

5. Based on the mesh generated in the previous step and the model equations provided in Section 4.3.5, the FE package ABAQUS was used to obtain the simulated tumor-induced deformation. Simulations were performed with different values of P and e, and of the material parameter values.

Table 2. Optimal Values of Parameters P and e for the Minimum Mean Error

	DC1	DC2	DC3	HC
P, Pa	8000	7000	15000	8000
e	0.3	0.15	0.4	0.3
Num. Landmarks	25	21	20	21
Land. Deform., mm	2.16/3.9/1.06	1.77/2.83/0.58	1.82/3.04/0.78	4.53/6.09/0.9
Land. error, mm	1.11/2.5/0.73	1.13/2.1/0.42	1.19/2.24/0.52	1.7/3.09/0.77
Tum. vol. (true/sim.) cm^3	0.496/0.509	0.996/1.25	0.514/0.555	1.734/1.842

Optimal values of parameters P and e for MME in landmark point coordinates are reported for each case in the used dataset. Results are for $v = 0.485$. The number of landmarks, landmark deformation statistics (mean, maximum, and standard deviation), and the model residual errors (mean, max, and standard deviation) for the landmark points are reported. A comparison between the tumor volume in the real images (obtained via manual segmentation) and in the simulated images is also provided.

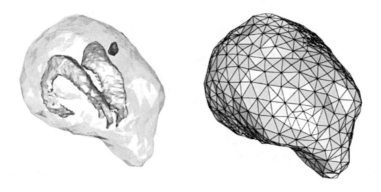

Figure 15. Two views of the FE mesh generated for DC1. Left: outer brain surface mesh; right: translucent outer brain surface and colored surfaces of the tumor and the ventricles. See attached CD for color version.

6. The deformation map resulting from each FE simulation was used to deform the starting image and the locations of the landmark points in this image. Errors between the simulated deformed landmark coordinates and rater's determined coordinates for these points in the target scan were computed.

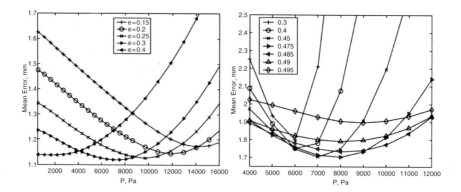

Figure 16. Example curves of the mean errors in the displacement of landmark points for two cases in the dataset. (a) Curves for DC1 at different values of P and e, and for $v = 0.49$. (b) Curves for HC at different values of P and v, and $e = 0.3$.

4.3.7.3. Material Stiffness   Values of the brain tissue's stiffness reported in the literature range over several orders of magnitude. For example, the asymptotic shear modulus at small strains predicted by Prange and Margulies [93] for human gray matter was $\mu_o \approx 60.3$ Pa, which translates into an equivalent Young's modulus of $E_o = 181$ Pa at small strains. On the other hand, a value of $E_o = 180$ kPa was used by Kyriacou et al. [79] for gray matter.

Since the loads in the proposed mass-effect model are in the form of a pressure, P, and a prescribed strain e, the resulting deformation will depend on the ratio P/E_o and on e, but not on the value of P alone. Therefore, choosing different values for E_o, but the same value of P/E_o, will provide the same deformation for a certain value of e. However, the generated stresses at a certain strain value will depend on the value of E_o used for the brain tissues. This observation was confirmed through actual FE simulations. Accordingly, we adopted the value of $\mu = 842$ Pa found by Miller and Chinzei for the used hyerpelastic material model [92]. For a perfectly incompressible material, this translates into $E_o = 2526$ Pa.

4.3.7.4. Material Compressibility   For each case in the dataset, simulations were performed to determine the values of P and e according to the following sequence. With $v = 0.49$ [94] (which implies $E_o = 2109$ Pa, $D_1 \approx 4.75 \times 10^{-5}$ Pa, e, and P were varied for each case, and the mean error in model predictions of the landmark locations was computed. Values of e for minimum error were recorded for each case. Representative error curves for cases DC1 are shown in Figure 16a.

With the value of e determined for each case, simulations were then run for $v \in [0.3, 0.499]$ and $P \in [1, 16]$ kPa. FE tetrahedra with special formulation for incompressibility were used for all simulations. Representative mean error curves for HC are shown in Figure 16b. For all tumor cases, the minimum mean error

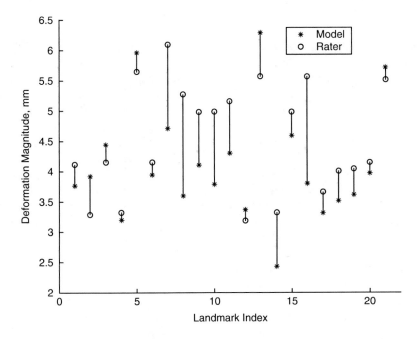

Figure 17. Comparison of the magnitude of deformations of landmarks predicted by the model and the rater for the HC tumor case.

occurs at $v \in [0.475, 0.499]$, which is in agreement with the almost-incompressible behavior reported in the brain biomechanics literature. Therefore, in subsequent simulations, we adopted the value $v = 0.485$ — near the middle of this range.

4.3.7.5. Validation Experiments With $v = 0.485$ and the values of e determined above, the optimal value of P for each tumor case was recorded. These values of P and e and the corresponding residual errors in the model predictions are reported in Table 2. Statistics on the errors and landmark deformations are also reported in the same table.

In Figure 17 we compare the magnitude of the landmark deformations for the HC case predicted by the model to those found by a rater. For most of the landmark points, the model seems to be underestimating the magnitude of the deformation. For this case, the smallest percentage residual error compared to the rater's magnitude of deformation (landmark point 6) and was equal to 15.31%. The deformation of that landmark point as predicted by the rater was 4.15 mm. On average, the model is able to predict more than 62% of the deformation for HC.

Since the coordinates of the landmarks were treated as ground truth, quantification of the accuracy of the rater's placement of these landmark points in the target images was evaluated. For DC1, landmark points selected in the starting image were found by two independent raters in the target images and the inter-rater variability was evaluated. The mean inter-rater variability in this case was 1.1176 mm, with a maximum of 3.2783 mm, which are similar to the respective values of the residual deformation errors. Further, a t-test was performed between the model residual errors (distances between the model-predicted landmark locations and the corresponding locations determined by the rater, averaged over the two raters) and the inter-rater distances. The two distributions were found to be statistically indistinguishable (p-value = 0.98 at a 0.05 significance level). It is also interesting to note that the mean residual errors reported in Table 2 were found to be highly correlated with the resolutions of the used MRI scans ($\rho = 0.9993$ for the cross-sectional resolutions, and $\rho = 0.9625$ for the inter-slice spacings). These observations indicate that residual errors likely arise from the inaccuracies in the rater's tracking of the landmark points as well as other errors that are related to the voxel size, such as rigid registration and manual segmentation errors.

Using the optimal values of all parameters, simulated target images of the used dataset are compared to real ones in Figure 18. Image intensities in the tumor and a small peri-tumor region are different between the simulated and target images – perhaps an indication of tumor infiltration or edema spread between the starting and target images, which was not accounted for in the definition of regions T_r and D_r. Despite such signal differences inside and in the vicinity of the tumor, the results indicate that for the optimal values of the model parameters the model can reproduce the true deformation caused by tumor growth in the brain tissues with sufficient accuracy and therefore can serve as a good forward model for this deformation.

4.3.7.6. Simulations From Normal Brain Images   Model simulations with different values of the four model parameters $\mathbf{c}_t$, r_t, r_e, and P will be used in Section 4.4.1 to generate a large number of example brain anatomies deformed by tumors of different locations, sizes, and varying degrees of spread of the associated peri-tumor edema. As argued above, in these simulations, the value of the edema expansion strain will be fixed at $e = 0.35$. Here, example results from two such model simulations for the same human subject but for different model parameters are presented. These simulations demonstrate the role of remeshing in simulating large tumors.

A volumetric T1-weighted MR scan of a healthy elderly subject is used in the simulations presented here. The image was segmented into brain tissue and ventricles CSF. Figure 19 presents the results of application of the presented model with parameter values $r_t = 5$mm and $P = 9000$ Pa are presented. No peri-tumor edema was assumed in this case, and the tumor center was chosen in an arbitrary location in the white matter. Without the use of remeshing, the simulation terminates before reaching the final P value because of severe distortion of some tetrahedral mesh elements in vicinity of the tumor. With one-time use of adaptive

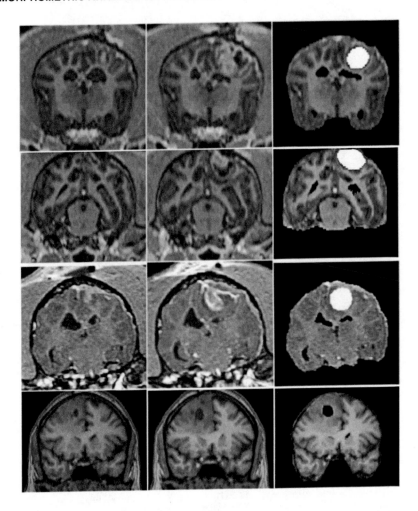

Figure 18. Example cross-sectional images from the starting (left column) and target (middle column) 3D images for all four tumor cases are compared to the deformed images obtained via the optimal parameter values (right column). Rows 1–4 are for DC1, DC2, DC3, and HC, respectively. Tumors in the dog cases are painted white in order to aid visual comparison to the gadolinium-enhanced final images. For HC, the tumor is assigned black.

remeshing halfway through the application of the full pressure, the simulation terminates at the desired value of P. The final volume of the tumor at termination of the simulation was approximately 37 cc (equal to the volume of a sphere with radius ≈ 2.07 cm) compared to 4.6 cc without remeshing (equal to the volume of a sphere with radius ≈ 2.07 cm). As observed in the resulting images, since

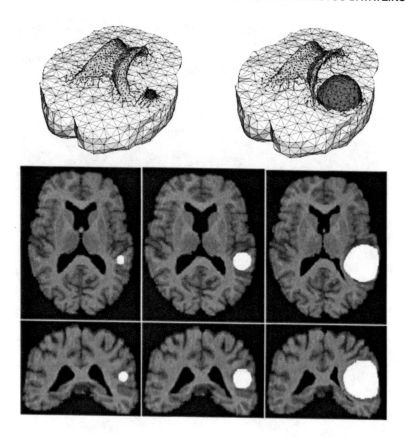

Figure 19. The top row shows a clipped view of an FE mesh generated from volumetric images of a healthy human subject. Surfaces of the ventricles (cyan) and tumor (red) are added. The left image illustrates the mesh at the beginning of the simulation, and the right image illustrates the mesh at termination. The bottom two rows provide transaxial (middle row) and coronal (bottom row) 2D slices of the volumetric images at the beginning of the simulation (left) and at termination (right). One-time remeshing was used halfway through application of pressure P. The middle column shows images from a simulation in which remeshing was not used. This simulation terminated before reaching the final value of P. See attached CD for color version.

the tumor is elastically constrained by the stresses in the surrounding brain tissue, the final tumor shape is not perfectly spherical. For the simulation in Figure 19, the initial mesh had 50,865 elements, with a minimum quality of 0.0235. Before remeshing, 1837 tetrahedra had $q_T \leq 0.02$. After remeshing, 3 elements had $q_T \leq 0.02$, with a minimum quality of $q_T \approx 0.02$. This, however, did not prevent completion of the simulation.

4.4. Statistical Estimation of Mass-Effect Model Parameters

Now, with the availability of the biomechanical model of the brain tumor mass-effect described in Section 3, it is possible to apply such a model to the atlas image in order to produce a version of the atlas image with a tumor. This atlas image will hopefully look more similar to that of the patient, which will make the deformable registration between the two images easier. However, in order to use the biomechanical model, values of this model's parameters Θ that correspond to the patient must be estimated. This is achieved through a statistical estimator as follows.

4.4.1. Statistical model training

The goal of this step is to create a statistical model for the deformation φ_f, which will aid in estimation of Θ for a particular tumor image. First, the deformation maps φ_{c_i}, $i = 1, ..., n_s$, between the atlas and MR images of n_s normal subjects are obtained using HAMMER, a deformable image registration approach designed for normal-to-normal brain image registration [52]. Simulations of the mass-effect of tumor growth are then conducted for each subject i for values Θ_j, $j = 1, ..., n_m$, covering a range of the model parameters to produce the deformations $\varphi_{d_{i,j}}$, $i = 1, ..., n_s$, $j = 1, ..., n_m$.

A problem preventing the collection of statistics on $\varphi_{d_{i,j}}$ directly is that the domains of these maps are different for different values of i and j. This precludes the point-to-point comparison of these deformation maps. To overcome this problem, for all tumor model simulations, regions T_{A_j} and D_{A_j} are defined in the atlas space based on Θ_j and mapped to each subject's space via φ_{c_i}, $i = 1, ..., n_s$. Next, for $\mathbf{X}_A \in A\backslash T_{A_j}$, $i = 1, ..., n_s$, $j = 1, ..., n_m$, define the displacement maps

$$\mathbf{u}_{d_{i,j}}(\mathbf{X}_A) \equiv \varphi_{f_{i,j}}(\mathbf{X}_A) - \varphi_{c_i}(\mathbf{X}_A) \tag{12}$$
$$\equiv \varphi_{d_{i,j}}(\varphi_{c_i}(\mathbf{X}_A)) - \varphi_{c_i}(\mathbf{X}_A), \tag{13}$$
$$\mathbf{u}_{c_{i,j}}(\mathbf{X}_A) \equiv \varphi_{c_i}(\mathbf{X}_A) - \mathbf{X}_A, \tag{14}$$
$$\mathbf{u}_{f_{i,j}}(\mathbf{X}_A) \equiv \varphi_{f_{c_i}}(\mathbf{X}_A) - \mathbf{X}_A, \tag{15}$$

which implies

$$\mathbf{u}_{f_{i,j}}(\mathbf{X}_A) = \mathbf{u}_{c_i}(\mathbf{X}_A) + \mathbf{u}_{d_{i,j}}(XA). \tag{16}$$

For different $i = 1, ..., n_s$ but the same $j = 1, ..., n_m$, the domains of $\mathbf{u}_{d_{i,j}}$ are the same. An example of a tumor model simulation and the involved displacement maps is shown in Figure 20.

Discrete versions of the displacement maps $\mathbf{u}_{c_i}$ and $\mathbf{u}_{d_{i,j}}$ are constructed by sampling their Cartesian components for all voxels in the atlas with coordinates $X_{A_k} \in B_A\backslash M_A$, $k = 1, ..., n_p$, to yield the $3n_p \times 1$ vectors $\mathbf{U}_{c_i}$ and $\mathbf{U}_{d_{i,j}}$, respectively. It is possible to see that the vectors $\mathbf{U}_{c_i}$ act as displacement-based

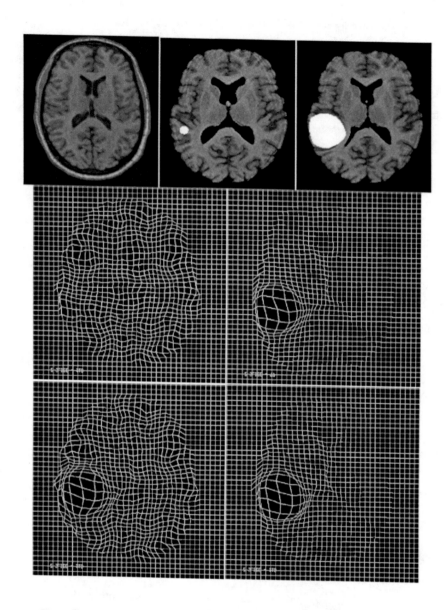

Figure 20. Illustration of a tumor mass-effect simulation and the associate displacement maps. Top row (left to right): atlas image, normal subject's MR image with an introduced small tumor, and resulting image after simulation of tumor mass-effect. Middle row: displacement map $\mathbf{u}_c$ (left) and displacement map $\varphi_d - \mathbf{X}_S$ (right). Bottom row: displacement map $\mathbf{u}_d$ (left) and displacement map $\mathbf{u}_c$ (right). Copyright ©2006, Elsevier B. V.

representations for the undeformed brain shapes of subjects $i = 1, ..., n_s$. Similarly, the vectors $\mathbf{U}_{c_i} + \mathbf{U}_{d_{i,j}}$ are representations of the deformed brain shapes of subjects $i = 1, ..., n_s$ for values of the tumor model parameters $\Theta_j, j = 1, ..., n_m$.

Assuming that $\mathbf{U}_{c_i}, i = 1, ..., n_s$, are independent realizations of a Gaussian random vector, principal component analysis (PCA) is applied to these vectors to yield the mean $\boldsymbol{\mu}_c$ and the $3n_p \times m_c$ matrix $\mathbf{V}_c$ whose columns are the first m_c principal components ($m_c \leq n_s - 1$). Next, we compute the component of $\mathbf{U}_{d_{i,j}}$ in the subspace orthogonal to the columns of $\mathbf{V}_c$ as

$$\mathbf{U}'_{d_{i,j}} = \mathbf{U}_{d_{i,j}} - \mathbf{V}_c \mathbf{V}_c^T \mathbf{U}_{d_{i,j}}$$

Further, assuming that for each j, $\mathbf{U}'_{d_{i,j}}, j = 1, ..., n_s$, are independent realizations of a Gaussian random vector, PCA is performed on these vectors to yield the mean $\boldsymbol{\mu}_{d_j}$ and the $3n_p \times m_{d_j}$ matrices $\mathbf{V}_{d_j}$ whose columns are the first m_{d_j} principal components associated with eigenvalues $\lambda_{d_j,l}, l = 1, ..., m_{d_j}$ ($m_{d_j} \leq n_s - 1$). It is now possible to approximate the discrete displacement map $\mathbf{V}_f$ between the atlas and a subject with a simulated tumor with parameters Θ_j, $j = 1, ..., n_m$, as follows:

$$\mathbf{U}_f \approx \boldsymbol{\mu}_c + \mathbf{V}_c \mathbf{a} + \boldsymbol{\mu}_{d_j} + \mathbf{V}_{d_j} \mathbf{b}_j.$$

Each of the vectors $\mathbf{a}$ and $\mathbf{b}_j = \begin{bmatrix} b_{j,1}, ..., b_{j,m_{d_j}} \end{bmatrix}^T$ follows a Gaussian distribution with decorrelated components, with that of $\mathbf{b}_j$ explicitly stated here as

$$f_j(b_j) = \frac{1}{\displaystyle\prod_{l=1}^{m_{d_j}} \sqrt{2\pi\lambda_{d_j,l}}} \exp\left(-0.5 \sum_{l=1}^{m_{d_j}} \frac{b_{j,l}^2}{\lambda_{d_j,l}}\right)$$

for $j = 1, ..., n_m$.

4.4.2. Statistical estimation

Given an approximate deformation map $\tilde{\varphi}_f$ (between a real tumor patient's image and the atlas image) obtained by the direct use of deformable image registration, the goal of the methods presented here is to obtain an estimate $\hat{\Theta}$ of the tumor model parameters. The displacement map $\tilde{\mathbf{u}}_f$ defined in a similar manner to Eq. (15) is also discretized over all the atlas voxels in $B_A \backslash M_A$ and represented by a vector $\tilde{\mathbf{U}}_f$. Owing to the orthogonality of $\mathbf{V}_{d,j}$ to $\mathbf{V}_c$ for all j, the component of this displacement that is caused by the tumor can be found by

$$\tilde{\mathbf{U}}_d = \tilde{\mathbf{U}}_f - \boldsymbol{\mu}_c \mathbf{V}_c \tilde{\mathbf{a}},$$

where $\tilde{a} = V_c^T (U_f - \mu_f)$. The likelihood that $\tilde{U}_d = \tilde{U}_f - \mu_c - V_c\tilde{a}$ is generated with tumor model parameters Θ_j is defined as

$$L_j \equiv f\left(\tilde{b}_j\right),$$

where

$$\tilde{b}_j^T = V_{d,j}\left(U_d - \mu_{d,j}\right)$$

for $j = 1, ..., n_m$. The estimate of the tumor model parameters is given by

$$\hat{\Theta} = \frac{\sum\limits_{j=1}^{n_m} L_j\Theta_j}{\sum\limits_{j=1}^{n_m} L_j}.$$

4.5. Registration Results

Results of applying the approach described above are reported here for two tumor cases. The first is an MR image of a patient with a glioma and a large region of peri-tumor edema. The second is a simulated tumor image obtained by applying the mass-effect model described in Section 4.3 to an MR image of a normal subject. Both images are registered to an anatomical brain atlas that is composed of a T1-weighted MR scan of a normal subject and an associated manual segmentation of 106 cortical and subcortical brain structures. Both subject's images are also T1-weighted MR scans. The atlas image dimensions are $256 \times 256 \times 198$, and the voxel size is $1 \times 1 \times 1$ mm. The real and simulated tumor images are both of dimension $256 \times 256 \times 124$ and voxel size $0.9375 \times 0.9375 \times 1.5$ mm.

The FE tumor mass-effect model simulations comprise the most computationally intensive step of the presented approach. In order to make the statistical training step tractable, tumor simulations were performed on $n_s = 20$ MR brain images of normal subjects. For each subject $n_m = 64$ simulations were performed, with two values of each of the six model parameters covering the range expected for the real tumor case. The parameter values were $r_t \in [3, 5]$ mm, $r_e \in [20, 27]$ mm, $P \in [2, 5]$ kPa, and corners of a cube in the atlas for the simulated tumor center locations.

The simulations were carried out using the FE software ABAQUS [96]. The average time needed to perform one simulation was about 35 minutes on a 900-MHZ processor Origin 300 SGI processor machine with 4Gb of RAM. For the results reported here, all principal components of the displacement U_c were retained and $m_{d_j} = 1, j = 1, ..., n_m$, was used.

Modeling the statistical properties of shape and deformation over the whole of the atlasl domain except for M_A requires the use of a very high-dimensional space to represent these shapes or deformations. Beside the limitation imposed by

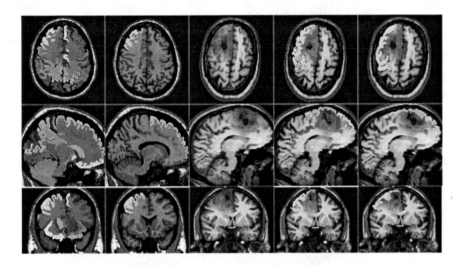

Figure 21. Three orthogonal 2D images of the atlas and the real tumor patient before and after deformable registration. Some labels associated with the atlas image are warped and superimposed on the patient's images. Left to right: atlas image with all labels; atlas image with five selected labels near the tumor area; patient's image; patient's image with superimposed labels warped from the atlas via direct deformable registration between the two images; and the patient's image with superimposed labels warped from the atlas via the proposed approach. The five selected labels are: the right middle frontal gyrus (green), the right medial frontal gyrus (dark green), the right superior frontal gyrus (cyan), the right cingulate region (magenta), and the left cingulate region (brown). Copyright ©2006, Elsevier B. V. See attached CD for color version.

the available computer memory size, with the relatively small number of available training samples, statistical models constructed using PCA are sensitive to data noise and may be unable to generalize to valid shape or deformation instances not used during training. Here, to deal with this problem, the statistical properties of only a part of the atlas domain immediately outside M_A was modeled. This region was obtained by several iterations of morphological dilation of region M_A followed by subtraction of M_A from the resulting region. The number of voxels in the modeled region of the atlas domain was typically a few thousand voxels (≈ 5000).

In Figure 21, the results of applying the proposed approach to register the image of the real tumor subject to the atlas is demonstrated. With the use of deformable registration to directly register the (normal) atlas image to the patient's MR image, the warping result is innaccurate in the tumor area. Gray matter from the right cingulate region and adjacent cortical CSF in the atlas were stretched to match the intensity of the tumor and the surrounding edema in the patient's image. The area M_A where the registration is inaccurate was outlined manually.

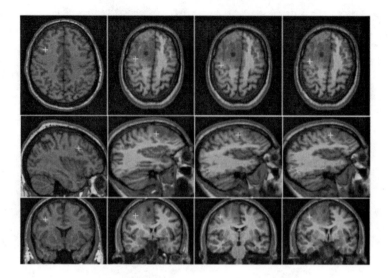

Figure 22. Locations of one manually selected landmark point in three orthogonal 2D images of the atlas and the patient before and after deformable registration. The landmark point is marked with a green cross. Left to right: atlas image, patient's image with the manually selected landmark point; patient's image with the warped landmark point from the atlas with direct use of deformable registration; and the patient's image with the warped landmark point from the atlas with the proposed approach. Copyright ©2006, Elsevier B. V. See attached CD for color version.

The estimated tumor model parameters were $\hat{\mathbf{c}}_t = (109, 86, 126)$, $\hat{r}_t = 3.9$ mm, $\hat{r}_e = 24$ mm, and $\hat{P} = 3.55$ Pa. In order to quantitatively assess the improvement in registration accuracy due to the proposed approach, 21 landmark points were selected around the tumor area in the patient's images and corresponding points were identified by an expert in the atlas. The point coordinates were mapped through the resulting deformation map with direct deformable registration, and with the approach described above. The location of one landmark point in the atlas image and the patient's image before and after registration are shown in Figure 22. The results for all 21 points are presented in Table 3. The maximum error was reduced by 71% via the use of the presented approach while the mean error was reduced by 57.6%.

Similar deformable registration experiments were performed on a simulated tumor case based on an MR scan of a normal subject. Using the biomechanical model described in Section 4.3, a simulation was performed on the image of the normal subject with simulation parameters $\mathbf{c}_t = (106, 86, 128)$, $r_t = 4.5$ mm, $r_e = 21$ mm, and $P = 4.5$ kPa. Using the approach described above, the estimated values of these parameters were $\hat{\mathbf{c}}_t = (109, 85, 128)$, $\hat{r}_t = 4.1$ mm, $\hat{r}_e = 23$ mm, and $\hat{P} = 3.6$ kPa. The warping of some labels associated with the atlas to the subject's image near the tumor area are shown in Figure 23.

Table 3. Deformable Registration Error Statistics
for Landmark Points in the Real Tumor
(RT) and Simulated Tumor (ST) Cases

	Minimum	Mean	Maximum	Standard Deviation
RT no Model, mm	1.06	8.70	24.87	6.19
RT with Model, mm	0.47	3.69	7.19	1.83
ST no Model, mm	2.54	6.39	10.91	2.62
ST with Model, mm	0.61	3.90	7.79	2.01

For each case, the errors are provided for the direct deformable image registration to the atlas (no model), and the registration using the approach described in this work (with model). 21 landmark points were used for RT and 25 for ST.

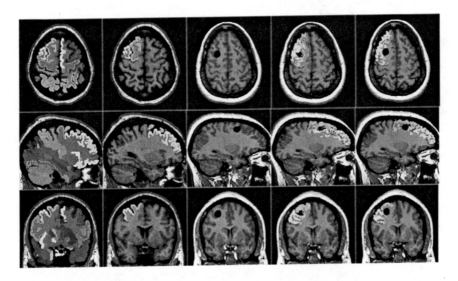

Figure 23. Three orthogonal 2D images of the atlas and the simulated tumor subject before and after deformable registration. Some labels associated with the atlas image are warped and superimposed on the subject's images. Left to right: atlas image with all labels; atlas image with five selected labels; subject's image; subject's image with superimposed labels warped from the atlas via direct deformable registration between the two images; and the subject's image with superimposed labels warped from the atlas via the proposed approach. The five selected labels are the same as those shown in Figure 21 for the real tumor case. Copyright ©2006, Elsevier B. V. See attached CD for color version.

To evaluate the registration error in this case, 25 points were selected arbitrarily in the area around the simulated tumor, and their corresponding coordinates (found through $\varphi_d \circ \varphi_c$, which is available in this case) were computed in the atlas image and treated as ground truth. The errors for the direct deformable registration and that obtained by the proposed approach are also presented in Table 3. The maximum error was reduced by 29% using the proposed approach and the corresponding average error was reduced by 39%.

4.6. Discussion and Future Work

We have here presented an approach for the deformable registration of normal anatomical atlases to brain tumor images. The approach utilizes a 3D biomechanical FE model of tumor-induced deformation to introduce and simulate the tumor mass-effect in the atlas image. HAMMER [52], a readily available deformable image registration method, is then used to find the map between the atlas with the simulated tumor and the patient's image. To solve the inverse problem of determining the parameters of the biomechanical model, a statistical approach is used. This approach relies on decomposition of the desired deformation map (between the atlas and the tumor-bearing patient's image) into the sum of two maps in orthogonal subspaces, defined on the same domain, but with different statistical properties. The first deformation map is from the atlas to another normal brain image. The second is the deformation map from the normal brain image to one that is deformed by the biomechanical model of tumor mass-effect. The statistical properties of both of these deformation maps are learned via PCA from a number of training samples. Owing to the orthogonality of the two components of the modeled deformation map, an initial rough estimate of this deformation map is projected on the subspace representing tumor-induced deformation and is used to estimate the tumor mass-effect model parameters.

The results of applying the proposed approach on a real tumor case and a simulated one indicate significant reduction in the registration error. These experiments should be regarded as a proof-of-concept study. More validation experiments are needed to assess the viability of the proposed approach for a variety of tumor cases of different grades, types, and sizes. In addition, the sensitivity of the statistical estimator of the model parameters to the number of used principal components and the number of training samples also present important directions for future investigations. Another possible extension to the approach presented here is to iteratively refine the estimate of the tumor model parameters, based on the latest available deformation map (iterate through steps 2 to 5 in the procedure in Section 4.2).

HAMMER, the used deformable registration method, was designed to deal with images of two normal subjects. The presence of the tumor and edema in the images present a significant challenge to the image matching, especially since these regions may not be exactly matching in two images. An image registration method that takes into account such differences between the images is expected to further improve the final deformable registration result.

Another complication associated with the deformable registration of brain tumor images is the significant signal changes associated with edema in MR images. Edema typically causes hypointensity changes in T1-weighted images, which makes it difficult to discern cortical sulci in the affected brain regions. It is therefore not possible to obtain an accurate deformable registration in these regions based on image matching alone. The coordinates of brain structures masked by edema, however, may be estimated from the known structures (outside the edema region) through a statistical estimation approach [98].

Dealing with the small sample size problem for statistical learning in very high-dimensional spaces is another challenging problem that needs to be addressed in future work. This problem made it necessary to collect statistics over part, and not the whole, of the atlas domain outside M_A. Rather than restricting the region of the atlas space where statistics are collected, an alternative approach to dealing with statistical learning problem in high-dimensional spaces from a small sample size was presented in [103]. This approach collects the statistics via PCA over subspaces constructed from a wavelet packet basis, and that correspond to different levels of detail of the analyzed shape or deformation.

5. CONCLUSION

Voxel-based morphometric analysis provides an unbiased way of examining high-dimensionality image data, in that it does not rely on any a priori hypotheses regarding the regions of interest to be examined, but it analyzes the entire image dataset and identifies regions in which morphological measurements are of interest (e.g., regions in which volumetric measurements differ between normal controls and patients, or between two serial scans). There is a plethora of voxel-based morphometric analysis methods [104], each of which has merits and limitations.

In the first part of this chapter, we described a technique based on high-dimensional elastic warping of brain images, formulated in a mass-preserving framework so that tissue volumes are properly preserved and measured in this process. We also discussed advantages of high-dimensional pattern classification and multivariate analysis over voxel-based (mass-univariate) methods, since the former capture complex associations among image measurements in different parts of the brain. We also presented a few representative studies in which tissue density statistical analysis was used as a means for volumetric analysis.

In the second part of this chapter, we presented an approach for deformable registration of brain tumor images. Solving this deformable registration problem makes available methods for brain image morphometry able to assist in quantifying and understanding changes in brain structure due to the presence of a brain tumor. In addition, deformable registration between brain tumor images and a brain template will facilitate the construction of statistical brain tumor atlases that will be instrumental in neurosurgery and radiotherapy planning, and in the study of brain cancer.

Future work in the field of voxel-based morphometry is certain to pursue better methods for accurately warping one anatomical image to another, as well as powerful methods for multivariate analysis, which is a particularly difficult task in view of the huge dimensionality of spatiotemporal image measurements.

6. ACKNOWLEDGMENTS

The authors would like to thank Dr. James Anderson and Ms. Carolyn Magee, of the Johns Hopkins University School of Medicine, and Dr. Edward Herskovits of the University of Pennsylvania School of Medicine for planning and executing the procedures of the dog tumor model. The authors also extend their gratitude to Dr. Nick Fox at University College London for providing the serial scans of the studied human case. This work was supported in part by the National Science Foundation under Engineering Research Center grant EEC9731478, and by National Institutes of Health grant R01NS42645.

7. REFERENCES

1. Davatzikos C, Resnick SM. 2002. Degenerative age changes in white matter connectivity visualized in vivo using magnetic resonance imaging. *Cereb Cortex* **12**:767–771.

2. Davatzikos C, Genc A, Xu D, Resnick SM. 2001. Voxel-based morphometry using the Ravens maps: methods and validation using simulated longitudinal atrophy. *NeuroImage* **14**:1361–1369.

3. Resnick SM, Pham DL, Kraut MA, Zonderman AB, Davatzikos C. 2003. Longitudinal magnetic resonance imaging studies of older adults: a shrinking brain. *J Neurosci* **23**:3295–3301.

4. Shen D, Liu D, Liu H, Clasen L, Giedd J, Davatzikos C. 2004. Automated morphometric study of brain variation in xxy males. *NeuroImage* **23**:648–653.

5. Bobinski M, de Leon MJ, Convit A, De Santi S, Wegiel J, Tarshish CY, Saint Louis LA, Wisniewski HM. 1999. MRI of entorhinal cortex in mild Alzheimer's disease. *Lancet* **353**:38–40.

6. Convit A, De Leon MJ, Tarshish C, De Santi S, Tsui W, Rusinek H, George A, 1997. Specific hippocampal volume reductions in individuals at risk for Alzheimer's disease. *Neurobiol Aging* **18**:131–138.

7. Cuenod CA, Denys A, Michot JL, Jehenson P, Forette F, Kaplan D, Syrota A, Boller F. 1993. Amygdala atrophy in Alzheimer's disease: an in vivo magnetic resonance imaging study. *Arch Neurol* **50**:941–945.

8. De Santi S, de Leon MJ, Rusinek H, Convit A, Tarshish CY, Roche A, Tsui WH, Kandil E, Boppana M, Daisley K, Wang GJ, Schlyer D, Fowler J. 2001. Hippocampal formation glucose metabolism and volume losses in MCI and AD. *Neurobiol Aging* **22**:529–539.

9. deToledo-Morrell L, Sullivan MP, Morrell F, Wilson RS, Bennett DA, Spencer S. 1997. Alzheimer's disease: in vivo detection of differential vulnerability of brain regions. *Neurobiol Aging* **18**:463–438.

10. Dickerson BC, Goncharova I, Sullivan MP, Forchetti C, Wilson RS, Bennett DA, Beckett LA, deToledo-Morrell L. 2001. MRI-derived entorhinal and hippocampal atrophy in incipient and very mild Alzheimer's disease. *Neurobiol Aging* **22**:747–754.

11. Du AT, Schuff N, Amend D, Laakso MP, Hsu YY, Jagust WJ, Yaffe K, Kramer JH, Reed B, Norman D, Chui HC, Weiner MW. 2001. Magnetic resonance imaging of the entorhinal cortex and hippocampus in mild cognitive impairment and Alzheimer's disease. *J Neurol Neurosurg Psychiatry* **71**:441–447.

12. Frisoni GB, Beltramello A, Weiss C, Geroldi C, Bianchetti A, Trabucchi M. 1996. Linear measures of atrophy in mild Alzheimer disease. *Am J Neuroradiol* **17**:913–923.

13. Jack Jr CR, Petersen RC, Xu YC, Waring SC, O'Brien PC, Tangalos EG, Smith GE, Ivnik RJ, Kokmen E. 1997. Medial temporal atrophy on MRI in normal aging and very mild Alzheimer's disease. *Neurology* **49**:786–794.

14. Jack CR, Petersen RC, Xu YC, O'Brien PC, Smith GE, Ivnik RJ, Boeve BF, Waring SC, Tangalos E, Kokmen E. 1999. Prediction of AD with MRI-based hippocampal volume in mild cognitive impairment. *Neurology* **52**:1397–1403.

15. Killiany RJ, Moss MB, Albert MS, Sandor T, Tieman J, Jolesz F. 1993. Temporal lobe regions on magnetic resonance imaging identify patients with early Alzheimer's disease. *Arch Neurol* **50**:949–954.

16. Killiany RJ, Gomez-Isla T, Moss M, Kikinis R, Sandor T, Jolesz F, Tanzi R, Jones K, Hyman. BT, Albert MS. 2000. Use of structural magnetic resonance imaging to predict who will get Alzheimer's disease. *Ann Neurol* **47**:430–439.

17. Krasuski JS, Alexander GE, Horwitz B, Daly EM, Murphy DG, Rapoport SI, Schapiro MB. 1998. Volumes of medial temporal lobe structures in patients with Alzheimer's disease and mild cognitive impairment (and in healthy controls). *Biol Psychiatry* **43**:60–68.

18. Laakso MP, Soininen H, Partanen K, Helkala EL, Hartikainen P, Vainio P, Hallikainen M, Hanninen T, Riekkinen Sr PJ. 1995. Volumes of hippocampus, amygdala and frontal lobes in the MRI-based diagnosis of early Alzheimer's disease: correlation with memory functions. *J Neural Transm Park Dis Dement Sect* **9**:73–86.

19. Laakso MP, Hallikainen M, Hanninen T, Partanen K, Soininen H. 2000. Diagnosis of Alzheimer's disease: MRI of the hippocampus vs delayed recall. *Neuropsychologia* **38**:579–584.

20. Lehericy S, Baulac M, Chiras J, Pierot L, Martin N, Pillon B, Deweer B, Dubois B, Marsault C. 1994. Amygdalohippocampal MR volume measurements in the early stages of Alzheimer disease. *Am J Neuroradiol* **15**:929–937.

21. Rosen AC, Prull MW, Gabrieli JD, Stoub T, O'Hara R, Friedman L, Yesavage JA, deToledo-Morrell L. 2003. Differential associations between entorhinal and hippocampal volumes and memory performance in older adults. *Behav Neurosci* **117**:1150–1160.

22. Xu Y, Jack Jr CR, O'Brien PC, Kokmen E, Smith GE, Ivnik RJ, Boeve BF, Tangalos RG, Petersen RC. 2000. Usefulness of MRI measures of entorhinal cortex versus hippocampus in AD. *Neurology* **54**:1760–1767.

23. Bookstein FL. 1989. Principal warps: thin-plate splines and the decomposition of deformations. *IEEE Trans Pattern Anal Machine Intell* **11**:567–585.

24. Miller MI, Christensen G, Amit Y, Grenander U. 1943. Mathematical textbook of deformable neuroanatomies. *Proc Natl Acad Sci USA* **90**:11944–11948.

25. Davatzikos C, Vaillant M, Resnick S, Prince JL, Letovsky S, Bryan RN. 1996. A computerized approach for morphological analysis of the corpus callosum. *J Comput Assist Tomogr* **20**:88–97.

26. Sandor S, Leahy R. 1997. Surface-based labelling of cortical anatomy using a deformable atlas. *IEEE Trans Med Imaging* **16**:41–54.

27. Thompson PM, MacDonald D, Mega MS, Holmes CJ, Evans A, Toga AW. 1997. Detection and mapping of abnormal brain structure with a probabilistic atlas of cortical surfaces. *J Comput Assist Tomogr* **21**:567–581.

28. Ashburner J, Hutton C, Frackowiak RSJ, Johnsrude I, Price C, Friston KJ. 1998. Identifying global anatomical differences: deformation-based morphometry. *Hum Brain Mapp* **6**:348–357.

29. Golland P, Grimson WEL, Kikinis R. 1999. Statistical shape analysis using fixed topology skeletons: corpus callosum study. In *Lecture notes in computer science*, Vol. 1613, pp. 382–387. New York: Springer.

30. Pizer S, Fritsch DS, Yushkevich PA, Johnson VE, Chaney EL. 1999. Segmentation, registration and measurement of shape variation via image object shape. *IEEE Trans Med Imaging* **18**:851–865.

31. Golland P, Grimson WEL, Shenton ME, Kikinis R. 2001. Deformation analysis for shape based classification. In *Lecture notes in computer science*, Vol. 2082, pp. 517–530. New York: Springer.

32. Rexilius J, Warfield SK, Guttman CRG, Wei X, Benson R, Wolfson L, Shenton ME, Handels H, Kikinis R. 1999. A novel nonrigid registration algorithm and applications. In *Proceedings of the international conference on medical image computing and computer-assisted intervention (MICCAI'98)*, pp. 202–209.

33. Christensen G, Rabbitt RD, Miller RI. 1994. 3D brain mapping using a deformable neuroanatomy. *Phys Med Biol* **39**:609–618.

34. Joshi S, Pizer S, Fletcher PT, Thall A, Tracton G. 2001. Multi-scale 3-D deformable model segmentation based on medial description. In *Lecture notes in computer science*, Vol. 2082, pp. 64–77. New York: Springer.

35. Szekely G, Kelemen A, Brechbuhler C, Gerig G. 1996. Segmentation of 2-D and 3-D objects from MRI volume data using constrained deformations of flexible Fourier contour and surface models. *Med Image Anal* **1**:19–34.

36. Styner M, Gerig G. 2001. Medial models incorporating object variability for 3d shape analysis. In *Lecture notes in computer science*, Vol. 2082, pp. 502–516. New York: Springer.

37. Freeborough PA, Fox NC. 1998. Modeling brain deformations in Alzheimer's disease by fluid registration of serial 3D MR images. *J Comput Assist Tomogr* **22**:838–843.

38. Collins L, Peters TM, Dai W, Evans AC. 1992. Model-based segmentation of individual brain structures from MRI data. *Proc SPIE* **1808**:10–23.

39. Thompson DW. 1917. *On growth and form*: Cambridge: Cambridge UP.

40. Grenander U. 1983. *Tutorial in pattern theory: a technical report*. Providence: Brown University.

41. Davatzikos C, Resnick SM. 1998. Sex differences in anatomic measures of interhemispheric connectivity: correlations with cognition in men but not in women. *Cereb Cortex* **8**:635–640.

42. Lorenzen P, Davis B, Joshi S. 2005. Unbiased atlas formation via large deformations metric mapping. In *Proceedings of the international conference on medical image computing and computer-assisted intervention (MICCAI'2005). Lecture notes in computer science*, Vol. 2717, pp. 411–418. New York: Springer.

43. Park H, Peyton HB, Hero III AO, Meyer CR. 2005. Least biased target selection in probabilistic atlas construction. In *Proceedings of the international conference on medical image computing and computer-assisted intervention (MICCAI'2005). Lecture notes in computer science*, Vol. 3750, pp. 419–426. New York: Springer.

44. Christensen GE, Johnson HJ. 2001. Consistent image registration. *IEEE Trans Med Imaging* **20**:568–582.

45. Collins DL, Neelin P, Peters TM, Evans AC. 1994. Automatic 3D intersubject registration of MR volumetric data in standardized Talairach space. *J Comput Assist Tomogr* **18**:192–205.

46. Rueckert D, Sonoda LI, Hayes C, Hill DLG, Leach MO, Hawkes DJ. 1999. Non-rigid registration using free-form deformations: application to breast MR images. *IEEE Trans Med Imaging* **18**:712–721.

47. Thirion JP. 1996. Non-rigid matching using deamons. In *Proceedings of the IEEE international conference on computer vision and pattern recognition (CVPR)*, pp. 245–151. Washington, DC: IEEE Computer Society.

48. Ferrant M, Warfield S, Guttman CRG, Mulkern RV, Jolesz F, Kikinis R. 1999. 3D image matching using a finite element based elastic deformation model. In *Proceedings of the international conference on medical image computing and computer-assisted intervention (MICCAI'98). Lecture notes in computer science*, Vol. 1679. pp. 202–209. New York: Springer.

49. Friston KJ, Ashburner J, Frith CD, Poline JB, Heather JD, Frackowiak RSJ. 1995. Spatial registration and normalization of images. *Hum Brain Mapp* 2:165–189.

50. Chung MK, Worsley KJ, Paus T, Cherif C, Collins DL, Giedd JN, Rapoport JL, Evanst AC. 2001. A unified statistical approach to deformation-based morphometry. *Neuroimage* 14:595–606.

51. Christensen GE. 1999. Consistent linear-elastic transformations for image matching. In *Proceedings of the international conference on medical image computing and computer-assisted intervention (MICCAI'98). Lecture notes in computer science*, vol. 1613, pp. 224–237. New York: Springer.

52. Shen D, Davatzikos C. 2002. HAMMER: hierarchical attribute matching mechanism for elastic registration. *IEEE Trans Med Imaging* 21:1421–1439.

53. Viola P, Wells III WM. 1997. Alignment by maximization of mutual information. *Int J Comput Vision* 24(2):133–154.

54. Wells WM III, Viola P, Kikinis R. 1995. Multi-modal volume registration by maximization of mutual information. In *Proceedings of the second international symposium on medical robotics and computer assisted surgery*, pp. 55–62. New York: Wiley.

55. Davatzikos C. 1996. Spatial normalization of 3D images using deformable models. *J Comput Assist Tomogr* 20:656–665.

56. Thompson P, Toga AW. 1996. A surface-based technique for warping three-dimensional images of the brain. *IEEE Trans Med Imaging* 15:402–417.

57. Wang Y, Staib LH. 1999. Elastic model-based non-rigid registration incorporating statistical shape information. In *Proceedings of the international conference on medical image computing and computer-assisted intervention (MICCAI'98). Lecture notes in computer science*, Vol. 1496, pp. 1162–1173. New York: Springer.

58. Wang Y, Peterson BS, Staib LH. 2003. 3D brain surface matching based on geodesics and local geometry. *Comput Vision Image Understand* 89:252–271.

59. Rangarajan A, Chui H, Bookstein FL. 1997. The softassign procrustes matching algorithm. In *Proceedings of the 15th international conference on information processing in medical imaging. Lecture notes in computer science*, Vol. 1230, pp. 29–42. New York: Springer.

60. Chui H, Rangarajan A. 2003. A new point matching algorithm for non-rigid registration. *Comput Vision Image Understand* 89:114–141.

61. Shen DG, Davatzikos C. 2003. Very high resolution morphometry using mass-preserving deformations and HAMMER elastic registration. *NeuroImage* 18:28–41.

62. Shen D. 2004. 4D image warping for measurement of longitudinal brain changes. In *Proceedings of the IEEE international symposium on biomedical imaging*, Vol. 1, pp. 904–907. Washington, DC: IEEE Computer Society.

63. Xue Z, Shen D, Davatzikos C. 2003. Correspondence detection using wavelet-based attribute vectors. In *Proceedings of the international conference on medical image computing and computer-assisted intervention (MICCAI 2003). Lecture notes in computer science*, Vol. 2870, pp. 762–770. New York: Springer.

64. Xue Z, Shen D, Davatzikos C. 2006. Determining correspondence in 3D MR brain images using attribute vectors as morphological signatures of voxels. *IEEE Trans Med Imaging* 25(5):626–630.

65. Johnson HJ, Christensen G. 2001. Landmark and intensity-based consistent thin-plate spline image registration. In *Proceedings of the international conference on information processing in medical imaging. Lecture notes in computer science*, Vol. 2081, pp. 329–343. New York: Springer.

66. Davatzikos C. 2001. Measuring biological shape using geometry-based shape transformations. *Image Vision Comput* **19**:63–74.

67. Ashburner J, Friston KJ. 2000. Voxel-based morphometry: the methods. *Neuroimage* **11**:805–821.

68. Good CD, Scahill RI, Fox NC, Ashburner J, Friston KJ, Chan D, Crum WR, N. Rossor M, Frackowiak RSJ. 2002. Automatic differentiation of anatomical patterns in the human brain: Validation with studies of degenerative dementias. *Neuroimage* **17**:29–46.

69. Goldszal AF, Davatzikos C, Pham D, Yan M, Bryan RN, Resnick SM. 1998. An image processing protocol for the analysis of MR images from an elderly population. *J Comput Assist Tomogr* **22**:827–837.

70. Davatzikos C. 1998. Mapping of image data to stereotaxic spaces. *Hum Brain Mapp* **6**:334–338.

71. Shen D, Davatzikos C. 2004. Measuring temporal morphological changes robustly in Brain MR images via 4-dimensional template warping. *NeuroImage* **21**:1508–1517.

72. Lao Z, Shen D, Xue Z, Karacali B, Resnick SM, Davatzikos C. 2003. Morphological classification of brains via high-dimensional shape transformations and machine learning methods. *Neuroimage* **21**:46–57.

73. Gerig G, Styner M, Lieberman J. 2001. Shape versus size: improved understanding of the morphology of brain structures. In *Proceedings of the international conference on medical image computing and computer-assisted intervention (MICCAI 2001). Lecture notes in computer science*, Vol. 2208, pp. 24–32. New York: Springer.

74. Braak H, Braak E, Bohl J, Bratzke H. 1998. Evolution of Alzheimer's disease related cortical lesions. *J Neural Transm* (suppl) **54**:97–106.

75. Moffat SD, Szekely CA, Zonderman AB, Kabani NJ, Resnick SM. 2000. Longitudinal change in hippocampal volume as a function of apolipoprotein E genotype. *Neurology* **55**:134–136.

76. Resnick SM, Goldszal A, Davatzikos C, Golski S, Kraut MA, Metter EJ, Bryan RN, Zonderman AB. 2000. One-year age changes in MRI brain volumes in older adults. *Cereb Cortex* **10**:464–472.

77. Dawant BM, Hartmann SL, Gadamsetty S. 1999. Brain atlas deformation in the presence of large space-occupying tumours. In *Proceedings of the international conference on medical image computing and computer-assisted intervention (MICCAI'99). Lecture notes in computer science*, Vol. 1679, pp. 589–596. New York: Springer.

78. Cuadra MB, Pollo C, Bardera A, Cuisenaire O, Villemure J-G, Thiran J-P. 2004. Atlas-based segmentation of pathological MR brain images using a model of lesion growth. *IEEE Trans Med Imaging* **23**:1301–1314.

79. Kyriacou S, Davatzikos C, Zinreich S, Bryan R. 1999. Nonlinear elastic registration of brain images with tumor pathology using a biomechanical model. *IEEE Trans Med Imaging* **18**:580–592.

80. Kansal AR, Torquato S, Harsh IGR, Chiocca EA, Deisboeck TS. 2000. Simulated brain tumor growth dynamics using a three-dimensional cellular automaton. *J Theor Biol* **203**:367–382.

81. Wasserman R, Acharya R. 1996. A patient-specific in vivo tumor model [review]. *Math Biosci* **136**:111–140.

82. Greenspan HP. 1976. On the growth and stability of cell cultures and solid tumors. *J Theor biol* **56**:229–242.

83. Kuroiwa T, Ueki M, Suemasu H, Taniguchi I, Okeda R. 1997. Biomechanical characteristics of brain edema: the difference between vasogenic-type and cytotoxic-type edema. *Acta Neurochir Suppl (Wien)* **60**:158–161.

84. Nagashima T, Tamaki N, Takada M, Tada Y. 1994. Formation and resolution of brain edema associated with brain tumors: a comprehensive theoretical model and clinical analysis. *Acta Neurochir Suppl (Wien)* **60**:165–167.

85. Skrinjar O, Nabavi A, Duncan J. 2002. Model-driven brain shift compensation. *Med Image Anal* **6**:361–373.

86. Ferrant M, Warfield S, Nabavi A, Macq B, Kikinis R. 2000. Registration of 3D intraoperative MR images of the brain using a finite element biomechanical model. In *Proceedings of the international conference on medical image computing and computer-assisted intervention (MICCAI 2000). Lecture notes in computer science*, Vol. 1935, pp. 19–28. New York: Springer

87. Hagemann A, Rohr K, Stiehl HS. 2002. Coupling of fluid and elastic models for biomechanical simulations of brain deformations using FEM. *Med Image Anal* **6**:375–388.

88. Clatz O, Sermesant M, Bondiau P-Y, Delingette H, Warfield SK, Malandain G, Ayache N. 2005. Realistic simulation of the 3D growth of brain tumors in MR images coupling diffusion with mass effect. *IEEE Trans Med Imaging* **24**:1334–1346.

89. Takizawa H, Sugiura K, Baba M, Miller JD. 1994. Analysis of intracerebral hematoma shapes by numerical computer simulation using the finite element method. *Neurol Med-Chir* **34**:65–69.

90. Mendis KK, Stalnaker R, Advani SH. 1995. A constitutive relationship for large-deformation finite-element modeling of brain tissue. *J Biomech Eng* **117**:279–285.

91. Miller K, Chinzei K. 1997. Constitutive modelling of brain tissue: experiment and theory. *J Biomech* **30**:1115–1121.

92. Miller K, Chinzei K. 2002. Mechanical properties of brain tissue in tension. *J Biomech* **35**:483–490.

93. Prange MT, Margulies SS. 2002. Regional, directional, and age-dependent properties of the brain undergoing large deformation. *J Biomech Eng* **124**:244–252.

94. Miga M, Paulsen K, Kennedy FE, Hartov A, Roberts D. 1999. Model-updated image-guided neurosurgery using the finite element method: incorporation of the falx cerebri. *IEEE Trans Med Imaging* **18**(10):866–874.

95. Miga M, Paulsen K, Kennedy FE, Hoopes J, Hartov A, Roberts D. 1998. Initial in-vivo analysis of 3d heterogeneous brain computations for model-updated image-guided neurosurgery. In *Proceedings of the international conference on medical image computing and computer-assisted intervention (MICCAI'98). Lecture notes in computer science*, Vol. 1496, pp. 743–752. New York: Springer.

96. ABAQUS, Version 6.1. 2000. Warwick, RI: Hibbitt, Karlsson, and Sorensen Inc.

97. Mohamed A. 2005. *Combining statistical and biomechanical models for estimation of anatomical deformations*. PhD dissertation. Baltimore: Johns Hopkins University.

98. Mohamed A, Kyriacou SK, Davatzikos C. A statistical approach for estimating brain tumor induced deformation. In *Proceedings of the IEEE workshop on mathematical methods in biomedical image analysis (MMBIA'01)*, pp. 52–57. Washington, DC: IEEE Computer Society.

99. Mohamed A, Davatzikos C. 2004. Finite element mesh generation and remeshing from segmented medical images. In *Proceedings of the IEEE workshop on mathematical methods in biomedical image analysis (MMBIA'04)*, Vol. 1, pp. 420–423.

100. Rivara MC. 1997. New longest-edge algorithms for the refinement and/or improvement of unstructured triangulations. *Int J Num Methods Eng* **40**:3313–3324.

101. Wodinsky I, Kensler C, Roll D. 1969. The induction and transplantation of brain tumors in neonatal beagles. *Proc Am Assoc Cancer Res* **10**:99.

102. Studholme C, Hill DLG, Hawkes DJ. 1999. An overlap invariant entropy measure of 3d medical image alignment. *Pattern Recognit* **32**:71–86.

103. Mohamed A, Davatzikos C. 2004. Shape representation via best orthogonal basis selection. In *Proceedings of the international conference on medical image computing and computer-assisted intervention (MICCAI 2000). Lecture notes in computer science*, Vol. 3216, pp. 225–233.

104. Ashburner J, Csernansky JG, Davatzikos C, Fox NC, Frisoni GB, Thompson PM. 2003. Computer-assisted imaging to assess brain structure in healthy and diseased brains. *Lancet (Neurol)* **2**:79–88.

13

EFFICIENT KERNEL DENSITY ESTIMATION
OF SHAPE AND INTENSITY PRIORS
FOR LEVEL SET SEGMENTATION

Daniel Cremers

Department of Computer Science,
University of Bonn
Bonn, Germany

Mikael Rousson

Department of Imaging and Visualization
Siemens Corporate Research,
Princeton, New Jersey, USA

We propose a nonlinear statistical shape model for level set segmentation that can be efficiently implemented. Given a set of training shapes, we perform a kernel density estimation in the low-dimensional subspace spanned by the training shapes. In this way, we are able to combine an accurate model of the statistical shape distribution with efficient optimization in a finite-dimensional subspace. In a Bayesian inference framework, we integrate the nonlinear shape model with a nonparametric intensity model and a set of pose parameters that are estimated in a more direct data-driven manner than in previously proposed level set methods. Quantitative results show superior performance (regarding runtime and segmentation accuracy) of the proposed nonparametric shape prior over existing approaches.

1. INTRODUCTION

Originally proposed in [1, 2] as a means to propagate interfaces in time, the level set method has become increasingly popular as a framework for image

---

Address all correspondence to: Daniel Cremers, Department of Computer Science, University of Bonn, Bonn, Germany. Phone: (49)228-734380; Fax: (49)228-734382. dcremers@cs.uni-bonn.de.

segmentation. The key idea is to represent an interface $\Gamma \subset \Omega$ in the image domain $\Omega \subset \mathbb{R}^3$ implicitly as the zero level set of an embedding function $\phi : \mathbb{R}^3 \to \Omega$:

$$\Gamma = \{x \in \Omega \mid \phi(x) = 0\}, \tag{1}$$

and to evolve Γ by propagating the embedding function ϕ according to an appropriate partial differential equation. The first applications of this level set formalism for the purpose of image segmentation were proposed in [3, 4, 5]. Two key advantages over explicit interface propagation are the independence of a particular parameterization and the fact that the implicitly represented boundary Γ can undergo topological changes such as splitting or merging. This makes the framework well suited for the segmentation of several objects or multiply connected objects.

When segmenting medical images, one commonly has to deal with noise, and missing or misleading image information. For certain imaging modalities such as ultrasound or CT, the structures of interest do not differ much from their background in terms of their intensity distribution (see Figure 1). Therefore, they can no longer be accurately segmented based on the image information alone. In recent years, researchers have therefore proposed to enhance the level set method with statistical shape priors. Given a set of training shapes, one can impose information about which segmentations are *a priori* more or less likely. Such prior shape information was shown to drastically improve segmentation results in the presence of noise or occlusion [6, 7, 8, 9, 10, 11]. Most of these approaches are based on the assumption that the training shapes, encoded by their signed distance function, form a Gaussian distribution. This has two drawbacks: First, the space of signed distance functions is not a linear space; therefore, the mean shape and linear combinations of eigenmodes are typically no longer signed distance functions. Second, even if the space were a linear space, it is not clear why the given set of sample shapes should be distributed according to a Gaussian density. In fact, as we will demonstrate in this work, they are generally not Gaussian distributed. Recently, it was proposed to use nonparametric density estimation in the space of level set functions [8] in order to model nonlinear distributions of training shapes. (The term *nonlinear* refers to the fact that the manifold of permissible shapes is not merely a linear subspace.) While this resolves the above problems, one sacrifices the efficiency of working in a low-dimensional subspace (formed by the first few eigenmodes) to a problem of infinite-dimensional optimization.

In the present chapter, we propose a framework for knowledge-driven level set segmentation that integrates three contributions.[1] First, we propose a statistical shape prior that combines the efficiency of low-dimensional PCA-based methods with the accuracy of nonparametric statistical shape models. The key idea is to perform kernel density estimation in a linear subspace that is sufficiently large to embed all training data. Second, we propose to estimate pose and translation parameters in a more data-driven manner. Thirdly, we optimally exploit the intensity information in the image by using probabilistic intensity models given by kernel density estimates of previously observed intensity distributions.

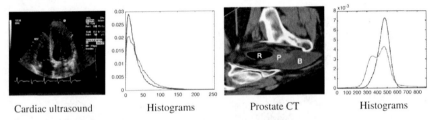

| Cardiac ultrasound | Histograms | Prostate CT | Histograms |

Figure 1. Segmentation challenges and estimated intensity distributions. The two curves on the right correspond to the empirical probability of intensities inside and outside the left ventricle (for the ultrasound image) and the prostate (for the CT image). The region-based segmentation of these structures is a challenging problem, because objects and background have similar histograms. Our segmentation scheme optimally exploits the estimated probabilistic intensity models. See attached CD for color version.

2. LEVEL SET SEGMENTATION AS BAYESIAN INFERENCE

The goal of level set segmentation can be formulated as the estimation of the optimal embedding function $\phi \colon \Omega \to \mathbb{R}$ given an image $I \colon \Omega \to \mathbb{R}$. In the Bayesian framework, this can be computed by maximizing the posterior distribution

$$\mathcal{P}(\phi \,|\, I) \propto \mathcal{P}(I \,|\, \phi)\,\mathcal{P}(\phi). \tag{2}$$

The maximization of (2) results in a problem of infinite-dimensional optimization. Given a set of training shapes encoded by their signed distance functions $\{\phi_i\}_{i=1\ldots N}$, Tsai et al. [7] proposed reducing the segmentation problem to one of finite-dimensional optimization by constraining the optimization problem to the finite-dimensional subspace spanned by the training shapes.

In this chapter we make use of this compact representation of the embedding function. Given the distance d on the space of signed distance functions defined by $d^2(\phi_1, \phi_2) = \int_\Omega (\phi_1(x) - \phi_2(x))^2 \, dx$, we align the set of training shapes with respect to translation and rotation. Subsequently, we constrain the level set function ϕ to a parametric representation of the form:

$$\phi_{\boldsymbol{\alpha},h,\theta}(x) = \phi_0(R_\theta x + h) + \sum_{i=1}^{n} \alpha_i\,\psi_i(R_\theta x + h), \tag{3}$$

where $\phi_0(x) = \frac{1}{N}\sum_{i=1}^{N}\phi_i(x)$ represents the mean shape, $\{\psi_i(x)\}_{i=1\ldots n}$ are the eigenmodes of the distribution, and $n < N$ is the dimension of the subspace spanned by the N training shapes. The parameter vector $\boldsymbol{\alpha} = (\alpha_1, \ldots, \alpha_n)$ models shape deformations, while the parameters $h \in \mathbb{R}^3$ and $\theta \in [0, 2\pi]^3$ model translation and rotation of the respective shape. In our applications, where the scale of objects is known, a generalization to larger transformations groups (e.g., similarity or affine) did not appear useful.

The infinite-dimensional Bayesian inference problem in Eq. (2) is therefore reduced to a finite-dimensional one where the conditional probability,

$$\mathcal{P}(\alpha, h, \theta \mid I) \propto \mathcal{P}(I \mid \alpha, h, \theta) \, \mathcal{P}(\alpha, h, \theta), \tag{4}$$

is optimized with respect to the shape parameters α, and the transformation parameters h and θ. In the following, we will assume a uniform prior on these transformation parameters, i.e., $\mathcal{P}(\alpha, h, \theta) = \mathcal{P}(\alpha)$. In the next section we will discuss three solutions to model this shape prior.

3. EFFICIENT NONPARAMETRIC STATISTICAL SHAPE MODEL

Given a set of aligned training shapes $\{\phi_i\}_{i=1...N}$, we can represent each of them by their corresponding shape vector $\{\alpha_i\}_{i=1...N}$. In this notation, the goal of statistical shape learning is to infer a statistical distribution $\mathcal{P}(\alpha)$ from these sample shapes. Two solutions that have been proposed are based on the assumptions that the training shapes can be approximated by a **uniform distribution** [7, 9]: $\mathcal{P}(\alpha) = \text{const.}$, or by a **Gaussian distribution** [6]:

$$\mathcal{P}(\alpha) \propto \exp\left(-\alpha^\top \Sigma^{-1} \alpha\right), \quad \text{where} \Sigma = \frac{1}{N} \sum_i \alpha_i \, \alpha_i^\top. \tag{5}$$

In the present chapter we propose to make use of nonparametric density estimation [12] to approximate the shape distribution within the linear subspace. We model the shape distribution by the **kernel density estimate**:

$$\mathcal{P}(\alpha) = \frac{1}{N\sigma^n} \sum_{i=1}^{N} K\left(\frac{\alpha - \alpha_i}{\sigma}\right), \quad \text{where } K(u) = \frac{1}{(2\pi)^{n/2}} \exp\left(-\frac{u^2}{2}\right). \tag{6}$$

There exist various methods to automatically estimate appropriate values for the width σ of the kernel function, ranging from the kth nearest neighbor estimates to cross-validation and bootstrapping. In this work, we simply set σ to be the average nearest neighbor distance: $\sigma^2 = \frac{1}{N} \sum_{i=1}^{N} \min_{j \neq i} |\alpha_i - \alpha_j|^2$.

In the context of level set-based image segmentation, the kernel density estimator (6) has two advantages over the uniform and Gaussian distributions:

- The assumptions of uniform distribution or Gaussian distribution are generally not fulfilled. In Figure 3, we demonstrate this for a set of silhouettes of sample shapes. The kernel density estimator, on the other hand, is known to approximate arbitrary distributions. Under mild assumptions, it was shown to converge to the true distribution in the limit of infinite sample size [13].

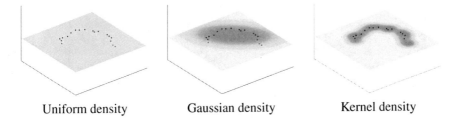

Uniform density   Gaussian density   Kernel density

Figure 2. Schematic plots of different density estimates within a subspace. Darker shading indicates areas of high probability density for the respective models. The kernel density estimator adapts to the training data more flexibly since it does not rely on specific assumptions about the shape of the distribution.

- The space of signed distance functions is known to not be a linear space. Therefore, neither the mean shape ϕ_0 nor a linear combination of eigenmodes as in (3) will in general be a signed distance function. As a consequence, the functions $\phi(x)$ favored by the uniform or the Gaussian distribution cannot be expected to be signed distance functions. The kernel density estimator (6), on the other hand, favors shape vectors α, which are in the vicinity of the sample shape vectors α_i. By construction, these vectors correspond to signed distance functions. In fact, **in the limit of infinite sample size, the distribution inferred by the kernel density estimator (6) converges toward a distribution on the manifold of signed distance functions.**

Figure 2 shows schematic plots of the three methods for a set of sample data spanning a two-dimensional subspace in $\mathbb{R}^3$. The kernel density estimator clearly captures the distribution most accurately. As we shall see in Section 5, constraining a level set-based segmentation process by this nonparametric shape prior will allow to compute accurate segmentations even for rather challenging image modalities.

Figure 3 shows a 3D projection of the estimated shape density computed for a set of silhouettes of a walking person. The bottom row shows shape morphing by sampling along geodesics of the uniform and the kernel density. These indicate that the kernel estimator captures the distribution of valid shapes more accurately.

In analogy to shape learning, we make use of kernel density estimation to learn the conditional probability for the intensity function I in (4) from examples. A similar precomputation of intensity distributions by means of mixture models was proposed in [14]. Given a set of presegmented training images, the kernel density estimate of the intensity distributions p_{in} and p_{out} of object and background are given by the corresponding smoothed intensity histograms. This has two advantages. First, the kernel density estimator does not rely on specific assumptions about the shape of the distribution. Figure 1 shows that the intensity distributions for ultrasound and CT images are not well approximated by Gaussian or Lapla-

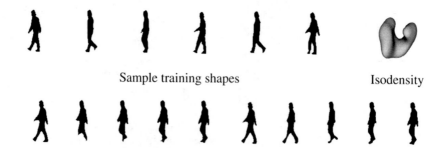

Figure 3. Linear versus nonlinear shape interpolation. The upper row shows 6 out of 49 training shapes and a 3D projection of the isosurface of the estimated (48-dimensional) shape distribution. The latter is clearly neither uniform nor Gaussian. The bottom row shows a morphing between two sample shapes along geodesics induced by a uniform or a kernel distribution. The uniform distribution induces a morphing where legs disappear and reappear and where the arm motion is not captured. The nonlinear sampling provides more realistic intermediate shapes. We chose human silhouettes because they exhibit more pronounced shape variability than most medical structures we analyzed.

cian models. Second, in contrast to the joint estimation of intensity distributions (cf. [15]), this simplifies the segmentation process, which no longer requires an updating of intensity models. Moreover, we found the segmentation process to be more robust to initialization in numerous experiments.

4. ENERGY FORMULATION AND MINIMIZATION

Maximizing the posterior probability in (2), or equivalently minimizing its negative logarithm, will generate the most probable segmentation of a given image. With the nonparametric models for shape and intensity introduced above, this leads to an energy of the form

$$E(\alpha, h, \theta) = -\log \mathcal{P}(I|\alpha, h, \theta) - \log \mathcal{P}(\alpha). \tag{7}$$

The nonparametric intensity model permits to express the first term, and equation (6) gives exactly the second one. With the Heaviside step function H and the short hand $H_\phi = H(\phi_{\alpha,h,\theta}(x))$, we end up with

$$E(\alpha, h, \theta) = -\int_\Omega H_\phi \log p_{\text{in}}(I) + (1 - H_\phi) \log p_{\text{out}}(I) dx - \log\left(\frac{1}{N\sigma} \sum_{i=1}^{N} K\left(\frac{\alpha - \alpha_i}{\sigma}\right)\right).$$

With $e(x) = \left[\log \frac{p_{\text{out}}(I(x))}{p_{\text{in}}(I(x))} \right]$, $K_i = K\left(\frac{\alpha - \alpha_i}{\sigma} \right)$, and $\psi = (\psi_1, \ldots, \psi_n)$, we obtain the following system of coupled gradient descent equations:

$$\begin{cases} \dfrac{d\alpha}{dt} = \displaystyle\int_\Omega \delta(\phi_{\alpha,h,\theta}(x))\, \psi(R_\theta x + h)\, e(x)\, dx + \dfrac{1}{\sigma^2} \dfrac{\sum_{i=1}^N (\alpha_i - \alpha) K_i}{\sum_{i=1}^N K_i}, \\[4mm] \dfrac{dh}{dt} = \displaystyle\int_\Omega \delta(\phi_{\alpha,h,\theta}(x))\, \nabla\phi_{\alpha,h,\theta}(x)\, e(x)\, dx, \\[4mm] \dfrac{d\theta}{dt} = \displaystyle\int_\Omega \delta(\phi_{\alpha,h,\theta}(x))\, (\nabla\phi_{\alpha,h,\theta}(x) \cdot \nabla_\theta R x)\, e(x)\, dx. \end{cases} \qquad (8)$$

In all equations, the Dirac delta function δ appears as a factor inside the integrals over the image domain Ω. This allows to restrict all computations to a narrow band around the zero crossing of ϕ. While the evolution of translation and pose parameters h and θ are merely driven by the data term $e(x)$, the shape vector α is additionally drawn toward each training shape with a strength that decays exponentially with the distance to the respective shape.

5. EXPERIMENTAL RESULTS AND VALIDATION

5.1. Heart Segmentation from Ultrasound Images

Figures 4–6 show experimental results obtained for the segmentation of the left ventricle in 2D cardiac ultrasound sequences, using shape priors constructed from a set of 21 manually segmented training images.

The segmentation in Figure 4 was obtained by merely imposing a small constraint on the length of the segmenting boundary. As a consequence, the segmentation process leaks into all darker areas of the image. The segmentation of the left ventricle based on image intensities and purely geometric regularity constraints clearly fails.

The segmentation in Figure 5 was obtained by constraining the shape optimization to the linear subspace spanned by the eigenmodes of the embedding function of the training set. This improves the segmentation, providing additional regularization and reducing the degrees of freedom for the segmentation process. Nevertheless, even within this subspace there is some leakage into darker image areas.

The segmentation in Figure 5 was obtained by additionally imposing a nonparametric statistical shape prior within this linear subspace. While the subspace allows for efficient optimization (along a small number of eigenmodes), the nonparametric prior allows to accurately constrain the segmentation process to a submanifold of familiar shapes (see also Figure 2). This prevents any leakage of the boundary and enables the segmentation of the left ventricle despite very limited and partially misleading intensity information.

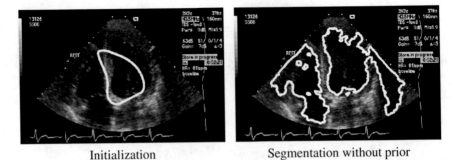

Initialization   Segmentation without prior

Figure 4. Segmentation without prior. Since there is no shape constraint imposed upon the contour — other than a small length constraint present in the Chan-Vese model — the boundary gradually separates brighter from darker areas. This indicates that intensity information is insufficient to induce the desired segmentation.

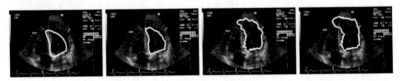

Figure 5. Boundary evolution for an ultrasound segmentation with uniform shape prior. By constraining the level set evolution to the linear subspace spanned by the first few eigenmodes computed from a set of training shapes, one can improve the segmentation of the given image (see, e.g., [7]). Nevertheless, in our application, the uniform shape prior does not sufficiently constrain the segmentation process, permitting the boundary to leak into darker image areas.

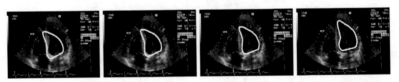

Figure 6. Boundary evolution for an ultrasound segmentation with nonparametric shape prior. Imposing a non-parametric shape prior within the eigenspace spanned by the training shapes leads to a segmentation process that is sufficiently constrained to enable an accurate segmentation of the left ventricle. In contrast to the uniform prior (see Figure 5, the nonparametric one does suppress leaking of the boundary), because it constrains the level set function to a well-defined submanifold around the training shapes (see also Figure 2).

As a quantitative evaluation we computed the percentage of correctly classified object pixels and that of misclassified ones. During energy minimization, the percentage of correctly classified pixels increases from 56 to 90%, while the percentage of false positives decreases from 27 to 2.7% by using the kernel prior. Using the uniform prior, we attain 92% correctly classified, yet the percentage of

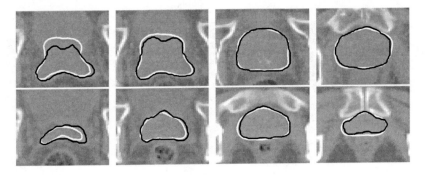

Figure 7. Prostate segmentation for two patients with the same shape model. Each row shows axial slices of the same segmentation for one patient. The manual segmentation is in black and the automatic one white.

false positives increases to 42%. Merely constraining the boundary evolution to the linear subspace spanned by the training shapes is insufficient to provide for accurate segmentation results.

5.2. Prostate Segmentation from 3D CT Images

5.2.1. A single statistical shape model for different patients?

Segmentation of the prostate from CT images is an important and challenging problem in radiotherapy. It may help to avoid the exposure to radiation of vital organs that are not infected by the cancer. In this image modality, the prostate appears with an intensity level very close to the one of adjacent organs like the bladder. The key assumption of our work is that the shape of the prostate in a given segmentation task is statistically similar to prostate shapes observed in a training set. Most related works on prostate segmentation are indeed model-based [7, 10, 11]. In contrast to existing works, we will show that a single (sufficiently sophisticated) statistical shape model can be applied to the segmentation of different patients.

To this end, we built a nonparametric 3D shape model of the prostate using 12 manually extracted prostates (with seminal vesicles) collected from two different patients.

We employed a leave-one-out strategy by removing the image of interest from the training phase. Figure 7 shows 2D cuts of a few results obtained using this strategy. With a one-click initialization inside the organ, the algorithm led to a steady-state solution in less than 10 seconds. We obtained 86% successfully classified organ voxels and 11% misclassified organ voxels. This compares favorably to the intra-patient results reported in [11]. One should note that these quantitative evaluations underestimate the quality of our results since the "ground-truth" seg-

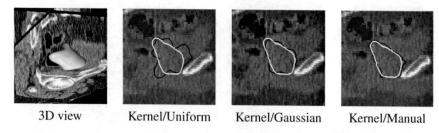

| 3D view | Kernel/Uniform | Kernel/Gaussian | Kernel/Manual |

Figure 8. Comparison of the segmentations obtained with the kernel prior (white) and with alternative approaches (black).

mentations are in general not perfect. Figure 7 provides qualitative comparisons to the manual segmentation, as well as to the segmentations obtained with uniform and Gaussian approximations of the shape distribution.

5.2.2. Quantitative analysis of segmentation accuracy

To further quantify the segmentation accuracy, we consider three different criteria: the Dice coefficient, the average surface distance, and the centroid distance. The Dice coefficient is defined as

$$DSC = \frac{2|S_{\text{manual}} \cap S_{\text{auto}}|}{|S_{\text{manual}}| + |S_{\text{auto}}|}, \tag{9}$$

where $|S_{\text{manual}}|$ and $|S_{\text{auto}}|$ are the volumes of the manual and automatic segmentations, and $|S_{\text{manual}} \cap S_{\text{auto}}|$ is the volume of their intersection. This coefficient can be expressed directly with the level set representations:

$$DSC = \frac{2 \int_{\Omega} H(\phi_{\text{manual}}) H(\phi_{\text{auto}}) \, dx}{\int_{\Omega} H(\phi_{\text{manual}}) \, dx \, \int_{\Omega} H(\phi_{\text{auto}}) \, dx}. \tag{10}$$

In general, a value of DSC superior to 0.7 is considered a good agreement. The other two criteria can also be expressed in similar manner. The average surface distance is given by

$$D_{surface} = \frac{1}{2} \left(\frac{\int_{\Omega} |\nabla H(\phi_{\text{manual}})| |\phi_{\text{auto}}| \, dx}{\int_{\Omega} |\nabla H(\phi_{\text{manual}})| \, dx} + \frac{\int_{\Omega} |\nabla H(\phi_{\text{auto}})| |\phi_{\text{manual}}| \, dx}{\int_{\Omega} |\nabla H(\phi_{\text{auto}})| \, dx} \right). \tag{11}$$

Essentially, this quantity amounts to averaging the distance of each contour point on one contour to the nearest contour point on the other contour (and vice versa).

The centroid distance is the distance between the centers of mass:

$$c_{\text{manual/auto}} = \frac{\int_{\Omega} x \, H(\phi_{\text{manual/auto}}) \, dx}{\int_{\Omega} H(\phi_{\text{manual/auto}}) \, dx}.$$

Table 1. Quantitative Validation on 26 CT Images

	DSC	$D_{surface}$ (mm)	$D_{centroid}$ (mm)
Average	0.8172	3.38	2.86
Standard deviation	0.0807	1.11	1.63
Minimum	0.6573	2.07	0.50
Maximum	0.9327	5.42	5.75

One should point out, however, that the centroid distance has only a very limited capacity to quantify shape differences. Obviously, it cannot distinguish between any two segmentations that share the same centroid.

Table 1 gives the average value of all three criteria computed for the entire dataset in the leave-one-out strategy mentioned above. In addition, we displayed the standard deviation, minimum, and maximum value of each criterion. Overall, these values show that our segmentations typically agree well with the manual ground truth.

5.2.3. Robustness to initialization

The level set method for image segmentation and also its implementation with nonparametric statistical shape priors are *local* optimization methods. As a consequence, experimental results will depend on the initialization. This aspect is a common source of criticism, it is generally believed that *local* indicates that segmentations can only be obtained if contours are initialized in the vicinity of the desired segmentation. Yet, this is not the case for the region-based segmentation schemes like the one developed in this work. The segmentation without shape prior in Figure 4 shows a drastic difference between initial and final boundary: clearly contours can propagate over large spatial distances from the initialization to the "nearest" local minimum.

In order to quantify the robustness of our method to initialization, we translated the initialization by a certain distance in opposite directions and subsequently computed the accuracy of the resulting segmentation process with nonparametric shape prior. Table 2 shows that the accuracy is quite robust with respect to displacements of the initialization up to 10mm in each direction.

5.2.4. Robustness to noise

The prostate CT images are in themselves rather challenging, since prostate and surrounding tissue have fairly similar intensities (see Figure 1, right side). The combination of statistically learned nonparametric models of both the intensity

Table 2. Robustness to Initialization

X Translation (mm)	-10	-5	0	5	10
DSC	0.9287	0.9297	0.9327	0.9289	0.9300
$D_{surface}$ (mm)	2.1358	2.0910	2.0673	2.1080	2.1105
$D_{centroid}$ (mm)	1.3942	1.4657	1.4826	1.4685	1.5481

distribution and the distribution of the shape embedding functions nevertheless allows to compute the desired segmentation. Yet, one may ask where the limitations of our model are. At what point does segmentation accuracy break down?

To investigate this, we artificially added noise to the images, computing at each time the segmentation accuracy. Figure 9 shows both the Dice coefficient defined in (10) and the average surface distance defined in (11) of the final segmentation as a function of the noise. While the segmentation is rather good over a large range of noise values, it does decay at very large values of noise.

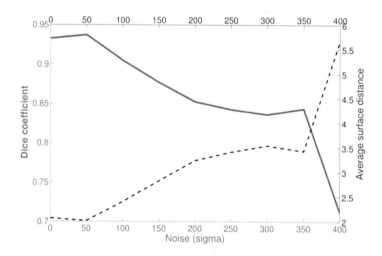

Figure 9. Robustness to noise. See attached CD for color version.

5.2.5. Efficiency versus accuracy: How many eigenmodes are needed?

The efficiency of our implementations arises because we solve the level set computation in the low-dimensional linear subspace spanned by the training shapes. Given N training shapes, this will typically amount to an optimization of $N - 1$ parameters.

Table 3. Segmentation Accuracy for Different Numbers of Modes

	DSC	$D_{surface}$ (mm)	$D_{centroid}$ (mm)
3 modes	0.8015	3.55	3.32
10 modes	0.8172	3.38	2.86
25 modes	0.8173	3.46	2.95

While there exist many ways to parameterize this subspace, the representation in terms of principal components (eigenshapes of the embedding function) has the additional advantage that the principal components associated with the largest eigenvalues by definition capture the largest variation of the embedding function. Hence, one could further reduce the dimensionality of the problem, by using merely the first few eigenmodes.

To quantify the loss in segmentation accuracy when using fewer eigenmodes in the optimization, we show in Table 3 the values of the Dice coefficient, the surface distance, and the centroid distance obtained when using 3, 10, and 25 eigenmodes. The reported quantities are averages computed for each of the 25 test images. As expected, the higher-order eigenmodes contain very little additional shape information, so that the accuracy increases only by a little amount when going from 10 to 25 eigenmodes, while the computation time scales linearly with the number of eigenmodes considered.

6. CONCLUSION

We proposed herein an efficient and accurate statistical shape prior for level set segmentation that is based on nonparametric density estimation in the linear subspace spanned by the level set surfaces of a set of training shapes. In addition, our segmentation scheme integrates nonparametric estimates of intensity distributions and efficient optimization of pose and translation parameters.

We reported quantitative evaluation of segmentation accuracy and speed for cardiac ultrasound images and for 3D CT images of the prostate. In particular, we quantitatively validated that the proposed segmentation scheme is robust to the initialization and robust to noise. Furthermore, we demonstrated that one can increase efficiency by reducing the number of eigenmodes considered in the optimization while losing a little accuracy of the average segmentation results. These results indicate that the proposed nonparametric shape prior outperforms previously proposed shape priors for level set segmentation.

7. ACKNOWLEDGMENTS

We thank Christophe Chefd'hotel for fruitful discussions. We thank Marie-Pierre Jolly for providing us with image and training data for the ultrasound sequences.

8. NOTES

1. A preliminary version of this work was presented in [16].

9. REFERENCES

1. Dervieux A, Thomasset F. 1979. A finite element method for the simulation of Rayleigh-Taylor instability. In *Approximation methods for Navier-Stokes problems*, pp. 145–158. Ed R Rautmann. Berlin: Springer.

2. Osher SJ, Sethian JA. 1988. Front propagation with curvature dependent speed: algorithms based on Hamilton-Jacobi formulations. *J Comput Phys* **79**:12–49.

3. Caselles V, Catté F, Coll T, Dibos F. 1993. A geometric model for active contours in image processing. *Num Math* **66**:1–31.

4. Malladi R, Sethian JA, Vemuri BC. 1994. A topology independent shape modeling scheme. In *Proceedings of the SPIE conference on geometric methods in computer vision*, Vol. 2031, pp. 246–258. Bellingham, WA: SPIE.

5. Kichenassamy S, Kumar A, Olver PJ, Tannenbaum A, Yezzi AJ. 1995. Gradient flows and geometric active contour models. In *Proceedings of the fifth international conference computer vision (ICCV'95)*, pp. 810–815. Washington, DC: IEEE Computer Society.

6. Leventon M, Grimson W, Faugeras O. 2000. Statistical shape influence in geodesic active contours. In *Proceedings of the IEEE international conference on computer vision and pattern recognition (CVPR)*, Vol. 1, pp. 316–323. Washington, DC: IEEE Computer Society.

7. Tsai A, Yezzi AJ, Willsky AS. 2003. A shape-based approach to the segmentation of medical imagery using level sets. *IEEE Trans Med Imaging*, **22**(2):137–154.

8. Cremers D, Osher SJ, Soatto S. 2006. Kernel density estimation and intrinsic alignment for shape priors in level set segmentation. *Int J Comput Vision*. **69**(3):335–351.

9. Rousson M, Paragios N, Deriche R. 2004. Implicit active shape models for 3d segmentation in MRI imaging. In *Proceedings of the international conference on medical image computing and computer-assisted intervention (MICCAI 2000). Lecture notes in computer science*, Vol. 2217, pp. 209–216. New York: Springer.

10. Dam EB, Fletcher PT, Pizer S, Tracton G, Rosenman J. 2004. Prostate shape modeling based on principal geodesic analysis bootstrapping. In *Proceedings of the international conference on medical image computing and computer-assisted intervention (MICCAI 2003). Lecture notes in computer science*, Vol. 2217, pp. 1008–1016. New York: Springer.

11. Freedman D, Radke RJ, Zhang T, Jeong Y, Lovelock DM, Chen GT. 2005. Model-based segmentation of medical imagery by matching distributions. *IEEE Trans Med Imaging* **24**(3):281–292.

12. Rosenblatt F. 1956. Remarks on some nonparametric estimates of a density function. *Ann Math Stat* **27**:832–837.

13. Silverman BW. 1992. *Density estimation for statistics and data analysis*. London: Chapman and Hall.

14. Paragios N, Deriche R. 2002. Geodesic active regions and level set methods for supervised texture segmentation. *Int J Comput Vision* **46**(3):223–247.

15. Chan LA Vese TF. 2001. Active contours without edges. *IEEE Trans Med Imaging*, **10**(2):266–277.

16. Rousson, M., Cremers, D., 2005. Efficient Kernel Density Estimation of Shape and Intensity Priors for Level Set Segmentation, *International conference on medical image computing and computed-assisted intervention (MICCAI 2005)*, **2**: 757–764.

14

VOLUMETRIC MRI ANALYSIS OF DYSLEXIC SUBJECTS USING A LEVEL SET FRAMEWORK

H. Abd El Munim, R. Fahmi, N. Youssry El-Zehiry, and A. A. Farag

Computer Vision and Image Processing Laboratory
Department of Electrical and Computer Engineering
University of Louisville, Louisville, Kentucky, USA

M. Casanova

Department of Psychiatry and Behavioral Sciences,
University of Louisville, Louisville, Kentucky, USA

The minicolumn is considered as an elementary unit of the neocortex in all mammalian brains. It is believed that enlargement of the cortical surface occurs as a result of the addition of minicolumns, not a single neuron. Hence, a modern trend to analyze developmental disorders such as dyslexia and autism is to investigate how the minicolumns in the brains of dyslexic and autistic patients vary from the minicolumns in normal brains mapping this variation into a noninvasive imaging framework such as Magnetic Resonance Imaging. This chapter provides the status of an investigation of the differences between the brains of normal control cases and dyslexic patients through an analysis of brain Magnetic Resonance Images. It will be shown that there exists a discriminant difference in the total volume of the white matter between the normal control cases and the dyslexic ones. The major objective of this study is to investigate the correlation between the pathological findings represented by the number of minicolumns, their widths, their arrangements, etc., and the MRI findings that may be represented by volumetric measures of the white and gray matter in different brain compartments. Since the pathological findings found a smaller number of minicolumns in patients with dyslexia, we hypothesize that the volume of the whole white matter in the

Address all correspondence to: Dr. Aly A. Farag, Professor of Electrical and Computer Engineering, University of Louisville, CVIP Lab, Room 412, Lutz Hall, 2301 South 3rd Street, Louisville, KY 40208, USA. Phone: (502) 852-7510, Fax: (502) 852-1580. farag@cvip.uofl.edu.

brains of such patients, as well as the volume of their outer compartments, are smaller than the corresponding items in normal control cases. This study aimed at proving whether this is true or not. For this purpose, white matter, for both normal and dyslexic cases, is first segmented, and then volumes are calculated and compared. The segmentation is performed within a novel level set framework. Furthermore, the white matter will be subdivided into inner and outer compartments to find out exactly which part affects the change in total volume.

1. INTRODUCTION

Developmental brain disorders represent one of the most interesting and challenging research areas in neuroscience. Dyslexia and autism are two of the most complicated developmental brain disorders that affect the behavior and learning abilities of children. Dyslexia is characterized by the failure to develop age-appropriate reading skills despite normal intelligence levels and adequate reading instruction [1], whereas autism is characterized by qualitative abnormalities in behavior and higher cognitive functions [2]. One of the major causes of developmental disorders is that some parts of the communications network in the brain fail to perform their tasks properly, and this may result from a malfunction of the structure of the minicolumns. Buxhoeveden et al. [3] presented a discussion of minicolumn structure and their organization in the brain. One of the most effective tools for the analysis and diagnosis of anatomical changes in brain is Magnetic Resonance Imaging (MRI). Brambilla et al. [2] introduced a review study that summarized morphometric brain investigations involving autistic patients in order to examine the brain anatomy and development in autistic brains. Palmen et al. [4] presented an article discussing the neuropathological findings in autistic brains and how they correlate with MRI findings. Eliez et al. [5] published an MRI study that investigated the morphological alteration of temporal lobe gray matter in dyslexia. One major advantage of using MR imaging in brain studies is the ability to extract several brain regions such as the cerebral cortex, corpus callosum, sulci, and white/gray matters, and then calculate some parameters for these parts (e.g., width, surface area, and volume), and use this information to discriminate between different diseases or to address a certain disease.

Segmentation of the cerebral cortex and isolating the deep structures (such as the corpus callosum, brain stem, and ventricles) has always been one of the most challenging and essential tasks in the pipeline of brain functional analysis. Over the last decade, deformable models and level sets have shown superiority in the analysis and quantification of the different brain structures [6–10]. Duncan et al. [11] presented a volumetric segmentation approach based on level sets in which two surfaces are evolving simultaneously, each driven by its own image-derived information while marinating the coupling until a representation of the two bounding surfaces is obtained, and then the layer is segmented. The approach has been applied in the segmentation of the gray matter of the brain and proved to be very promising. Deformable models proposed in [6, 12, 13] depend on evolving an initial co-dimensional object (curve in 2D or surface in 3D) under certain constraints until it covers the structure of interest. Although this approach is very flexible in its initialization, it requires tuning of a large number of parameters. Baillard et al. [7] presented an approach that does not require that any parameters be tuned. The proposed algorithm controls the evolution of the surface by taking into consideration probabilistic region information. The designed level set model is based on the estimated density functions using the stochastic expectation maximization. But this method can only work for bimodal images, and this may be too restrictive for many applications. Farag et al. [9] generalized the previously discussed approach to be applied to multimodal images. Xu et al. [14] introduced a method for reconstruction of the cerebral cortex from MR imaging based on fuzzy segmentation and deformable models. This chapter will utilize the advanced level set techniques used for brain segmentation and analysis to develop an integrated system that will be used in the analysis and quantification of brain developmental disorders, and especially dyslexia, which is the main focus of this chapter. Unlike the previously published approaches, we will focus on investigating the relationship between the microscopic findings that have been investigated through the minicolumnar structures of autistic and dyslexic brains [3, 15] and the Magnetic Resonance Images employing level sets. We will present this subject matter in the following order:

The neuroanatomy background: This will handle the definition of the minicolumns, and how they relate to the developmental brain disorders of interest. The hypotheses made to quantify these diseases either using Magnetic Resonance Imaging or Diffusion Tensor Imaging will be included.

Problem statement, dataset description: This will introduce a description of the data, the data collection procedure, and the MRI protocol, as well as the basic pipeline for the approach used to analyze the data.

Volumetric MRI analysis of dyslexic subjects using a level set framework: This section will introduce the details of the approach used in the analysis and the results on both synthetic and real MRI data.

Concluding remarks: This section will present the conclusion of the work and propose possibilities for future work.

2. THE NEUROANATOMY BACKGROUND

Brain function research suggests that the minicolumns, not individual neuronal cells, are the basic operational units in the brain. For instance, Mountcastle [17] reported that the effective unit of operation in the human brain is not the single neuron and its axon, but groups of cells with similar functional properties and anatomical connections. The most highly acclaimed neurobiology textbooks consider the vertical organization of the cortex to be a basic concept of neurobiology, commonly referring to it as the columnar hypothesis [3]. Minicolumns are defined as vertical organizations of neurons arranged in the neocortex. They grow in the gray matter and communicate through the white matter. Minicolumns, rather than the neurons, are believed to be the basic units of the brain in the sense that the enlargement of the neocortex, in the phase of the brain development, is characterized by an increase in the number of minicolumns rather than that of single neurons. In the aging phase, the neocortex loses whole minicolumns, not randomly scattered neurons. This is clearly illustrated in Figure 1, where the minicolumnar structure for a 9-year-old child and a 67-year-old adult are depicted. It is quite obvious that the neurons are lost within columns, not randomly. Any disturbance in the number, structure, or organization of minicolumns will affect the development of the brain and, as a result, its functionality. According to this, we hypothesize that the brain developmental disorders and aging disorders can be diagnosed and analyzed in terms of an analysis of the number as well as organization of the minicolumns in the neocortex. These changes are expected to be captured *at a different scale* by the Magnetic Resonance Images or the Diffusion Tensor Images. Consequently, level sets and deformable models play a major role in analyzing the structural changes of minicolumns, which allows one to draw conclusions and perform measurements regarding disease analysis and diagnosis. On one hand, there have been several MRI studies in this field [5, 18, 19]. For example, Herbert et al. [18] conducted a study to analyze autism and developmental language disorder through the volumes of the white matter in several brain regions: the frontal lobe, parietal lobe, temporal lobe, and occipital lobe (for the superficial layer), the corpus callosum, cingulum, basal forebrain, and internal capsule (for the deep structures). Eliez et al. [5] studied morphological alteration of temporal lobe gray matter in dyslexia, and they also made some volumetric analysis for the whole brain tissues as well as for different lobes. Chung et al. [19] recently presented analysis of cortical thickness in autism studies. On the other hand, Diffusion Tensor Magnetic Resonance Imaging (DT-MRI) has recently emerged as a noninvasive imaging modality that can yield rich information about the white matter structure in the human brain and aid in inferring the architecture of the underlying structure [20, 21]. The DT-MRI technique was first introduced in the mid1980s [22, 23]. As of today it is the unique noninvasive technique capable of probing and measuring the anisotropic diffusion properties of water molecules in living tissues like brain or muscles [24]. The Diffusion Tensor (DT) provides information about the intensity of water diffusion in any direction at a certain point. In the specific case of the brain, the cellular organization, in particular axonal cell membrane and myelin sheath, highly affects water mobility. Hence, the measured DT becomes highly anisotropic and oriented in areas of compact nerve fiber organization, providing an indirect method for fiber tract identification. Motivated by this advantage of DT-MRI over traditional MRI, numerous works have addressed the study of white matter diseases (such as

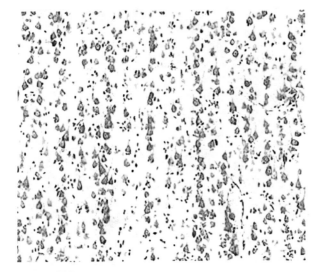

9-year-old human

67-year-old human

Figure 1. Differences between the minicolumnar structure in 9- and 67-year-old human brains. The bottom picture illustrates that in aging stage the brain loses whole minicolumns and not randomly scattered neurons, which supports the fact that the minicolumn is the basic unit of the human cortex. See attached CD for color version.

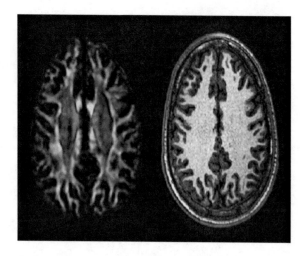

Figure 2. A diffusion tensor image that shows the white matter bundles and the corresponding MRI slice. See attached CD for color version.

multiple sclerosis and dyslexia). Recently, Lenglet et al. [21] proposed a global approach to white matter connectivity mapping through global modeling of the white matter as a Riemannian manifold, and used the diffusion information to infer its geometry and compute its geodesics, which correspond to diffusion pathways. The level set method was used in that work to compute the signed distance and for geodesic estimation. Goraly et al. [25] conducted a study to investigate the values of the fractional anisotropy of the DTI in seven autistic children.

Some studies have been conducted to analyze developmental dyslexia through Diffusion Tensor Imaging [26], but we propose a novel method to investigate DTI in analyzing dyslexia by analyzing the fiber tracts of the white matter in the outer compartment and analyzing the relationship between the geometrical structures of these fiber tracts that directly reflect the manner of communications between minicolumns.

3. PROBLEM STATEMENT, DATASET DESCRIPTION AND PROPOSED APPROACH

One of the major causes of developmental disorders is that some parts of the communication network of the brain fail to perform their tasks properly. Hence, most of the previous MRI studies [2, 4, 5] focused on investigating morphometric brain changes in certain structures such as the corpus callosum, brain stem, and other structures. In this study we analyze the morphometric changes in the normal

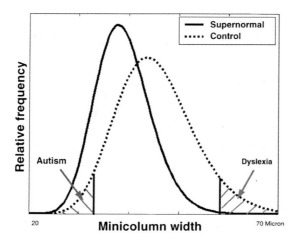

Figure 3. Histogram of the minicolumn width in human brain with the dyslexic and autistic regions illustrated. The Figure demonstrates that the minicolumns in the normal brain have a normal width distribution, whereas in autism all the minicolumns are of smaller width and in dyslexia all the minicolumns are of larger width. See attached CD for color version.

and dyslexic brain through an investigation of the minicolumnar organization rather than looking at changes in brain structures, as was done in the studies listed above.

3.1. The Hypothesis

The analysis is based on the fact that the failure to develop proper communication between the different parts of the brain can be caused by a disturbance in the minicolumns. Meanwhile, postmortem studies have shown that common features to both dyslexia and autism include minicolumnar abnormalities [15]. These studies indicate that within the general population, dyslexia and autism exist as opposite tail ends within the normal distribution of the minicolumnar widths [15]. Figure 3 illustrates this idea.

More precisely, the brains of dyslexic subjects have minicolumns with larger widths compared to normal control cases. It has been proven pathologically that dyslexics have fewer numbers of minicolumns. Conversely, the presence of a minicolumnopathy in the brains of autistic patients, i.e., a reduction in the width of pyramidal cell arrays, has been corroborated by the results presented in [15]. Bearing in mind that in a normal brain the minicolumnar interconnectivity is of the order of 1000 [27] and that the minicolumns communicate through the white matter, the following hypothesis can be posed: The brain of a dyslexic patient has fewer numbers of minicolumns, and then a smaller white matter volume compared to a normal brain. The contrary is then assumed to be true for autistic cases. Proving (or verifying) this hypothesis is the major focus of the present study. We will also prove, through white matter parcellation into inner and outer compartments, that an increment or decrement in white matter volume occurs respectively in the outer compartment, where the communication between minicolumns takes place.

In addition to the volumetric study of white matter, the study of cortical thickness, the geometrical difference in gyrification between normals and dyslexics, as well as surface area and gray matter volume are of major importance, and will be included in our future attempts to investigate the relationship between the MRI and changes in minicolumnar structures. The level set representation for the gray matter surface will play a major role in characterizing the geometry of the cortex and analyzing the gyration window through the curvature at the different points. Moreover, the wavelet transform will be applied on different sub-images as an attempt to transfer the images to a different domain in which some information about the temporal and frequency content of the images can be inferred.

3.2. Dataset Description

Sixteen right-handed dyslexic men, aged 18 to 40 years, and a group of 14 controls matched for gender, age, educational level, socioeconomic background, handedness, and general intelligence participated in the present study. All subjects were physically healthy and free of any history of neurological disease, head injury, significant uncorrected sensory deficit, severe psychiatric disorder, and chronic substance abuse, as determined by medical history, a physical examination, laboratory testing, and a structured psychiatric interview. Subjects currently under treatment for attention deficit disorders were excluded. Dyslexic patients with a childhood history of significant reading impairment were subject to intervention, which ranged from tutoring to full-time special education. Despite their significant reading disability, all had graduated from high school, several were in college, and three had completed postdoctoral degrees. All met DSM-IV (American Psychiatric Association, 1994) criteria for developmental reading disorder. All had at least average intelligence and good spoken language skills (Wechsler Full Scale, Verbal, and Performance IQs $\geq$ 90) but showed persistent reading deficits. Passage (decoding) scores, reflecting a combination of reading rate and accuracy, on the Gray Oral Reading Test, third edition (GORT-3), were 8 or lower using norms for the ceiling of the test at a 12.9 grade level and an age of 18 years, 11 months. This cutoff score is 0.67 of an SD below average for high school seniors. Using the GORT-3, all but one dyslexic subject read at a level that was, at the time of study, at least 1 SD lower than his Full Scale IQ. Thus, this group generally met both absolute and discrepancy-based criteria for dyslexia. Single-word recognition scores (Wide Range Achievement Test, third edition, WRAT-3) were less sensitive to the reading deficits. Ten out of 16 scored within an average range on a test of single-word recognition (WRAT-3 Reading: 90–110), whereas the others were deficient on this measure as well (range 73–88). Based on subject interviews and reviews of childhood records, only one subject had a history of a clinically significant delay in acquisition of spoken language suggestive of a developmental language disorder. This subject spoke well by the time he entered school and, at the time of study, showed good spoken language, with an average Verbal IQ, and excellent reading comprehension, much like our other subjects, and thus was not excluded. Controls (all right-handed males) were free of any history of developmental disorder, attention deficit disorder, special education, and reading decoding or spelling deficits. All scored well within an average range or above on reading measures. All but one had additional psychometric testing (one was not tested because of his familiarity with some of the tests, a factor that would invalidate his scores). The controls were matched to the dyslexic group with respect to gender, age, educational level, socioeconomic status, handedness, and estimated IQ, obtained with a short form of the WAIS-R. The dyslexic sample and 13 of the 14 controls reported here participated in a study of planum temporale asymmetry reported in [5, 28]. Fourteen of the 16 dyslexic men and 11 of the 14 controls studied here also participated in functional brain imaging studies [5, 28, 29] that suggested functional variations in left and right temporal and inferior parietal cortex in the dyslexic men.

3.3. Magnetic Resonance Imaging Protocol

All images were acquired with the same 1.5-T Signa MRI scanner (General Electric, Milwaukee, WI) using a 3D spoiled gradient recall acquisition in the steady state (time to echo = 5 ms; time to repeat = 24 ms; flip angle = 45; repetition = 1; field of view = 24 cm^2). Contiguous axial slices, 1.5 mm in thickness (124 per brain), were acquired. The images were collected in a 192×256 acquisition matrix and were 0-filled in k-space to yield an image of 256×256 pixels, resulting in an effective voxel resolution of approximately $0.9375.0 \times 0.9375 \times 1.5$ mm.

4. PROPOSED APPROACH

The proposed approach consists mainly of four steps, as shown in Figure 4. First, a brain extraction algorithm is applied to remove all the non-brain tissues from the images. Second, brain segmentation is performed to isolate the white matter. Third, white matter parcellation is performed to parcel the white matter into inner and outer compartments, and, finally, volumetric measures of the whole white matter as well as the outer compartment are recorded. Tests of the hypothesis are then performed to investigate if there exists a significant difference between the groups or not in terms of volume changes. The following subsections will provide a detailed description of each of the previously mentioned steps.

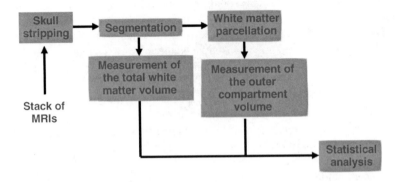

Figure 4. Block diagram of the proposed approach. See attached CD for color version.

4.1. Brain Extraction

Brain extraction, also known as *skull stripping*, consists in removing all non-brain tissues (such as skull, eyes, and fat) from brain MRI scans. For this purpose the MRICro program (free software available at www.sph.sc.edu/comd/rorden /mricro.html) has been used to extract brain tissues and exclude all other artifacts. Figure 5 shows the results of applying this program to an MRI slice in a normal case. Figure 6 shows the results of applying MRICro on a more complicated MRI slice that contains larger parts of the skull and eyes, so as to show the reliability of the program when applied on different brain slices.

4.2. Segmentation

In this section we present the framework used to extract the white matter from the dataset described earlier. Recall that the datasets at hand consist of brain grayscale MR images. The following sections describe the adaptive multi modal image segmentation approach using level sets [9]. The curve evolution representation is given in addition to the partial differential equation that is related to the region information.

4.2.1. Introduction to level set segmentation

3D segmentation of anatomical structures is very important for various medical applications. Due to image noise and inhomogeneities as well as the complexity of anatomical structures, the segmentation process remains a tedious and challenging one. Therefore, this process cannot rely only on image information, but has to involve prior knowledge of the shapes and other properties of the objects of interest. In many applications, 3D segmentation is performed using deformable

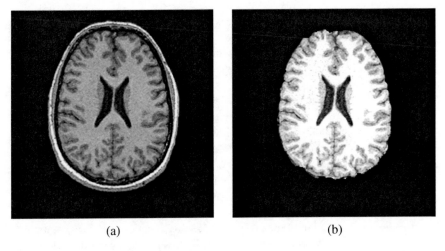

(a)   (b)

Figure 5. Skull Stripping using MRICro software: (a) MRI slice 71; (b) result of skull stripping.

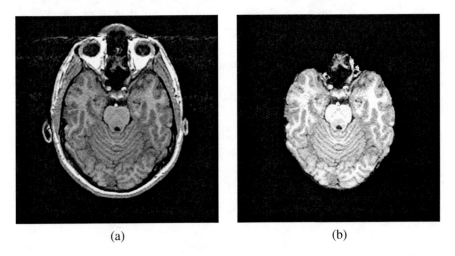

(a)   (b)

Figure 6. Skull Stripping using MRICro software: (a) MRI slice 42, (b) result of skull stripping. The Figure illustrates the efficiency of the software when applied to a complicated brain slice and its ability to remove the eyes and skull.

models. Such a model iteratively evolves toward the relevant anatomy according to global energy minimization. The functional energy represents the confluence of physics and geometry. The latter represents an object shape and the former places constraints on how the shape may vary over space and time. For these models to produce accurate results, the initial contour should be close to the desired boundaries. Coping with the topological changes is another limitation of the deformable models.

The level set-based segmentation techniques overcome the limits of the classical deformable models [31, 13, 6, 30]. These techniques handle efficiently topological changes (curve breaking and merging) during the course of curve evolution. In addition, the initial curve needs not be close to the desired solution, and its initialization can be either manual or automatic. However, since the level set models evolve using gradient descent, a proper initialization is required for accurate segmentation. The chosen initialization needs an accurate estimate of the parameters for each class. The Stochastic Expectation Maximization (SEM) algorithm is used to give initial estimates of class parameters. During the level sets evolution, these parameters are iteratively re-estimated in order to obtain more accurate segmentation. Our work differs from that in [7] by its suitability for multimodal images and due to adaptive estimation of the probability density functions. The segmentation model as a partial differential equation will be given in detail in the following section.

Curve/surface evolution has two main representations: explicit and implicit forms. For each form a partial differential equation is derived to control the evolution. The details of these approaches are as follows.

4.2.2. Curve and surface evolution theory

In this section we present a brief overview of curve evolution theory. For a more comprehensive presentation, the interested reader can refer to [32, 33], among others.

For the sake of simplicity, we formulate the equations of motion of planar propagating curves. The extension to surfaces in 3D is straightforward. Let $C(p, t) : S^1 \times [0, \mathcal{T}) \to \mathbb{R}^2$ denote a family of planar closed curves, where S^1 denotes the unit circle, t parameterizes the family, and p parameterizes the curve. Assume that the motion of this family of curves obeys the following partial differential equation (PDE):

$$\frac{\partial C}{\partial t} = \alpha \cdot \overrightarrow{T} + \beta \cdot \overrightarrow{N}, \text{ and } C(p, 0) = C_0(p), \tag{1}$$

where $\alpha = \alpha(p, t)$ and $\beta = \beta(p, t)$ denote the tangential and normal velocities, respectively; $\overrightarrow{T} = \overrightarrow{T}(p, t)$ is the unit tangent vector, and $\overrightarrow{N} = \overrightarrow{N}(p, t)$ is the unit inward normal vector.

Following the result of Epstein and Gage [34], if the normal velocity β does not depend on the parametrization (we say in this case that β is a geometric intrinsic characteristic of the curve), then the solution to equation (2) is identical to the solution of the following equation of motion:

$$\frac{\partial C}{\partial t} = \beta \cdot \overrightarrow{N}, \text{ and } C(p, 0) = C_0(p). \tag{2}$$

It is this equation that we will consider for further analysis.

Now, let us represent $\mathcal{C}(p, t)$ as the zero level set of a smooth embedding function $\phi : \mathbb{R}^2 \times [0, \mathcal{T}) \rightarrow \mathbb{R}$:

$$L_0(t) = \{X \in \mathbb{R}^2 / \phi(X, t) = 0\}, \tag{3}$$

whereas the initial curve $\mathcal{C}_0$ is represented by an initial function ϕ_0.

Since $\mathcal{C}(p, t)$ is implicitly represented as the zero level set of ϕ, then $\phi(\mathcal{C}, t) = 0$. By differentiation w.r.t. t, using the chain rule, we find,

$$\nabla\phi(\mathcal{C}, t) \cdot \frac{\partial \mathcal{C}}{\partial t} + \frac{\partial \phi}{\partial t}(\mathcal{C}, t) = 0,$$

$$\Rightarrow \nabla\phi(\mathcal{C}, t) \cdot (\beta \overrightarrow{N}) + \frac{\partial \phi}{\partial t}(\mathcal{C}, t) = 0.$$

where ∇ denotes the gradient operator.

Using the fact that the unit normal vector is given, at each instant t, as $\overrightarrow{N} = -\frac{\nabla\phi}{\|\nabla\phi\|}$, we get,

$$\nabla\phi(\mathcal{C}, t) \cdot \beta(-\frac{\nabla\phi}{\|\nabla\phi\|}) + \frac{\partial\phi}{\partial t}(\mathcal{C}, t) = 0,$$

which results in the general motion form in the level set framework, namely:

$$\frac{\partial\phi}{\partial t} = \beta \|\nabla\phi\|. \tag{4}$$

Depending on the problem to be solved, one can design the appropriate velocity term β. Among several formulations proposed in the literature (see, e.g., [36, 35]), we have chosen the following formulation:

$$\beta = \nu - \epsilon\kappa, \tag{5}$$

where $\nu = \pm 1$ controls the motion direction, $\epsilon \ll 1$ is a positive real number, and κ is the local curvature of the front defined in the 2D case as follows:

$$\kappa = \frac{\phi_{xx}\phi_{yy}^2 - 2\phi_x\phi_y\phi_{xx} + \phi_{yy}\phi_x^2}{\|\nabla\phi\|^3}. \tag{6}$$

The latter term in (5) acts as a regularization term.

4.2.3. Our level set model

It is worth mentioning that several evolution models were proposed for segmentation purposes, but most of them depend on a large number of parameters to be tuned in order to guarantee the success of the process. Examples of these parameters include, but are not limited to, the iteration step, speed terms, time step, etc.

In [7] a more efficient 3D segmentation technique was proposed. In that work, where almost no parameter setting is required, surface evolution is controlled by current probabilistic region information. Probability density functions for the object and the background are estimated using SEM. The resulted level set model is based on these density functions. However, the proposed model works only for bimodal images, and this may be too restrictive for many applications.

In [9] we proposed a novel and robust level set-based segmentation technique. A statistical model of regions is explicitly embedded into partial differential equations describing the evolution of the level sets. SEM is used to estimate the initial values of class parameters. The probability density function for each region is modeled by a Gaussian with adaptive parameters. These parameters and the prior probability of each region are automatically re-estimated at each iteration of the process. The designed level set model depends on these density functions. The region information over the image is also taken into account. Our proposed model differs from that in [7] due to its suitability for multimodal images and due to adaptive estimation of the probability density functions. Our experiments in 3D segmentation of MR images demonstrate the accuracy of the algorithm.

4.2.4. Curve/surface modeling by level sets

Within the level set formalism [37], the evolving surface is a propagating front embedded as the zero level of a higher-dimensional scalar function $\phi(x, t)$. This hypercurve/surface is usually defined as a signed distance function: positive inside the region enclosed by the evolving interface, negative outside, and zero on the boundary of the enclosed region. As we have seen earlier, the continuous change of ϕ can be described by the following PDE:

$$\frac{\partial \phi(x, t)}{\partial t} + F \parallel \nabla \phi(x, t) \parallel = 0, \tag{7}$$

where F is a scalar velocity function depending on the local geometric properties (e.g., local curvature) of the front and on the external parameters related to the input data, e.g., image gradient. The function ϕ deforms iteratively according to F, and the position of the 2D/3D front is given at each iteration step by the equation $\phi(x, t) = 0$.

The design of the velocity function F plays a major role in the evolutionary process. In our formulation, we have chosen the formulation given by (5), that is, $F = \nu - \epsilon \kappa$, where the local curvature κ of the front is defined in the 3D case as follows:

$$\kappa = \quad (\quad (\phi_{xx} + \phi_{yy})\phi_z^2 + (\phi_{xx} + \phi_{zz})\phi_y^2$$
$$+ \quad (\phi_{zz} + \phi_{yy})\phi_x^2 - 2\phi_x\phi_y\phi_{xy} - 2\phi_x\phi_z\phi_{xz}$$
$$- \quad 2\phi_z\phi_y\phi_{zy})/(2(\phi_x^2 + \phi_y^2 + \phi_z^2)^{3/2}). \tag{8}$$

With this representation, a single level set either contracts until vanishing or expands to cover all the space. To stop the evolution at the edge, F can be multiplied by a value that is a function of the image gradient [38]. However, if the edge is missed, the surface cannot propagate backward. Hence, relying mainly on the edge is not sufficient for an accurate segmentation and other information from the image should be used.

The segmentation partitions the image into regions, each belonging to a certain class. In our approach a separate level set function is defined for each class and automatic seed initialization is used. Given parameters of each class, the volume is initially divided into equal non-overlapped sub-volumes. For each sub-volume, the average gray level is used to specify the most probable class with the initial parameters estimated by SEM. Such initialization differs from the one in [39], where only the distance to the class mean is used. Then, a signed distance level set function for the associated class is initialized. Therefore, selection of the class parameters is very important for successful segmentation. The probability density function of each class is embedded into the velocity term of each level set equation. The parameters of each of these density functions are re-estimated at each iteration. The automatic seed initialization produces initially non-overlapped level set functions. The competition between level sets based on the probability density functions stops the evolution of each level set at the boundary of its class region.

Tracking the curve/surface with time needs a solution of the associated partial differential equations. Dealing with non-smooth data represents a challenge in this problem. More sophisticated numerical techniques are required. The details of the numerical solution used for getting the front at any time are presented below.

4.2.5. Numerical implementation for interface evolution

A standard numerical approach to modeling moving fronts results from discretizing the Lagrangian description of the problem (Eq. (7)) with a set of discrete marker particles lying on the moving front and whose positions at any time are used to reconstruct the front. This technique, known as the *marker particle technique* or the *strings method*, has several drawbacks, including amplification of the errors in the computed particle positions due to the curvature term. The absence of a smoothing curvature (*viscous*) term leads to development of singularities in the propagating front. In addition, managing the topological changes becomes very complex as the front breaks and/or merges. Finally, bookkeeping of removing, repositioning, and connecting markers is a tedious task, typically for higher-dimensional cases. Our aim in this section is to present numerical schemes for interface evolution problems. This presentation will be based on the link between Hamilton-Jacobi HJ equations and hyperbolic conservation laws (HCLs).

Although these two views are formally equivalent for only one dimensional case, multidimensional schemes are motivated using the 1D numerical methodology. We shall borrow the schemes designed for HCLs to motivate our schemes for HJ equations.

4.2.6. Hamilton-Jacobi equations

Definition An equation of the form

$$U_t + H(x, y, z, U_x, U_y, U_z) = 0 \tag{9}$$

is called a Hamilton-Jacobi equation. The function $H(\cdot)$ is called the Hamiltonian. Note that our level set equation (7) can be cast in the form of an HJ equation with

$$H(x, y, z, p, q, r) = F\sqrt{p^2 + q^2 + r^2}.$$

Let us focus on a one-dimensional version, that is, $U_t + H(U_x) = 0$. If we let $u = U_x$ and differentiate w.r.t. t, we get the following:

$$u_t = \frac{d}{dt}(U_x) = \frac{d}{dx}(U_t) \quad = \quad \frac{d}{dx}(-H(U_x)) = \frac{d}{dx}(-H(u)) = -[H(u)]_x$$
$$\Rightarrow \quad u_t + [H(u)]_x = 0, \tag{10}$$

which is an HCL. The corresponding flux function is equal to the Hamiltonian $H(\cdot)$. (Given an HCL $u_t + [G(u)]_x = 0$ and a discretized grid in space $\{x_0, x_1, \cdots, x_n\}$, a "numerical flux" function is a function g such that $g(u_{i-1}, u_i) \simeq G(u_{i-\frac{1}{2}}) \doteq G_{i-\frac{1}{2}}$, that is, g approximates the flux G at the half grid points.) Thus, in order to solve our Hamilton-Jacobi equation, we first formulate it as an HCL, borrow numerical flux schemes designed for an HCL [37], and then return back to the original equation.

Given that $u = U_x$, one can notice that the forward difference approximation $D^{+x}U_i^n = \frac{U_{i+1}^n - U_i^n}{\Delta x}$ to u_i^n is actually the central difference approximation to $u_{i+\frac{1}{2}}^n$. Likewise, the backward approximation $D^{-x}U_i^n = \frac{U_i^n - U_{i-1}^n}{\Delta x}$ is the central difference approximation to $u_{i-\frac{1}{2}}^n$. Moreover, from the definition of the numerical function, one can deduce that

$$g(u_{i-\frac{1}{2}}^n, u_{i+\frac{1}{2}}^n) \simeq H(u_i^n).$$

Hence, the equation $U_t + H(u) = 0$ yields the following scheme:

$$U_i^{n+1} = U_i^n - \Delta t g(D^{-x}U_i^n, D^{+x}U_i^n).$$

Remark: In the case of higher-dimensional HJ equations with symmetric Hamiltonians, numerical schemes can be built by replicating in each space variable what we did for the one-dimensional case. Hence, the following equation with convex (H is convex $\Leftrightarrow$ H smooth and $\frac{\partial^2 H(p)}{\partial p_i \partial p_j} \geq 0$ ($p = (p_1, p_2, \ldots, p_n)$) or $H(\lambda p + (1 - \lambda q)) \leq \lambda H(p) + (1 - \lambda)H(q), \forall 0 \leq \lambda \leq 1, \forall p, q \in \mathbb{R}$) Hamiltonian

$$U_t + H(U_x, U_y, U_z) = 0$$

can be approximated by

$$
\begin{aligned}
U_{i,j,k}^{n+1} &= U_{i,j,k}^n - \Delta t g(D^{-x} U_{i,j,k}^n, \\
&\quad D^{+x} U_{i,j,k}^n, D^{-y} U_{i,j,k}^n, D^{+y} U_{i,j,k}^n, D^{-z} U_{i,j,k}^n, D^{+z} U_{i,j,k}^n),
\end{aligned}
$$

where

$$D^{-x} U_{i,j,k}^n = \frac{U_{i-1,j,k}^n - U_{i,j,k}^n}{\Delta x}, \text{ and } D^{+x} U_{i,j,k}^n = \frac{U_{i-1,j,k}^n - U_{i,j,k}^n}{\Delta x}.$$

The same thing applies for the other space variables, with Δy and Δz the spacings in the y and z directions.

Example — first-order accuracy scheme: The 2D version of level set Eq. (7) can be approximated as

$$\phi_{i,j}^{n+1} = \phi_{i,j}^n - \Delta t(\max(F_{i,j}, 0)\nabla^+ + \min(F_{i,j}, 0)\nabla^-)^{\frac{1}{2}},$$

where

$$\nabla^+ = [\max(D_{i,j}^{-x}, 0)^2 + \min(D_{i,j}^{+x}, 0)^2 + \max(D_{i,j}^{-y}, 0)^2 + \min(D_{i,j}^{+y}, 0)^2]^{\frac{1}{2}},$$

$$\nabla^- = [\max(D_{i,j}^{+x}, 0)^2 + \min(D_{i,j}^{-x}, 0)^2 + \max(D_{i,j}^{+y}, 0)^2 + \min(D_{i,j}^{-y}, 0)^2]^{\frac{1}{2}}.$$

where we have used shorthand notation in which $D_{i,j}^{+\alpha} = D^{+\alpha}\phi_{i,j}$ with $\alpha = x, y$. Note that this scheme chooses the appropriate *"upwinding"* [37] direction depending on the sign of the speed fuction F.

Finally, all of the second-order curvature-dependent terms can be approximated, for instance, using central differences:

$$\frac{\partial^2 \phi}{\partial x^2} = \frac{\phi_{i+1,j}^n - 2\phi_{i,j}^n + \phi_{i-1,j}^n}{(\Delta x)^2},$$

$$\frac{\partial^2 \phi}{\partial x \partial y} = \frac{\phi_{i+1,j+1}^n + \phi_{i-1,j-1}^n - \phi_{i+1,j-1}^n - \phi_{i-1,j+1}^n}{4(\Delta x)^2}.$$

The same applies for the other derivatives and for higher dimensions. For more details on the numerical techniques for level sets, see [40, 41, 42]. Estimating the region parameters based on the level set function will be presented in the next section so that they can be placed in the main evolution equation.

4.2.7. Estimation of intensity probability density functions

A segmented image I consists of homogeneous regions characterized by statistical properties related to a visual consistency. The inter-region transitions are assumed to be smooth. Let $\Omega \subseteq \mathbb{R}^p$ be an open and bounded p-dimensional domain. Let $I : \Omega \to \mathbb{R}$ be the observed p-dimensional image data. We assume that the number of classes K is known. Let $p_i(I)$ be the intensity probability density function of class i. Each density function must represent the region information to discriminate between two different regions. In our experience, Gaussian models show satisfactory results in medical image segmentation. In this work, we use such density functions and associate the mean μ_i, variance σ_i^2, and prior probability π_i with each class i. The priors satisfy the obvious condition:

$$\sum_{i=1}^{K} \pi_i = 1. \tag{11}$$

In accordance with the estimation method in [30], the model parameters are updated at each iteration as follows:

$$\mu_i = \frac{\int_\Omega H_\alpha(\phi_i) I(x) dx}{\int_\Omega H_\alpha(\phi_i) dx}, \text{ and } \sigma_i^2 = \frac{\int_\Omega H_\alpha(\phi_i)(\mu_i - I(x))^2 dx}{\int_\Omega H_\alpha(\phi_i) dx}. \tag{12}$$

We propose the following equation to estimate the prior probability by counting the number of pixels in each region and dividing it by the total number of pixels:

$$\pi_i = \frac{\int_\Omega H_\alpha(\phi_i) dx}{\sum_{i=1}^{K} \int_\Omega H_\alpha(\phi_i) dx}. \tag{13}$$

Here, $H_\alpha(\cdot)$ is the Heaviside step function defined in [43] as a smoothed differentiable version of the unit step function. The function $H_\alpha(\cdot)$ changes smoothly at the boundary of each region. By the above equations, the model parameters are estimated based on the region information and the main equation.

4.2.8. Evolutionary curve/surface model

The term $\nu = \pm 1$ in Eq. (5) specifies the direction of front propagation. Several approaches were developed to make all fronts either contracting or expanding (see, e.g., [8]) in order to evolve in both directions and avoid overlaps between the regions. The problem can be reformulated as classification of each point at the evolving front. If the point belongs to the associated class, the front expands; otherwise, it contracts.

• *PDE System*: The classification decision is based on the Bayes decision [44] at point x as follows:

$$i^*(x) = \arg \max_{i=1,\cdots,K} (\pi_i p_i(I(x))). \tag{14}$$

The term (ν) for each point x is replaced by the function $\nu_i(x)$ so the velocity function is defined as

$$F_i(x) = \nu_i(x) - \epsilon \cdot k(x), \ \forall \ i = 1, \cdots, K, \tag{15}$$

where

$$\nu_i(x) = \begin{cases} -1 & \text{if} \quad i = i^*(x), \\ 1 & \text{otherwise.} \end{cases} \tag{16}$$

If the pixel x belongs to the front of the class $i = i^*(x)$ associated with the level set function ϕ_i, the front will expand; otherwise, it will contract. Now, we write Eq. (7) in the general form using the derivative $\delta_\alpha(\cdot)$ of the smeared version of the Heaviside function $H_\alpha(\cdot)$ [39], as follows:

$$\frac{\partial \phi_i(x, t)}{\partial t} = \delta_\alpha(\phi_i(x, t))(\epsilon \cdot k(x) - \nu_i(x)) \parallel \nabla \phi_i(x, t) \parallel. \tag{17}$$

The function $\delta_\alpha(\cdot)$ selects the narrow band (NB) points around the front. Solution of the PDEs such as 7) requires numerical processing at each point of the image or volume, which is a time-consuming process. Since we are interested only in the changes of the front, then the solution is important at the points around the front. Such NB points are selected in Eq. (17) thanks to the smeared delta function $\delta_\alpha(\cdot)$. Note that the width of the NB around the moving front is determined by the value of the parameter α. In practice, α is usually taken equal to 1.5, so the that the NB is 3 pixels wide. Points outside the NB are assigned large positive or large negative values in order to be excluded from the computation phase. This highly improves the speed of the numerical process.

4.2.9. Experimental results

Having obtained the skull-stripped MRI slices, the segmentation algorithm is to be applied to all the datasets to isolate the white matter. Applying the automatic seed initialization directly may result in misclassifying some pixels that share the graylevel range of the brain. This may lead to segmentation of the eye as the brain, for example. Therefore, gray levels only are not sufficient for good segmentation.

To solve this problem, the previously discussed level set segmentation with the stochastic Expectation Maximization algorithm for initialization has been used, and it has shown promising results. The results with the algorithm are shown in Figure 7. A 3D evolution of the (WM) surface is shown in Figure 8.

4.3. White Matter Parcellation

White matter parcellation aims at dividing the white matter into inner and outer compartments. Various studies have developed techniques to divide the white matter into radiating, bridging, and sagittal compartments so as to use these compartments for further analysis of different brain disorders [18, 16]. The methodology

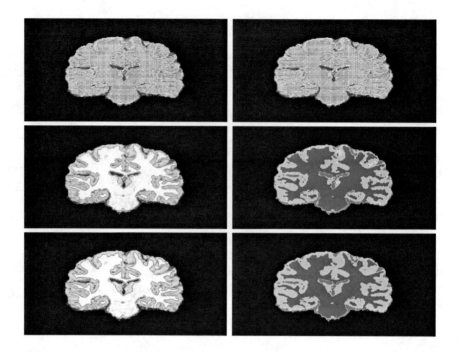

Figure 7. Three steps in the evolution of the three classes of segmentation of a T1-weighted MRI image in the coronal section. **Left column:** blue contour represents white matter region, green contour represents gray matter, and the CSF is marked in red. Associated adaptive regions are given in the right column. See attached CD for color version.

that we will be using here is the same as that discussed by Herbert et al. [18], where the cerebral white matter was divided into inner and outer zones based on a voxel-by-voxel basis according to an arbitrary distance from the white matter boundary. The arbitrary choice of the distance in the present study does make sense as long as it is sufficiently large to include the layer where communications between the minicolumns take place. In other words, the way we define the outer compartment of the white matter or the region of interest is the region where the axon ends and the synapses communicate to different dendrites to transfer information. Therefore, we have two choices to determine such a region: either to ask a neuroscientist to draw this boundary (between the inner and outer compartments) manually, which is very effort and time consuming, or to choose a distance that will be sufficiently large so that it is guaranteed that the communications between the minicolumns occur through it. Bearing in mind that if the chosen distance is larger than the actual one "that could be determined by a neuroscientest," this will just add a bias to the volumes, but the differential comparison will still be valid. In other words, the choice of distance will surely affect the volumes of individual

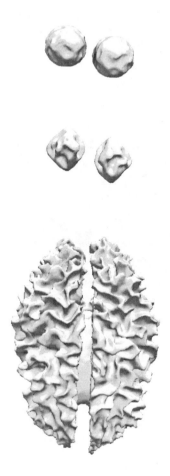

Figure 8. Several steps in a surface evolution to cover the white matter of the brain from an MRI dataset of size $256 \times 256 \times 124$. The top Figure shows initialization of the algorithm by two spheres inside the white matter; the middle illustration depicts an intermediate step that represents evolution; the bottom Figure represents the final result of the surface evolution. See attached CD for color version.

cases; however, it will be still feasible to make a gross comparison of the volumes of the dyslexic and normal brains.

The outer compartment is extracted by detecting the outer contour of the white matter and moving it inward to obtain a boundary between the inner and outer compartments. The reader may expect that moving inward for the same distance in all cases may not result in a significant difference in volumes, so we would like to draw your attention to the fact that a change in the geometry of each case (represented by the changes in structure of the gyrifications between normal and dyslexic, and changes between individuals as well) is expected to affect the volumetric measurements. Figure 9 illustrates the change in geometry. Thus, the basic goal of fixing the depth is to be able to study fairly the effect of these geometric changes (using the volume as a quantitative parameter) that is directly related to the number and width of minicolumns.

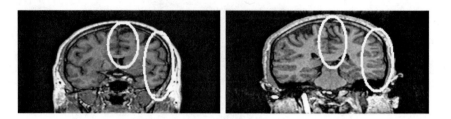

Figure 9. The difference in geometry between normal and dyslexic brains. The marked areas show that the gyrifications in the normal brain (right image) is much more complex than its corresponding part in the dyslexic brain.

The parcellation algorithm was designed and tested on both synthetic and MR images. The basic idea of the algorithm is to calculate the sign distance function ϕ from the boundary Γ (the outer contour of the white matter). This function has the following properties [45]:

$$\phi(x) = \begin{cases} d(x), \text{ if } x \text{ inside of } W \text{ (white matter point)}, \\ 0, \text{ if } x \in \Gamma, \\ -d(x), \text{ if } x \text{ outside of } W, \end{cases} \tag{18}$$

where

$$d(x) = \min_{y \in \Gamma}(|x - y|), \text{ and } W : \text{ the region enclosed by } \Gamma. \tag{19}$$

The boundary between the inner and outer compartments is obtained by detecting the set $X = \{x/d(x) = d_1\}$ of all points that are d_1 away from the boundary Γ, that is, the set X represents a contour that is distant from the outer contour by d_1 pixels. Figure 10 illustrates this idea, which simply consists of representing the outer contour as the zero level set that is the intersection of the plane $z = 0$ (the blue plane) with the signed distance function. Pushing the contour inward is done by getting the intersection of the plane $z = d_1$ (the green plane) with the signed distance function.

Figure 11 shows the result of applying the algorithm on a synthetic image of a circle, whereas Figure 12 shows the parcellation results on a real MRI slice.

After parcellating the white matter and isolating the outer compartment, the volumes of the whole white matter (V) as well as the volume of the outer com-

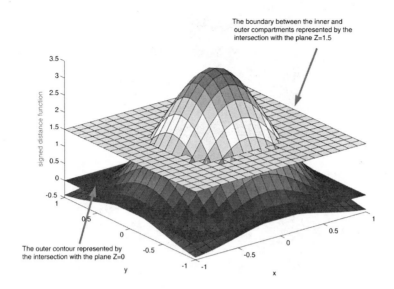

The boundary between the inner and outer compartments represented by the intersection with the plane Z=1.5

The outer contour represented by the intersection with the plane Z=0

Figure 10. This illustrates the idea of moving the outer contour using the signed distance function ϕ. Intersection of ϕ with plane $z = 0$ represents the original contour, and its intersection with plane $z = d_1$ represents the new boundary. See attached CD for color version..

partment (V_o) are calculated for both dyslexic patients and normal control cases. The obtained values are reported in Table 1. The means and standard deviations for each category were calculated as well.

4.4. Statistical Analysis

The brain extraction and segmentation represent the basic preliminary work that enables us to extract the white matter from each MRI stack. White matter parcellation helped in obtaining the region of interest. Having segmented and parcellated the white matter, the statistical analysis consists of the following steps:

1. The volumes of the whole white matter of all cases were calculated. The means (μ_{o_1} and μ_{o_2}) and standard deviations (σ_{w_1} and σ_{w_2}) for the normal and dyslexic groups, respectively, were calculated.

2. The volumes of the outer and inner compartments of the normal and control cases were calculated. The means (μ_{o_1}, μ_{i_1}, and μ_{o_2}, μ_{i_2}) as well as standard deviations (σ_{o_1}, σ_{i_1}, and σ_{o_2}, σ_{i_2}) were calculated.

3. Three hypotheses tests were performed to test the proposed concept.

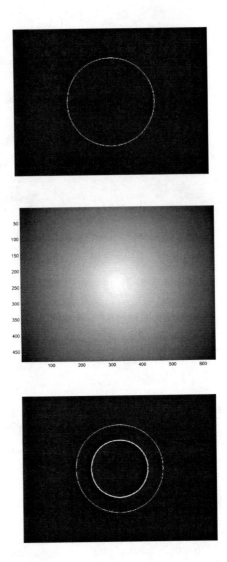

Figure 11. Parcellation results for a synthetic image of a circle. **Top**: original contour. **Middle**: signed distance map. **Bottom**: new boundary superimposed on the original image.

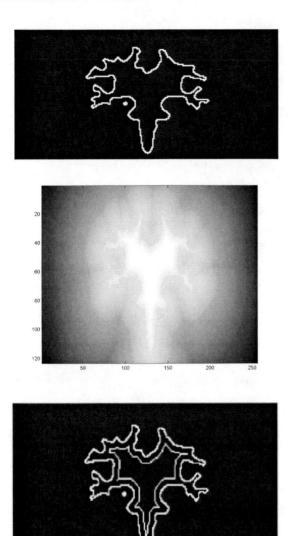

Figure 12. Parcellation results for an MRI slice: **Left**: original contour. **Middle**: signed distance map. **Right**: new boundary superimposed on the original MR image.

White Matter Parcellation Algorithm

SET NumberofSlices to 256

SET NumberofVoxels to 0

    FOR i=1 to NumberofSlices

        INPUT WhiteMatterImage

        SET FilledContour to RegionFill(WhiteMatter)

        SET Edge to Edge(FilledContour)

        CALCULATE DistanceMap(Edge)

        SET LowerLimit to d-0.5

        SET UpperLimit to d+0.5

            FOR k=size(Edge,1) do

                FOR l=size(Edge,2)do

                    IF WhiteMatterImage(k,l)=255 do

                        IF DistanceMap(k,l)> LowerLimit AND

                        DistanceMap(k,l)< UpperLimit do

                        SET NumberofVoxels = NumberofVoxels+1

                    END IF

                  END IF

                END FOR

            END FOR

    END FOR

INPUT Resolution

CALCULATE OuterCompartmentVol as Resolution* NumberofVoxels

Table 1. Volumetric Measures of the Outer Compartment
at a Parcellation distances $d = 5$ and $d = 7$

Normal Cases	V	$V_o(d_1 = 5)$	$V_1(d_1 = 7)$	Dyslexic Cases	V	$V_o(d_1 = 5)$	$V_1(d_1 = 7)$
1	615.375	469.4941	509.6487	1	540.5625	447.5553	477.312
2	650.8125	516.4356	560.2039	2	546.1875	446.7867	480.8070
3	699.1875	584.0372	638.4656	3	513.5625	419.5890	449.9455
4	626.0625	517.4468	561.6488	4	529.3125	441.1969	470.0294
5	604.1250	510.2974	548.1369	5	567.5625	447.6634	485.4542
6	599.0625	465.5905	505.0028	6	565.8750	453.4378	490.7065
7	665.4375	546.3848	592.2163	7	544.5000	437.8838	472.8335
8	609.7500	470.6741	504.0800	8	563.6250	449.2745	485.8665
9	567.5625	468.6702	507.7015	10	475.8750	382.3809	407.9558
10	546.7500	459.4852	503.2006	10	432.0000	365.0273	383.8285
11	560.2500	494.2015	531.7247	11	585.0000	470.3933	506.0193
12	480.3750	362.6372	390.7261	12	508.5000	409.7843	444.3069
13	637.3125	510.0851	549.2417	13	577.6875	471.4308	506.6007
14	640.1250	477.8618					
MEAN	607.2991	489.5215			534.6346	434.0311	

(a) Comparison between the volumetric measures of the total white matter volume to test if there is a significant difference in the volumes or not; the t test has the null hypothesis $\mu_{w_1} > \mu_{w_2}$

(b) Comparison between the volumetric measurement of the outer compartment to test that the increment of volume (if proved by the first test) is resulting from the increment of the outer compartment volume; the t test has the null hypothesis $\mu_{o_1} > \mu_{o_2}$.

(c) A third t test that has a null hypothesis of $\mu_{i_1} \neq \mu_{i_2}$ and is performed to test if the inner compartment played any role in the volumetric changes found between the different groups.

The results for these hypotheses tests were very promising. The first test was performed twice, once at a confidence level $\alpha = 0.05$ and again at a more restricted tolerance $\alpha = 0.01$, and both times the null hypothesis was accepted. The second test, as well, was performed with several combinations. It was done with the volumetric measures at different distances $d_1 = 5$ and $d_1 = 7$, as well as different confidence levels $\alpha = 0.05$ and $\alpha = 0.01$, and the null hypothesis that $\mu_{o_1} > \mu_{o_2}$ was accepted in all previous combinations. The third test was performed with similar combinations. The null hypothesis was accepted when $d_1 = 5$ and $\alpha = 0.01$, but it was rejected in all the remaining combinations.

5. CONCLUSION

This chapter has presented a novel method for investigating brain developmental disorders through minicolumnar structures. A hypothesis-driven work has been introduced by correlating pathological findings, represented by the number and width of minicolumns, to MRI findings, represented by volumetric measurement of the total white matter and the outer compartment of the white matter. A novel level set-based segmentation technique was used to segment the MR images for both dyslexic and control cases. Signed distance maps and front propagation have been utilized to parcel the white matter into inner and outer compartments. The pacellated images were then used to compute and compare the white matter volumes. Statistical hypotheses tests were performed to investigate the differences between the volumetric measurements in dyslexic patients and normal control cases. We concluded that the reduced number of minicolumns in the dyslexic brains directly affects the volume of the white matter. This work is considered a beginning of a series of studies of the effect of minicolumnar disturbance on the brain via MRI. We propose to investigate the relationship between pathological findings and the geometrical structures of the brain. This will be accomplished by analyzing the gyral window and bending in the gyrification of normal and dyslexic cases. Future work will also involve the use of diffusion tensor images to analyze white matter tracts and correlate it to the way in which minicolumns communicate. And, last but not least, texture analysis as well as scale representations will be used to extract more features that may help analyzing brain developmental disorders.

6. APPENDIX: PSEUDO CODE FOR THE SEGMENTATION ALGORITHM

Assume that we have an image $I : R^n \to R^+$ and K regions with initial means $\mu_1, ..., \mu_K$. Assign a level set function for each region $\phi_1, ..., \phi_K$. The main steps will be as follows:

1. Initialize the level set function using automatic seed initialization ($InitFunc$).

2. Calculate mean (μ_i), variance (σ_i^2), and prior probability (π_i) of each adaptive region ($ParamFunc$).

3. Mark the narrow band points ($NarrowBandFunc$).

4. Carry out Bayesian decision based on the above estimated parameters in each point in the narrow band to decide adding or removing the point from the associated region ($IterateFunc$).

5. Mark the front points to show contours in 2D. In case of 3D, regions can be visualized by means of binary values.

6. If the functions do not reach the steady state, go to step 2; otherwise, exit.

Pseudo Code for $InitFunc$

▪ Set all level set functions to zeros at every point in the domain.

▪ Divide the image into sub-blocks ($1...M$) equal in size based on a given window size.

▪ For j=1:M
Calculate the average gray level μ_j.
Calculate the index of the nearest mean $indx = \arg\min_{k=1,2,...,K}(|\mu_j - \mu_k|^2)$.
Set ϕ_{index} to 1 at every point in block j.

▪ End

Pseudo Code for $ParamFunc$

▪ Set $\mu_k = 0$, $\sigma_k = 0$, and $\pi_k = 0 \ \forall \ k \in [1, K]$

▪ For k=1:K
Set μ_k to the average gray level of pixels in the positive region of ϕ_k.
Set σ_k^2 to the variance of pixels in the positive region of ϕ_k.
Set π_k to the number of pixels in the positive region of ϕ_k.

▪ End

▪ Normalize priors to have the sum of one $\pi_k = \frac{\pi_k}{\sum_{i=1}^{K} \pi_i}$.

Pseudo Code for $NarrowBandFunc(\phi_k)$

▪ Set the narrow-band function NB_k to zero at every point in space.

▪ Mark the front points E.

▪ $\forall \ e \in E$, set $NB_k(f) = 1$ where $f \in B$ and B is the set of neighbor points of e (usually, we take the horizontal and vertical ones).

Pseudo Code for $IterateFunc$

- For k=1:K
  $\forall\, e \in\, NB_k.$
  —calculate $indx(e) = \arg\max_{i=1,\cdots,K}(\pi_i p_i(I(e)))$.
  —if $index(e) = k$, then $\phi_k(e) = 1$, else $\phi_k(e) = 0$.
  Smooth ϕ_k.

- End

7. REFERENCES

1. Pugh KR, Mencl WE, Jenner AR. 2000. Functional neuroimaging studies of reading and reading disability: (developmental dyslexia). *Ment Retard Dev Disabil Res Rev* **6**(3):207–213.
2. Brambilla P, Hardan A, Nemi SV. 2003. Brain anatomy and development in autism review of MRI studies. *Brain Res Bull* **61**(6):557–569.
3. Buxhoeveden DP, Casanova MF. 2002. The minicolumn and evolution of the brain: a review. *Brain Behav Evol* **60**(3):125–51.
4. Palmen S, Engeland H, Hof P, Schmitz C. 2004. Neuropathological findings in autism. *Brain*, **127**(12):2572–2583.
5. Eliez S, Rumsey JM, Giedd JN, Schmitt JE, Patwardhan AJ, Reiss AL. 2000. Morphological alteration of temporal lobe gray level matter in dyslexia: an MRI study. *J Child Psychol Psychiatry* **41**(5):637–44.
6. Goldenberg R, Kimmel R, Rivlin E, Rudzsky M. 2002. Cortex segmentation: a fast variational geometric approach. *IEEE Trans Med Imaging* **21**(2):1544–1551.
7. Baillard C, Barillot C. 2001. Robust 3D segmentation of anatomical structures with level sets. *Med Image Anal* **5**(3):185–94.
8. Zeng X, Staib LH, Schultz RT, Tagare H, Win L, Duncan JS. 1999. A new approach to 3D sulcal ribbon finding from MR images. In *Proceedings of the international conference on medical image computing and computer-assisted intervention (MICCAI'99). Lecture notes in computer science*, Vol. 1679, pp. 148–157. New York: Springer.
9. Farag AA, Hassan H. 2004. Adaptive segmentation of multimodal 3d data using robust level set techniques. In *Proceedings of the international conference on medical image computing and computer-assisted intervention (MICCAI'2004). Lecture notes in computer science*, Vol. 3216, pp. 143–150, New York: Springer.
10. Rousson M, Paragios N, and Deriche R. 2004. Implicit active shape models for 3d segmentation in mri imaging. In *Proceedings of the international conference on medical image computing and computer-assisted intervention (MICCAI'2004). Lecture notes in computer science*, Vol. 3216, pp. 209-216. New York: Springer.
11. Zeng X, Staib LH, Duncan JS. Volumetric layer segmentation using coupled surface propagation. In *Proceedings of the IEEE international conference on computer vision and pattern recognition*, pp. 708–715. Washington, DC: IEEE Computer Society.
12. Caselles V, Kimmel R, Sapiro G. 1997. Geodesic active contours. *Int J Comput Vision* **22**(1):61–79.
13. Zaho H-K, Chan T, Merriman B, Osher S. 1995. A variational level set approach to multiphase motion. *J Comput Phys* **127**:179-195.
14. Xu C, Pham D, Prince J. 1999. Reconstruction of the human cerebral cortex from magnetic resonance images. *IEEE Trans Med Imaging* **18**(6):467–480.
15. Casanova M, Switala A, Trippe J, Fobbs A. 2004. *Minicolumnar Morphometry: a report on the brains of Yakovlev, Meyer, And geschwind*. Technical Report, Department of Psychiatry and Behavior Science, University of Louisville, Louisville, Kentucky.

16. Makris N, Meyer JW, Bates JF, Yeterian EH, Kennedy DN, Caviness VS. 1999. MRI-based topographic parcellation of human cerebral white matter. *Neuroimage* **9**(1):18–45.

17. Mountcastle VB. 1997. The minicolumnar organization of the neocortex. *Brain* **120**:701–722.

18. Herbert MR, Zeigler DA, Markis N. 2004. Localization of white matter volume increase in autism and developmental language disorders. *Ann Neurol* **55**:530–540.

19. Chung M, Robbins S, Dalton K. 2005. Cortical thickness analysis in autism with heat kernel smoothing. *NeuroImage* **25**:1256–1265.

20. Jackowski M, Kao C, Qiu M, ConsTable R, Staib L. 2005. White matter tractography by anisotropic wavefront evolution and diffusion tensor imaging. *Med Image Anal* **9**:427–440.

21. Lenglet C, Deriche R, Faugeras O. 2003. *Diffusion tensor magnetic resonance imaging: brain connectivity mapping*. Research Report no. 4983, Institut National de Rechereche en informatique et automatique, Sophia-Antipolis, France.

22. Bihan D, Breton E. 1985. Imagerie de diffusion in vivi par resonance magnitique nucleaire. *CR Acad Sci Paris* **301**:1109–1112.

23. Merboldt K, Hanicke W, Frahm J. 1985. Self-diffusion NMR imaging using stimulated echoes. *J Magn Reson* **64**:479–486.

24. Bihan D, Mangin J, Poupon C. 2001. Diffusion tensor imaging: concepts and applications. *J Magn Reason Imag* **13**:534–546.

25. Goraly N, Kwon H, Eliez S. 2004. White matter structures in autism: preliminary evidence from diffusion tensor imaging. *Biol Psychiatry* 55 :323–326.

26. Eckert MA, Leonard CM, Wilke M, Eckert M, Richards T, Richards A, Berninger V. 2004. Anatomical signatures of dyslexia in children: unique information from manual and voxel based morphometry brain measures. *Cortex* **41**(3):304–315.

27. El-Zehiry N, Casanova M, Hassan H, Farag A. 2005. Structural MRI analysis of the brains of patients with dyslexia. In *Proceedings of the international conference on computer assisted radiology and surgery (CARS 2005)*, pp. 1291–1296. New York: Elsevier.

28. Rumsey JM, Donohue BC, Brady DR, Nace K, Giedd JN, Andreason P. 1997. A magnetic resonance study of planum temporale asymmetry in men with developmental dyslexia. *Arch Neuorol* **54**(12):1481–1489.

29. Rumsey JM, Nace K, Donohue BC, Wise D, Maisog JM, Andreason P. A positron emission tomographic study of impaired word recognition and phonological processing in dyslexic men. *Arch Neurol* **54**(5):562–573.

30. Chan T, Vese L. 2002. A multiphase level set framework for image segmentation using the mumford and shah model. *Int J Comput Vision* **50**(3):271–293.

31. Osher S, Paragios N. 2003. *Geometric level set methods in imaging, vision, and graphics.* New York: Springer.

32. Sapiro G. 2001. *Geometric partial differential equations and image analysis.* Cambridge: Cambridge UP.

33. Caselles V, Kimmel R, Sapiro G. 1997. Geodesics active contours. *Int J Comput Vision* **22**:61–97.

34. Epstein CL, Gage M. 1987. The curve shhortening flow. In *Wave motion: theory modeling and computation*, pp. 15–59. Ed A Chorin, A Majda. New York: Springer.

35. Paragios N, Deriche R. 1999. Unifying boundary and region-based information for geodesic active tracking. In *Proceedings of the IEEE international conference on computer vision and pattern recognition (CVPR'99)*, Vol. 2, pp. 300–305. Washington, DC: IEEE Computer Society.

36. Gomes J, Faugeras O. *Reconciling distance functions and Level Sets.* Technical Report no 3666, INRIA, Institut National de Rechereche en informatique et automatique, Sophia-Antipolis, France.

37. Sethian JA. 1999. *Level set methods and fast marching methods.* Cambridge: Cambridge UP.

38. Malladi R, Sethian J, Vemuri B. 1995. Shape modeling with front propagation: a level set approach. *IEEE Trans Pattern Anal Machine Intell* **17**(2):158–175.

39. Samson C, Blanc-Féraud L, Aubert G, Zerubia J. 1999. Multiphase evolution and variational image classification. Technical Report no. 3662, INRIA, Institut National de Rechereche en informatique et automatique, Sophia-Antipolis, France.

40. Osher S. UCLA Technical Report, available at http://www.math.ucla.edu/applied/cam/index.html.

41. Sethian JA. 1996. *Level set methods: evolving interfaces in geometry, fluid mechanics, computer vision and material sciences.* Cambridge: Cambridge UP.

42. Osher SJ, Sethian JA. 1988. Front propagation with curvature speed: algorithms based on Hamilton-Jacobi formulations. *J Comput Phys* **79**:12–49.

43. Chan T, Sandberg B, Vese L. 2000. Active contours without edges for vector valued images. *J Vis Commun Image Represent* **2**:130-141.

44. Duda R, Hart P, Stork D. 2001. *Pattern classification.* New York: John Wiley and Sons.

45. Osher S, Fedkiw R. 2003. *Level set methods and dynamic implicit surfaces.* New York: Springer.

15

ANALYSIS OF 4-D CARDIAC MR DATA WITH NURBS DEFORMABLE MODELS: TEMPORAL FITTING STRATEGY AND NONRIGID REGISTRATION

Nicholas J. Tustison and Amir A. Amini

Cardiovascular Image Analysis Laboratory,
Washington University
St. Louis, Missouri 63110, USA

We present research in which both left- and right-ventricular deformation is estimated from tagged cardiac mgnetic resonance imaging using volumetric deformable models constructed from nonuniform rational B-splines (NURBS). The four model types considered and compared for the left ventricle include two Cartesian NURBS models — one with a cylindrical parameter assignment and one with a prolate spheroidal parameter assignment. The remaining two are non-Cartesian, i.e., prolate spheroidal and cylindrical, each with their respective prolate spheroidal and cylindrical parameter assignment regime. These choices were made based on the typical shape of the left ventricle. For each frame subsequent to end-diastole, an NURBS model is constructed by fitting two surfaces with the same parameterization to the corresponding set of epicardial and endocardial contours from which a volumetric model is created. Using normal displacements of the three sets of orthogonal tag planes as well as displacements of contour/tag line intersection points and tag plane intersection points, one can solve for the optimal homogeneous coordinates, in a weighted least-squares sense, of the control points of the deformed NURBS model at end-diastole using quadratic programming. This allows for subsequent nonrigid registration of the biventricular model at end-diastole to all later time frames. After registration of the model to all later time points, the registered NURBS models are temporally lofted in order to create a comprehensive four-dimensional NURBS model. From the lofted model, we can extract 3D myocardial deformation fields and corresponding Lagrangian and Eulerian

Address all correspondence to: Amir Amini, Cardiovascular Image Analysis Laboratory, Schools of Engineering and Medicine, Washington University in St. Louis, Box 8086, 660 S. Euclid Avenue, St. Louis, MO 63110, USA. Phone: (314) 454-7408; Fax: (314) 454-5350. amini@cauchy.wustl.edu. http://www-cv.wustl.edu.

strain maps that are local measures of nonrigid deformation. The results show that, in the case of simulated data, the quadratic Cartesian NURBS models with the cylindrical and prolate spheroidal parameter assignments outperform their counterparts in predicting normal strain. The decreased complexity associated with the Cartesian model with the cylindrical parameter assignment prompted its use for subsequent calculations. Lagrangian strains in three sets of canine data, a normal human, and a patient with a history of myocardial infarction are presented. Eulerian strains for the normal human are also included.

1. INTRODUCTION

Noninvasive imaging techniques for assessing the dynamic behavior of the myocardial tissue, such as tissue tagging with magnetic resonance imaging (MRI), are invaluable in the characterization of heart disease [1]. The advantages of tagged MRI have encouraged significant research in the area of quantitative analysis of myocardial deformation via physical and mathematical models [2, 3]. While most relevant work has focused exclusively on the left ventricle, promising results have been obtained from myocardial tag analysis of the right ventricle [4–7]. Our coupled biventricular NURBS model is capable of providing comprehensive 3D analysis of both the left and right ventricles using tag and contour information from tagged MR images.

1.1. Magnetic Resonance Tagging

1.1.1. Overview

MR tagging methods allow for noninvasive measurement of intramural heart wall motion by combining the high spatiotemporal resolution of MRI with tissue tagging techniques [8, 9]. By altering the magnetization of the myocardial tissue with special RF and gradient pulses, planes of hypointense signal, or tag planes, are placed orthogonal to the image plane at end-diastole, producing a grid pattern in the short-axis (Figure 1a) or long-axis (Figure 1b) image planes.

The intersections of the image planes with the tag planes are known as tag lines. These tag lines deform in conjunction with the myocardial tissue facilitating the visualization of deformation (Figure 2). The tag plane geometry consists of a sequence of horizontal and a sequence of vertical tag planes placed orthogonal to the short-axis image planes. Since displacement information with these two sets of tag planes is only within the short-axis plane, a third set of tag planes is placed orthogonal to the longitudinal set of images to capture motion normal to the short-axis image plane. Thus, all three sets of tag planes are used to measure 3D motion.

1.1.2. Imaging protocol

For the canine studies presented in this chapter, the following imaging protocol was utilized on a 1.5-T Sonata (Siemens Medical Solutions, Erlangen, Germany)

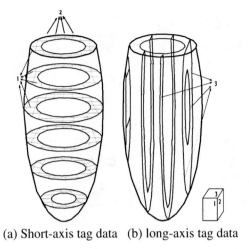

(a) Short-axis tag data   (b) long-axis tag data

Figure 1. The cube in the lower right illustrates the three orthogonal directions of the tag plane normals. The intersection of the short-axis image planes with the short-axis tag planes results in the tag lines marked '1' and '2.' Similarly, the tag lines marked '3' are formed from the intersection of the long-axis image planes with the long-axis tag planes.

with a slew rate of 200 mT/m/msec and a maximum gradient strength of 40 mT/m. A breath-hold, segmented k-space ECG-gated SPAMM pulse sequence with 100% k-space coverage, and five segments was used to collect multiple images in both short-axis and long-axis views of the entire heart without gaps. Immediately after the R-wave of the electrocardiogram, radio-frequency (RF) tagging pulses were applied in two orthogonal directions. The temporal resolution of the imaging sequence was 32.0 msec (note, however, that the real repetition time (TR) = 32.0/5 = 6.4 msec), the echo time (TE) was 2.8 msec, the RF pulse flip angle was 20°, the bandwidth was 184 Hz/pixel, and the time extent of RF tag pulses was 2.2 msec. Other imaging parameters were: field of View = 300 × 300 mm², in-plane resolution = 1.17 × 1.17 mm², and slice thickness = 8 mm. The tag spacing (grid tag pattern in the short-axis images and stripes in the long-axis images) was chosen to be 8 mm due to practical limitations in automated delineation of tags with smaller separation.

1.2. Relevant Work

Early techniques for evaluating myocardial deformation based on B-splines were restricted to 2D short-axis techniques [10, 11]. Although fast, such techniques did not take into account myocardial through-plane motion. Extension to more comprehensive 3D analysis was based on the geometrical configuration of the MR tag planes. This configuration is conducive to tag analysis using B-spline

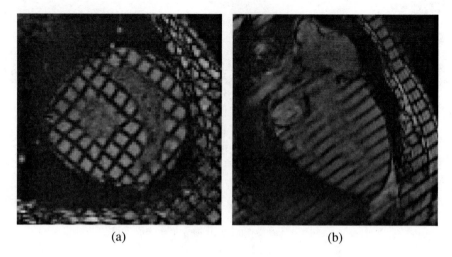

(a)   (b)

Figure 2. MR images from a canine study showing the left and right ventricles in both (a) the short- and (b) long-axis views.

cubic deformable models [12–16]. The construction in [13, 14, 16] interpolates each tag plane by an isoparametric surface of the cubic model (B-solid). The spatial extent of these cubic models extends past the myocardial contours, which yields nonzero strain values outside the myocardial region. Cylindrical B-spline models have also been employed that more closely match the shape of the left ventricle [17, 18]. However, these authors only considered cylindrical parameter assignments with uniform, nonrational, cylindrical B-splines. We demonstrate that Cartesian NURBS models that also employ cylindrical parameter assignments outperform the cylindrical NURBS models with cylindrical parameter assignments. The approach described herein constructs a model based on the morphology of the biventricular anatomical structure for each imaging study using the short- and long-axis contours in each image. This forces the spatial extent of the model to be confined within the myocardial boundaries. As an additional novelty, we improve the approximation capabilities of our model by extending the model bases from uniform nonrational B-splines to its superset; namely, nonuniform rational B-splines (NURBS). The models are constructed using Cartesian or non-Cartesian NURBS with both cylindrical and prolate spheroidal parameter assignment.

2. NURBS MODEL

2.1. Nonuniform Rational B-Splines

NURBS, an acronym for **no**nuniform **r**ational **B**-splines, have become the de facto standard for computational geometric representation [19, 20]. NURBS provide an additional parameter, the weighting of the control points, which can be varied for more accurate fitting over nonrational B-splines while maintaining all the favorable properties of nonrational B-splines.

An NURBS curve of degree d, $\mathbf{R}(u)$, consisting of n control points is defined by the equation

$$\mathbf{R}(u) = \frac{\sum_{i=1}^{n} N_{i,d}(u)\psi_i\mathbf{P}_i}{\sum_{i=1}^{n} N_{i,d}(u)\psi_i} \qquad 0 \leq u \leq 1, \qquad (1)$$

where $\mathbf{P}_i$ represents the coordinates of the ith control point and $N_{i,d}(u)$ is the corresponding B-spline basis function calculated at location parameter value u. The additional parameter, ψ_i, is the weight of the ith control point. Note that nonrational B-spline curves are a subset of NURBS with all weights equal to a nonzero constant value.

After defining a *knot vector* $\mathbf{U} = \{U_1, \ldots, U_m\}$ to be a sequence of non-decreasing real numbers, called *knots*, and selecting an appropriate degree, the B-spline basis functions are calculated using the Cox-deBoor recurrence relation

$$N_{i,d}(u) = \frac{u - U_i}{U_{i+d} - U_i} N_{i,d-1}(u)$$
$$+ \frac{U_{i+d+1} - u}{U_{i+d+1} - U_{i+1}} N_{i+1,d-1}(u), \qquad (2)$$

$$N_{i,0}(u) = \left\{ \begin{array}{ll} 1 & U_i \leq u < U_{i+1}, \\ 0 & \text{otherwise}, \end{array} \right. \qquad (3)$$

where $\frac{0}{0}$ is defined to be 0. The ith *knot span* is defined to be the interval of the curve $[\mathbf{R}(U_i), \mathbf{R}(U_{i+1}))$. The degree d (order $= d + 1$), number of knots, and the number of control points are related by the formula $m = n + d + 1$.

Two important properties of B-splines are

Locality Each span of the piecewise B-spline curve of degree d is influenced by the neighboring $d + 1$ control points. Similarly, moving a single control point on the same curve influences the placement of only $d + 1$ neighboring spans.

Continuity A d degree B-spline curve is C^{d-k} continuous at the knot locations (where k is the knot multiplicity) and is smooth elsewhere.

2.1.1. Cylindrical and prolate spheroidal-based NURBS

The conventional implementation of NURBS employs a Cartesian basis in which the B-spline basis functions smooth over the x, y, and z coordinates of the

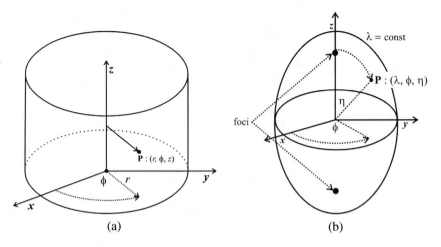

Figure 3. (a) Cylindrical coordinate system; (b) prolate spheroidal coordinate system used in constructing the NURBS model.

control points separately in the construction of the B-spline curve, surface, etc. However, we can use the same principles to construct both cylindrical and prolate spheroidal B-splines where the basis functions blend the location of control points in (r, ϕ, z) and (λ, ϕ, η), respectively. These two coordinate systems are illustrated by the diagrams located in Figure 3.

A point (x, y, z) has cylindrical coordinates (r, ϕ, z) given by the formulae

$$
\begin{aligned}
r &= \sqrt{x^2 + y^2}, \\
\phi &= \tan^{-1} \frac{y}{x}, \qquad 0 \le \phi < 2\pi, \\
z &= z.
\end{aligned}
\tag{4}
$$

The reciprocal conversion is

$$
\begin{aligned}
x &= r \cos \phi, \\
y &= r \sin \phi, \\
z &= z.
\end{aligned}
\tag{5}
$$

In addition, a point (x, y, z) has prolate spheroidal coordinates (λ, ϕ, η):

$$
\begin{aligned}
\lambda &= \cosh^{-1} \frac{r_1 + r_2}{2\delta}, \\
\phi &= \tan^{-1} \frac{y}{x}, \qquad 0 \le \phi < 2\pi, \\
\eta &= \cos^{-1} \frac{r_1 - r_2}{2\delta}, \qquad -\frac{\pi}{2} \le \eta \le \frac{\pi}{2},
\end{aligned}
\tag{6}
$$

where

$$r_1 = \sqrt{x^2 + y^2 + (z + \delta)^2},$$
$$r_2 = \sqrt{x^2 + y^2 + (z - \delta)^2}, \tag{7}$$

and δ is the distance from the origin to either focus. The reverse transformation is calculated from

$$x = \delta \sinh \lambda \sin \eta \cos \phi,$$
$$y = \delta \sinh \lambda \sin \eta \sin \phi, \tag{8}$$
$$z = \delta \cosh \lambda \cos \eta.$$

The B-spline basis functions determine the shape of the curve by smoothing, in a weighted fashion, over the coordinates of the control points. Thus, by changing the coordinates of the control points from a Cartesian to another description, the entire curve changes. This distinction is illustrated by the plots in Figure 4. The Cartesian B-spline curve is shown in Figure 4a. It was plotted on the Cartesian axes using the formulae

$$x(u) = \sum_{i=1}^{n} N_{i,d}(u) \mathbf{P}_i^x, \tag{9}$$

$$y(u) = \sum_{i=1}^{n} N_{i,d}(u) \mathbf{P}_i^y, \tag{10}$$

where $(\mathbf{P}_i^x, \mathbf{P}_i^y)$ is the Cartesian description of the ith control point. The non-Cartesian (polar) B-spline curve is plotted on the same Cartesian axes in Figure 4b. The curve is produced by the formulae

$$x(u) = r(u) \cos(\phi(u))$$
$$= \left(\sum_{i=1}^{n} N_{i,d}(u) \mathbf{P}_i^r \right) \cos \left(\sum_{i=1}^{n} N_{i,d}(u) \mathbf{P}_i^\phi \right), \tag{11}$$
$$y(u) = r(u) \sin(\phi(u))$$
$$= \left(\sum_{i=1}^{n} N_{i,d}(u) \mathbf{P}_i^r \right) \sin \left(\sum_{i=1}^{n} N_{i,d}(u) \mathbf{P}_i^\phi \right), \tag{12}$$

where $(\mathbf{P}_i^r, \mathbf{P}_i^\phi)$ is the polar coordinate of the ith control point.

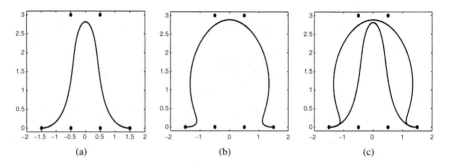

Figure 4. Cartesian versus non-Cartesian nonrational B-spline curves: order = 4; control point coordinates (x, y) — $\mathbf{P}_1 = (-1.5, 0)$, $\mathbf{P}_2 = (-0.5, 0)$, $\mathbf{P}_3 = (-0.5, 3)$, $\mathbf{P}_4 = (0.5, 3)$, $\mathbf{P}_5 = (0.5, 0)$, $\mathbf{P}_6 = (1.5, 0)$. Illustrated are (a) the Cartesian B-spline curve, (b) the polar-based B-spline curve, and (c) their superposition constructed from the control points.

2.1.2. Higher-dimensional NURBS objects

Equation (1) can be extended to create higher-order NURBS objects. A volumetric NURBS object, $\mathbf{S}(u, v, w)$, is defined by the equation

$$\mathbf{S}(u, v, w) = \frac{\sum_{i=1}^{l} \sum_{j=1}^{m} \sum_{k=1}^{n} N_{i,p}(u) N_{j,q}(v) N_{k,r}(w) \psi_{i,j,k} \mathbf{P}_{i,j,k}}{\sum_{i=1}^{l} \sum_{j=1}^{m} \sum_{k=1}^{n} N_{i,p}(u) N_{j,q}(v) N_{k,r}(w) \psi_{i,j,k}}, \quad (13)$$

which consists of a triple summation involving three sets of basis functions spanning the volume of the NURBS model for the u, v, and w location parameters, $l \times m \times n$ control points, and the corresponding weights, $\psi_{i,j,k}$. The respective degree in each of the three parametric directions is p, q, and r. Additionally, we can add a fourth B-spline basis function and parameter to compose a temporally varying NURBS volumetric object. The 4D model created in our methodology is constructed by *skinning* or *lofting* a temporal series of volumetric NURBS models representing each frame of data [20].

3. MATHEMATICAL PRELIMINARIES

One of the distinct attributes of the work presented in this chapter is the use of NURBS to model left- and right-ventricular deformation. The motivation for employing NURBS over uniform nonrational B-splines is that NURBS allow for variation of the knot vector and weighting of the control points in addition to the degree of the spline and the location and number of control points.

The degrees of freedom available in constructing the approximating model should be optimized to produce the most accurate results. To construct the initial model for subsequent registration one must select the knot vectors, number of control points, as well as the degree of spline. These parameters remain fixed for the registration process for each frame of data. This stems from the fact that material point correspondence is dictated by the parameterization of the model, and altering any one of these variables changes the parameterization. In choosing these initial parameters, we want to avoid oversmoothing of the data using a low degree of parametric complexity (underfitting) while avoiding undue influence of noise in our estimation (overfitting). This is the well-known underfitting/overfitting problem [21]. After the initial model construction, NURBS allow for two degrees of freedom for subsequent fitting — control point location and control point weighting. Nonrational B-splines only allow one degree of freedom (control point location). Additionally, due to the spatial configuration of displacement data, the number of spans of the volumetric B-spline model is limited (see the explanation of the *Schoenberg-Whitney* conditions in Section 3.1). Therefore, the control point weight variation inherent with NURBS is essential for increased accuracy over nonrational B-splines.

Ma and Kruth presented a method for free-form curve or surface fitting using NURBS in which the optimal homogeneous control point locations were found using quadratic programming [22]. They found that the ability to vary the control point weighting associated with NURBS allowed for more accurate fitting over nonrational B-splines for curves and surfaces with the same parameterization. We extend this methodology to our research involving volumetric NURBS models in which the optimal control point coordinates are calculated using tagged MR data. We give a brief overview of the least-squares method for curve fitting. We also describe the necessary modifications for fitting curve data to polar B-spline curves. Extension to surface or volumetric NURBS objects is straightforward.

3.1. NURBS Least-Squares Fitting with Measurement Confidences

Solving for the location of the control points of a B-spline curve or surface in a least-squares sense is a well-studied problem [20]. Suppose a set of s discrete points, denoted by the set $\mathcal{D} = \{\mathbf{p}_i = (x_i, y_i, z_i)^{\mathrm{T}} : i \in \{1, s\}\}$, is given representing a free-form curve (extension to volumetric NURBS objects is straightforward). If, in addition to the set $\mathcal{D}$, we have a corresponding set of weights $\mathcal{W} = \{w_i : i \in \{1, s\}\}$ that quantifies the relative confidence in the measurement of each corresponding point, the weighted least-squares error criterion, E_w, for the x coordinate is

$$E_w = \sum_{i=1}^{s} w_i \left(x_i - \frac{\sum_{j=1}^{n} N_{j,d}(u_i)\psi_j P_j^x}{\sum_{j=1}^{n} N_{j,d}(u_i)\psi_j} \right)^2, \tag{14}$$

where u_i is the precomputed parametric value corresponding to the point $\mathbf{p}_i$, and P_j^x is the x coordinate of the jth control point. Similar equations are used for the

y and z coordinates. Minimizing E_w with respect to each homogeneous control point coordinate yields the equivalent matrix formulation:

$$\mathbf{B}^\mathrm{T}\mathbf{WXB}\boldsymbol{\Psi} = (\mathbf{B}^\mathrm{T}\mathbf{WB})\mathbf{P}_x^\psi, \tag{15}$$

$$\mathbf{B}^\mathrm{T}\mathbf{WYB}\boldsymbol{\Psi} = (\mathbf{B}^\mathrm{T}\mathbf{WB})\mathbf{P}_y^\psi, \tag{16}$$

$$\mathbf{B}^\mathrm{T}\mathbf{WZB}\boldsymbol{\Psi} = (\mathbf{B}^\mathrm{T}\mathbf{WB})\mathbf{P}_z^\psi, \tag{17}$$

where the diagonal matrices $\mathbf{X}$, $\mathbf{Y}$, $\mathbf{Z}$, and $\mathbf{W}$ are formulated from the sets $\mathcal{D}$ and $\mathcal{W}$.

Combining the previous equations and performing certain matrix manipulations, the resulting system is derived:

$$\bar{\mathbf{B}} \cdot \bar{\mathbf{P}} = \mathbf{0}, \tag{18}$$

where $\bar{\mathbf{B}}$ is the $4n \times 4n$ block matrix

$$\begin{bmatrix} \mathbf{B}^\mathrm{T}\mathbf{W}^2\mathbf{B} & \mathbf{0} & \mathbf{0} & -\mathbf{B}^\mathrm{T}\mathbf{W}^2\mathbf{XB} \\ \mathbf{0} & \mathbf{B}^\mathrm{T}\mathbf{W}^2\mathbf{B} & \mathbf{0} & -\mathbf{B}^\mathrm{T}\mathbf{W}^2\mathbf{YB} \\ \mathbf{0} & \mathbf{0} & \mathbf{B}^\mathrm{T}\mathbf{W}^2\mathbf{B} & -\mathbf{B}^\mathrm{T}\mathbf{W}^2\mathbf{ZB} \\ \mathbf{0} & \mathbf{0} & \mathbf{0} & \mathbf{M} \end{bmatrix}, \tag{19}$$

$\mathbf{M}$ is the $n \times n$ matrix given by

$$\begin{aligned} \mathbf{M} =\ & \mathbf{B}^\mathrm{T}\mathbf{W}^2\mathbf{X}^2\mathbf{B} + \mathbf{B}^\mathrm{T}\mathbf{W}^2\mathbf{Y}^2\mathbf{B} + \mathbf{B}^\mathrm{T}\mathbf{W}^2\mathbf{Z}^2\mathbf{B} \\ & -(\mathbf{B}^\mathrm{T}\mathbf{W}^2\mathbf{XB})(\mathbf{B}^\mathrm{T}\mathbf{W}^2\mathbf{B})^{-1}(\mathbf{B}^\mathrm{T}\mathbf{W}^2\mathbf{XB}) \\ & -(\mathbf{B}^\mathrm{T}\mathbf{W}^2\mathbf{YB})(\mathbf{B}^\mathrm{T}\mathbf{W}^2\mathbf{B})^{-1}(\mathbf{B}^\mathrm{T}\mathbf{W}^2\mathbf{YB}) \\ & -(\mathbf{B}^\mathrm{T}\mathbf{W}^2\mathbf{ZB})(\mathbf{B}^\mathrm{T}\mathbf{W}^2\mathbf{B})^{-1}(\mathbf{B}^\mathrm{T}\mathbf{W}^2\mathbf{ZB}), \end{aligned} \tag{20}$$

and $\bar{\mathbf{P}}$ is the $4n \times 1$ vector $[\mathbf{P}_x^\psi, \mathbf{P}_y^\psi, \mathbf{P}_z^\psi, \boldsymbol{\Psi}]^\mathrm{T}$. A similar derivation follows from employing a non-Cartesian NURBS description.

In this form, calculation of the weights can be performed separately from calculation of the control points by first solving the homogeneous system $\mathbf{M} \cdot \boldsymbol{\Psi} = \mathbf{0}$. In general, the nontrivial solution can be solved using singular-value decomposition. However, this could lead to negative weights causing singularities in the B-spline model. Therefore, we look for an optimal solution consisting of strictly positive weights. This leads to the quadratic programming [23] formulation

$$\min_{\boldsymbol{\Psi}} \|\mathbf{M} \cdot \boldsymbol{\Psi}\|_2^2 \quad \text{subject to} \quad \{\psi_i \geq \psi_\circ : \forall \psi_i \in \Psi\}, \tag{21}$$

where $\psi_\circ$ is a positive constant. Since only the relative weighting of control points is important, and to be consistent with the formulation in the original publication [22], we choose $\psi_\circ = 1$.

Implicit in the assignment of parameter values to the points in set $\mathcal{D}$ is the necessity of satisfying the *Schoenberg-Whitney* conditions [24, ?] to ensure that the matrix $\mathbf{B}^{\mathsf{T}}\mathbf{B}$ is positive definite and well conditioned. Suppose that the knot vector of the fitting spline is given by $\mathbf{U} = \{U_1, U_2, \ldots, U_m\}$ and the parameterization assigned to the s sample points of $\mathcal{D}$ for least-squares fitting is $U_{\mathcal{D}} = \{u_1, u_2, \ldots, u_s\}$. Compliance with the Schoenberg-Whitney conditions implies that there exists a set $\bar{U}_{\mathcal{D}} = \{\bar{u}_1, \ldots, \bar{u}_m\} \subset U_{\mathcal{D}}$ such that

$$U_i < \bar{u}_i < U_{i+d+1} \qquad i = 1, \ldots, m - (d+1). \tag{22}$$

This requirement in the presence of knots with multiplicity $(d+1)$ is relaxed to

$$U_i \le \bar{u}_i < U_{i+d+1} \qquad U_i = \ldots = U_{i+d} < U_{i+d+1}, \tag{23}$$

$$U_i < \bar{u}_i \le U_{i+d+1} \qquad U_i < U_{i+1} = \ldots = U_{i+d+1}. \tag{24}$$

This requirement is easily extended to the case for higher-order NURBS objects [?].

3.2. Least-Squares Fitting with Polar NURBS

Closed periodic NURBS using the Cartesian formulation simply require repetition of the first d control points, where d is the degree of spline. However, straightforward application to the ϕ coordinate of the cylindrical or prolate spheroidal-based NURBS model would yield erroneous results because of the discontinuity at $\phi = -\pi$. This requires subtraction or addition of 2π to the appropriate control point ϕ coordinates when the ordered set of control points crosses over this discontinuity. Essentially, this is a type of *phase unwrapping* to ensure a smooth transition across the ϕ-coordinate.

From a set of sample points, one of which is denoted by $\mathbf{p}_i(r_i, \phi_i)$ $(-\pi \le \phi_i < \pi)$, with the corresponding parametric value u_i, one can construct a d-degree closed NURBS curve using polar coordinates consisting of n distinct control points. (The periodicity issue using both cylindrical and prolate spheroidal-based closed NURBS is illustrated using polar coordinates. Polar coordinates are simply the 2D analog of cylindrical coordinates and contain the ϕ coordinate inherent to both 3D coordinate systems.) Assume, without loss of generality, that $-\pi \le \mathbf{P}_1^\phi < \ldots < \mathbf{P}_n^\phi < \pi$, where $\mathbf{P}^\phi$ denotes the ϕ coordinate of the control point $\mathbf{P}$. Due to the local support property of B-splines, each sample point influences, at most, the location of $(d+1)$ control points. If this ordered set of control points, beginning with $\mathbf{P}_k$, crosses over the discontinuity at $\phi = -\pi$, a suiTable solution is to add or subtract 2π from the ϕ coordinate of the appropriate control points. This necessitates modifying the general equation for calculating $\phi_i(u_i)$ to

$$\phi_i(u_i) = \frac{\sum_{j=k}^{k+d} N_{h,d}(u_i)\psi_h \mathbf{Q}_j^\phi}{\sum_{j=k}^{k+d} N_{h,d}(u_i)\psi_h}, \tag{25}$$

where $h = (j - 1) \bmod n + 1$ with 'mod' as the modulo operator, and

$$
\mathbf{Q}_j^\phi = \begin{cases}
\mathbf{P}_h^\phi + 2\pi & n - d < k \le n - \lfloor 0.5d \rfloor \text{ and } j > n, \\
\mathbf{P}_j^\phi - 2\pi & n - \lfloor 0.5d \rfloor < j, k \le n, \\
\mathbf{P}_h^\phi & \text{otherwise.}
\end{cases}
\tag{26}
$$

Application to the method outlined in the previous section requires us to rewrite Eq. (25) as

$$
\sum_{j=k}^{k+d} \left(\phi_i(u_i) N_{h,d}(u_i) + 2\pi N_{j,d}^*(u_i) \right) \psi_h = \sum_{j=k}^{k+d} N_{h,d}(u_i) \psi_h \mathbf{P}_h^\phi,
\tag{27}
$$

where

$$
N_{j,d}^*(u) = \begin{cases}
-N_{h,d}(u) & n - d < k \le n - \lfloor 0.5d \rfloor \text{ and } j > n, \\
N_{h,d}(u) & n - \lfloor 0.5d \rfloor < j, k \le n, \\
0 & \text{otherwise.}
\end{cases}
\tag{28}
$$

This is equivalent to the matrix formulation

$$
\left(\mathbf{\Phi B} + 2\pi \mathbf{B}^* \right) \mathbf{\Psi} = \mathbf{B P}_\phi^\psi,
\tag{29}
$$

where $\mathbf{B}^*$ is the observation matrix composed of the evaluated basis functions $N_{j,d}^*$. This is incorporated into the methodology discussed in Section 3.1 to solve for the control point locations and corresponding weights.

4. MODEL FITTING AND NONRIGID REGISTRATION

4.1. Algorithm Overview

Having discussed the mathematical preliminaries involved in fitting an NURBS object to data, we present in Table 1 an algorithmic overview for fitting a biventric-ular NURBS model to 4D short-axis and 4D long-axis tagged MRI data consisting of $N + 1$ synchronized volumetric frames. The principles presented in Table 1 apply regardless of whether Cartesian or non-Cartesian B-splines are employed. Note that $\mathcal{R}$ denotes the reference frame at time $t = 0$ (end-diastole) and $\mathcal{R}_t$ de-notes a deformed frame later in the cardiac cycle at $t > 0$. Below, we describe the methodological components of the various steps.

4.2. Initialization: Construction of the Biventricular NURBS Model

To construct the initial model for subsequent registration, one must select the knot vectors, number of control points, as well as degree of spline. Following

Table 1. Algorithmic Synopsis for Fitting a 4D Biventricular
NURBS model to $N + 1$ Volumetric Short-Axis and
$N + 1$ Volumetric Long-Axis Tagged Data

---

0. Initialization: create an NURBS biventricular model for time $t = 0$ from short- and long-axis contour information by performing a least-squares fit to all contour points in all short- and long-axis slices (each such point is preassigned a (v, w) parametric value). From the resulting NURBS fit, construct the volumetric parameterization $S_L(u, v, w, t = 0)$ by placing control points linearly in the u direction.

for $i = 1, \ldots, N\{$

1. For time $t = i$ create a parameterized NURBS biventricular model from short- and long-axis contour information by performing a least-squares fit to the contour points (prior to least-squares, each contour point is assigned a (v, w) parametric value). Linearly place control points in the u direction to construct the volumetric parameterization $S_E(u, v, w, i)$.

2. Use 1D, 2D, and 3D displacement information to determine corresponding tag points between $t = i$ and $t = 0$ using the following sources of information: a) Tag plane normal distances (Figure **??**), b) contour/tag intersections (Figure **??**), and c) intersections of 3D tag planes. Assign identical parametric values to corresponding points at $t = 0$.

3. Perform NURBS weighted least-squares to determine control points and weights for the model at $t = 0$ (this is the Eulerian fit). The weights reflect confidences in the correspondences established in step 2. Couple the RV to the LV by assigning corresponding points on the RV/LV interface at $t = 0$ the same parameters as at $t = i$. Call the NURBS parameterization resulting from weighted least-squares at time $t = 0$ $S_E^i(u, v, w, 0)$.

4. Densely sample $S_E^i(u, v, w, 0)$. For each sample point $\mathbf{p}_j = S_E^i(u_j', v_j', w_j', 0)$ determine via conjugate gradient descent the (u_j, v_j, w_j) of $S_L(u, v, w, 0)$ (constructed in step 0) that corresponds to the same spatial point $\mathbf{p}_j$. Calculate the set of displacements $V_E(u_j', v_j', w_j') = S_E(u_j', v_j', w_j', i) - S_E^i(u_j', v_j', w_j', 0)$.

5. Perform the least-squares fit for the biventricular model at $t = i$, denoted by $S_L(u, v, w, i)$, from assigning the parameters (u_j, v_j, w_j) to the point $S_L(u_j, v_j, w_j, 0) + V_E(u_j', v_j', w_j')$ for all j. This is the Lagrangian fit.

$\}$

6. Since all models are registered in the common parametric coordinates (u, v, w), temporal smoothing of all models is now possible. Perform the temporal lofting — $S_L(u, v, w, t) = \sum_{l=0}^{N} S_L(u, v, w, l) N_{l,s}(t)$.

7. Lagrangian strain values between time points $t = 0$ and $t > 0$ can easily be determined from the displacements $V_L(u, v, w, t)$. Similarly, Eulerian strain values can be determined from the displacements $V_E(u, v, w, t)$. From the displacements the deformation gradient tensor, $\mathbf{F}$, is determined. Subsequently, for any point of interest within the LV wall or the RV free wall and direction $\mathbf{n}$, the Lagrangian strains in the reference configuration $\mathcal{R}$ can be calculated from $\frac{1}{2}\mathbf{n}^T(\mathbf{F}^T\mathbf{F} - \mathbf{1})\mathbf{n}$. The Eulerian strains in the direction $\mathbf{n}$ in the deformed configuration $\mathcal{R}_t$ may be calculated from $\frac{1}{2}\mathbf{n}^T(\mathbf{1} - (\mathbf{F}\mathbf{F}^T)^{-1})\mathbf{n}$.

the selection of these parameters, we construct the reference configuration (the left- and right-ventricular volumetric NURBS models) using contour data from the end-diastolic images. We denote this initial model as $S_L(u, v, w, t = 0)$. These parameters remain fixed for the nonrigid registration for each frame of data. For each time point $t > 0$ we construct a separate NURBS model from the contour data of that time point using the same parameters selected for constructing $S_L(u, v, w, t = 0)$. We denote this model as $S_E(u, v, w, t = i)$. This construction corresponds to Steps 0 and 1 in Table 1.

The basic principle is the same for formulation of all models: two parametrically identical surfaces are constructed that correspond to the epicardial and endocardial surfaces in the (v_{LV}, w_{LV}) or (v_{RV}, w_{RV}) parametric directions shown in Figure 5. The identical parameterization for both the endocardial and epicardial surfaces is required to create a volumetric NURBS model with a third set of control points creating the third parametric direction (u_{LV} or u_{RV}). The maximal apical extent of the left (right) ventricular model is limited by the most apical short-axis left (right) ventricular endocardial contour. The maximal basal extent of both ventricular models is similarly limited by the most basal short-axis image. A biventricular NURBS model constructed from a canine heart is shown in Figure 6. In addition to the limits imposed by the image locations, inclusion of the most apical portions of the ventricles is problematic in that it requires a degenerate condition of the tensor product volume at that location. Some possible remedies for future research are discussed in the Conclusions section.

4.2.1. B-spline parameterization of the LV and RV

Consider the biventricular parametric coordinates of Figure 5, examining the LV and the RV separately. The u_{LV} and w_{LV} directions require open, aperiodic parameterizations, whereas the v_{LV} direction requires periodic parameterization. There are several ways to achieve this. (1) We can use Cartesian NURBS with the constraints that for the v_{LV} direction periodic B-spline basis functions are used. This would be similar to taking the Cartesian B-spline model described in [13, 16, 26], attaching two opposite faces of the cubic model together, and ensuring continuity of the resulting topological torus at the connection interface through use of periodic B-spline basis functions in the v_{LV} direction. Note that in this scenario the B-spline control points are represented in the Cartesian coordinates. (2) We can use non-Cartesian (e.g., cylindrical and prolate spheroidal) B-splines. For these splines, the control points are represented in the cylindrical or prolate spheroidal coordinates, while aperiodic basis functions are used in the u_{LV} and w_{LV} directions, and periodic basis functions are used in the v_{LV} direction. In the case of the RV, all three parametric directions (u_{RV}, v_{RV}, w_{RV}) require use of open, aperiodic splines. Thus far, in our work, we have only used Cartesian B-Splines for modeling the RV.

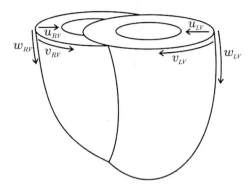

Figure 5. Parametric directions of the left- and right-ventricular NURBS model given by (u_{LV}, v_{LV}, w_{LV}) and (u_{RV}, v_{RV}, w_{RV}), respectively.

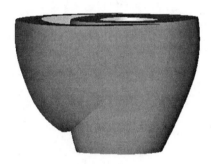

Figure 6. Initial NURBS model of a canine heart constructed from the left- and right-ventricular contours. See attached CD for color version.

4.2.2. Left-ventricular NURBS model

Using the concept of a *base surface* [?], we construct the left-ventricular model based on a cylindrical or prolate spheroidal parameter assignment. The selection of these two particular geometric primitives is a natural choice considering the shape of the left ventricle. Usage of the base surface concept permits the utilization of both short- and long-axis contour information in building the model. The origin of the coordinate system is defined as the center of the short-axis left-ventricular endocardial contour in the most basal short-axis image slice. The focus (for the prolate spheroidal parametrization) is placed along the central axis of the left ventricle at a distance equal to the radius of curvature of the apical point of the long-axis endocardial contour from the apex.

Table 2. NURBS Type and Parameter Assignment of Each
of the Four Models Used to Calculate Strain

	NURBS Type	**Parameter Assignment**
Model 1.1	Cartesian	Cylindrical
Model 1.2	Cartesian	Prolate
Model 2.1	Cylindrical	Cylindrical
Model 2.2	Prolate	Prolate

Left-ventricular geometry prescribes closed, periodic B-splines in the v_{LV} parametric direction and open, clamped B-splines in the u_{LV} and w_{LV} directions. Selecting the appropriate B-spline parameters (order, number of control points, knot vector, etc.), we first calculate the observation matrix. Given a sample point from one of the contours, we calculate its ϕ and η values in the prolate spheroidal coordinate system. Establishing a parameterization such that $0 \leq v \leq 1$ and $0 \leq w \leq 1$, the surface parameter values (v, w) corresponding to ϕ and η are simply $v = \frac{\phi}{2\pi}$ and $w = \frac{\eta}{\eta_{max}}$, where η_{max} is the maximal η extent of the model. The cylindrical parameter assignment is performed similarly except the w parameter value is given by $w = \frac{z}{z_{max}}$, where z_{max} is the maximal extent of the model in the z direction (Figure 3).

For the Cartesian-based models, we modify the parameterization in the v direction slightly by temporarily moving the origin to the center of the sample points of each short-axis endocardial contour for the specific purpose of assigning parameteric values to the contour samples. This adjustment is not required, but we found that such a shift provides a more evenly sampled parameterization in the v direction, especially for nonconcentric short-axis left-ventricular contours. Due to the discontinuity at $\phi = -\pi$, the shifting of the origin for each short-axis contour is not possible for the models with a non-Cartesian description.

4.2.3. Right-ventricular NURBS model

Since the morphology of the right ventricle precludes a simple assignment of parametric values to sample contour points based on base surfaces, we loft a set of open short-axis epicardial and endocardial B-spline curves to compose the corresponding surfaces spanned by the parametric directions (v_{RV}, w_{RV}) shown in Figure 5. Linear placement of control points between the epicardial and endocardial surface control points provides the third parametric direction. The right-ventricular model B-spline composition is similar to the left ventricle, except that open, clamped B-splines are employed in the v_{RV} parametric direction.

4.3. Coupling the Left- and Right-Ventricular Models

In order to couple the two ventricular models (as described in step 3 of Table 1, we determine the parametric values of the left-ventricular model where the right-ventricular model attaches corresponding to the anatomical ventricular junctions for each frame $t > 0$. We sample the two interfaces between the left and right ventricles. These surfaces are defined by the surface (u_{RV}, w_{RV}) at $v_{RV} = 0$ and (u_{RV}, w_{RV}) at $v_{RV} = 1$. For each sample point along those surfaces, we determine, via conjugate gradient descent [27], the parametric values of the left-ventricular model corresponding to that point. This information is used in conjunction with the tag and contour information to temporally fit the right ventricle at time $t > 0$ to time $t = 0$.

4.4. Temporal Nonrigid Registration of Models

This section comprises Steps 2–6 of the algorithm presented in Table 1. To nonrigidly register the initial model to subsequent frames of data, we define a mapping χ between the deformed frame at time $t > 0$, denoted by $\mathcal{R}_t$, and the reference frame, denoted by $\mathcal{R}$, such that $\chi : \mathcal{R} \to \mathcal{R}_t$. Within the NURBS volumetric model, a material point $\mathbf{p} \in \mathcal{R}$ and its image point $\mathbf{p}_t \in \mathcal{R}_t$ are related by the mapping $\chi(\mathbf{p}(u, v, w)) = \mathbf{p}_t(u, v, w)$, where u, v, and w are the parameter values of the NURBS model. This mapping allows us to use the theory developed in the previous section on NURBS fitting to reconstruct 3D deformation fields and corresponding strain maps.

4.4.1. Warping $\mathcal{R}_t \to \mathcal{R}$ (Steps 2 and 3 in Table 1)

The data that comprise the spatial displacement information include:

- the normal displacement of the tag planes,

- the intersections of the each triplet of tag planes, and

- the intersections of the contours and tag lines in both the short- and long-axis images,

which are illustrated in Figures 7 and 8. Using these data we can warp the model at each time frame $t = i$, denoted by $S_E(u, v, w, i)$, back to the reference frame. The resulting model we denote as $S_E^i(u, v, w, 0)$. This is the Eulerian fitting portion of the algorithm.

Each data type has an associated confidence value that is incorporated into our registration procedure using weighted least squares. The contour/tag line intersection displacements describe two components of motion versus the one component given by the normal displacements of the tag planes. Therefore, the relative confidence value ratio is 2:1 (actual values = 1.0 and 0.5). The displacement information

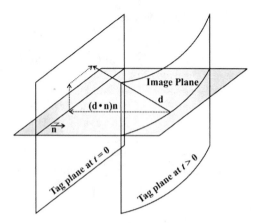

Figure 7. Diagrammatic representation of available measurements for model fitting. The only discernible measurement of the true displacement, **d**, is the orthogonal component at time $t > 0$ to the tag plane configuration at time $t = 0$.

provided by the intersections of the tag planes includes all three components of motion. We have empirically determined the optimal confidence values for tag plane intersections, contour/tag intersections, and tag plane normals. This is described in Section 6.1.

The tag line data are extracted using a previously published method explained in [13], where a maximum a posteriori framework was used to estimate the tag line locations based on a sampling of isoparametric surfaces of a cubic B-spline solid that model the tag surfaces. Once the tag line data are available, we loft the tag lines to create B-spline surfaces that represent each tag plane of the three sets of tag planes. The normal displacement of these tag plane surfaces are used in the model-fitting process. Contours are manually traced as part of the preprocessing step.

Tag plane data provide three sets of mutually orthogonal sample points corresponding to the two sets of short-axis tag planes and one set of long-axis tag planes. The true displacement of a point on a tag plane consists of both a normal and a tangential component (Figure 7). However, due to the *aperture problem* [28], only the normal component is discernible. Therefore, for each time point $t > 0$, the set of measurements from the tag planes for each time frame is

$$\mathbf{M}_{\mathrm{T}} = \{\mathbf{p}_i + (\mathbf{d}_i \cdot \mathbf{n})\mathbf{n}\}, \tag{30}$$

where $\mathbf{p}_i$ is the position of a sample point on one of the tag planes at $t > 0$, $\mathbf{n}$ is the normal to the undeformed tag plane, and $\mathbf{d}_i$ is the true displacement for the ith sample point at time $t > 0$.

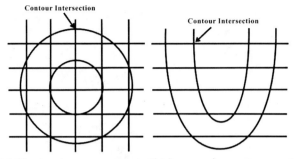

(a) Short-axis measurements (b) Long-axis measurements

Figure 8. Diagrammatic representation of additional measurements for model fitting consisting of the contour intersection points in the short- and long-axis views.

Each triplet of the lofted B-spline short- and long-axis tag plane surfaces intersects at a single point. True displacement is available from the tracking of each of these intersection points. This set of measurements is denoted as

$$\mathbf{M_I} = \{\mathbf{p}_i + \mathbf{d}_i\}, \tag{31}$$

where $\mathbf{p}_i$ is the position of an intersection point at $t > 0$, and $\mathbf{d}_i$ is the true displacement for the ith sample point at time $t = 0$. The tag plane intersections are calculated using the conjugate gradient descent algorithm [27].

The third set of measurements consists of the set of contour/tag line intersection points that provide displacement information along the epicardial and endocardial surfaces of the model (Figure 8), defined by

$$\mathbf{M_C} = \{\mathbf{p}_i + \mathbf{v}_i\}, \tag{32}$$

where $\mathbf{p}_i$ is the position of the contour/tag line intersection point at $t > 0$, and $\mathbf{v}_i$ is the component of the true displacement within the image plane for the ith sample point at time $t = 0$. The contour/tag line intersection points are calculated using the conjugate gradient descent algorithm.

In addition to knowledge of the absolute position of the sample points, least-squares fitting of B-splines also requires assigning parametric values to each sample point. Due to the mapping explained previously, each measurement value, $\mathbf{m}_i$, is assigned the identical parametric vector, (u_i, v_i, w_i), as the origination point, $\mathbf{p}_i$. These parametric vectors are calculated from the NURBS model at time $t > 0$ via conjugate gradient descent. The coordinates of the position of the measurement points contained in the sets $\mathbf{M_T}$, $\mathbf{M_I}$, and $\mathbf{M_C}$ for each time frame compose the diagonal matrices $\mathbf{\Gamma}_t$, $\mathbf{\Pi}_t$, and $\mathbf{\Omega}_t$. Their corresponding parametric vectors are used to formulate the observation matrices $\mathbf{B}_\gamma$, $\mathbf{B}_\pi$, and $\mathbf{B}_\omega$. For fitting the

NURBS model at time $t = 0$, the previously discussed registration strategy is employed, given by the following system:

$$\mathbf{B}_\gamma^T \mathbf{W} \mathbf{\Gamma}_t \mathbf{B}_\gamma \mathbf{\Psi}_t = (\mathbf{B}_\gamma^T \mathbf{W} \mathbf{B}_\gamma) \mathbf{P}_{\gamma,t}^\psi,$$

$$\mathbf{B}_\pi^T \mathbf{W} \mathbf{\Pi}_t \mathbf{B}_\pi \mathbf{\Psi}_t = (\mathbf{B}_\pi^T \mathbf{W} \mathbf{B}_\pi) \mathbf{P}_{\pi,t}^\psi, \quad (33)$$

$$\mathbf{B}_\omega^T \mathbf{W} \mathbf{\Omega}_t \mathbf{B}_\omega \mathbf{\Psi}_t = (\mathbf{B}_\omega^T \mathbf{W} \mathbf{B}_\omega) \mathbf{P}_{\omega,t}^\psi.$$

The generalization of the fitting strategy given above in using separate observation matrices reflects an additional modification to the NURBS fitting algorithm. The Cartesian coordinate system, used for the NURBS models with a Cartesian description, is aligned with the normals of the three sets of tag planes. Therefore, a single sample point normal displacement is limited to influencing only one of the three coordinate values of the control points. However, for the NURBS models with a prolate spheroidal control point description the normal displacement of a single sample point affects all three coordinate values. Similarly, the normal displacement of a sample point from a short-axis tag plane affects both the r and θ coordinate values, whereas the longitudinal displacement affects only the z coordinate value. This separation in the fitting strategy is an added advantage associated with the NURBS models with a Cartesian description.

4.4.2. Warping $\mathcal{R} \rightarrow \mathcal{R}_t$ (Steps 4–6 in Table 1)

After calculating the mapping $\mathcal{R}_t \rightarrow \mathcal{R}$ in the previous section, we obtain the models $S_E^i(u, v, w, t = 0)$ and $S_E(u, v, w, t = i)$. Spatial displacements between the two frames are easily found as

$$V_E(u, v, w) = S_E(u, v, w, i) - S_E^i(u, v, w, 0). \quad (34)$$

In order to construct a comprehensive 4D myocardial deformation model that includes temporal smoothing, one must use the spatial displacements, V_E, to construct a Lagrangian description of deformation. This is done by using the volumetric NURBS model constructed from the epicardial and endocardial contours at time $t = 0$. This model was denoted above by $S_L(u, v, w, 0)$. The displacement field, V_E, is densely sampled. For each point $\mathbf{p}_j = S_E^i(u_j', v_j', w_j', 0)$, conjugate gradient descent is used to find the parameters (u_j, v_j, w_j) in $S_L(u_j, v_j, w_j, 0)$ that correspond to $\mathbf{p}_j$. A least-squares fit is then performed to find the model $S_L(u, v, w, i)$ using the parameters (u_j, v_j, w_j) and the associated displacements $V_E(u_j', v_j', w_j')$. This is the Lagrangian fitting portion of the algorithm. Once this process is completed for all time frames, temporal lofting is possible.

5. LAGRANGIAN AND EULERIAN STRAIN MEASUREMENTS FROM AN NURBS MODEL

Lagrangian strain maps are produced from our model by describing the deformation of the left ventricle in the Lagrangian reference frame. If the spatial coordinates are represented by $\mathbf{X}$ at time $t = 0$ and by $\mathbf{x}$ at time $t > 0$ then, in the Lagrangian reference frame, the mapping $\chi(\mathbf{X})$ warps $\mathbf{X}$ into $\mathbf{x}$, that is, $\mathbf{x} = \chi(\mathbf{X}) = \mathbf{V}(\mathbf{X}) + \mathbf{X}$. The deformation gradient tensor can be written as $\mathbf{F} = \nabla\chi(\mathbf{X}) = \nabla\mathbf{V}(\mathbf{X}) + \nabla\mathbf{X}$. The elements of the deformation gradient tensor are

$$
\mathbf{F} = \begin{bmatrix} \frac{\partial x}{\partial X} & \frac{\partial x}{\partial Y} & \frac{\partial x}{\partial Z}, \\ \frac{\partial y}{\partial X} & \frac{\partial y}{\partial Y} & \frac{\partial y}{\partial Z}, \\ \frac{\partial z}{\partial X} & \frac{\partial z}{\partial Y} & \frac{\partial z}{\partial Z} \end{bmatrix},
$$
(35)

where the displacement field $\chi(\mu, \nu, \omega)$ relates the coordinates of a material point in the reference configuration $\mathbf{X}(X, Y, Z)$ with its coordinates at a later time point: $\mathbf{x}(x, y, z)$:

$$
\mu = x - X, \qquad \nu = y - Y, \qquad \omega = z - Z.
$$
(36)

In order to solve for each of the three partials of the components of the displacement field necessary for calculation of the deformation gradient tensor, $\mathbf{F}$, we calculate the following vector quantities:

$$
\frac{\partial \chi}{\partial u} = \frac{\partial \chi}{\partial X}\frac{\partial X}{\partial u} + \frac{\partial \chi}{\partial Y}\frac{\partial Y}{\partial u} + \frac{\partial \chi}{\partial Z}\frac{\partial Z}{\partial u},
$$
(37)

$$
\frac{\partial \chi}{\partial v} = \frac{\partial \chi}{\partial X}\frac{\partial X}{\partial v} + \frac{\partial \chi}{\partial Y}\frac{\partial Y}{\partial v} + \frac{\partial \chi}{\partial Z}\frac{\partial Z}{\partial v},
$$
(38)

$$
\frac{\partial \chi}{\partial w} = \frac{\partial \chi}{\partial X}\frac{\partial X}{\partial w} + \frac{\partial \chi}{\partial Y}\frac{\partial Y}{\partial w} + \frac{\partial \chi}{\partial Z}\frac{\partial Z}{\partial w},
$$
(39)

where (u, v, w) are the parametric directions of the NURBS model. This yields the following linear system:

$$
\frac{\partial(\mu, \nu, \omega)}{\partial(u, v, w)} = \begin{bmatrix} \mu_X & \mu_Y & \mu_Z \\ \nu_X & \nu_Y & \nu_Z \\ \omega_X & \omega_Y & \omega_Z \end{bmatrix} \begin{bmatrix} X_u & X_v & X_w \\ Y_u & Y_v & Y_w \\ Z_u & Z_v & Z_w \end{bmatrix}.
$$
(40)

Considering the relationships in (36), the following linear system is derived:

$$
\mathbf{F} = \begin{bmatrix} 1 + \mu_X & \mu_Y & \mu_Z \\ \nu_X & 1 + \nu_Y & \nu_Z \\ \omega_X & \omega_Y & 1 + \omega_Z \end{bmatrix} = \begin{bmatrix} x_u & x_v & x_w \\ y_u & y_v & y_w \\ z_u & z_v & z_w \end{bmatrix} \begin{bmatrix} X_u & X_v & X_w \\ Y_u & Y_v & Y_w \\ Z_u & \omega_v & \omega_w \end{bmatrix}^{-1}.
$$
(41)

Therefore, for calculation of the deformation gradient tensor, the partial derivatives of the model with respect to its parameterization in the Cartesian coordinate system need to be known. For NURBS models using Cartesian coordinates, this is derived analytically directly from the model. For cylindrical coordinates, this is found by differentiating the relationships in Eq. (5):

$$\frac{\partial x}{\partial(u,v,w)} = \frac{\partial r}{\partial(u,v,w)}\cos\phi - r\sin\phi\frac{\partial\phi}{\partial(u,v,w)}, \tag{42}$$

$$\frac{\partial y}{\partial(u,v,w)} = \frac{\partial r}{\partial(u,v,w)}\sin\phi + r\cos\phi\frac{\partial\phi}{\partial(u,v,w)}, \tag{43}$$

$$\frac{\partial z}{\partial(u,v,w)} = \frac{\partial z}{\partial(u,v,w)}. \tag{44}$$

Similar results are obtained for the case of prolate spheroidal coordinates (Eq. (8)):

$$\frac{\partial x}{\partial(u,v,w)} = \delta\cosh\lambda\sin\eta\cos\phi\frac{\partial\lambda}{\partial(u,v,w)}$$
$$+\delta\sinh\lambda\cos\eta\cos\phi\frac{\partial\eta}{\partial(u,v,w)} \tag{45}$$
$$-\delta\sinh\lambda\sin\eta\sin\phi\frac{\partial\phi}{\partial(u,v,w)},$$

$$\frac{\partial y}{\partial(u,v,w)} = \delta\cosh\lambda\sin\eta\sin\phi\frac{\partial\lambda}{\partial(u,v,w)}$$
$$+\delta\sinh\lambda\cos\eta\sin\phi\frac{\partial\eta}{\partial(u,v,w)} \tag{46}$$
$$-\delta\sinh\lambda\sin\eta\cos\phi\frac{\partial\phi}{\partial(u,v,w)},$$

$$\frac{\partial z}{\partial(u,v,w)} = \delta\sinh\lambda\cos\eta\frac{\partial\lambda}{\partial(u,v,w)}$$
$$-\delta\cosh\lambda\sin\eta\frac{\partial\eta}{\partial(u,v,w)}. \tag{47}$$

The Lagrangian strain tensor, $\mathbf{E}$, is then given by $\mathbf{E} = \frac{1}{2}(\mathbf{F}^T\mathbf{F} - \mathbf{1})$, where $\mathbf{1}$ is the identity matrix. Similarly, we can use the Eulerian displacements found in step 4 of Table 1 to calculate the deformation gradient tensor, $\mathbf{F}$, which is used to calculate the Eulerian strain tensor, $\mathbf{G} = \frac{1}{2}(\mathbf{1} - (\mathbf{F}\mathbf{F}^T)^{-1})$. From the strain tensors we can calculate the various normal, shear, and principal strain values that describe the local deformation of the myocardium.

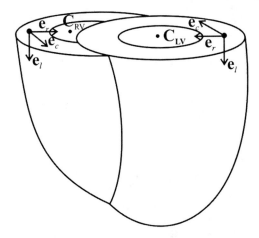

Figure 9. Strain calculation directions for both the left and right ventricles given by the orthonormal basis $\{e_r, e_c, e_l\}$. The centers of the left and right ventricles are shown by the points C_{LV} and C_{RV}, respectively.

Directional strains are calculated and regionally averaged based on myocardial geometry consistent with clinical reporting [29]. The recommendation presented divides the left ventricle into seventeen regions. The division along the midventricular axis consists of four layers: basal, mid-cavity, apical, and apex. The top three layers (basal, mid-cavity, and apical) encompass the endocardial cavity region. Based on the locations of the LV/RV junctions, the basal and mid-cavity portions of the left ventricle are each further divided into six regions in the short-axis view: antero-septal, anterior, lateral, posterior, inferior, and infero-septal. Similarly, the apical portion is divided into four regions anterior, lateral, inferior, and infero-septal. The apex comprises the seventeenth region. We follow the division utilized in [5] for regional analysis of the right ventricle. Similar to the left ventricle, the right ventricle is divided into basal, mid-cavity, and apical layers. Each layer is further divided into anterior, mid, and inferior regions.

The orthonormal basis for calculating directional strain is given by $\{e_r, e_c, e_l\}$ (Figure 9). The center of the left ventricle, C_{LV}, used to calculate directional strain values, is the same point as the origin of the coordinate system calculated from the center of the short-axis endocardial contour of the most short-axis basal image slice. C_{RV} is derived from the right-ventricular NURBS model for each w_{RV} parametric value by fitting a circle to the curve of constant w_{RV} value with $u_{RV} = 0.5$. As this process is dependent upon the curvature of the right ventricle, it is possible that C_{RV} is not inside the right-ventricular cavity. However, this is not important since C_{RV} is only used to derive the orthonormal basis $\{e_r, e_c, e_l\}$ for calculating the right-ventricular normal strains.

Table 3. Thirteen k-Parameters of the Cardiac Simulator

k_1	Radially dependent compression
k_2	Left-ventricular torsion
k_3	Ellipticalization in long-axis planes
k_4	Ellipticalization in short-axis planes
k_5	Shear in x direction
k_6	Shear in y direction
k_7	Shear in z direction
k_8	Rotation about x axis
k_9	Rotation about y axis
k_{10}	Rotation about z axis
k_{11}	Translation in x direction
k_{12}	Translation in y direction
k_{13}	Translation in z direction

6. RESULTS

6.1. System Performance

An environment based on a 13-parameter kinematic model of Arts et al. [30] has been implemented, as described in [31], for simulating a time sequence of tagged MR images at arbitrary orientation. Based on user-selected discretization of the space between two concentric shells and by varying the canonical parameters of the model, both a sequence of tagged MR images as well as "ground truth" strains are available.

A pair of prolate spheroids represent the endocardial and epicardial left-ventricular surfaces, and provide a geometric model of the left ventricle. The motion model involves application of a cascade of incompressible linear transformations describing rigid as well as nonrigid motions. Once a discretization step is assumed and a mesh for tessellating the 3D space is generated, the linear matrix transformations are applied in a sequence to all the mesh points so as to register the reference model. The parameters of the motion model, referred to as k-parameters, and the transformations to which they correspond are stated in Table 3. In order to simulate MR images, an imaging plane intersecting the geometric model is selected, and tagged spin echo imaging equations are applied for simulating the in vivo imaging process.

To determine the model type and associated parameters to apply to real data, the model parameters were varied within specific limits dictated by Eq. (22) and previous research [32]. The resulting models were applied to simulated image data derived from Arts' left-ventricular analytical model. The parameter variation was as follows: order = $\{3, 4\}$, spans in the u_{LV} direction = $\{1\}$, spans in the v_{LV} direction = $\{$order, order + 1, order + 2, order + 3$\}$, and spans in the w_{LV} direction = $\{1, 2, 3, 4\}$, with the additional constraint that the span lengths in each direction have similar Euclidean lengths. In addition, we varied the confidence value for the tag plane intersections from the set $\{1, 1.5, 2, 2.5, 5, 10, 50\}$. This variation led to 224 model variants for strain analysis. The governing parameters of Arts' analytical model were varied so that the resulting analytical normal strains, i.e., radial, circumferential, and longitudinal strains, followed the same systolic evolutionary pattern in the basal and midventricular regions as those reported in [33]. The simulated data consisted of eleven frames of eight short-axis images and seven long-axis images. Sample images are shown in Figure 10.

The variation in the computational time is partly dependent upon the number of control points and the number of data points. Associated with the data points is the computational time to find the corresponding parametric values in the model that are found via conjugate gradient descent. Associated with both the data points and the number of control points is the matrix inversion involving the observation matrix, which, as previously noted, is of size $s \times n$, where s is the number of data points and n the number of control points. For the models described in the previous paragraph, the computational time took anywhere from 30 minutes and 1 hour and 15 minutes on a Sun Blade 100.

Bland-Altman methodology [34] was used for determining which model was the optimal predictor of circumferential strain. The circumferential strains were chosen for comparison due to the greater quantity of data in that direction as compared with the radial and longitudinal directions. The strains predicted by our model were averaged over 12 basal regions and 12 mid-cavity regions, and compared with the corresponding strains predicted by Arts' model. This division incorporated the previous segmentation described earlier (Section 5) with the additional regional division separating the endocardium and epicardium as illustrated in Figure 11. The apical regions were not included since the model does not extend sufficiently along the left-ventricular long-axis to encompass the entire apical region. This division translates into $24 \times 9 = 216$ points for analysis of each model from a total of eleven frames (only nine frames are available since the very first and very last frames are identical and have zero strains everywhere). For each of the 224 models we calculated the standard deviation and the mean of the difference between Arts' model and the analyzed model. We then ranked the 224 models by the equation

$$\frac{|\mu|}{|\mu|_{max}} + \frac{\sigma}{\sigma_{max}}, \tag{48}$$

where μ and $sigma$ are the mean and standard deviation of the difference, respectively. The use of this ranking measure is motivated by two factors used in assessing predictive modelling — the need for accurate measurement and the minimization of variability in that measurement. The latter component is arguably the

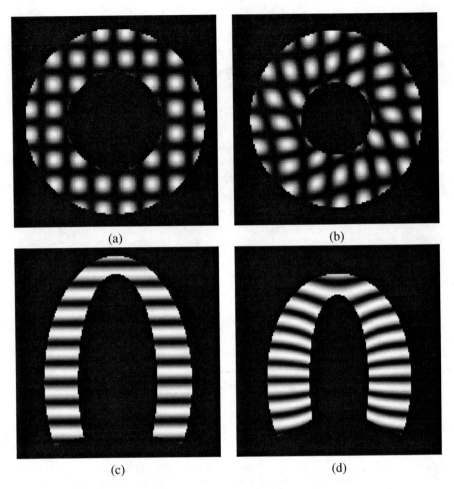

(a)   (b)

(c)   (d)

Figure 10. Simulated images generated from Arts' left-ventricular analytical model. A basal short-axis image is shown at (a) end-diastole and (b) end-systole. Similarly, long-axis images at (c) end-diastole and (d) end-systole are also illustrated.

most important when one considers the two extreme cases: (1) $|\mu| = 0$, $\sigma > 0$, and (2) $|\mu| > 0$, $\sigma = 0$. The second situation is preferable to the first since a mean of zero could be derived from largely varying data, producing little confidence in its predictive value, whereas a measurement with perfect confidence could rectify a nonzero mean value simply by the introduction of an offset. Our results lie somewhere between the two extreme cases. Relative weighting of the two components could fine-tune the ranking. However, we found that such ad hoc adjustments did not provide additional insight or warrant their use.

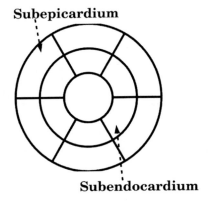

Figure 11. Diagrammatic representation of the regional division for analysis using Arts' model for a basal or mid-cavity short-axis view. The arrows point to one of six subendo-cardial or subepicardial regions.

Table 4. Optimal Confidence Values for the Four Models Shown in Figure 12

| | **Optimal Confidence Values** | | |
	Normals	Plane Inters.	Contour/Tag Inters.
Model 1.1	0.5	50.0	1.0
Model 1.2	0.5	50.0	1.0
Model 2.1	0.5	50.0	1.0
Model 2.2	0.5	50.0	1.0

In Figure 12 we give Bland-Altman plots for each of the four models' top performer. Each plot has the same scale for both the abscissa and ordinate values. The plots illustrate that the two Cartesian models (models 1 and 2) outperform the cylindrical and prolate spheroidal parameterized models with non-Cartesian B-spline descriptions (models 3 and 4, respectively).

Due to ease of implementation associated with the Cartesian models and the requirement for a focus for the prolate spheroidal parameterized models, we used the Cartesian B-splines with cylindrical parameter assignment for in vivo analysis. This third-order model has one span in the radial direction (three control points), four spans in the circumferential direction (four distinct control points), and two spans in the longitudinal direction (four control points).

We also show the strain prediction variation over the best performing 112 models (top 50%) (many of the models below the 50% level exhibited ill-conditioned

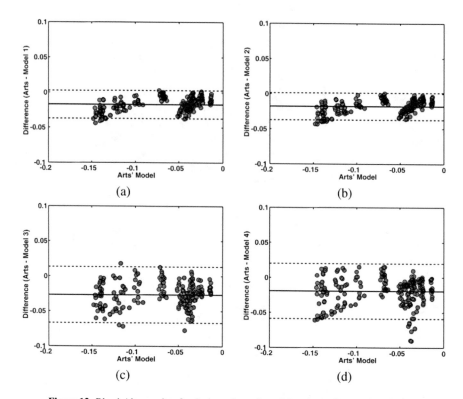

Figure 12. Bland-Altman plots for the best circumferential strain predictors of each model type. Plotted are the difference between Arts' model and the best performer from each model type of the 224 total models. Also included are the mean of the difference (solid line) and the 95% limits of agreement (dashed lines). (a) Cartesian-based cylindrical-parameterized NURBS model (order = 3, number of control points in $(u_{LV}, v_{LV}, w_{LV}) = (3, 4, 4)$). (b) Cartesian-based prolate spheroidal-parameterized NURBS model (order = 3, number of control points in $(u_{LV}, v_{LV}, w_{LV}) = (3, 4, 4)$). (c) Cylindrical-based cylindrical-parameterized NURBS model (order = 3, number of control points in $(u_{LV}, v_{LV}, w_{LV}) = (3, 3, 3)$). (d) Prolate spheroidal-based prolate spheroidal-parameterized NURBS model (order = 3, number of control points in $(u_{LV}, v_{LV}, w_{LV}) = (3, 5, 5)$). See attached CD for color version.

fitting results, which led to exclusion of the lower 50%). This is illustrated by plotting the temporal mean and standard deviation of these models for the radial (Figures 13 and 14), circumferential (Figures 15 and 16), and longitudinal (Figures 17 and 18) strains along with the ground truth predicted by Arts' model.

These plots show that, for this dataset, the NURBS models generally overpredict the subepicardial radial strain values, underestimate the subendocardial radial strain values, accurately calculate the circumferential strains, and vary for the longitudinal strain values. As discussed earlier, we can partially attribute this phe-

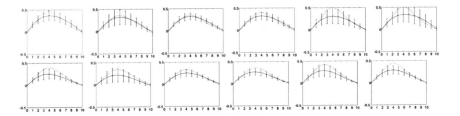

Figure 13. Average subendocardial radial strain plots across 112 NURBS model variants showing the mean (solid line) and standard deviation (error bars) for the predicted strain values for the six basal (top row) and six mid-cavity (bottom row) regions. The dashed line represents the ground truth strain value predicted by the analytical model.

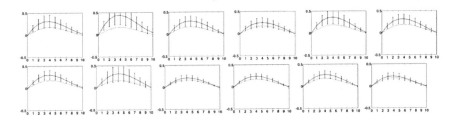

Figure 14. Average subepicardial radial strain plots across 112 NURBS model variants showing the mean (solid line) and standard deiation (error bars) for the predicted strain values for the six basal (top row) and six mid-cavity (bottom row) regions. The dashed line represents the ground truth strain value predicted by the analytical model.

nomenon to the amount of data available for fitting in each of the three parametric directions. In the radial direction there is a paucity of tag line data compared with the circumferential direction. The variability in longitudinal strains for a number of regions is due to the motion dictated by the large k_1 parameter values used for this deformation, which provided the requisite circumferential strains but generated slightly abnormal radially dependent deformation in the long-axis images. Increasing the number of tag lines within the myocardium is likely to increase the strain accuracy in all three directions.

After finding the tags and contours for the three dog studies, we apply the Cartesian-based cylindrical parameterized NURBS model described in the previous section and calculate the strain values for each dog. After registering all models to $t = 0$, the resulting registered 3D volumetric NURBS models at each time point were then temporally lofted (order = 4 with 6 temporal control points) to formulate a single 4D NURBS model for each dog study. This allows us to normalize all dogs in terms of the temporal length of the cardiac cycle. The normal systolic strains were then averaged over the twelve regions described earlier. These values were averaged across all three dog studies and plotted in Figures 20 and 21.

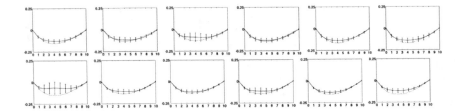

Figure 15. Average subendocardial circumferential strain plots across 112 NURBS model variants showing the mean (solid line) and standard deviation (error bars) for the predicted strain values for the six basal (top row) and six mid-cavity (bottom row) regions. The dashed line represents the ground truth strain value predicted by the analytical model.

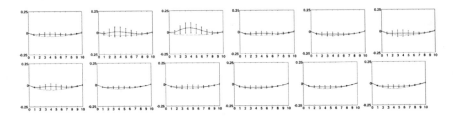

Figure 16. Average subepicardial circumferential strain plots across 112 NURBS model variants showing the mean (solid line) and standard deviation (error bars) for the predicted strain values for the six basal (top row) and six mid-cavity (bottom row) regions. The dashed line represents the ground truth strain value predicted by the analytical model.

For all plots, end-diastole is assumed to occur at time $t = 0$ and is considered the reference undeformed state for calculating Lagrangian strains. Since the plots only demonstrate strain values during systole, peak strain is typically achieved at the last time point shown. As compared with circumferential and longitudinal directions, please note that there is a large variance in the radial direction for the computed strains. This is likely due to lack of sufficient data points in the radial direction.

6.2. In Vivo Canine Data: Left Ventricle

Assessment of our methodology for in vivo data incorporates both the residual values from the least-squares fitting (e.g., Eq. (14)) as well as the average Jacobian of the model. For subsequent analysis, we only show the residuals for the Eulerian fits since those fits involve the data derived directly from the images (i.e., Eqs. (30), (31), and (32)). Additionally, the Jacobian plots are derived from the Lagrangian fits since we illustrate the capability of our model by plotting the Lagrangian strains. The only exception is the case of the normal human volunteer for which

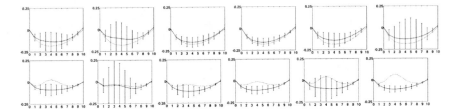

Figure 17. Average subendocardial longitudinal strain plots across 112 NURBS model variants showing the mean (solid line) and standard deviation (error bars) for the predicted strain values for the six basal (top row) and six mid-cavity (bottom row) regions. The dashed line represents the ground truth strain value predicted by the analytical model.

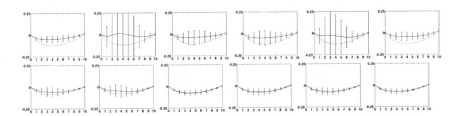

Figure 18. Average subepicardial longitudinal strain plots across 112 NURBS model variants showing the mean (solid line) and standard deviation (error bars) for the predicted strain values for the six basal (top row) and six mid-cavity (bottom row) regions. The dashed line represents the ground truth strain value predicted by the analytical model.

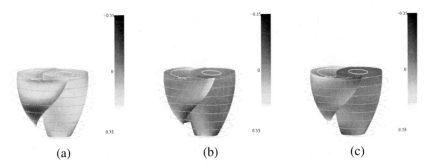

(a)　　　　　　　　(b)　　　　　　　　(c)

Figure 19. Qualitative peak strain results for a midventricular surface for the left ventricle ($u_{LV} = 0.5$) and right ventricle ($u_{RV} = 0.5$) of one dog study (Dog 3). Illustrated strains include (a) the radial strain, (b) the circumferential strain, and (c) the longitudinal strain. See attached CD for color version.

we also show the average Jacobian values calculated from the Eulerian fits. The least-squares residuals for the systolic portion of the cardiac cycle for all three dog studies are shown in Figure 22. Myocardial incompressibility [2] implies that the

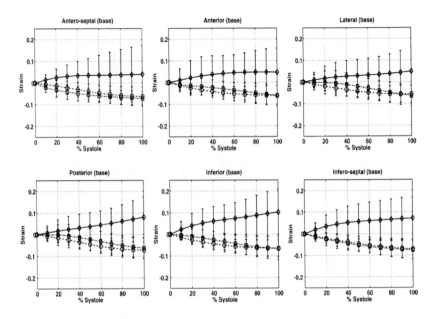

Figure 20. Average Lagrangian normal strain plots across three normal canine datasets for the six basal regions of the left ventricle. The different geometric shapes (diamond, circle, and square) represent the radial, circumferential, and longitudinal strain values, respectively. The x axis marks the time point during systole.

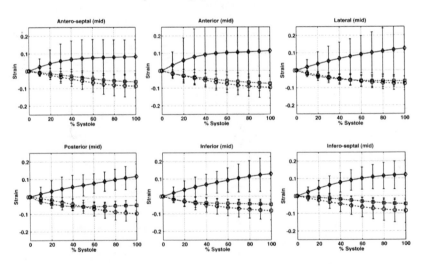

Figure 21. Average Lagrangian normal strain plots across three normal canine datasets for the six mid-cavity regions of the left ventricle. The different geometric shapes (diamond, circle, and square) represent the radial, circumferential, and longitudinal strain values, respectively. The x axis marks the time point during systole.

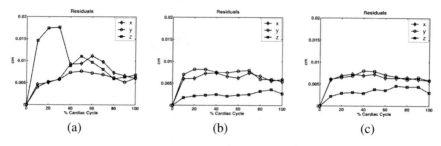

(a)   (b)   (c)

Figure 22. Average residuals per sample point for all three coordinates for $\mathcal{R}_t \rightarrow \mathcal{R}$ model registration for (a) Dog 1, (b) Dog 2, and (c) Dog 3. The y axis has dimension of centimeters.

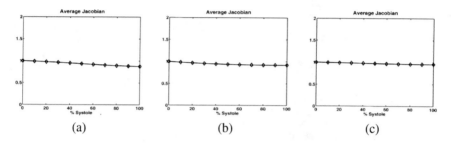

(a)   (b)   (c)

Figure 23. Average Jacobian (Lagrangian) over the twelve left-ventricular regions for (a) Dog 1, (b) Dog 2, and (c) Dog 3.

Jacobian (the determinant of the deformation gradient tensor (Eq. (35)) is equal to unity everywhere. The time plots of the average Jacobian for all three dog studies are shown in Figure 23.

6.3. In Vivo Canine Data: Right Ventricle

To our knowledge, there is no analytical model with which to optimize the parameters governing the right-ventricular NURBS model. However, the same factors that dictated our selection of parametric values for the left-ventricular model also directed our choice of parametric values for the right-ventricular model. These parameters include: order = 3, spans in $u_{RV} = 1$, spans in $v_{RV} = 2$, and spans in $w_{RV} = 2$. In addition, the model is lofted temporally (order = 4 with six control points). In Figure 24 strain plots for one dog (Dog 3) are shown. The assessment measures for this model are given in Figure 25.

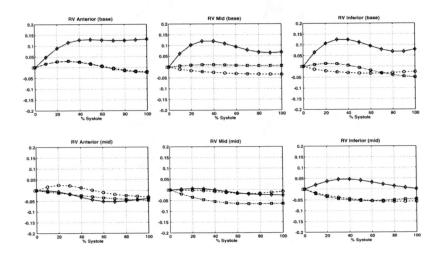

Figure 24. Average Lagrangian normal strain plots for one dog study (Dog 3) for the six basal and mid-cavity regions of the right ventricle. The different geometric shapes (diamond, circle, and square) represent the radial, circumferential, and longitudinal strain values, respectively. The x axis marks the time point during systole.

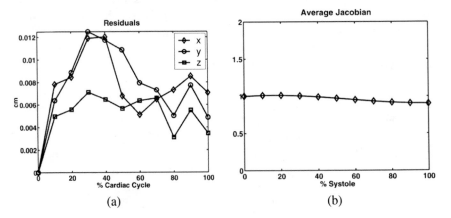

Figure 25. Assessment of a NURBS right-ventricular model for Dog 3 showing both (a) the average residual per sample point for all three coordinates for $\mathcal{R}_t \rightarrow \mathcal{R}$ model fitting and (b) the average Jacobian over systole.

Table 5. Peak Systolic Principal Strains (E_3) for Six Right-Ventricular Regions of Dog 3

	Base	Mid-Cavity
Anterior	-0.12 ± 0.004	-0.22 ± 0.018
Mid	-0.10 ± 0.001	-0.16 ± 0.008
Inferior	-0.20 ± 0.007	-0.18 ± 0.007

6.4. In Vivo Human Data

Also included in this analysis is an illustration of the application of our method to systolic human datasets. One dataset is from a normal human volunteer (Figures 26, 28, and 29) and one dataset is from a patient with a history of myocardial infarction (Figures 27 and 30). For each human study we have included the average Jacobian over 12 left-ventricular regions as well as the weighted least-squares residuals of the fitting algorithm. For each case, we also illustrate the left ventricular radial, circumferential, and longitudinal strains.

6.5. Interpretation of Results

6.5.1. Canine data

Normal LV strains, i.e., average radial, circumferential, and longitudinal strains, are given in Figures 20 and 21. The radial strains remain positive for most of the twelve regions, indicative of the systolic thickening of the left ventricle. Both the circumferential and longitudinal strains are negative. Circumferential

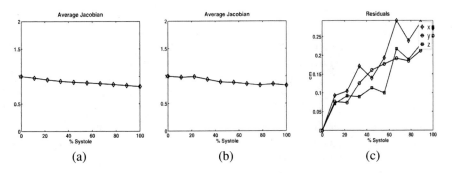

(a)   (b)   (c)

Figure 26. Metrics for the left ventricle of a normal human volunteer illustrated by (a) the Jacobian for the Lagrangian fit, (b) the Jacobian for the Eulerian fit that registers $\mathcal{R}_t \rightarrow \mathcal{R}$, and (c) the residuals for fitting $\mathcal{R}_t \rightarrow \mathcal{R}$.

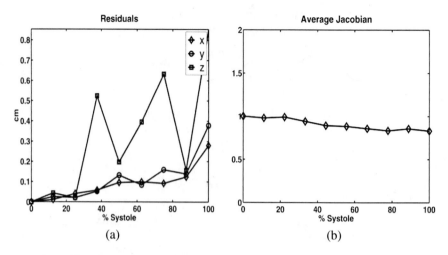

Figure 27. Metrics for the left ventricle of a patient with a history of myocardial infarction illustrated by (a) the Jacobian for the Lagrangian fit that registers $\mathcal{R} \rightarrow \mathcal{R}_t$, and (b) the residuals for fitting $\mathcal{R}_t \rightarrow \mathcal{R}$.

shortening during left-ventricular contraction results in the negative strain values in the circumferential direction, while compression in the longitudinal direction results in negative longitudinal strains. These results are comparable with other relevant work ([2, 33]). Qualitative strain results for one dog study are shown in Figure 19. Strain maps are reconstructed on the midventricular surfaces of the biventricular model. The RV surface ($u_{RV} = 0.5$) exhibits circumferential shortening (Figure 19b), consistent with the segmental shortening seen in [5, 6, 7]. Regional peak principal strains (E_3) are given in Table 5 and are consistent with those given in [4].

6.5.2. Human data

The general strain patterns seen in the canine data, i.e., positive radial strains and negative circumferential and longitudinal strains, are also seen in the normal human volunteer data (Figure 28). These strain patterns have similar physiological interpretations. Comparison with Table 2 from Moore et al.'s work [33] demonstrates that the three strain values in the LV are consistent with the range of strain values in previous findings. The Eulerian strains depicted in Figure 29 are not as smooth as their Lagrangian counterparts. This is to be expected since temporal lofting is not performed for the Eulerian fits.

The strains from the clinical data (Figure 30) are more difficult to interpret. While some of the regional plots are similar to their counterparts of the normal human data, some of the plots demonstrate disparate behavior. Additional insight

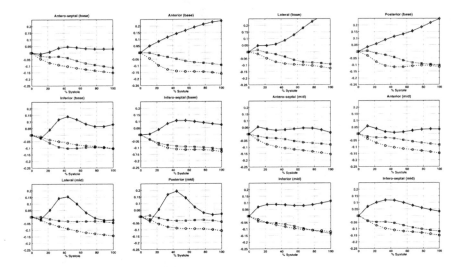

Figure 28. Average Lagrangian normal strain plots for the twelve basal and mid-cavity regions of the left ventricle of a normal human volunteer. The different geometric shapes (diamond, circle, and square) represent the radial, circumferential, and longitudinal strain values, respectively. The x axis marks the time point during systole.

is needed to formulate a physiological explanation for the abnormal strain patterns. The observant reader will notice that the residuals are close to an order of magnitude larger for the human data relative to the canine data. Applying our parametrically optimal model to different datasets provides no guaranteed upper bounding of the residuals, but rather the resulting residuals will naturally vary depending on the complexity of the deformation of the tag lines.

7. CONCLUSIONS

Our 4D NURBS model is capable of producing comprehensive myocardial strain calculations for assessing local myocardial contraction in both the left and right ventricles by reconstructing 3D deformations fields based on available tag and contour information. The contribution of this research includes the extension of the model basis from uniform nonrational B-splines to NURBS, the comparison Cartesian-based NURBS models with a cylindrical and prolate spheroidal parameter assignment with their non-Cartesian counterparts, and construction of a biventricular model based on the short- and long-axis contours at end-diastole. These four model types were not meant to exhaust all possible combinations of parameter assignment and coordinate system, for one could certainly imagine other plausible combinations. However, considering the shape of the left ventricle, the

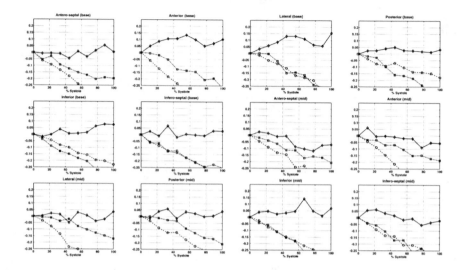

Figure 29. Average Eulerian normal strain plots for the twelve basal and mid-cavity regions of the left ventricle of a normal human volunteer. The different geometric shapes (diamond, circle, and square) represent the radial, circumferential, and longitudinal strain values, respectively. The x axis marks the time point during systole.

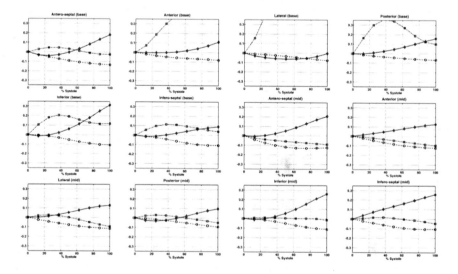

Figure 30. Average Lagrangian normal strain plots for the twelve basal and mid-cavity regions of the left ventricle of a patient with a history of myocardial infarction. The different geometric shapes (diamond, circle, and square) represent the radial, circumferential, and longitudinal strain values, respectively. The x axis marks the time point during systole.

chosen geometric primitives for parameter assignment as well as the selected co-ordinate systems were the most obvious.

The results show that, in the case of simulated data, the quadratic Cartesian-based NURBS models either with a cylindrical or a prolate spheroidal parameter assignment outperformed their counterparts in predicting normal strain. The decreased complexity associated with the cylindrical-parameterized model prompted its use for subsequent calculation of Lagrangian and Eulerian strains for in vivo data. We illustrated the capabilities of the methodology with results from three canine studies, a normal human, and a patient with a history of myocardial infarction. The resulting strain values were plotted over the systolic phase of the cardiac cycle. Qualitative results from right-ventricular analysis were also demonstrated by displaying midventricular strain maps.

While a rigourous analysis explaining the disparity in performance between the models is beyond the scope of this work, we posit that such a disparity is to be expected based on the tagging pattern geometry. A significant portion of the displacement data for nonrigidly registering the models is derived from the tag plane normals in the three orthogonal directions (in addition to the tag plane intersections and tag line/contour intersections). These three normal directions are aligned with the Cartesian axes of the fitting coordinate system. For the Cartesian models, this implies that each coordinate of the control points is solved from a single set of tag plane normals, i.e., the x-value of each control point location is solved only using the set of tag plane normals aligned in the x-direction and the same for the y and z-values. However, for the non-Cartesian models, the geometries of the tag plane normals and coordinate values of the control points are not aligned, which, we believe, leads to a degradation in performance. For example, the r-values of the control point locations of the cylindrical models are solved using normal displacements from the two sets of tag plane normals that are aligned along the x and y axes. A future area of possible research would be to apply our approach to other MR tagging patterns (radial tags [9] and circular ring tags [35]), and look at discrepancies in performance between the different model formulations.

There are several additional areas for possible future development. As noted previously, the current biventricular NURBS model does not encompass the most apical regions of the LV/RV nor the outflow tracts, which would be important for a more comprehensive analysis of myocardial deformation. One could perhaps solve the degeneracy issue at the apical tip by clamping the B-spline volume at the apex. However, that would impose certain limitations on the model's ability to deform at the apex.

RV deformation analysis is challenging considering the sparseness of tag data in the myocardial wall. Even in the LV, where the myocardial wall is thicker, measurement of the radial strains is less tenable due to the paucity of displacement information in the radial direction. This can be readily seen in Figure 30, where the computed radial strains display unexpected irregularities. Increasing the density of tag lines in both the LV and RV could provide for more accurate radial strains, although in that case one would be faced with increased challenges in terms of accurate tag line delineation. In addition to tagging density considerations, one must also be cautious in ensuring the fidelity of the MR images. Potential problems include motion artifacts (e.g., related to breath-holds) and misalignment of the short- and long-axis images due to variabilities in heart motion. These are not issues restricted to this study, but concern all cardiac MR applications. In general, however, with increased acquisition speed, particularly in the use of parallel imaging techniques, these issues may become less of a concern. We note that our canine studies involved manual breath-holds, and so issues related to breathing motion artifacts were not encountered. In human studies the subjects underwent training prior to the actual imaging session so that the breath-holds always took place at end-inspiration and subjects were cued as to when they could breathe (duration of all breath-holds remained the same across acquisition of all images for a given study). In a few instances for both human and canine imaging, misalignments were observed, and these were resolved by ensuring consistency between corresponding myocardial regions in short- and long-axis images.

Alternative and complementary techniques for tagged MRI have been developed for greater spatial resolution such as DENSE [36] and HARP [37, 38], from which dense displacement information could be inferred. The NURBS methodology should prove helpful in spatiotemporal filtering of data from these alternate motion tracking methods and can lead to accurate estimates of 4D myocardial kinematics.

In addition to further development of the technical aspects of our research, current applications are directed to a variety of disease pathophysiologies. We have looked at patient data exhibiting ischemic heart disease and LV hypertrophy, and plan to apply our technique to RV hypertrophic models.

8. REFERENCES

1. S. Masood, Yang G-Z, Pennell DJ, Firmin DN. 2000. Investigating intrinsic myocardial mechanics: the role of MR tagging, velocity phase mapping, and diffusion imaging. *J Magn Reson Imaging* **12**:873–883.

2. Amini AA, Prince JL, eds. 2001. *Measurement of cardiac deformations from mri: physical and mathematical models*. Dordrecht: Kluwer Academic

3. Frangi AF, Niessen WJ, Viergever MA. 2001. Three-dimensional modeling for functional analysis of cardiac images: a review. *IEEE Trans Med Imaging* **20**(1):2–25.

4. Haber I, Metaxas DN. 2000. Three-dimensional motion reconstruction and analysis of the right ventricle using tagged MRI. *Med Image Anal* **4**:335–355.

5. Klein SS, Graham TP, Lorenz CH. 1998. Noninvasive delineation of normal right ventricular contractile motion with magnetic resonance imaging myocardial tagging. *Ann Biomed Eng* **26**:756–763.

6. Naito H, Arisawa J, Harada K, Yamagami H, Kozuka T, Tamura S. 1995. Assessment of right ventricular regional contraction and comparison with the left ventricle in normal humans: a cine magnetic resonance study with presaturation myocardial tagging. *Br Heart J* **74**:186–191.

7. Young A, Fayad ZA, Axel L. 1996. Right ventricular midwall surface motion and deformation using magnetic resonance tagging. *Am J Physiol* **271**:H2677–H2688.

8. Axel L, Dougherty L. 1989. MR imaging of motion with spatial modulation of magnetisation. *Radiology* **171**:841–845.

9. Zerhouni E, Parish D, Rogers W, Yang A, Shapiro E. 1988. Human heart: tagging with MR imaging: a method for noninvasive assessment of myocardial motion. *Radiology* **169**:59–63.

10. Amini AA, Chen Y, Curwen RW, Mani V, Sun J. 1998. Coupled B-snake grids and constrained thin-plate splines for analysis of 2-D tissue deformations from tagged MRI. *IEEE Trans Med Imaging* **17**(3):344–356.

11. Wang Y-P, Chen Y, Amini AA. 2001. Fast LV motion estimation using subspace approximation techniques. *IEEE Trans Med Imaging* **20**(6):499–513.

12. Chandrashekara R, Mohiaddin RH, Rueckert D. 2002. Analysis of myocardial motion in tagged MR images using nonrigid image registration. *Proc SPIE* **4684**:1168–1179.

13. Chen Y, Amini AA. 2002. A MAP framework for tag line detection in SPAMM data using Markov random fields on the B-spline solid. *IEEE Trans Med Imaging* **21**(9):1110–1122.

14. Huang J, Abendschein D, Dávila-Román V, Amini A. 1999. Spatiotemporal tracking of myocardial deformations with a 4D B-spline model from tagged MRI. *IEEE Trans Med Imaging* **18**(10):957–972.

15. Ozturk C, McVeigh ER. 1999. Four dimensional b-spline based motion analysis of tagged cardiac mr images. *Proceedings SPIE* **3660**:46–56.

16. Radeva P, Amini AA, Huang J. 1997. Deformable B-solids and implicit snakes for 3D localization and tracking of SPAMM MRI data. *Comput Vision Image Understand* **66**(2):163–178.

17. Chandrashekara R, Mohiaddin RH, Rueckert D. 2003. Analysis of myocardial motion and strain patterns using a cylindrical B-spline transformation model. In *Proceedings of the international symposium on surgery simulation and soft tissue modeling (IS4TM). Lecture notes in computer science*, vol. 2673, pp. 88–99. New York: Springer.

18. Deng X, Denney Jr TS. 2002. 3D myocardial strain reconstruction from tagged MR image data using a cylindrical B-spline model. In *Proceedings of the IEEE international symposium on biomedical imaging*, pp. 609–612. Washington, DC: IEEE Computer Society.

19. Piegl L. 1991. On NURBS: a survey. *IEEE Comput Graphics Appl* **10**(1):55–71.

20. L. Piegl, Tiller W. 1997. *The NURBS book*. New York: Springer.

21. Figueiredo MAT, Letão JMN, Jain AK. 2000. Unsupervised contour representation and estimation using B-splines and a minimum description length criterion. *IEEE Trans Image Process* **9**(6):1075–1087.

22. Ma W, Kruth JP. 1994. Mathematical modelling of free-form curves and surfaces from discrete points with NURBS. In *Curves and surfaces in geometric design*, pp. 319–326. Ed PJ Laurent, A Le Méhauté, LL Schumaker. Wellesley, MA: A.K. Peters,

23. Gertz EA, Wright S. 2001. *OOQP user guide*. Argonne, IL: Argonne National Laboratory. http://www.cs.wisc.edu/ swright/ooqp/.

24. Schoenberg IJ, Whitney A. 1953. On Pólya frequency functions, III: the positivity of translation determinants with an application to the interpolation problem by spline curves. *Trans Am Math Soc* **74**:246–259.

25. Ma W, Kruth JP. 1995. Parameterization of randomly measured points for least-squares fitting of B-spline curves and surfaces. *Comput Aided Design* **27**(9):663–675.

26. Tustison NJ, Dávila-Román VG, Amini AA. 2003. Myocardial kinematics from tagged MRI based on a 4-D B-spline model. *IEEE Trans Biomed Eng* **50**:1038–1040.

27. Press WH, Flannery BP, Teukolsky SA, Vetterling WT. 1988. *Numerical recipes in C: the art of scientific computing*. Cambridge: Cambridge UP.

28. Horn B, Schunck B. 1981. Determining optical flow. *Artif Intell* **17**:185–203.

29. Cerqueira MD, Weissman NJ, Dilsizian V. 2002. Standardized myocardial segmentation and nomenclature for tomographic imaging of the heart: a statement for healthcare professionals from the Cardiac Imaging Committee of the Council on Clinical Cardiology of the American Heart Association. *Circulation* **105**:539–542.

30. Arts T, Hunter WC, Douglas A, Muijtjens AMM, Reneman RS. 1992. Description of the deformation of the left ventricle by a kinematic model. *J Biomech* **25**:1119–1127.

31. Waks E, Prince JL, Douglas AS. 1996. Deformable Fourier models for surface finding in 3D images. *Proceedings of the IEEE workshop on mathematical methods in biomedical image analysis (MMBIA'96)*, pp. 182-191. Washington, DC: IEEE Computer Society.

32. Suter D, Chen F. 2000. Left ventricular motion reconstruction based on elastic vector splines. *IEEE Trans Med Imaging* **19**(4):295–305.

33. Moore C, Lugo-Olivieri C, McVeigh E, Zerhouni E. 2000. Three-dimensional systolic strain patterns in the normal human left ventricle: characterization with tagged MR imaging. *Radiology* **214**(2):453–466.

34. Bland JM, Altman DG. 2003. Applying the right statistics: analyses of measurements studies. *Ultrasound Obstet Gynecol* **22**:85–93.

35. Spiegel M, Luechinger R, Weber O, Scheidegger M, Schwitter J, Boesiger P. 2000. Ring-Tag: assessment of myocardial midwall motion in volunteers and patients with myocardial hypertrophy. *Proc ISMRM* **6**:1607.

36. Aletras AH, Balaban RS, Wen H. 1999. High-resolution strain analysis of the human heart with fast-DENSE. *J Magn Reson Imag* **140**:41–57.

37. Osman NF, McVeigh ER, Prince JL. 2000. Imaging heart motion using harmonic Phase MRI. *IEEE Trans Med Imaging* **19**(3):186–202.

38. Kuijer JPA, Jansen E, Marcus JT, van Rossum AC, Heethaar RM. 2001. Improved harmonic phase myocardial strain maps. *Magn Reson Med* **46**:993–999.

ROBUST NEUROIMAGING-BASED CLASSIFICATION TECHNIQUES OF AUTISTIC VS. TYPICALLY DEVELOPING BRAIN

Rachid Fahmi, Ayman El-Baz*, Hossam Abd El-Munim,
Alaa E. Abdel-Hakim, and Aly A. Farag

Computer Vision and Image Processing Laboratory,
Department of Electrical and Computer Engineering,
*and *Bioengineering Department, University of Louisville,*
Louisville, Kentucky, USA

Manuel F. Casanova

Department of Psychiatry and Behavioral Sciences,
University of Louisville, Louisville, Kentucky, USA

Autism is a developmental disorder characterized by social deficits, impaired communication, and restricted and repetitive patterns of behavior (American Psychiatry Association, 2000). Various neuropathological studies of autism have revealed abnormalities in several brain regions. Increased head size was the first observed characteristic in children with autism. According to the published studies, different anatomical structures of the brain have been identified as being involved in the abnormal neurodevelopment associated with autism. Classical neuropathological studies as well as MRI structural findings are consistent with respect to some brain structures, while observations with respect to other structures have differed among studies. This lack of consistency may be due to the sample size as well as to the failure to account for significant confounding factors (e.g., age, sex, IQ, handedness). However, there is an increasing agreement from structural imaging studies on the abnormal anatomy of the white matter (WM) in autistic brains. In addition, deficits

Address all correspondence to: Dr. Aly A. Farag, Professor of Electrical and Computer Engineering, University of Louisville, CVIP Lab, Room 412, Lutz Hall, 2301 South 3rd Street, Louisville, KY 40208, USA. Phone: (502) 852-7510, Fax: (502) 852-1580. aafaraol@louisville.edu.

in the size of the corpus callosum (CC) and its subregions in patients with autism relative
to controls are well established. In this work, we aim at using the reported abnormalities
of the WM and the CC, in order to devise robust classification methods of autistic vs.
normal subjects through analyzes of their respective MRIs. To overcome the limitations
and shortcomings of the volumetric studies, our analysis is based on shape descriptions and
geometric models. A novel technique is used to compute the 3D distance map as a shape
descriptor of the WM. The distribution of this distance map is then used as a statistical
feature that allows discrimination between the two groups. Furthermore, we use our newly
proposed nonrigid registration technique based on scale space and curve evolution theories
to devise a new classification approach by analyzing the deformation fields (DF) generated
from registering CCs onto each others. For each group (autistic and control), we pick a
number of segmented CC datasets, one of which is chosen as reference and the remaining
ones registered to this reference using our registration method. The generated DFs are
averaged, and their distributions are computed to represent the changes of the magnitudes
of each group. Given a subject to be classified, we register its MR dataset, once to the
chosen control reference and then to the chosen autistic reference. The two corresponding
DFs are statistically compared to the two average DFs, representing each class, in order to
indicate the class to which the tested subject belong. The accuracy of our techniques was
tested on postmortem and in-vivo brain MR data. The results are very promising and show
that, contrary to traditional methods, the proposed techniques are less sensitive to age and
volume effects.

1. INTRODUCTION

Autism is a complex developmental disability that typically appears during
the first three years of life and is the result of a neurological disorder that affects the
normal functioning of the brain, impacting development in the areas of social interaction and communication skills. Both children and adults with autism typically
show difficulties in verbal and nonverbal communications, social interactions, and
leisure or play activities. Autism is a spectrum disorder and it affects each individual differently and at varying degrees, with milder forms like Asperger syndrome,
in which intellectual ability is high but social interaction is low, and with the most
severe cases typified by unusual, self-injurious, and aggressive behaviors. Such
behaviors may persist throughout life and may inflict a heavy burden on those who
interact with autistic persons. Cognitive impairments may also last over time and
often result in mental retardation in the majority of individuals with autism [1].
Nowadays, doctors prefer the term Autistic Spectrum Disorder (ASD) to refer to
autism.

Autism is not a rare disorder, as once was thought. According to the Centers
for Disease Control and Prevention (CDC), about 1 in 166 American children
fall somewhere within the autistic spectrum [4]. Although the cause of autism
is still largely not clear, researchers have suggested that genetic, developmental,
and environmental factors may be the cause or the predisposing effects toward
developing autism [5, 6, 7]. No current cure is specifically designed for autism.
However, there are some therapies or interventions designed to remedy specific
symptoms in each individual. These therapies are educational, behavioral, or skill-

oriented, and they often result in substantial improvement, especially when started at an early age.

During the past two decades, the study of autism's neuropathology has dramatically intensified. Most studies have reported alterations in some regions of the brain in autistic individuals compared to typically developing ones. Increased head size was the first observed characteristic in children with autism 60 years ago in a study by Kanner [8]. Since then, several studies have reported enlarged brain size and head circumference (HC) in autistic patients. Postmortem studies have revealed evidence of increased brain weight, while bigger brain volume and macrocephaly, defined as HC above the 97th percentile, were reported by several clinical and neuroimaging studies [9–16]. In particular, Courchesne et al. [13, 17] showed that while children with autism have ordinary size brains at birth, they experience an acceleration of brain growth, resulting, between 2 and 4 years of age, in increased brain volume relative to controls. By adolescence and adulthood, differences in mean brain size between the two groups diminish largely as a result of increased relative growth in the normal control group. Indeed, no differences in brain volume between the two groups were reported in[12, 17, 18].

The rest of this section will briefly survey the neuropathological and neuroimaging literature on autism and will discuss the findings that have emerged. Different studies have focused on different parts of the brain in order to identify the structures that are involved in the abnormal neurodevelopment associated with autism. Alterations of different brain regions have been reported by these studies in autistic subjects relative to controls.

Limbic System

The limbic system, known as the center of emotions, includes many cortical and subcortical brain structures. These structures are involved in emotion, and emotional associations with the memory. Examples of these structures are the amygdale, the hypothalamus, the orbito-frontal cortex, and the subiculum. Kemper and Bauman [19] were the first to report an increase in cell packing and reduced cell size in the hypocampus, amygdale, subiculum, and other structures as the result of a comparative study between six autistic cases (9–29 years of age) and six age- and sex-matched controls. Gurin et al. [20] have reported a thin corpus callosum (CC) in a 16-year-old female with autism and severe mental illness. Microscopically, however, no alterations were observed in the limbic structures.

A number of MRI-based studies have reported that the corpus callosum, which is the largest commisure in the brain that allows neural communications between the two hemispheres, has a reduced size in autistic subjects [21, 22]. However, findings are inconsistent as to which segment of the CC is abnormal. Most studies have reported reduction in the size of the body and the posterior subregions of the CC in autistic patients [21, 23–25], whereas other studies have found that the reduction was limited to the body and the anterior segment of the CC [20, 26].

Recently, a two-dimensional voxel-based morphometric study, accounting for an age effect, has reported significant white matter deficiency in the splenium of the CC, but showed no significant difference in the middle body [27]. Sixteen autistic and 12 control subjects, all right-handed males with one ambidextrous subject, participated in this study. The average age for autistic boys is 16.1 ± 4.5 and for controls 17.1 ± 2.8. A later study by Waiter et al. [28] reported reductions in the isthmus and the splenium of the CC in autistic patients. In addition, abnormalities of fractional anisotropy, "*a measure derived from diffusion tensor data that is sensitive to developmental changes and pathological differences in axonal density, size, myelination, and the coherence of organization of fibers within a voxel,*" in the anterior CC were noted in a study using diffusion tensor imaging (DTI) by Barnea-Goraly et al. [29]. Most recently, computational mapping methods were used in an MRI study by Vidal et al. [30] to investigate CC abnormalities in male patients with autism. Twenty-four boys with autism (age 10 ± 3.3 years; range 6–16 years) and 26 healthy boys (age 11.0 ± 2.5 years; range 6–16 years) participated in that study. Contrary to the traditional volumetric studies that have reported a significant reduction in the total callosal area and the anterior subregion of the CC in patients with autism, this study revealed significant reductions in both the splenium and genu of the CC in autistic sufferers relative to controls. Similarly, MRI studies of the hippocampus and the amygdale have reported inconsistent findings. The volume of these structures was found to be increased, decreased, or similar in autistic patients relative to control cases [31].

Cerebellum

The cerebellum is a part of the human brain located in the lower back of the brain. This structure plays a major role in the integration of sensory perceptions and motor output through neural connections with the motor cortex. Most neuropathological studies of autistic individuals agree on the decreased number of Perkinje cells in cerebellar hemispheres, vermis, and cerebellum. Williams et al. [32] were the first to examine cortical and subcortical structures and the cerebellum in four autistic individuals (three males, 12, 27, and 33 years old, and a 3-year-old female, all mentally retarded and two with seizures). They reported a reduction of the Perkinje cell density in one case. Lately, Ritvo et al. [33] reported a decreased number of Perkinje cells in the cerebellar hemisphere and the vermis, in a study involving three mentally retarded autistic males and none with seizures, and three male controls. Other studies have followed and showed the same results [34, 35]. However, few studies reported no abnormalities in the cerebellum of some autistic patients [20].

The first MRI study to examine the cerebellum was conducted by Courchesne et al. [36]. This study showed a reduction in the area of the neocerebellar vermis, which is consistent with the pathological studies noting reduced Perkinje cell density in autism. Other MRI studies have reported an increased volume in cerebellar white matter of young children with autism, relative to control subjects [17]. However, this same group found that the cerebellar gray matter volume in autistic young children did not differ from control subjects, but this difference was noticed in older patients. Additionally, a functional MRI (fMRI) study has examined the cerebellum, and has found that abnormalities of cerebellar development in autism may have different implications for motor and attentional functioning [37].

Recently, a computer image analysis study, based on the analysis of the configuration of minicolumns ("*the basic functional unit of the brain that organizes neurons in cortical space* [38, 39]"), provided evidence of diminished width for pyramidal cell arrays in the neocortex of autistic patients [40]. This study showed that diminution was greatest within the peripheral neuropil space of the minicolumn. A second study using the Gray Level Index (GLI) corroborated these findings [41]. This study showed diagnosis-dependent effects in distance between adjacent local maxima in the GLI. The tighter packing of cortical modules suggests increased cellular density. This increase in the total number of minicolumns in autism requires a scale increase (roughly a 3/2 power law) in white mater to maintain modular interconnectivity [42]. This additional white matter takes the form of short-range connections that make up the bulk of intracortical connections [42]. More recent analysis of intra and inter-cluster distances using Delaunay triangulation indicates that reported increased cellular density in autism is the result of an increased number of minicolumns rather than an increase in the total number of cells per minicolumn [43]. Furthermore, the pyramidal neurons that populate the cell minicolumns in autism appear smaller and have reduced nucleolar size [43].

Nucleolar size in pyramidal cells reflects metabolic demand. Large nucleoli are seen in correspondingly large pyramidal cells. These neurons provide for long projections, e.g., cortical efferent axons to spinal cord motor neurons. On the other hand, small nucleoli are seen primarily in smaller pyramidal cells. These neurons are characterized by short intracortical projections. The findings in autism suggest a metabolic bias that makes short corticocortical connections efficient at the expense of longer association and commisural connections. Anatomically the results can be seen in structural MRI studies as an increase in the outer radiate compartment of white matter [44]. This compartment is made up of late myelinating short association fibers. Contrariwise, five out of eight structural MRI studies of the corpus callosum have reported reduction in its total area and/or one of its subdivisions [45]. The findings explain why autistics excel in performance in tasks that require information processing within a given brain area (e.g., visual discrimination) but otherwise perform poorly in those that require inter-areal integration (e.g., joint attention, language).

Brainstem

Like some of the other brain regions, inconsistencies exist between pathological findings related to the brainstem in autism. In a study by Bauman et al.

[46, 47], it was reported that the neurons in the inferior olive were large in young autistic individuals (9–12 years of age), whereas these neurons were small and pale in older cases (>22 years). More recently, Bailey et al. [35] have reported olivary abnormalities in five autistic patients.

According to these reviewed studies, different anatomical structures of the brain have been identified as being involved in the abnormal neurodevelopment associated with autism. Classic MRI structural findings are consistent with respect to some brain structures, while observations with respect to other structures have differed among studies. This lack of consistency may be due, at least in part, to the unavailability of larger sample sizes and closely matched control groups. The failure to account for significant confounding factors (e.g., age, sex, IQ, socioeconomic status, mental retardation, handedness) may also play a major role in causing these uncertainties and inconsistencies. The reported structural MRI findings, on the other hand, cannot be directly correlated to the neuropathological findings in autism. However, several important and consistently replicated results suggest an elevated brain volume in autism, particularly in young children. Other regions of the brain were identified, perhaps with less certainty, as being directly involved in the abnormal neurodevelopment associated with autism, particularly the white matter and the CC.

Consequently, more studies are needed to narrow the gap between the neuroimaging and neuropathological researches in autism. Challenges for future studies also include an understanding of how the brain grows and changes over time in autism, and how these changes are related to clinical manifestations and impairments. Longitudinal studies are hence necessary to track the course of brain development in autism. In addition, autism may benefit a great deal from the new imaging modalities such as diffusion tensor imaging (DT-MRI). This imaging modality offers a good opportunity to learn about white matter in autism. Some studies that use DT-MRI to probe white matter differences in several developmental disorders including autism have already been published, as mentioned above (e.g., see [29] for DT-MRI use in autism).

It is worth noting at this point that it remains unclear as to whether the interconnectivity findings are the cause of autism or its result.

Our Contributions

In this work, we aim at using the reported abnormalities in some brain regions in order to devise a way that permits the classification of autistic vs. normal subjects by analyzing their respective magnetic resonance images (MRIs). To overcome the limitations and shortcomings of the volumetric studies, we base our analyzes on shape descriptions and geometric models. We focus on analysis of the WM and the CC since these two brain structures were extensively studied and have been shown to provide coherent discriminatory measurements between autistic and normal subjects.

A novel technique is used to compute the 3D distance map as a shape descriptor of the WM. The distribution of this distance map is then used as a statistical feature that allows the discrimination between the two groups. The preliminary results were very promising and motivated us to push the shape analysis even further and for more specific brain structures, particularly for the CC.

We also use our new nonrigid registration technique, which is based on scale space and curve evolution theories [69], to devise a new classification approach by analyzing the deformation fields generated from registering CCs onto each others.

The remainder of this chapter is organized as follows. Section 2 describes the data sets and how they were collected, as well as the MRI protocol. The image processing approaches used in the analysis and the results are introduced in Section 3. Finally, we present our results and conclude with a discussion section.

2. SUBJECTS AND IMAGE ACQUISITION

Two types of brain data are used in this study: postmortem proton density (PD)-weighted MRI data, and in-vivo T1-weighted MRI metadata. The latter will be referred to as the *savant data* in this chapter.

Data and Specimens

Postmortem brains were obtained from the Autism Tissue Program (ATP). Diagnosis for each patient was established by the Autism Diagnostic Interview-Revised (ADIR). Postmortem brains from 14 autistic patients (mean interval between death and autopsy: 25.8 hours) and from 12 controls (mean interval between death and autopsy: 20.4 hours) were used in this study.

Data Collection

A quick description of the postmortem MRI data used in this study is presented in this section. For more details, one can refer to [48]. In order to optimize white–gray matter substance contrast in formalin-fixed brains, a PD-weighted imaging sequence was used. The method employed a 1.5-Tesla GE MRI system to scan brains that were placed within a special device that avoids dehydration during the scanning procedure. The scan time lasted an average of 50 minutes and 29 seconds. A Fast Spin Echo (FSE) technique with a long Repetition time (TR) of 6700 ms and a short Echo time (TE) of 8.23 ms and an Echo train of 4 render coronal images with excellent gray–white matter contrast. The technique allows the full coverage of brains with 114 slices, 1.6 mm thick, with no inter-slice gap. A high-resolution K-space dataset consisting of 256 points in the phase and Zero-fill interpolation (ZIP) 512 points in the frequency both encode direction. An in-plane resolution of 625 microns $\times$ 312.5 microns, a field of view of 16×16 cm^2, and a number of repeated excitations (NEX) of 7 with a bandwidth of 62.5 were used.

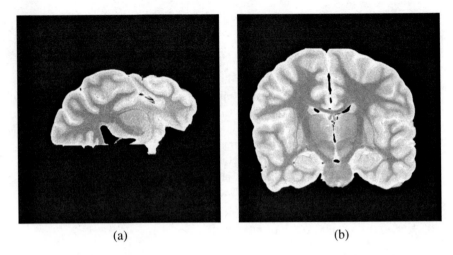

(a)   (b)

Figure 1. Sample postmortem coronal slices: (a) slice 50 from half-brain of a control case;
(b) slice 60 from whole brain of an autistic subject.

These techniques demonstrate good results in samples fixed for from 6 weeks to
15 months [48]. All images were acquired with the same 1.5-T Signa MRI scanner
(General Electric, Milwaukee, WI) using a 3D spoiled gradient recall acquisition
in the steady state (time to echo, 5 ms; time to repeat, 24 ms; flip angle, 45°;
repetition, 1; field of view, 24 cm^2). Contiguous axial slices 1.5 mm thick (124
per brain), were obtained. The images were collected in a 192×256 acquisition
matrix and were 0-filled in the k space to yield an image of 256×256 pixels^2,
resulting in an effective voxel resolution of approximately $1.0 \times 1.0 \times 1.5$ mm^3.

The acquired datasets are PD-weighted volumes of size $512 \times 512 \times 114$.
Each slice is 1.6 mm thick with an in-plane resolution of 0.625×0.3125 mm^2, on
which the WM appears dark, the GM appears light, and the fluid appears brighter.
Due to different factors including removal of the brain from the skull and fixation
problems, distortions such as large deep cuts commonly occur and are revealed in
the MRI scans. Sample slices of the postmortem data are shown in Figure 1.

The savant datasets were acquired with the same 1.5-T Signa MRI scanner
(General Electric, Milwaukee, WI) using a 3D spoiled gradient recall acquisition
in the steady state (time to echo, 5 ms; time to repeat, 24 ms; flip angle, 45°;
repetition, 1; field of view, 24 cm^2). Contiguous axial slices (1.5 mm thick)
or coronal slices (2 mm thick) were obtained, 124 per brain. The images were
collected in a 192×256 acquisition matrix and were 0-filled in the k space to yield
an image of 256×256 pixels, resulting in an effective voxel resolution of 0.9375
$\times$ 0.9375 $\times$ 1.5 mm^3 (or 0.9375 $\times$ 0.9375 $\times$ 2 mm^3). Subject placement was
standardized. A total of 30 normals and 15 autistic brain datasets were collected.

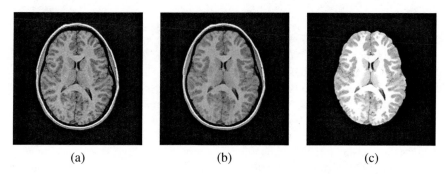

(a)   (b)   (c)

Figure 2. Smoothing and skull stripping results using the BET2/FSL software: (a) slice from original dataset: (b) smoothing results using the anisotropic filter: (c) skull stripping result. The slice is from the savant dataset corresponding to a normal female, 25 years of age.

3. IMAGE PROCESSING AND ANALYSIS

The data at hand undergo a series of preprocessing steps. First, all datasets are smoothed using the anisotropic diffusion filter, which is known to preserve the image edges. Then a brain extraction algorithm is applied to get rid of the non-brain tissues in the savant images. Finally, all datasets are segmented into three classes: white matter (WM), gray matter (GM), and cerebrospinal fluid (CSF).

3.1. Brain Extraction

Brain extraction, also known as skull stripping, is the process of removing the non-brain tissues (e.g., skull, eyes, fat) from the MRI scans. The Brain Extraction Tool (BET2) as implemented in the FSL package (free package at http://www.fmrib.ox.ac.uk/fsl/) is used in this work to isolate the brain tissues and get rid of all other artifacts. Figure 2 shows the result of applying the BET tool on a T1-weighted MRI scan.

3.2. Image Segmentation

Three-dimensional segmentation of anatomical structures is very important for various medical applications. Due to image noise and inhomogeneities, as well as the complexity of anatomical structures, the segmentation process remains a tedious and challenging process. Therefore, this process can not rely only on image amounts of information, but has to involve prior knowledge of the shapes and other properties of the objects of interest.

Deformable models have been extensively used for 3D image segmentation. Such a model evolves iteratively toward the objects of interest by minimizing a global energy. The functional energy represents the confluence of physics and geometry. The latter represents an object shape and the former puts constraints on how the shape may vary over space and time. Deformable models-based segmentation approaches have many limitations, including their sensitivity to initialization, the handling of the topological changes (curve breaking and merging) during the course of evolution, and their dependence on a large number of tuning parameters. The level set-based segmentation techniques offer a solution to some of the limitations of the classical deformable models [49, 50, 51, 52]. These techniques, for which the evolving curve is represented as the zero level set of a higher-dimensional function, handle efficiently the topological changes. In addition, curve initialization can be either manual or automatic, and needs not be close to the desired solution. However, an accurate initial estimation of each class parameters is needed to ensure accurate segmentation.

In this work, we use our level set based-adaptive multimodal image segmentation approach [53, 54] to segment the images into WM, GM, and CSF. In [53], we have proposed a novel and robust level set-based segmentation approach suitable for both 2D and 3D medical applications. We build a statistical Gaussian model with adaptive parameters for each region to be segmented, and we explicitly embed these models into the partial differential equations (PDEs) governing the curves evolution. The parameters of each region are initially estimated using the Stochastic Expectation Maximization (SEM) algorithm and are automatically re-estimated at each iteration step. Our method differs from the one proposed in [55] in the sense that it is more suitable for multimodal images and allows for re-estimation of the probability density functions representing each class. The robustness and accuracy of our technique were demonstrated through our work on MR images and angiography [53]. Figure 3 shows the results of extracting the WM from a stack of MR images using our evolution model, while Figure 4 shows some results of our segmentation technique when applied to T1-weighted MRI scans to extract the WM, GM, and CSF.

3.3. Distance Map and Shape Description

Distance map $D(\mathbf{x})$, also known as a distance transform, assigns to each point in a given image (2D or 3D) a minimal distance from a locus of points (usually object boundaries) as shown in Figure 5.

The exact computation of $D(\mathbf{x})$) is very time consuming, especially for large datasets. Therefore, $D(\mathbf{x})$ can be discretely approximated using the Chamfer metric [56], or continuously approximated by solving a special first order, nonlinear partial differential equation, known as the eikonal equation. Several methods have been proposed to solve the eikonal equation [57, 58, 59, 60, 61, 62], the most stable and consistent of which is the fast marching method (FMM), which is applicable to both Cartesian [61, 63] and triangulated surfaces [64, 65]. The FMM combines entropy satisfying upwind schemes and fast sorting techniques to find the solution in one pass algorithm. Although the FMM is the most stable and consistent method

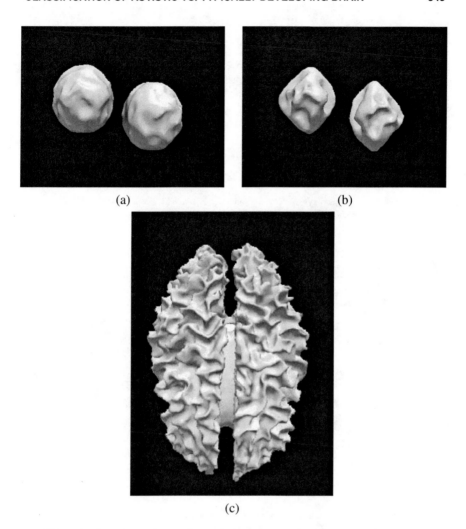

Figure 3. Several steps in a surface evolution to extract the white matter of the brain from an MRI scan: (a) initialization of the algorithm by two spheres inside the WM; (b) intermediate evolution step; (c) final result of the surface evolution representing the extracted WM volume.

for solving the eikonal equation, it lacks accuracy along diagonal directions and its computational complexity is not optimal. Recently, we proposed an improved version of the FMM that is highly accurate on Cartesian domains. This new method is called multi-stencils fast marching (MSFM), and it computes the solution at each point by solving the eikonal equation along several stencils and then picks the solution that satisfies the fast marching causality relationship. The stencils are

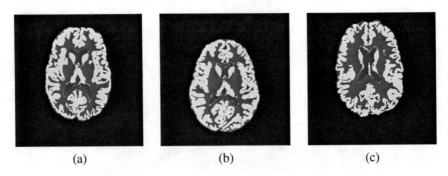

(a)   (b)   (c)

Figure 4. Some 2D displays of segmentation results (into WM, GM, CSF). Slice 69 from MRI scan of (a) an 68-year-old autistic female; (b) a 4-year-old autistic male; (c) a 34-year-old healthy male. See attached CD for color version.

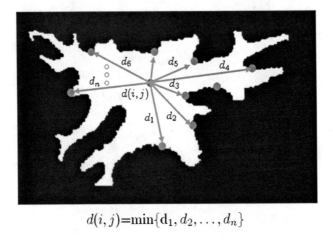

$$d(i,j) = \min\{d_1, d_2, \ldots, d_n\}$$

Figure 5. Distance map concept. See attached CD for color version.

centered at each point and cover its entire nearest neighbors. In 2D space, two stencils cover the 8-neighbors of the point as shown in Figure 6. For those stencils that are not aligned with the natural coordinate system, the eikonal equation is derived using directional derivatives and then solved using a higher-order finite difference scheme [66]. Figure 7 shows the distance maps inside the segmented white matter corresponding to two 2D typical slices from the postmortem data at hand. These distances were computed using the proposed method MSFM.

In order to use the distance map, $D(\cdot)$, of a given object, Ω_1 as a discriminatory feature that distinguishes it from other objects, e.g., Ω_2, and we compute the Cumulative Distribution Function (CDF) of $D(\cdot)$ inside of Ω_1 and compare it to that

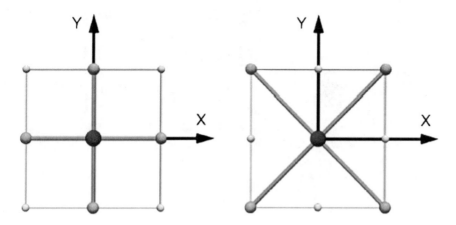

Figure 6. Proposed stencils for 2D Cartesian domain. See attached CD for color version.

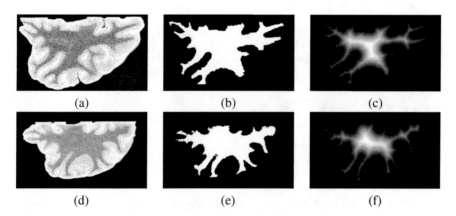

(a)   (b)   (c)

(d)   (e)   (f)

Figure 7. Left to right: 1st column = two typical MR slices from postmortem data; 2nd column = segmented white matter; 3rd column = distance maps inside the WM.

corresponding to Ω_2. Figure 8 shows the CDFs of distance maps corresponding to different objects with different shapes, areas, and orientations. It is clear from the CDF plots that the distance map provides a good comparative feature to represent a shape.

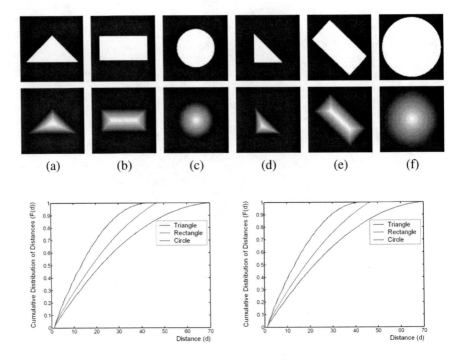

Figure 8. Illustration examples of using the cumulative distribution to discriminate between different shapes. From top to bottom: 1st row = six different objects; 2nd row = their corresponding distance maps computed by the proposed MSFM technique; 3rd row = CDFs of the left three shapes and those of the right three shapes. See attached CD for color version.

3.4. Image Registration

Registration is a major component in many medical image analysis applications. Registration techniques can be categorized into two main families: feature-based and intensity-based techniques. The feature-based methods rely on extracting and matching salient anatomical structures from images (edges, contours line intersections, corners, etc.). The intensity-based methods are used directly to match image intensities without any attempt to detect distinctive objects. A major disadvantage of such methods is their sensitivity to intensity changes introduced by noise, illumination variations, etc. Another limitation of intensity-based methods is their inability to directly solve the problem of anatomical correspondences, as image similarity does not necessarily imply accurate registration of the underlying anatomy. This may be the case when registering brain images where large areas (e.g. gray matter) have practically uniform intensity which makes it hard to define correspondence and then results in false alignment. To cope with some of the drawbacks of the area-based techniques, Shen and Davatzikos [67] proposed a new deformable registration for brain images, known as "HAMMER." This method utilizes an attribute vector, which reflects the geometric characteristics of the underlying anatomical structures, as a signature for each point instead of using only the image intensity. Part of each attribute vector is a number of geometric moment invariants (GMIs) calculated locally around each point. We do not intend to give a comprehensive survey on image registration, but the interested reader may refer to [68] for such a survey.

Recently, we proposed a new nonrigid registration technique that combines ideas from the feature-based and the intensity-based registration approaches [69]. Given two images (2D or 3D), $I_s(\mathbf{x})$ and $I_t(\mathbf{x})$, of the same anatomical organs, taken from different patients or from the same patient over a period of time, our method performs matching between these two images in two main steps and outputs a spatial transformation $\mathbf{T} : \mathbb{R}^n \rightarrow \mathbb{R}^n$ ($n = 2 \text{ or } 3$), such that the similarity between the intensities $I_s(\mathbf{x})$ and $I_t(\mathbf{T}(\mathbf{x}))$ is optimized. The first step of the introduced approach consists in globally aligning the two images. This corresponds to finding the optimal global transformation $T_{\text{global}} : \mathbf{x} \mapsto \mathbf{x}'$, which maps any point in one image into its corresponding point in the other image. In 3D space, the global motion can be modeled, for example, by a 12-parameter affine transformation that can be written as

$$T_{\text{global}}(x, y, z) = \begin{pmatrix} a_{11} & a_{12} & a_{13} \\ a_{21} & a_{22} & a_{23} \\ a_{31} & a_{32} & a_{31} \end{pmatrix} \cdot \begin{pmatrix} x \\ y \\ z \end{pmatrix} + \begin{pmatrix} a_{14} \\ a_{24} \\ a_{34} \end{pmatrix}. \quad (1)$$

The parameters a_{ij}, $i, j = 1, \cdots, n$, of T_{global} represent rotation, scaling, shearing, and translation. In this work, these parameters are determined through a minimization of the mean squared positional error between matched features. The scale space theory plays a major role here in extracting and matching these features. A novel approach to build robust and efficient 3D local invariant feature descriptors is introduced.

The second step of the proposed approach is to find the optimal transformation, T_{local}, to model the local deformations of the imaged anatomy. The basic idea is to deform an object by evolving equispaced contours/surfaces in the target image $I_t(\cdot)$ to match those in the source image $I_s(\cdot)$. These iso-surfaces are generated using fast marching level sets, where the built local invariant feature descriptors are used as voxel signatures. Finally, we combine the local and global transformations to produce our registration transformation $T(\mathbf{x}) = T_{\text{global}}(\mathbf{x}) + T_{\text{local}}(\mathbf{x})$. The following sections present a description of the main components of our nonrigid registration technique.

3.4.1. 3D local invariant features for voxel-based similarity measure

Building a good invariant feature descriptor starts from the selection of the points that are less affected by geometrical variations. Hence, distinct characteristics, which also should be invariant to different imaging changes, are carefully collected to build the feature descriptor. Finally, matching these feature descriptors is performed to find the correspondent pairs of control points.

Interest point detection: Interest points are usually selected in highly informative locations such as edges, corners, or textured regions. In the context of feature invariance, interest points should be selected so that they achieve the maximum possible repeatability under different imaging conditions.

The most challenging point is the invariance with respect to scale changes. Scale-space theory offers the main tools for selecting the most robust feature locations, or the interest points, against scale variations. Indeed, given a signal $f : \mathbb{R}^n \rightarrow \mathbb{R}$, where $n = 3$ in the case of volumetric data, the scale-space representation $L : \mathbb{R}^n \times \mathbb{R}^+ \rightarrow \mathbb{R}$ is defined as the following convolution:

$$L(\mathbf{x}, t) = g(\mathbf{x}, t) * f(\mathbf{x}), \tag{2}$$

where $L(\mathbf{x}, 0) = f(\mathbf{x}), \forall \mathbf{x} \in \mathbb{R}^n$, and $g(\mathbf{x}, t)$ denote the scale-space kernel that is proven to be Gaussian with $t = \sigma^2$ [70]. Note that as t increases, the scale-space representation $L(\mathbf{x}, t)$ of the signal tends to coarser scales [70].

Normalization of the Laplacian of Gaussian $\nabla^2 g$ with factor $\sigma^2 = t$ is necessary for true scale invariance, as proven by Lindeberg [70]. Later, Mikolajczyk and Schmid [71] proved experimentally that the extrema (maxima and minima) of $\sigma^2 \nabla^2 g$ produce the most stable image features:

$$\sigma^2 \nabla^2 g \approx \sigma \frac{g(\vec{x}, k\sigma) - g(\vec{x}, \sigma)}{k\sigma - \sigma},$$
$$\Rightarrow g(\vec{x}, k\sigma) - g(\vec{x}, \sigma) \approx (k-1)\sigma^2 \nabla^2 g,$$

which shows that the σ^2 normalization of the Laplacian of Gaussian can be approximated by the Difference-of-Gaussian (DoG). In other words, the locations of the extrema in the DoG hyperpyramid, i.e., scale-space levels, correspond to the most stable features with respect to scale changes.

In this work, the scale-space representation of an input 3D signal f is generated as follows. First, let's define

$$L_0 = g(\mathbf{x}, t_0) * f(\mathbf{x}), \text{ and } L_1 = g(\mathbf{x}, t_1) * f(\mathbf{x}), \ t_1 = C.t_0, \tag{3}$$

where $C > 1$ is a real number, and

$$g(\mathbf{x}, t) = \frac{1}{(2\pi t)^{\frac{3}{2}}} \exp(\frac{-\mathbf{x}^T \mathbf{x}}{2t}).$$

The first level of the DoG hyperpyramid is obtained by subtracting L_0 from L_1. Then, L_1 is sub-sampled to a smaller scale ($\frac{1}{2}$ of L_1 is used). The convolution and subtraction process is repeated for L_1 to generate the second level of the hyper-pyramid. The whole procedure is repeated recursively to generated the consecutive levels.

The interest points are detected at the local extrema of the DoG hyperpyramid. This is performed by checking every voxel in the current level. If the checked voxel is a local extremum, then it is compared with its neighbors in the upper and the lower levels. The location of the voxel is selected as an interest point if it is also an extremum with respect to its local neighborhood in the upper and the lower levels of the DoG hyperpyramid.

3.4.2. Descriptor building and matching

We build our descriptor in 3D space using gradient orientations histograms with 2D polar-coordinate bins for neighboring cells that consist of voxels in the current level-neighborhood of every interest point. This method was previously used in [72] for 2D medical applications and was proven to be efficient with respect to rotation and affine transformations in other applications [74, 73]. The gradient magnitude of each voxel in the neighborhood of an interest point is calculated as

$$r = \sqrt{G_x^2 + G_y^2 + G_z^2}, \tag{4}$$

where G_x, G_y and G_z are the gradient components in the x, y and z directions, respectively. The gradient orientations in the polar coordinate system are given by

$$\theta = \tan^{-1}\frac{G_y}{G_x}, \text{ and } \phi = \sin^{-1}\frac{\sqrt{G_x^2 + G_y^2}}{r} = \cos^{-1}\frac{G_z}{r}. \tag{5}$$

To successfully describe the neighborhood of an interest point, the closer voxel should have a larger influence on the descriptor's entries. Therefore, Gaussian weights are assigned to every voxel in the neighborhood of the interest point, and are used with mean at the interest point itself to guarantee a distance-weighted contribution to the gradient orientation histogram. Moreover, this gives the built descriptor a robustness with respect to skew distortions [70].

According to [70, 74], one way to achieve rotation invariance is to describe all the descriptor entries relative to a canonical orientation. This orientation can be set to the dominant gradient orientation in the interest point neighborhood, which corresponds to the histogram bin with the maximum value. Therefore, the 2D histogram bin (ϕ_i, θ_i) for the ith feature is updated by adding the term $r(\mathbf{x}_i) \cdot g(\mathbf{x}_i, \sigma^2)$. The considered bin for update is calculated as $\theta_r = \theta - \theta_c$, and $\phi_r = \phi - \phi_c$, where θ_c, ϕ_c are the components of the canonical orientation of the interest point, and θ, ϕ are the components of the gradient orientation referred to

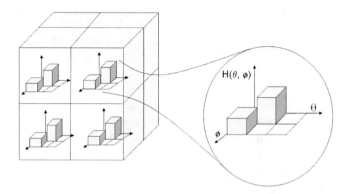

Figure 9. Structure of the 3D feature descriptor. Only eight samples of neighboring cells and six histogram bins are shown in the Figure for illustration purposes. See attached CD for color version.

the zero-axes of the coordinate system, as calculated above. The final descriptor is built as shown in Figure 9. This vector is normalized to reduce the effect of linear intensity changes [74]. In this work, we use neighborhoods of $8 \times 8 \times 8$ for both canonical gradient orientation and descriptor's entries, and cells of $4 \times 4 \times 4$, which means that eight cells are used for building the entries of the descriptor. For each cell, we use eight and four histogram bins for ϕ and θ, respectively. So, the descriptor is of size $8 \times 8 \times 4 = 256$, and after adding the overhead of the original location, pyramid level, and the canonical orientation, the total descriptor size becomes $256 + 6 = 262$.

Finally, given a descriptor feature F_1 in the first image, its match, F_2, in the second image is found when the following condition is satisfied:

$$\frac{D(F_1, F_2)}{\min(D(F_1, F_2'))} < Threshold < 1, \forall F_2' \neq F_1, \text{and} F_2' \neq F_2, \tag{6}$$

where $D(\cdot, \cdot)$ is the Euclidean distance. Other distances may be used as well.

3.4.3. Global and Local Motion Modeling

To model the global motion between the two images $I_t(\cdot)$ and $I_s(\cdot)$, we build the 3D feature descriptor as described in Section 3.4.1, and then we match the features of the reference image to those of the transformed image. The matched pairs are used to estimate a 3D global transformation through the gradient descent minimization of the mean squared positional error between the corresponding points. In this work, a 9 DOF affine transformation model is adopted.

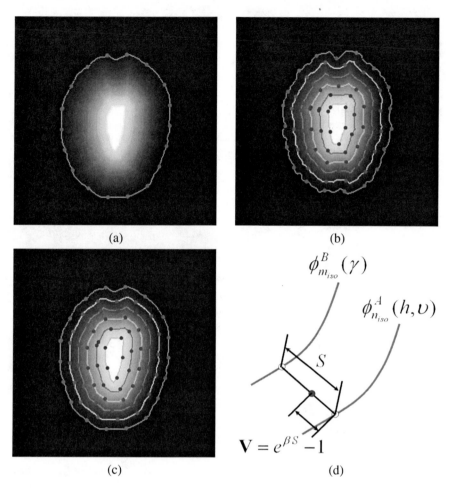

(a)   (b)

(c)   (d)

Figure 10. Cross-sectional views of generated distance map and iso-surfaces before (a) and after (b,c) deformation. The evolution scenario is depicted in (d). See attached CD for color version.

To handle local deformations undergone by the imaged organ, we propose a new approach based on deforming the organ over evolving closed and equispaced surfaces (iso-surfaces) to closely match the prototype. The evolution of the iso-surfaces is guided by an exponential speed function in the directions minimizing distances between corresponding voxel pairs on the iso-surfaces on both images. The proposed 3D local invariant feature descriptor (see Section 3.4.2) is built for each point of each iso-surface after discretization. These descriptors, which are invariant to the image deformations, are used for an image similarity measure.

The first step of our approach is to generate the distance map inside the brain images as shown in Figure 10a. The second step is to use this distance map to generate iso-surfaces as shown in Figure 10b–c. Note that the number of iso-surfaces, which is not necessarily the same for both images, depends on the accuracy and speed required by the user. The third step consists is finding the correspondences between the iso-surfaces. The final step is evolution of the iso-surfaces. Here, our goal is to deform the iso-surfaces in the first dataset (target image $I_t(\cdot)$) to match the iso-surfaces in the second dataset (source image $I_s(\cdot)$). Before stating the evolution equation, let us define the following:

- $\phi^{I_t}_{n_{\mathrm{iso}}}(\cdot, \nu)$ are the iso-surfaces on the target image $I_t(\cdot)$, with $n_{\mathrm{iso}} = 1, \ldots, N_{\mathrm{iso}}$ being the index of the iso-surfaces and ν the iteration step,

- $\phi^{I_s}_{m_{\mathrm{iso}}}(\cdot)$ are the iso-surfaces on the source image $I_s(\cdot)$, where $m_{\mathrm{iso}} = 1, \ldots, M_{\mathrm{iso}}$ is the index of the iso-surfaces,

- $S(h, \gamma_h)$ denotes the Euclidean distance between an iso-surface voxel h on $I_t(\cdot)$, and its corresponding iso-surface voxel γ_h on $I_s(\cdot)$; γ_h is searched for within a local window centered at the position of h in $I_s(\cdot)$; note also that γ_h may be the same for different h,

- $S^{I_t}_{n_{\mathrm{iso}},n_{\mathrm{iso}}-1}(h)$ is the Euclidian distance between $\phi^{I_t}_{n_{\mathrm{iso}}}(h, \nu)$ and $\phi^{I_t}_{n_{\mathrm{iso}}-1}(h, \nu)$ at each iteration ν,

- $V(\cdot)$ is the propagation speed function.

One major step in the propagation model is selection of the propagation speed function V. This selection must satisfy the following conditions:

$$V(h) = 0, \text{ if } S(h, \gamma_h) = 0, \tag{7}$$
$$V(h) \leq \min(S(h, \gamma_h), S^{I_t}_{n_{\mathrm{iso}},n_{\mathrm{iso}}-1}(h), S^{I_t}_{n_{\mathrm{iso}},n_{\mathrm{iso}}+1}(h)), \text{ if } S(h, \gamma_h) \neq 0. \tag{8}$$

The latter condition, known as the smoothness constraint, prevents the current point from cross-passing the closest neighbor surfaces, as shown in Figure 10d. Note that the function

$$V(h) = \exp(\beta(h) \cdot S(h, \gamma_h)) - 1 \tag{9}$$

satisfies the above conditions, where $\beta(h)$ is the propagation term such that, at each iso-surface point $h \in I_t$,

$$\beta(h) \preceq \frac{\ln[\min(S(h, \gamma_h), S^{I_t}_{n_{\mathrm{iso}},n_{\mathrm{iso}}-1}(h), S^{I_t}_{n_{\mathrm{iso}},n_{\mathrm{iso}}+1}(h)) + 1]}{S(h, \gamma_h)}. \tag{10}$$

Based on this speed function, the evolution process is governed by the following equation:

$$\phi_{n_{\mathrm{iso}}}^{I_t}(h, \nu + 1) = \frac{V(h)}{S(h, \gamma_h)} \phi_{m_{\mathrm{iso}}}^{I_s}(\gamma_h) + \frac{S(h, \gamma_h) - V(h)}{S(h, \gamma_h)} \phi_{n_{\mathrm{iso}}}^{I_t}(h, \nu), \quad (11)$$

where $h = 1, \ldots, \mathcal{H}$ denotes the iso-surface points on image $I_t(\cdot)$, and γ_h is its corresponding iso-surface point on $I_s(\cdot)$. We have tested our proposed deformable registration technique on various 2D and 3D medical images (e.g., kidney, lung, brain). In this work, we present some results corresponding to the application of our registration technique on two T1-weighted brain MRIs of the same patient acquired at different times ($\approx$ 1 year apart). Each of the two datasets is of size 256×200, with a voxel size of $1 \times 1 \times 1$ mm^3.

The performance of our approach was assessed qualitatively and compared to our own implementation of the free form deformation technique [75]. For a quantitative assessment of our method's accuracy, we proposed a validation framework using finite-elements methods (see [69] for more details). For a visual assessment of the quality of our approach, we fused the two registered volumes in a checkerboard visualization, as shown in Figure 11. One can clearly see that the connectivity between the two volumes is smoother both at the edges and inside the brain region.

4. PROPOSED CLASSIFICATION APPROACHES

The main objective of the present work is to devise new techniques that allow the classification of autistic subjects vs. typically developing ones by analyzing their respective brain MR images. To this end, we aim at taking advantage of the abnormalities of some brain regions, in autistic patients relative to controls, as reported in the neuropathological and neuroimaging literature. We will focus on analyzing the white matter (WM) and the corpus callosum (CC) using the image-processing tools presented in previous sections. For the WM analysis, both the postmortem and savant datasets will be used, while, due to geometric distortions in the postmortem data, only the savant MRI scans will be used to investigate the discriminatory measures that the CCs may reveal. To overcome the limitations of the traditional techniques, which mainly depend on volumetric descriptions of different brain structures, and hence are sensitive to the segmentation results as well as to selection of the confounding parameters such as age and sex, our approaches are based on shape descriptions and geometrical models. In the following sections we present a description of our approaches followed by the corresponding results and discussions.

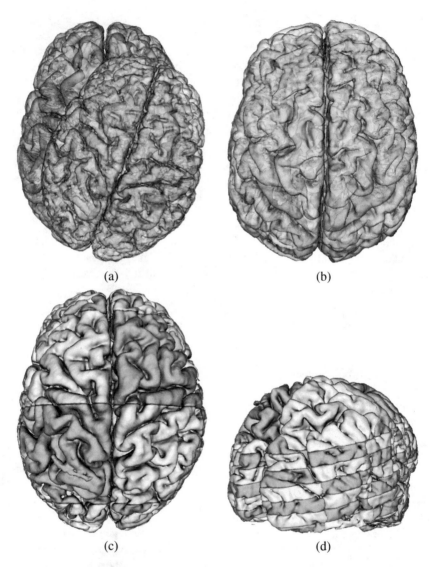

(a)

(b)

(c)

(d)

Figure 11. (a) The two volumes before alignment: (b) rigid alignment; (c,d) two different views after applying our nonrigid registration method [69]. See attached CD for color version.

4.1. White Matter Analysis

There is increasing agreement among structural imaging studies on the abnormal anatomy of the white matter in autistic brains. Asymmetry of the WM was reported by Herbert et al. [44] in a morphometric analysis of postmortem brain tissue. In addition, volumetric studies of the WM have reported early overgrowth of WM in autistic children, followed by a reduction in adulthood [17, 44, 28]. In autism, the WM grows normally during the first nine months, then by 2 years excessive WM is found in some brain areas, such as the frontal lobes and the cerebellum [44].

Beyond measurement of the volume of WM, diffusion tensor imaging (DTI) studies have reported that the fractional anisotropy (FA), which provides an index of structural WM integrity, is reduced in the WM of autistic children relative to controls. More recently, another DTI study showed that these reductions of FA in the WM persist into adulthood in several cortical regions of the autistic brain [76].

This coherent finding related to the anomalies in the WM of autistic brains relative to healthy ones is one of the main motivations behind our study. We intend to use the difference in WM anatomy in order to develop a classification approach that separates the two groups based on MRI analyzes.

First, we believe that the reported WM anomalies explain the difference in folds and gyrifications of the WM between autistic and typical brains, which we have observed on the data at hand, as shown in Figure 12. Note that the WM was segmented using our level set-based segmentation technique as explained in Section 3.2.

For classification purposes, we use the distance map inside of the segmented WM as a shape representation of the WM structure. We first computed the distance maps inside the WM of four autistic brains, and that inside the WM of six healthy brains from the postmortem data, and we did the same for 4 autistic and 16 healthy brains from the savant data. Second, we compute the corresponding cumulative distribution functions of these distance maps as shown in Figure 13a for the postmortem data, and in Figure 13b for the savant data. It is clear from these figures that the two classes, autistic and normal, are completely separable, which encourages us to use the CDFs of distance maps as a discrimination measure between the two classes. Furthermore, in order to remove the volume effect, these CDFs are normalized between 0 and 1, and then averaged, as shown in Figure 14.

Finally, given the brain MRI scan of a subject to be classified, we compute and normalize, in similar way, the CDF of the distance map inside of its segmented white matter and compare this CDF to the two average CDFs (autistic and normal) using the Levy distance. The smallest Levy distance indicates the class to which the test subject belongs. Figure 15 shows the classification results of two test subjects from the savant datasets. Both subjects were classified successfully. This classification method was tested on the two types of datasets. Table 1 summarizes the performance of the proposed classification method.

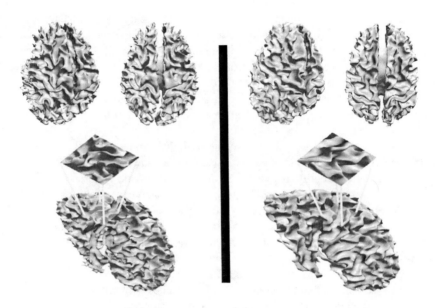

Figure 12. Different views of segmented white matter for autistic and normal subjects (savant data). Left, autistic; right, normal. Note that the gyrifications in autistic WM are thinner than those in normal WM. The zooms illustrate this difference in WM gyrification between the two groups. See attached CD for color version.

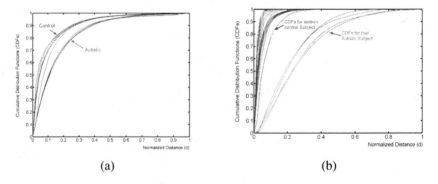

(a)   (b)

Figure 13. (a) From postmortem data: distance map CDFs inside the WM of four autistic subjects and six controls. (b) From savant data: distance map CDFs inside the WM of four autistic subjects and sixteen controls. See attached CD for color version.

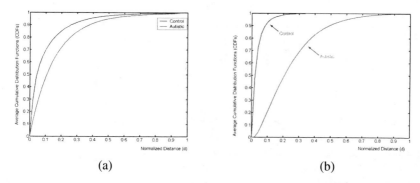

(a)   (b)

Figure 14. Average cumulative distribution functions inside the WM of four autistic subjects and six controls: (a) from postmortem data; (b) from savant data.   See attached CD for color version.

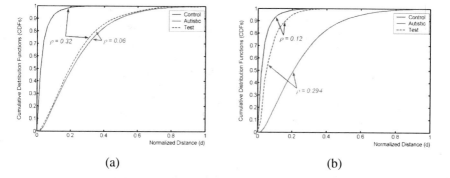

(a)   (b)

Figure 15. Illustration of using the proposed classification approach: (a) green CDF is classified as normal; (b) green CDF is classified as autistic. The parameter ρ denotes the Levy distance.   See attached CD for color version.

Table 1. Performance of the Classification Approach, Based on Analysis of the WM, When Applied to Postmortem and Savant Datasets

Confidence Rate	Autistic		Normal	
	Postmortem	Savant	Postmortem	Savant
85%	14/14	13/15	12/12	30/30
90%	13/14	12/15	12/12	30/30
95%	13/14	11/15	11/12	28/30

4.2. Corpus Callosum Analysis

According to the reviewed literature, the deficits in the size of the corpus callosum and its subregions in patients with autism relative to controls is well established (see, e.g., [30]). This finding motivates the analysis presented in this section. The main goal is to use the difference in the CC anatomy in order to devise a classification technique between the two groups. Unlike the traditional approaches, which are sensitive to the segmentation ouputs as well to the effect of volume, we propose a novel classification approach based on analyzing the displacement fields generated from the nonrigid registration of different corpus callosums. The details of this approach are summarized below.

Due to the distortions from which the postmortem images suffer and which made the segmentation of the CC for these data very challenging, results corresponding to the savant datasets are presented in this part of the chapter. For these data, the CCs are extracted manually from the segmented brain images.

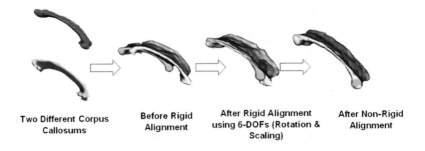

Two Different Corpus Callosums   Before Rigid Alignment   After Rigid Alignment using 6-DOFs (Rotation & Scaling)   After Non-Rigid Alignment

Figure 16. 3D registration of CC datasets using our nonrigid registration technique. See attached CD for color version.

For each group (autistic and normal), we randomly picked four CC datasets, one of which is chosen as the reference, and the remaining ones are registered to it using our deformable registration method (Section 3.4). During these registration steps, a deformation field is generated for each alignment with the reference (total of 3 for each group), as shown in Figure 18a. These deformation fields are then averaged, and the cumulative distribution functions are computed to represent the changes of the magnitudes of each one of these two averaged deformation fields, as shown in Figure 18b.

Given a subject to be classified, we register it, once to the chosen control reference and then to the chosen autistic reference. Two deformation fields are then generated and, as we did before, a CDF is computed for each one of these deformation fields. Finally, we compute the Levy distance between each of these deformation fields and the average CDFs of deformation fields representing each

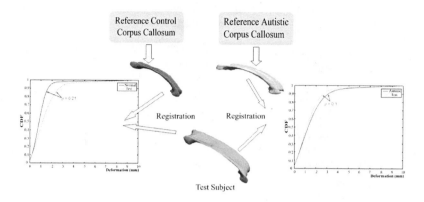

Figure 17. Illustration of CC registration-based classification approach. Parameter ρ denotes the Levy distance chosen to measure the difference between CDFs. See attached CD for color version.

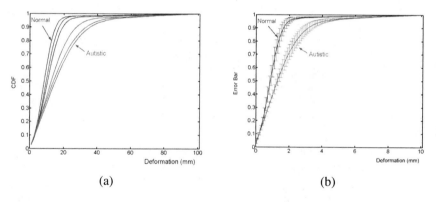

(a)   (b)

Figure 18. (a) Cumulative distribution of displacement fields resulting from registration of 3 subjects to the reference within each group. (b) Error analysis showing the averages CDFs for each group. See attached CD for color version.

class. This outputs two distances, the smallest of which indicates the class to which the tested subject belongs. This scenario is illustrated in Figure 17.

This approach has been applied on a set of eight 30 normal and 15 autistic datasets. Table 2 summarizes the classification performances for each group. Note that this approach did not provide good results on the postmortem brains due to the large distortions caused by the acquisition procedure, as explained earlier. These results are not presented herein.

Table 2. Performance of the Classification Approach Based on
analysis of the CC, when Applied to Savant Datasets

Confidence Rate	Autistic		Normal	
	Postmortem	Savant	Postmortem	Savant
85%	–	10/15	–	29/30
90%	–	9/15	–	29/30
95%	–	7/15	–	25/30

Note that this approach was not tested on the postmortem datasets because of geometric distortions.

5. DISCUSSION

In this study, we proposed two neuroimaging-based approaches to discriminate between autistic and typically developing brain. These approaches exploit the reported anomalies of the white matter and the deficit in the area of the corpus callosum in the autistic brain in order to extract geometrically based features that can be used as accurate discriminating measures between the two groups. Unlike traditional approaches, which mainly depend on volumetric descriptions of different brain structures, the proposed classification techniques are less sensitive to the selection of ages as well as to segmentation methods.

Research on the pathology of autism lacks consistency between findings. This may be explained by the unavailability of larger sample sizes and closely matched control groups, along with the failure to account for such confounding factors as age, sex, IQ, socioeconomic status, mental retardation, and handedness. The use of the distribution of the distance map inside the white matter, and the anatomical features that the corpus callosum reveals through nonrigid registration, as explained in this work, may provide for a biomarker in autism that allows to evaluate the validity among varied studies.

Different brain structures will be investigated in order to follow the development and variations of the autistic brain over time. This investigation will not be limited to the white matter region but will also include gray matter studies. The approach will be tested on postmortem datasets for more results and validation.

Eventually, a study needs to be established in which patients are scanned according to a defined protocol. Typical T1- and T2-weighted MRI scans as well as DTI need to be obtained. In addition, fMRI, MEG, as well as EEG may be used in our future work.

6. REFERENCES

1. Minshew NJ, JB Payton. 1988. New perspectives in autism, part I: the clinical spectrum of autism. *J Curr Probl Pediatr* **18**:561–610.
2. Yeargin-Allsop M, Rice C, Karapurkar T, Doernber N, Boyle C, Murphy C. 2003. Prevalence of autism in a US metropolitan area. *JAMA* **289**:48–55.
3. Tidmarsh L, Volkmar FR. 2003. Diagnosis and epidemiology of autism spectrum disorders. *Can J Psychiatry* **48**(8):517–525.
4. Wallis C. 2006. Inside the autistic mind. *Time* **167**(20):43–51.
5. Bolton P, Macdonald H, Pickles A, Rios P, Goode S, Crowson M, Bailey A, Rutter M. 1994. A case-control family history study of autism. *J Child Psychol Psychiatry* **35**:877–900.
6. Minshew NJ, Payton JB. 2003. New perspectives in autism, part II: the differential diagnosis and neurobiology of autism. *Curr Probl Pediatr* **18**:613–694.
7. Stevens MC, Fein DA, Dunn M, Allen D, Waterhouse LH, Feinstein C, Rapin I. 2000. Subgroups of children with autism by cluster analysis: a longitudinal examination. *J Am Acad Child Adolesc Psychiatry* **39**:346–352.
8. Kanner L. 1943. Autistic disturbances of affective contact. *J Nervous Child* **2**:250–250.
9. Bailey A, Luthert P, Bolton P, Le Couteur A, Rutter M, Hardin B. 1993. Autism and megalencephaly. *Lancet* **341**:1225–1226.
10. Davidovitch M, Patterson B, Gartside P. 1996. Head circumference measurements in children with autism. *J Child Neurol* **11**:389–393.
11. Miles JH, Hadden LL, Takahashi TN, Hillman RE. 2000. Head circumference is an independent clinical finding associated with autism. *Am J Med Gen* **95**:339–350.
12. Aylward EH, Minshew NJ, Field K, Sparks BF, Singh N. 2002. Effects of age on brain volume and head circumference in autism. *Neurology* **59**(2):175–183.
13. Courchesne R, Carper R, Akshoomoff N. 2003. Evidence of brain overgrowth in the first year of life in autism. *JAMA* **290**:337–344.
14. Steg JP, Rapoport JL. 1975. Minor physical anomalies in normal, neurotic, learning disabled, and severely disturbed children. *J Autism Dev Disord*, **5**(4):299–307.
15. Walker HA. 1997. Incidence of minor physical anomaly in autism. *J Autism Child Schizophr* **7**(2):165–176.
16. Woodhouse W, Bailey A, Rutter M, Bolton P, Baird G, Le Couteur A. 1996. Head circumference in autism and other pervasive developmental disorders. *J Child Psychol Psychiatry* **37**(6):665–671.
17. Courchesne E, Karns CM, Davis HR, Ziccardi R, Carper RA, Tigue ZD, Chisum HJ, Moses P, Pierce K, Lord C, Lincoln AJ, Pizzo S, Schreibman L, Haas RH, Akshoomoff NA., Courchesne RY. 2001. Unusual brain growth patterns in early life in patients with autistic disorder: an MRI study. *Neurology* **57**(2):245–254.
18. Sparks B, Friedman S, Shaw D, Aylward E, Echelard D, Artru A, Maravilla K, Giedd J, Munson J, Dawson G, Dager S. 2002. Brain structural abnormalities in young children with autism spectrum disorder. *Neurology* **59**(2):184–192.
19. Kemper TL, Bauman ML. 1993. The contribution of neuropathologic studies to the understanding of autism. *J Neurol Clin* **11**(1):175–187.
20. Guerin P, Lyon G, Barthelemy C, Sostak E, Chevrollier V, Garreau B, Lelord G. 1996. Neuropathological study of a case of autistic syndrome with severe mental retardation. *Neurology* **38**(3):203–211.
21. Egaas B, Courchesne E, Saitoh O. 1995. Reduced size of corpus callosum in autism. *J Arch Neurol* **52**(8): 794–801.
22. Hardan AY, Minshew NJ, Keshavan MS. 2000. Corpus callosum size in autism. *Neurology* **55**:1033–1036.

23. Piven J, Bailey J, Ranson BJ, Arndt S. 1997. An MRI study of the corpus callosum in autism. *Am J Psychiatry* **154**(8):1051–1056.

24. Haas R, Townsend J, Courchesne E, Lincoln A, Schreibman L, Yeung-Courchesne R. 1996. Neurologic abnormalities in infantile autism. *J Child Neurol* **11**(2):84–92.

25. Saitoh O, Courchesne E, Egaas B, Lincoln A, Schreibman L. 1995. Crosssectional area of the posterior hippocampus in autistic patients with cerebellar and corpus callosum abnormalities. *Neurology* **45**(2):317–324.

26. Manes F, Piven J, Vrancic D, Nanclares V, Plebst C, Starkstein S. 1999. An MRI study of the corpus callosum and cerebellum in mentally retarded autistic individuals. *J Neuropsychiatry Clin Neurosci* **11**(4):470–474.

27. Chung M, Dalton K, Alexander A, Davidson R. 2004. Less white matter concentration in autism: 2D voxel-based morphometry. *Neuroimage* **23**:242–251.

28. Waiter G, Williams J, Murray A, Gilchrist A, Perrett D, Whiten A. 2005. Structural white matter deficits in high-functioning individuals with autistic spectrum disorder: a voxel-based investigation. *Neuroimage* **24**(2):455–461.

29. Barnea-Goraly N, Kwon H, Menon V, Eliez S, Lotspeich L, Reiss A. 2004. White matter structure in autism: preliminary evidence from diffusion tensor imaging. *Am J Biol Psychiatry* **55**:323–326.

30. Vidal C, Nicolson R, DeVito T, Hayashi K, Geaga J, Drost D, Williamson P, Rajakumar N, Sui Y, Dutton R, Toga A, Thompson P. 2006. Mapping corpus callosum deficits in autism: an index of aberrant cortical connectivity. *J Biol Psychiatry* **60**(3):218–225.

31. Cody H, Pelphrey K, Piven J. 2002. Structural and functional magnetic resonance imaging of autism. *Int J Dev Neurosci*, **20**:421–438.

32. Williams R, Hauser S, Purpura D, DeLong G, Swisher C. 1980. Autism and mental retardation: neuropathologic studies performed in four retarded persons with autistic behavior. *J Arch Neurol*, **37**(12):749–753.

33. Ritvo E, Freeman B, Scheibel A, Duong T, Robinson H, Guthrie D, Ritvo A. 1986. Lower Purkinje cell counts in the cerebella of four autistic subjects: initial findings of the UCLA-NSAC autopsy research report. *Am J Psychiatry* **143**:862–866.

34. Lee M, Martin-Ruiz C, Graham A, Court J, Jaros E, Perry R, Iversen P, Bauman M, Perry E. 2002. Nicotinic receptor abnormalities in the cerebellar cortex in autism. *Brain* **125**(7):1483–1495.

35. Bailey A, Luthert P, Dean A, Harding B, Janota I, Montgomery M, Rutter M, Lantos P. 1998. A clinicopathological study of autism. *Brain* **121**(5):889–905.

36. Courchesne E, Yeung-Courchesne R, Press G, Hesselink J, Jernigan T. 1988. Hypoplasia of cerebellar vermal lobules VI and VII in autism. *N Engl J Med* **318**(21):1349–1354.

37. Allen G, Courchesne E. 2003. Autism and mental retardation: neuropathologic studies performed in four retarded persons with autistic behavior. *Am J Psychiatry* **160**: 262–273.

38. Mountcastle VB. 1997. The minicolumnar organization of the neocortex. *Brain* **120**:701–722.

39. Mountcastle VB. 2003. Introduction: computation in cortical columns. *J Cereb Cortex* **13**(1):2–4.

40. Casanova MF, Buxhoeveden D, Switala A, Roy E. 2002. Minicolumnar pathology in autism. *Neurology* **58**:428–432.

41. Casanova MF, Buxhoeveden D, Switala A, Roy E. 2002. Neuronal density and architecture (gray level index) in the brains of autistic patients. *J Child Neurol*, **17**:515–521.

42. Casanova MF. 2004. White matter volume increases and minicolumns in autism. *Ann Neurol* **56**(3):453.

43. Casanova MF, Van Kooten I, Switala A, van Engeland H, Heinsen H, Steinbusch H, Hof PR, Trippe J, Stone J, Schmitz C. 2006. Minicolumnar abnormalities in autism. *Acta Neuropathol*. In press. Available online.

44. Herbert M, Ziegler D, Makris N, Filipek P, Kemper T, Normandin J, Sanders HA, Kennedy D, Caviness VJ. 2004. Localization of white matter volume increase in autism and developmental language disorder. *Ann Neurol* **55**:530–540.

45. Lainhart JE, Lazar M, Bigler E, Alexander A. 2005. The brain during life in autism: advances in neuroimaging research. In *Recent advances in autism research*, pp. 57–108. Ed MF Casanova. New York: NOVA Biomedical.

46. Bauman ML, Kemper TL. 1990. Limbic and cerebellar abnormalities are also present in an autistic child of normal intelligence. *Neurology* **40**:359.

47. Bauman ML, Kemper TL. 1994. Neuroanatomic observations of the brain in autism. In *The neurobiology of autism*, pp. 119–145. Ed ML Bauman, TL Kemper TL. Baltimore: Johns Hopkins UP.

48. Schumann CM, Buonocore HM, Amaral DG. 2001. Magnetic resonance imaging of the postmortem autistic brain. *J Autism Dev Disord* **31**(6):561–568.

49. Osher S, Sethian J. 1988. Fronts propagating with curvature speed: algorithms based on Hamilton-Jacobi formulations. *J Comput Phys* **79**:12–49.

50. Chan T, Sandberg B, Vese L. 2000. Active contours without edges for vector valued images. *J Vis Commun Image Represent*, **2**:130–141.

51. Zaho H-K, Chan T, Merriman B, Osher S. 1996. A variational level set approach to multiphase motion. *J Comp Phys* **127**:179–195.

52. Zeng X, Staib LH, Duncan JS. 1998. Volumetric layer segmentation using coupled surface propagation. In *Proceedings of the IEEE conference on computer vision and pattern recognition (CVPR)*, pp. 179–195. Washington, DC: IEEE Computer Society.

53. Farag AA, El-Baz A, Gimelfarb G. 2004. Precise image segmentation by iterative em-based approximation of empirical gray level distribution with linear combination of gaussians. In *IEEE international workshop on learning in computer vision and pattern recognition*, pp. 121–129. Washington, DC: IEEE Computer Society.

54. Farag AA, Hassan H. 2004. Adaptive segmentation of multi-modal 3d data using robust level set techniques. In *Proceedings of the 7th international conference on medical image computing and computer-assisted intervention (MICCAI'2004). Lecture notes in computer science*, Vol. 2306, pp. 169–176. New York: Springer.

55. Goldenberg R, Kimmel R, Rivlin E, Rudzsky M. 2002. Cortex segmentation: a fast variational geometric approach. *IEEE Trans Med Imaging* **21**(2):1544–1551.

56. Geusebroek M, Burghouts G, Smeulders A. 2005. The Amsterdam library of object images. *Int J Comput Vis* **61**(1):103–112.

57. Cerveny V. 1995. Ray synthetic seismograms for complex two- and three-dimensional structures. *Am J Geophys* **58**:2–26.

58. Vidale JE. 1990. Finite-difference calculation of traveltimes in three dimensions. *Geophysics* **55**:521–526.

59. Van Trier J, Symes WW. 1991. Upwind finite-difference calculation of traveltimes. *Geophysics* **56**:812–821.

60. Podvin P, and Lecomte I. 1991. Finite-difference computation of traveltimes in very contrasted velocity models: a massively parallel approach and its associated tools. *Geophys J Int* **105**:271–284.

61. Adalsteinsson D, and Sethian J. 1995. A fast level set method for propagating interfaces. *J Comput Phys* **118**:269–277.

62. Kim S. 1999. ENO-DNO-PS: a stable, second-order accuracy eikonal solver. *J Soc Explor Geophys* **28**:1747–1750.

63. Sethian J. 1999. *Level sets methods and fast marching methods: evolving interfaces in computational geometry, fluid mechanics, computer vision, and materials science*, 2nd ed. Cambridge: Cambridge UP.

64. Kimmel R, and Sethian JA. 1998. Fast marching methods on triangulated domains. *Proc Natl Acad Sci USA* **95**(11):8341–8435.

65. Sethian JA, Vladimirsky A. 2000. Fast methods for the eikonal and related Hamilton-Jacobi equations on unstructured meshes. *Proc Natl Acad Sci USA* **97**(11):5699–5703.

66. Hassouna MS, Farag AA. 2006. Accurate tracking of monotonically advancing fronts. In *Proceedings of the IEEE conference on computer vision and pattern recognition (CVPR)*, pp. 355–362, Washington, DC: IEEE Computer Society.

67. Shen D, Davatzikos C. 2002. Hammer: hierarchical attribute matching mechanism for elastic registration. *IEEE Trans Med Imaging* **21**(11):257–270.

68. Zitova B, Flusser J. 2003. Image registration methods: a survey. *Image Vision Comput* **21**(21):977–1000.

69. Fahmi R., Farag A. A., El-Baz A. 2006. New deformable registration technique using scale space and curve evolution theory and a finite element based validation framework. In *Proceedings of the 28th IEEE EMBS annual international conference*, pp. 3041–3044. Washington, DC: IEEE Computer Society.

70. Lindeberg T. 1994. *Scale-space theory in computer vision*. New York: Kluwer Academic.

71. Mikolajczyk K, Schmid C. 2002. An affine invariant interest point detector. In *Proceedings of the European conference on computer vision (ECCV'02). Lecture notes in computer science*, Vol. 2350, pp. 128–142. Ed A Heyden. New York: Springer.

72. Abdel-Hakim A., Farag A. A. 2005. "CSIFT: a SIFT Descriptor with Color Invariant Characteristics", Proc. of IEEE Conf. on Computer Vision and Pattern Recognition (CVPR-06), pp. 1978–1983, June 2006, Los Alamitos, CA, USA.

73. Mikolajczyk K, and Schmid C. 2005. A performance evaluation of local descriptors. *IEEE Trans Pattern Anal Machine Intell* **27**(10):1615–1630.

74. Lowe D. 2004. Distinctive image features from scale-invariant key points. *Int J Comput Vision* **60**(2):91–110.

75. Rueckert D, Sonoda L, Hayes C, Hill D, Leach M, Hawkes D. 1999. Nonrigid registration using free-form deformations: application to breast mr images. *IEEE Trans Med Imaging* **18**(8):712–721.

76. Keller T, Kana R, Just M. 2006. A developmental study of the structural integrity of white matter in autism. *NeuroReport*. In press.

INDEX

Printed in the USA

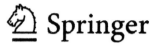